MARITIME QU

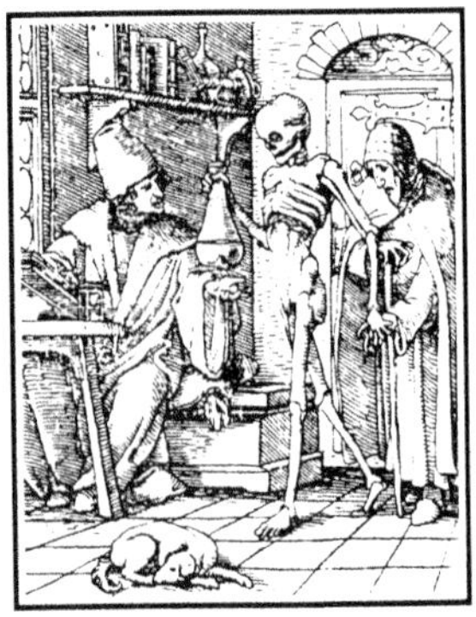

The History of Medicine in Context

Series Editors: Andrew Cunningham and Ole Peter Grell

Department of History and Philosophy of Science
University of Cambridge

Department of History
The Open University

Titles in this series include

With Words and Knives
Learning Medical Dispassion in Early Modern England
Lynda Payne

Medicine and Religion in Enlightenment Europe
Edited by Ole Peter Grell and Andrew Cunningham

The Making of Addiction
The 'Use and Abuse' of Opium in Nineteenth-Century Britain
Louise Foxcroft

Melancholy and the Care of the Soul
Religion, Moral Philosophy and Madness in Early Modern England
Jeremy Schmidt

Hospital Politics in Seventeenth-Century France
The Crown, Urban Elites and the Poor
Tim McHugh

Maritime Quarantine

The British Experience, *c.*1650–1900

JOHN BOOKER
Independent Scholar

Routledge
Taylor & Francis Group
LONDON AND NEW YORK

First published 2007 by Ashgate Publishing

Published 2016 by Routledge
2 Park Square, Milton Park, Abingdon, Oxfordshire OX14 4RN
711 Third Avenue, New York, NY 10017, USA

First issued in paperback 2016

Routledge is an imprint of the Taylor & Francis Group, an informa business

British Library Cataloguing in Publication Data
Booker, John
Maritime Quarantine: the British Experience, c.1650–1900. – (The History of Medicine in Context)
1. Quarantine – History. 2. Quarantine – Great Britain - History.
I. Title
614.4'6'09

Library of Congress Cataloging-in-Publication Data
Booker, John, 1941-
Maritime Quarantine: the British Experience, c.1650–1900 / John Booker.
p. cm. – (The History of Medicine in Context)
Includes bibliographical references.
1. Quarantine – Great Britain – History. 2. Communicable diseases – Great Britain – Prevention – History. 3. Naval hygiene – Great Britain – History. I. Title. II. Series.
[DNLM: 1. Quarantine – history – Great Britain. 2. History, 17th Century – Great Britain. 3. History, 18th Century – Great Britain. 4. History, 19th Century – Great Britain. 5. Naval Medicine – history – Great Britain. WA 11 FA1 B5987m 2007]
RA644.P7B6694 2007
614.4'60941--dc22 2007007394

ISBN 13: 978-1-138-27412-9 (pbk)
ISBN 13: 978-0-7546-6178-8 (hbk)

Contents

Appendices

List of Illustrations

Illustrations 8.2–4 are reproduced by courtesy of the Sir John Soane's Museum; Illustrations 5.1, 8.1, 10.1, and 12.1 are by courtesy of the British Library; and Illustration 16.1 is by courtesy of the National Library of Malta.

List of Maps

List of Tables

Preface

Maritime quarantine, in the unbeatable precision of Sir Peter Froggatt, is 'the enforced detention and segregation of vessels, persons, and merchandise, believed to be infected with certain epidemic diseases, for specified periods at or near ports of disembarkation'.[1] The word itself is a corruption of the Italian for 40, *quaranta*, as that number of days was the usual detention period. The derivation underlines the Venetian origins of the developed system, although quarantine against leprosy was not unknown in biblical times. Indeed the 40-day duration was a recognition of various religious precedents, and superstition ensured its permanence. At every point in the history of quarantine from the fourteenth century until its virtual abandonment nearly six hundred years later, 40 days remained the standard tariff of quarantine unless there were specific reasons for its increase or reduction.

This book is a history of maritime quarantine as it affected Great Britain, Ireland and British possessions in the Mediterranean until 1896, when Westminster legislation ensured quarantine was ousted (although not totally) by the parallel system of medical inspection. The point of including Gibraltar, Malta, Minorca and the Ionian Islands is that they were exposed not only to the most feared source of infection (the Levant) but also to the critical gaze of sanitary establishments in Italy and France which claimed to manage quarantine better than anyone else. The diseases most feared were what Ackerknecht has called the 'big three' – that is, bubonic plague, yellow fever and cholera. It is true that only the first-named was endemic in the Levant, but the fear of plague was ancient and persistent, whereas yellow fever did not alarm Europe until the very late eighteenth century, and cholera nearly 40 years after that. In every century the northern Mediterranean ports took the lead in quarantine management, and plague never left the minds of their health officials even when other diseases threatened more immediate mortality.

In 1853 Dr Gavin Milroy thought it unfortunate that not a single work existed, as far as he knew, 'to which any one seeking for detailed and trustworthy information upon the subject of quarantine can be referred'. Over 40 years later Dr Charles Creighton apologized for not filling the gap. Both authors could offer no other source than the article in the *Encyclopaedia Britannica*. Creighton had intended to include a history of quarantine in his two-volume treatise on British epidemics but could 'find no convenient context' for its inclusion. This lack of convenience, or some other discouragement, has been equally manifest in later literature where quarantine is mentioned obliquely, spasmodically, and with little understanding of its long development or the legal process that underpinned it.

But if quarantine has lacked a comprehensive history, articles have not been wanting. In the second half of the twentieth century, quarantine in Britain attracted the attention of medical historians, several of them American, but their focus on episodes

1 P. Froggatt, 'The Chetney Hill lazaret', *Archaeologia Cantiana*, 79 (1964), 1.

or eras ran the risk of distorting the overall picture. There were also problems of accuracy. Mullett called the work of his compatriot McDonald 'regrettably careless', and that stricture could be applied to others. Even the research of British writers, who at least understood their national geography, has been less than comprehensive. For instance, there are scholarly discussions by two unconnected authors on the abortive lazaretto in Kent, but each work has important sources unmentioned in the other. Ironically, the most sustained enthusiasm for international quarantine has been demonstrated by postal historians with their journal named *Pratique*. The main interest in that context is the fumigation of letters, and the franking marks, slits and discolouring which followed the passage of mail through a lazaretto.

Why has quarantine been overlooked for a definitive history? It was, after all, frequently a subject of national debate which taxed and alarmed both Parliament and the Privy Council. Doctors and intellectuals riled against it. For Dr Russell it was 'an oppressive empty form'; for Dr Maclean it was 'perhaps, without exception, the most gigantic, extraordinary, and mischievous superstructure, that has ever been raised by man, upon a purely imaginary foundation'. Sir Thomas Maitland, Governor of Malta, swore that quarantine had given him 'more plague and vexation than anything else'. Although he meant plague in a figurative sense, bad quarantine practice involved Malta in a plague which was all too real. Underpinning the discontent in Britain was the equivocal status of quarantine as a responsibility for the Privy Council, implementing a royal prerogative in which Parliament dabbled and trespassed with little understanding and less enthusiasm. In a practical sense, quarantine embarrassed travellers and infuriated merchants. Ships lay idle, cargoes rotted, and scheduled voyages were cancelled and delayed. Surely there has been enough meat in all this to provide historians with a notable dinner.

The problem has been that the subject is just too diverse. In his history of the Levant Company, A.C. Wood mentioned the danger of falling between the stools of economic and diplomatic history, exposing himself to the charge of inadequacy and irrelevance from specialists in either sphere. The historian of quarantine risks an even greater bridge between disciplines. As quarantine was against disease, it would seem a subject for the medically trained. But the epidemiology of plague and the other disorders takes no account of the constitutional, political, economic and social dimensions which give the study of quarantine its historical depth. Given the impossibility of writing a history which covers all aspects equally, this enquiry has approached the topic from only two of the possible standpoints. These are the constitutional and the economic. Medical issues are not neglected, but introduced only as far as necessary to explain why quarantine was introduced, altered and finally abandoned. Much has been written by medical historians about the tussle between those who believed that plague and other diseases were or were not contagious. It has sometimes been necessary to continue this discussion because quarantine was founded on the doctrine of contagion (that is, that disease was transmitted literally by touch), and its efficacy was challenged or confirmed as the argument swung this way and that.

As regards constitutional and economic history, it will be shown they were intertwined. The Privy Council had a long and monopolistic role which they never felt inclined or empowered to delegate, although the complexities of shipping and international trade were no more within members' understanding than the medical debates. If the Council were vulnerable on those points, their stand was further weakened by the need to be constantly nice to the mercantile lobby. Free-trade arguments carried weight with politicians and the press, and if quarantine caused any impediment to the normal intercourse between merchants and dealers, then the Council could be sure of an uncomfortable response. Surprisingly seldom did the councillors take shelter behind their own offshoot, the Board of Trade. It says much for their moral courage that, by and large, they stuck to the received wisdom of quarantine as a defence against infection at the risk of upsetting the City of London and, later, the northern textile barons who imported raw materials from countries where plague was endemic. Usually some compromise was arrived at with merchants whereby the vigour of quarantine, in response to some scare, was progressively reduced. But the Council did not hesitate to detain ships if members had reason to believe the public were at risk. Another factor continually to influence their judgement was the realization that European Mediterranean powers would inflict punitive quarantine on British ships if London were judged neglectful in the international line of defence.

If medical historians have been less than adequate in their analysis of quarantine, historians in other disciplines have been equally disappointing. Among works on the Privy Council, quarantine is mentioned but with no suggestion of the relentless pressure which it put on councillors for nearly two centuries, to the extent that at some meetings there was no other topic on the agenda. It will be apparent from the many references in this study to the Levant Company that quarantine was a key issue for its members, but Wood refers to it only as an incidental contribution to the Company's decline. Among economic historians generally it is difficult to find any reference whatsoever to the impact or even existence of quarantine, except briefly in the context of Levantine cotton. It might be argued that this was because the impact of quarantine on the national economy was minimal, and it has been impossible in this study to produce meaningful figures, beyond vague estimates occasionally bandied before Parliament, that the opposite was the case.

But that is not to say that the impact on mercantile and shipping interests was also minimal. It was a matter of where trade was conducted. An East India merchant, for instance, knew of quarantine only by hearsay; whereas anyone trading within the Mediterranean, or at certain times to the Baltic, found quarantine only slightly less troublesome than war. The destruction of vessels and cargoes in 1721, 1754 and 1800, although relieved by compensation from the public purse, was a horrid reminder to shipowners and importers that a policy of quarantine could occasionally involve extreme measures beyond the normal detentions. Not that those detentions could be treated lightly. Quarantine, for various reasons, might extend beyond the normal 40 days to 60 or even longer. Crews needed paying and victualling, cargoes were damaged by compulsory airing, and fees were payable at many stages, not least for the privilege of eventual release. Wherever possible this study produces statistics – often compiled from Privy Council registers – of numbers of ships detained, along with their origins, cargoes and quarantine stations. It is still difficult to quantify absolute damage, for instance whether quarantine forced any shipowners out of business, but the sheer volumes involved and the diversity of cargoes suggest a consequential effect on prices and availability. There is room for an academic study to examine such issues in more depth.

It cannot be argued that the lack of an earlier history of British quarantine is explained by any dearth of sources. In fact, the amount of evidence available is overwhelming, in so far as the administration of quarantine is concerned. Privy Council registers, until the second decade of the nineteenth century, are brimful of decisions regarding individual ships, procedures and policy. Treasury books and papers are useful for earlier years, and parliamentary blue books for later ones. Acts of Parliament, parliamentary journals and records of debates are easily accessed; likewise, there are any number of pamphlets, treatises and books, many discussing quarantine in relation to the contagious properties of plague, to keep the historian abreast of contemporary thinking. Often one episode can be approached from a number of angles. For instance in 1766, when the merchants of Leghorn wished to trade with England free of quarantine restrictions, the story unfolds in the Privy Council register as well as in the journal (published) of the Commissioners for Trade and Plantations, while the representation itself is in Privy Council papers. Furthermore, the episode is mentioned in anonymous pamphlets on the nature of quarantine and the need for a British lazaretto. For several British ports, Customs papers are useful, although the London Custom House fire in 1814 deprived the maritime historian of much important material at a central level. The main gap in knowledge, however, concerns business records of merchants and shipowners. Only from a sustained series of these would it be possible to analyse the real effect of quarantine on the mercantile community, and they are virtually non-existent.

Quarantine in Scotland is discussed in some detail, but the position in Ireland could certainly be enhanced by a more detailed examination. While the destruction of Irish records has meant significant losses, an historian resident on the island of Ireland could undoubtedly add much to the rather sketchy coverage in this study. The official quarantine stations in Ireland have been difficult to establish at any given date, but perhaps that is of no great consequence as ships usually used the first safe haven from Atlantic storms. Undoubtedly, a lot more could also be written on quarantine by a local historian in the Channel Islands. In contrast to these weaknesses, it is hoped that the position on Malta has been examined very thoroughly. The literature on Maltese quarantine replicates the position in England. That is to say there is a thorough medical history which deals with quarantine incidentally, and there is an article specifically on quarantine which is notably stronger at some periods than others. The totality of the subject has not been covered, and while broader historical and economic studies touch upon the relevance of quarantine to the Maltese economy, they do it only at periods and intervals within the limits of the author's enquiry.

As regards source material, quarantine on Malta is even better covered than it is in Britain, at least from the period of control from London. Colonial Office papers in the National Archives at Kew are a rich seam, and the fortunate survival of minutes, letter books and other records in the island's repositories adds a valuable local dimension. Equally useful are the records of the Board of Health at Marseilles. If this port was not always the acknowledged leader in the hierarchy of Mediterranean quarantine, it was never ranked lower than second. The Board corresponded meticulously with colleagues at other ports, and in-letters (sometimes still noxious from fumigation two centuries earlier) survive in neat and comprehensive bundles. These provide a view of Maltese quarantine from the outside looking in, and the series extends to Gibraltar and the Ionian Islands. Much could be written about quarantine in British possessions elsewhere, but there is no scope for such diversity in a work already so extended.

It will be the aim of this study to show that Britain found quarantine impossibly difficult. A system suited to autocratic control could never sit comfortably in a nation proud of democratic and parliamentary traditions. The fact that quarantine was an issue for the Crown made it all the more difficult to impose a regime which was democratically acceptable and legally binding. Parliament laboured to find reasons to intervene, never wanting to make quarantine a pretext for constitutional debate. Within this basic dichotomy lay other problems of bureaucracy and demarcation. Quarantine was administered by the Customs service but instructions from the Privy Council were received through the Treasury. In comparison to these complications, the position at, say, Leghorn or Marseilles could hardly be simpler. Whatever theoretical control existed over Boards of Health in the Mediterranean basin, they did what they pleased: they formulated their own policies and employed those responsible for the operation of quarantine. They were accountable to no one and made others, including health authorities elsewhere, accountable to themselves. They had no literary journals, no self-opinionated doctors, and no maverick politicians to challenge either their arrogance or their unquestioning confidence in the doctrine of contagion. These points become especially interesting in relation to Malta, where the British agreed reluctantly to the establishment of a Board of Health to avoid punitive quarantine at ports where such institutions were judged essential. But the British-run Board was, for many decades, little more than a front for the autocratic decisions of the Governor (or Lieutenant-Governor), taking advice from the Chief Secretary to Government and the Superintendent of Quarantine. The Privy Council did not intervene in Maltese quarantine and the island Board, ironically, was even less democratic within itself than its counterparts on the Continent.

It is hoped, at a broader level, that quarantine will now be recognized as one of the last neglected topics of national historical importance. If its multifaceted identity has made researchers fight shy of a comprehensive analysis, perhaps that same characteristic will encourage historians of specific disciplines to build on the new base and expose the impact of quarantine on, for example, medical issues, the British and Irish constitutions, commerce, the Post Office, steam power and especially tourism. The quarantine experiences of Grand Tourists and travellers could fill a book on their own, and perhaps give the subject a degree of public notoriety to which a general history can hardly aspire. It was possible to do a Grand Tour as far as Italy and not be affected by quarantine, but any return from Greece, unless it was entirely overland and between epidemics, meant almost certain detention in one port or another. Even from Italy, Horace Walpole discovered to his dismay that valuable artefacts, if the timing were particularly bad, could be delayed as long as people. Of course, some travellers' experiences of quarantine were markedly more comfortable than others'; much depended on the location, the climate and the season. But the overwhelming consensus of opinion was that quarantine was an expensive and vexatious impediment to freedom of movement, based on old-fashioned (even corrupt) motives and of dubious value. It will be suitable to end on that note with a laconic quotation from Henry Matthews, a traveller detained in one of the Leghorn lazarettos in the autumn of 1817. He made reference to Johnson's observation that no man ever does anything for the last time without some feeling of regret. 'The last day of quarantine', Matthews commented, 'might form an exception'.[2]

JOHN BOOKER
Little Braxted, Essex

2 H. Matthews, *The Diary of an Invalid being the Journal of a Tour in Pursuit of Health in Portugal Italy Swizerland and France in the Years 1817 1818 and 1819*, 2nd edn (London, 1820), p. 36.

Acknowledgements

My first thanks are due to the Wellcome Trust for a generous grant towards research over more than two years at the Public Record Office (PRO), since renamed the National Archives. The PRO provided a vast corpus of material central to my enquiry, especially the Register Books of the Privy Council and Colonial Office papers. Second only in importance to the PRO has been the British Library where the several departments have provided printed and documentary material covering many centuries and all aspects of my research, and the staff have been constantly helpful with advice and facilities for copying. Elsewhere in London, Susan Palmer of Sir John Soane's Museum guided me to draft drawings of lazaretto designs, and Carol Morgan in the Archives of the Institution of Civil Engineers made available the papers of John Rennie. The librarians of the Wellcome Trust have most helpfully produced rare material which it was difficult or impossible to find in other centres. I must also thank the staff of the Caird Library in the National Maritime Museum, and especially the London Library, probably the most congenial centre of knowledge anywhere.

Around England, I am grateful to the obliging staff in Hull City Archives, the Tyne and Wear Archive Service in Newcastle, and the Staffordshire Record Office. In York, Professor David Palliser received me very kindly in the archives of the Company of Merchant Adventurers. In Scotland, I found useful advice and material at the National Archives, housed in the West Register Office, while staff at Archbishop Marsh's Library in Dublin sent me useful sources via the Internet.

Abroad, I am particularly grateful to Maroma Camilleri of the National Library of Malta in Valletta, who introduced me to invaluable sources, both manuscript and printed, and to Charles Farrugia, Head of the National Archives of Malta at Rabat, who directed me to the letter-books of the Board of Health. Godfrey Monreal of the University of Malta Library copied for me an article unobtainable in England, and the whole experience of research on Malta has been a delight. I am equally enthusiastic about the Archives départmentales des Bouches-du-Rhône at Marseilles, which deserves a much wider attendance by British researchers. Also at Marseilles, the Département du patrimoine culturel of the Chambre de commerce et d'industrie is a wonderful storehouse of quarantine material, although within the limited terms of my research it was difficult to do it justice.

For maps and design advice, I have once again to thank Leo Maggs. For encouragement, patience and companionship in travels to Malta and Marseilles I am deeply obliged to my wife, Pam, who made no fuss when I disappeared all day into academic retreats and has helped me with medical aspects of my enquiry. Generally, all comments, opinions and mistakes are my own responsibility, and I would solicit the reader's indulgence for this foray into areas where others, no doubt very sensibly, have found it unwise to dabble.

Chapter One

The Seventeenth Century

England

> The plague, it seems, grows more and more at Amsterdam. And we are going upon making of all ships coming from thence and Hambrough, or any other infected places, to perform their Quarantine (for 30 days as Sir Rd. Browne expressed it in the Order of the Council, contrary to the import of the word; though in the general acceptation, it signifies now the thing, not the time spent in doing it) in Holehaven – a thing never done by us before.

This is an extract from the diary of Samuel Pepys dated 26 November 1663[1] and as Pepys was Clerk of the Acts to the Navy Board he is a reliable source. Indeed, the *Oxford English Dictionary* cites this extract as its first reference to the word quarantine. But it would be wrong to assume that maritime quarantine in England began in 1663. What Pepys appears to be saying is that this was the first instance of quarantine at Hole Haven, which is the estuary of an Essex creek where it meets the Thames by Canvey Island. It would also seem that this was the first occasion when the word quarantine was used in any Order or Proclamation in England; Pepys does not spell this out, but the novelty of the term is partly the reason for the lengthy parenthesis.

Quarantine in England can be traced back almost a century before Pepys was writing. G. Hadley, the eighteenth-century historian of Hull, referred to an outbreak of plague there in 1576: 'quarantine not being strictly performed, it [plague] was brought by seamen into this Town'.[2] This presumably means that detention measures were in place, though badly enforced. Four years later the Lord Treasurer ordered officers of the port of London to stop ships from plague-stricken Lisbon coming up the river, 'lymiting them a certen place of their staie until ther merchandises shold be ayred for the avoyding of further danger'.[3] The Privy Council thought fit to let the Lord Mayor of London know this, asking him to assist the port authority with similar measures for suspect ships and cargoes from anywhere else, especially 'from Plymouth at this presente visited [with plague]'.[4] It is not clear how long ships were detained, or how long the embargo was maintained.

---

1 R. Latham and W. Matthews (eds), *The Diary of Samuel Pepys* (9 vols, London, 1970–83), vol. 4, p. 399.

2 G. Hadley, *A New and Complete History of the Town and County of ... Kingston-upon-Hull* (Hull, 1788), p. 95.

3 *Acts of the Privy Council* [*APC*], *New Series (1580–81)* (London, 1896), p. 61.

4 Ibid.

In the early seventeenth century, Europe was rife with disease and the Privy Council took action from time to time when the threat seemed particularly great. It will become noticeable in this study that England and Scotland had different views as to the places whence danger was strongest. In 1629 London and specified outports were ordered to be on their guard against ships arriving from places as far apart as Amsterdam, Brittany and La Rochelle. Nothing and no one was to come ashore, and no one was to go on board until the goods had been aired for such time 'as may give hope and lykelyhood' that all was well.[5] No indication was given of the number of days this would take. In 1634 even the airing of goods was felt to be inadequate against reports of the plague at Rouen. The Council, via the Lord Treasurer, absolutely prohibited any goods from there to be landed at London or outports.[6] A ship from Rouen, with two dead men aboard, was to be detained by Customs officers wherever she might be intercepted.[7]

Plague was also reported at The Hague, Amsterdam and Leyden, and the Privy Council were sufficiently worried to ask the Lord Mayor of London for advice about what to do. This request, in a letter of 9 October 1635, implied that the Lord Mayor could himself initiate countermeasures, 'wherein if neede required we shall be readie to assist you from tyme to tyme wth the Arme of this Board.'[8] The opportunity for direct action was not heeded and it took nearly two weeks for the mayor to give his recommendations: there should be a Proclamation against the landing of men or goods from infected places without licence from Customs officers; no liberty to land should be given 'till some certain days be overpassed'; and waiters or guardians should be put aboard each suspected ship on its arrival.[9] The Privy Council agreed and on 1 November 1635 a Proclamation was issued in similar terms against vessels from infected places in France and Holland. The days to be 'overpassed' were given as 20.[10] Here, then, was the first national imposition of maritime quarantine for a stated period, although the word quarantine was not used. It was also the first time that a Proclamation to this effect had been issued in England; it will be seen later that Proclamations in both Scotland and Ireland were issued earlier – in Scotland much earlier.

France and Holland were not the only worry. Even before the Proclamation was issued, several ships began arriving at The Downs from the Straits of Gibraltar (where the plague was 'verie hott') having lost masters and crewmen during the voyage.[11] But this dramatic development warranted no more than a letter from the Privy Council to the farmers of the Customs. Until further order, the ships (unnamed) were not to enter the Thames, no person was to go aboard or come ashore, and no goods were to be landed.[12] It would seem that ships from

5 *APC* (1629–30), p. 160.

6 National Archives [NA] PC 2/44/182.

7 NA PC2/45/132–3.

8 NA PC2/45/148.

9 *Calendar of State Papers, Domestic Series* [*CSPD*] (1635), pp. 443–4.

10 Bibliotheca Lindesiana, vol. 5: *A Bibliography of Royal Proclamations of the Tudor and Stuart Sovereigns and of Others ... England and Wales* (Oxford, 1910), p. 205.

11 NA PC 2/45/184–5.

12 Ibid.

the Straits were judged too infrequent to merit the constitutional weaponry of Order and Proclamation. In any event, potential danger from the Mediterranean was soon eclipsed by more problems across the Channel. In March 1638, Morlaix in Brittany was adjudged 'exceedingly infected wth ye plague', so that two linen ships making for London were to come no closer than Tilbury; in May the Lord Mayor of London and Customs officers stopped all linen ships from Morlaix unloading 'untill they have remayned upon ye River full fortie daies.'[13] A week later the Mayor and Customs officers at Exeter were authorized to allow a vessel from Morlaix carrying linen and wine to unload, also after 40 days.[14] Thus it was in 1638 that quarantine in England was first practised, to a very limited extent, for the duration of its literal meaning.[15]

The episode mentioned by Pepys was the next real test of the English defences. The plague was particularly bad at Amsterdam, carried there by an Algerian warship, and letters to Clarendon from Sir George Downing, English Resident at The Hague, relayed the brutal statistics of death.[16] Plague was also reported at Hamburg. Pepys noted on 19 October 1663 that the King was planning to keep all ships from infected ports out of the Thames.[17] Charles adopted the traditional tactic of asking the Lord Mayor of London for advice, this time via Secretary Morice.[18] The Lord Mayor responded very quickly that vessels from infected places should come no nearer to London than roughly Gravesend, at which point, following practice in other countries, 'some Repositories may be appointed after the manner of Lazaretoes, into wch the Shipps may be discharged & the Goods lye to be Aired for the space of 40 dayes after the unlading'.[19] The initial reaction of the Privy Council, on 23 October, was to agree, with the lazaretto to be no nearer than Tilbury Hope, at such precise location as the City should agree with the farmers of Customs.[20]

The lazaretto evidently proved too difficult to site, as no more is heard of it. On 6 November the Privy Council set up a committee to consider the Lord Mayor's recommendations; it reported a week later with some ideas of its own, which were implemented.[21] The Postmaster General was to ensure that no passenger 'be permitted to be wafted over into England' in the packet boats from Holland, and two small warships, each with two Customs' officials, were to be stationed

13 NA PC 2/49/28, 182.

14 NA PC 2/49/187.

15 The *Speedwell* from Morlaix was allowed to dock at London after 'almost two months' in good health, but what proportion of that time had been spent in the voyage is not stated (NA PC 2/49/94–5).

16 *Calendar of the Clarendon State Papers Preserved in the Bodleian Library* [*CCSP*], vol. 5 (1660–1726) (Oxford, 1970), pp. 351, 369, 376, etc. In February 1664 Downing reported 200–300 deaths a week, but towards the end of the year the numbers were four times as many.

17 Latham & Matthews (eds), *The Diary of Samuel Pepys*, vol. 4, p. 340.

18 NA PC 2/56/592.

19 Ibid.

20 Ibid.

21 NA PC 2/56/607, 610–12.

at the mouth of the river to interrogate every ship.[22] Those from Amsterdam or Hamburg, or any other infected place, had either to turn back or perform 30 days' quarantine at Hole Haven, where a ketch with six men would keep an eye on the detainees.[23] Ships from uninfected places were to be given a pass and allowed to proceed up to London, showing their passes on the way to the commanders of blockhouses at Gravesend or Tilbury Fort.[24] For the period of detention at Hole Haven, Privy Council minutes used the novel word 'Triantane', an infelicity which has escaped the dictionary.[25] It can be deduced from Pepys's quotation that it was not used in the phrasing of the Order.

Correspondence from The Hague suggests that Downing was slow to grasp the English end of the crisis. In February and March 1664, he was still suggesting to Clarendon what quarantine precautions were advisable, while Pieter Cunaeus, Dutch secretary in London, was reporting to the States General the latest de facto restrictions.[26] These were the broadening of detention to cover ships from the Maes (to prevent Amsterdam goods arriving via Rotterdam), and later (May) from Zealand, with 'triantane' requirements extended to all outports of the kingdom.[27] Outports were presumably included in the initial Order of 11 November but the minutes of the Privy Council meeting do not make that clear. On 13 May detention was increased to 40 days, and so the term quarantine became literally relevant.[28] The reason was the increasing sickness at Amsterdam '& the heat of weather approaching, which renders the Contagion more dangerous'.[29] Quarantine against Hamburg had earlier been relaxed, but in July it was 'strictly & inviolably' reinstated, for the full 40 days.[30]

The Dutch took quarantine very badly. Relations between England and Holland were in any case markedly difficult. Neither Charles nor Clarendon wanted another trial of strength, but a war lobby in England was straining at the leash, while the merchants of Holland were snarling at the latest Navigation Act.[31] Quarantine was seen as an over-reaction – just another English ploy against Dutch trade. On 30 March the States General had sent a resolution to Charles asking for quarantine to be repealed.[32] Cunaeus reported that the King and Privy Council seemed inclined to suspend it, although the resolution was never formally discussed, or at least minuted, in the Council's business.[33] In late April, Cunaeus

22 NA PC 2/56/610–11.

23 NA PC 2/56/611.

24 NA PC 2/56/611.

25 At one point (NA PC 2/56/612) the word 'triantane' was entered over a deletion of 'quarantine'.

26 *CCSP*, vol. 5, pp. 369, 375–6.

27 *CCSP*, vol. 5, pp. 375, 394; NA PC 2/57/89.

28 NA PC 2/57/93.

29 Ibid.

30 NA PC 2/56/688; 2/57/164.

31 J.F. Bense, *Anglo-Dutch Relations from the Earliest Times to the Death of William the Third* (Oxford and The Hague, 1925), pp. 176–8.

32 *CCSP*, vol. 5, p. 386.

33 *CCSP*, vol. 5, p. 392; NA PC 2/57 is silent.

was writing more dismally to the States General that nothing had changed.[34] Then came the increased detention from 30 days to 40, stinging the Dutch into formal protest. Their ambassador complained in July that vessels from the United Provinces were being stopped 'under pretence' of infection, by which means 'the Freedome of Trade & Passage' was obstructed.[35] He insisted that the strictness be relaxed. Charles replied expressing sorrow for the affliction, but pointed out that England had been the last neighbour of the United Provinces to make restrictions, and commerce would now have to be suspended altogether.[36] Thus another Dutch plea for mitigation was greeted by a precisely opposite response.

In the forefront of defensive nations had been France, and news reached Holland in mid-August that France was so alarmed at the mortality in Amsterdam (another 905 people died in the first week of that month) that all Dutch ships were to be barred from French ports until December.[37] On 31 August Charles followed suit: quarantine times for ships already in detention were to continue, but no more ships from Holland, Zealand or any other part of the United Provinces were to enter any port in his kingdom until 1 December.[38] The Dutch were incensed; the Admiralty proposed a retaliatory quarantine against shipping of all nations that had imposed it on them, but anger against England was to some extent deflected by events in Spain, where Admiral de Ruyter had been refused pratique to the chagrin of the Dutch Grand Pensionary, Jan de Witt.[39] In fact, the considered reply of the States General to Charles's memorial was surprisingly plaintive: could he please permit commerce with places not actually infected?[40] That was late September, and news of the loss of New Amsterdam would not yet have reached de Witt's ears. With outrage to follow humiliation, the prognosis of war was inescapable. In the anxiety of open conflict, and with London soon suffering a catastrophic plague of its own, the quarantine orders against Holland withered gently to a natural extinction. Quarantine against Hamburg was lifted on 30 November 1664.[41]

The efficacy of these measures is very much open to question. Defoe, in his *Journal of the Plague Year*, linked the London epidemic to the outbreak in Holland, but how the two Frenchmen who appear to have imported the disease in late 1664 came into the country is unexplained. Defoe, of course, may not have been correct about the Frenchmen, and another writer, on 'irrefrigable Authority', believed the plague was imported, certainly from Holland, but in trans-shipped bales of Turkish cotton or silk.[42] Detention at Hole Haven, the only quarantine harbour to be named by the Privy Council, netted three merchant ships and one warship

34 *CCSP*, vol. 5, p. 394.

35 NA PC 2/57/199.

36 Ibid.; *CCSP*, vol. 5, p. 412.

37 *CCSP*, vol. 5, pp. 351, 414.

38 NA PC 2/57/199; *CCSP*, vol. 5, p. 421.

39 *CCSP*, vol. 5, p. 424.

40 *CCSP*, vol. 5, pp. 425–6.

41 NA PC 2/57/305.

42 N. Hodges, *Loimologia* ... (London, 1720), p. 30.

as early as 18 November 1663.[43] They were then destined to stay there another 14 days; as quarantine at that time was 30 days, they would seem to have arrived about 2 November, but that date is earlier than the Order. Because the ships had come from the island of Texel, perhaps they were considered relatively 'safe'. The haven held 18 vessels in early September 1664, with more expected daily, but by 1 November it was reported empty of ships, 'their time having expired'.[44] As quarantine was then 40 days, the new daily arrivals clearly never materialized. This was presumably the result of Charles's total embargo against Dutch ships, announced on 31 August.

Whatever period of quarantine was inflicted on ship and crew, there were always people who, or cargo which, for one reason or another escaped the restrictions. An early problem was caused by barrels of fish destined for London in Lent, and lying in five ships at Hole Haven in February 1664.[45] Clearly this was a most perishable cargo, and encouraged by a statement from the Lord Mayor 'of the great want ... in this season', and relying on the strength of certificates of good health from Rotterdam (which they might in other cases have ignored), the Privy Council allowed the fish to be trans-shipped up the river.[46] And reasons could always be found for allowing small personal items ashore if the owner were well-enough connected: thus the Danish Resident in London could retrieve a trunk, portmanteau and some linen sent from Hamburg; and the Countess of Chesterfield could receive effects from Flushing.[47] Both these concessions concerned ships under quarantine at Hole Haven.

Some individuals fared especially well. In May 1664 the wife and maid of Nicholas Oudart were allowed to land at Harwich from The Hague, performing no quarantine at all; Sir William Killigrew and his servant, travelling between the same two ports, enjoyed the like privilege in June.[48] In the same month a gentleman and his servant were allowed out of Hole Haven to deliver a present for the King from a German prince.[49] The weak justification was that he had travelled through Holland to embark, but had not stayed there. In July, Lieutenant-Colonel Cromwell came ashore at Harwich without quarantine, and Lady Davidson and family did likewise a little later.[50] In October a pregnant Mrs Martha Watson, travelling from Hamburg, was permitted on shore near Rochester with a maidservant, under certain conditions.[51]

43 NA PC 2/56/624.

44 *CSPD* (1664–65), pp. 3, 51.

45 NA PC 2/57/23.

46 Ibid.

47 *CSPD* (1664–65), pp. 15, 17.

48 *CSPD* (1664–65), pp. 580, 605.

49 NA PC 2/57/108. The bearer was Nicholas Bowman.

50 *CSPD* (1663–64), pp. 634, 647.

51 NA PC 2/57/235.

Sir John Hebdon, an envoy to Russia, was allowed to land in September 1664 'so he may be enabled the sooner to give an Account to his Matie of his Service'.[52] It was not even known where Hebdon would land, but his son petitioned the Privy Council because he was expected 'hourly'.[53] Hebdon had been driven on shore in the Baltic before reaching The Sound, near Elsinore; this had forced him overland to Hamburg, from where Sir William Swan would certify that he had been in no infected house.[54] But Hebdon tarried in diseased Hamburg long enough for his son to learn all this by post, for a petition to be written and presented, for the Privy Council to inform the farmers of Customs, and for the farmers to notify outports.

In two cases a partial exemption was made for horses. Sixteen from Friesland, ordered by the Duke of Albermarle for the King's service, were allowed to complete their quarantine in a meadow near Hole Haven, having been 14 days on board 'to their greate prejudice by reason of the faintness of the Weather.'[55] The justification was that Friesland was from free of disease (although Schiedam, the port of departure, was not). Similarly there was a concession for Lord Wotton to land six horses from The Brill at Hole Haven, provided they kept their distance from 'other cattle' ashore; his lordship's servants could also land after four days in good health.[56]

More significant were the exemptions for naval stores. In July 1664 the Duke of York, as Lord High Admiral, told the Privy Council of cordage 'whereof there is a great Want at p^{re}sent', arrived at Yarmouth from Holland, and destined for the King's service at Portsmouth.[57] When this could be unloaded immediately, it was the cue for the fishing lobby at Yarmouth to argue successfully for cordage to be discharged for their herring fleet.[58] There was a useful argument here, as 'the Nature of Tarred-Cordage is rather a preservative against Infection, then Apt to convey It'.[59] Later, it became routine to allow ships at Yarmouth to unload cordage without quarantine.[60] Sir William Warren, the biggest naval contractor of the era, warned the Privy Council that a new 50-gun ship for the Turkey Company could not be completed unless cordage and cables imported from East Friesland in a Dutch ship were allowed ashore.[61] A further inducement for the Council's indulgence were the glazed tiles on the same vessel destined for the royal palace

52 NA PC 2/57/220. Hebdon suggested the Russians as potential providers of naval stores.

53 Ibid.

54 Ibid.

55 NA PC 2/57/132.

56 *CSPD* (1663–64), p. 618. The Brill was the English name for Briel near Rotterdam.

57 NA PC 2/57/139.

58 NA PC 2/57/177.

59 Ibid.

60 For example *CSPD* (1664–65), pp. 7, 11 for three ships permitted to unload by Secretary Bennet.

61 NA PC 2/57/218–9. Warren presented his case 'doubting a warr might happen at sea'.

under construction at Greenwich.[62] In October 1664 the Privy Council listened to a petition from Denis Gauden, Surveyor General of his Majesty's marine victuals.[63] Gauden was responsible for providing pipestaves (used in barrel making) and hogshead staves for naval use. With constraints on cutting timber in Ireland, Gauden relied on supplies from the Baltic and Hamburg. But Hamburg ships could not unload for 40 days. Not only was the shortfall of supplies affecting the navy, but shipowners were too 'discouraged' to hire out their vessels.[64] The Privy Council, of course, gave immediate exemption.

The total embargo on vessels from Holland, instituted on 31 August 1664, brought inevitable problems for ships which had sailed before news of the ban had reached them. The first petition, in late September, was from the owners and freighters of the *Sampson* of London, which had arrived at Amsterdam from the Straits, taken in a cargo, and then gone north to Texel before the embargo had been issued or received.[65] The arguments for compassion were based on patriotic sentiment: the ship was English and so were the crew (therefore the Navigation Act was being observed) and the cargo was destined for his Majesty's subjects; the petitioners, rather vaguely, were 'desirous to withdraw their Estates from those parts in this juncture of time'; and worst of all the ship was too leaky to put back to sea. Could she, please, be allowed to proceed to Hole Haven to do quarantine?[66] The Privy Council could scarcely have objected. In October merchants at Plymouth found themselves in the same curious situation of petitioning for a gross inconvenience which was simply the lesser of two evils.[67] Other petitions came from Colchester and London, the former worrying about bills of exchange drawn for the goods, the latter pointing out that the ship carried cordage suitable for the navy.[68] All these petitions were successful, in that quarantine rather than exclusion was the resulting remedy.

Although the Privy Council did not reject outright any petition (at least, any minuted petition) which came their way, they were far from complacent about the way quarantine as a whole was managed. The authorities at Yarmouth were never sure where they stood, at one point praised for their 'Circumspeccon to p^{re}vent the feared Infection of the Pestilence', and then warned that persons and goods were landing illegally, 'which neglect is no waies suitable to that care you ought to have of the Health & Welfare of his Maties Subjects, nor to the Obedience you owe to the Commands of this Board, and which for the future will be more exactly expected from you.'[69] This rider was added to the Yarmouth version of a circular letter to London and all outports dated 17 June 1664.[70] The burden of this

62 Ibid.

63 NA PC 2/57/237.

64 Ibid.

65 NA PC 2/57/230–31.

66 Ibid.

67 NA PC 2/57/242.

68 NA PC 2/57/245, 278–9.

69 NA PC 2/56/676; 2/57/127. In January 1636 the Yarmouth authorities had been formally warned for letting a man ashore from Rotterdam (PC 2/45/401–2).

70 NA PC 2/57/126–8.

letter was that no goods were to be received from the United Provinces without a Customs certificate that quarantine had been performed. If this were disobeyed, then the house of an offender was to be 'shut up' as if it were harbouring plague. London and 27 outports received a virtually identical text. Other than Yarmouth, the only outport to receive a tailored letter was Harwich: the mayor and corporation were told of 'a generall neglect or Connivance in the severall Out Ports of this Kingdome', reminded to observe the restrictions, and told to inform the master of the packet boat from Holland that he was to land no one in England.[71]

There is certainly some evidence of problems in the outports. In May 1664, Customs officers at Topsham, the port for Exeter, reported that a sailor from Amsterdam had disobeyed quarantine and come ashore with his family.[72] A far more serious incident arose at Whitby a few months later.[73] Five ships from Holland arrived on the same day, but they would not be moored together to facilitate surveillance, and some seamen went ashore. The authorities ordered the houses which received them to be shut up, but this provoked the rest of the crews, and some inhabitants, to threaten to release them by force. The Customs officers, finding the men were local and the town was on their side, 'resorted to good words', which at least got the offenders back on board. But the Customs officers warned that the situation was untenable: either commerce with infected places had to be suspended, or trained bands were needed to supervise the arrivals. As this report was made to the farmers of Customs, and not to the Privy Council, and as the records of the Customs service have generally not survived, it can easily be imagined that the position at Whitby was by no means unique.

While London suffered from plague in 1665, and attempted to fight the Dutch, naval stores like hemp and rope yarn arrived at Portsmouth from St Malo.[74] But the French reacted to the English affliction as they had to the Dutch, prohibiting all commerce between those Channel ports for the duration of the plague, and for six months afterwards.[75] The Baltic supply route remained open, but the hard lesson was being taught, if not learnt, that in a state of war disease found various ways to side with the enemy. It was also being made clear to the English that quarantine could have an absolute and dispassionate application. There was little sign of the French making the kind of concessions, even for their own dignitaries, as had weakened the English defences. When the French ambassadors were recalled from England, they sat out their quarantine at St-Valéry.[76] Similarly, the Spanish summarily stopped all trade with England, Scotland and Ireland, partly in response to a botched attempt at smuggling to breach their quarantine rule.[77]

71 NA PC 2/57/127.

72 Ibid.

73 *CSPD* (1663–64), p. 670, from which remaining references in this paragraph are taken.

74 *CSPD* (1664–65), p. 499.

75 Ibid.

76 *CSPD* (1665–66), p. 63.

77 *CSPD* (1665–66), p. 38.

When plague returned to northern France in 1668, England's response was directed only at places judged to be the greatest risk. The Privy Council ordered all ports to prevent ships from Rouen and Caen unloading until quarantine (presumably 40 days) had been completed.[78] A sloop, HMS *Emsworth*, was ordered to the mouth of Hole Haven, to direct ships from Normandy to the quarantine station.[79] Up to a point, this worked: in February 1669 there were seven ships detained there, but in earlier months many others had got through.[80] The *Emsworth*'s captain complained rather pathetically that the Thames was wide, the nights were dark, and the ships could be obstinate[81]. At Hull, however, there were signs of confidence, with the Customs officers taking it upon themselves to keep ships from Ostend (not in the suspect area) out of the harbour until they had given a satisfactory account of their journey.[82]

England's last brush with quarantine in the seventeenth century involved danger from a new direction. In terms of the origin of the disease, the ports initially at risk, and the nature of the infection (which was never openly discussed), England was unprepared. On 1 July 1692 Secretary of State Lord Nottingham wrote to the Treasury, conveying the Queen's concern about mortality in Barbados and the Leeward Islands, of which news had very recently reached Bideford in Devon.[83] While quarantine from those areas was being introduced, the Customs Commissioners discovered that two ships had recently reached Penzance from Jamaica, one confessing five deaths on the voyage, the other admitting nothing but testifying that Jamaica was very sickly.[84] On 27 July the Treasury accepted a recommendation from the Customs Commissioners that quarantine should be extended to ships from Jamaica.[85] The Commissioners were already considering a revival of the previous quarantine station, but ships from the West Indies were significantly larger than those trading with the near Continent and Hole Haven was judged too cramped.[86] The Commissioners recommended, therefore, that ships should do quarantine at The Hope – that is, in the river itself – and the Treasury agreed that a naval ketch, supported by two boats from the Customs service, should patrol between the Essex and Kent shores.[87]

On 1 August 1692 the Queen, through the Privy Council, formally ordered quarantine to take place, but with no holding ground for ships going anywhere other than London.[88] There was also a curious concession: if a ship had put in at Ireland, Scotland, the Isles of Scilly, or the Isle of Man on the way to London,

78 NA PC 2/60/444–5.

79 Ibid.

80 *CSPD* (1668–69), pp. 2, 162, 193.

81 *CSPD* (1668–69), p. 2.

82 *CSPD* (1667–68), p. 580.

83 NA T1/19/1; *Calendar of Treasury Papers* [*CTP*] (1556/57–1696), p. 245

84 *Calendar of Treasury Books* [*CTB*] (1689–92), p. 1708; *Acts of the Privy Council, Colonial Series* [*APCCS*] *(1680–1720)*, p. 213.

85 NA T1/19/71; *CTB* (1689–92), pp. 1739–40.

86 *APCCS (1680–1720)*, pp. 213–15.

87 Ibid.; NA T1/19/71/73.

88 *APCCS (1680–1720)*, pp. 214–15; *CTB* (1689–92), p. 1762.

and spent some time there (of which 'divers instances ... daily happen'), that same time should be deducted from the quarantine.[89] No thought was apparently given to the possibility of disease striking these extremities of the kingdom. Final release from quarantine could only be secured by a certificate from the appropriate Customs officer that he had frequently mustered the men during the detention; and by the oath of the master that all on board were healthy.[90] These stipulations had been put by the Customs Commissioners to the Treasury as no more than points for their consideration.

As in earlier decades, quarantine induced a variety of petitions for the Privy Council to ponder. But this time the subjects were new: a naval captain was rude to the Mayor of Plymouth; press gangs were taking men from potentially infected ships; and owners and freighters were coming up with ingenious reasons why quarantine should not apply to their vessels.[91] London merchants petitioned that two ships in The Hope from Barbados should perform only half-quarantine 'as is usuall in such Cases [i.e. the crew were all well], the Shipps lyeing at Extraordinary Charges'.[92] The exact reasons for another merchant ship to be exempt are not recited,[93] but the master of the sloop *Neptune* had a winning formula. The ship had come rapidly from Jamaica with official despatches about an earthquake that had occurred there on 7 June.[94] He and two seamen testified to the good health of the island when they left, and showed the need for an equally rapidly return, bearing news of what aid could be expected.[95] On 18 August 1692, on the strength of this message, quarantine from Jamaica was summarily removed.[96] The lifting of quarantine generally occurred in November.[97] The decision was taken quickly, for no obvious reason, almost as though the Privy Council were looking for an excuse: a ship's master from the West Indies petitioned for entry, claiming that his vessel, the *Coronation*, was 'one of the most healthy ... that ever went and came from thence' and no crewman had even been ill on board, let alone died, for the last four months.[98] In allowing the ship to unload, quarantine generally was lifted as a kind of rider to the ad hoc decision. A significant factor was that most of the crew had recently been impressed, and any application of quarantine would logically have extended to the warships.

The West Indies, and Barbados in particular, continued to cause periodic concern. Governor Russell lost his wife and ten servants to rampant fever, while ships, undermanned at the outset, were barely operational through sickness.[99]

89 *APCCS (1680–1720)*, pp. 214–15; NA PC 2/74/455–6.

90 Ibid.

91 *APCCS (1680–1720)*, pp. 215–16; NA PC 2/74/464, 496; T1/19/71, 107.

92 NA T1/19/105, 107.

93 This ship was the *East India Merchant* from Jamaica. The Privy Council minutes (NA PC 2/74/459) refer only to the petition and 'the reasons therein contained'.

94 NA PC 2/74/465 (*APCCS (1680–1720)*, p. 215).

95 Ibid.

96 NA PC 2/74/467.

97 *APCCS (1680–1720)*, p. 216; *CTB* (1689–92), p. 1891.

98 Ibid.

99 *Calendar of State Papers, Colonial Series* [*CSPC*] (1693–6), pp. 362, 386, 445.

In September 1693 another order for quarantine at The Hope was made against arrivals from Barbados, but this petered out very quickly.[100]

England, at the close of the seventeenth century, was like a nervous householder, rushing between the front and back doors, locking them at a whim against deadly intrusion from east or west, but knowing that if the doors stayed locked for too long, the household itself could not function. One solution, the house being big enough, was to employ specialist janitors, but England was still a very long way from the Continental model.

Policy in embryo

Among the measures of the seventeenth century, most of the later characteristics of British quarantine policy can be seen at a formative stage. The imposition of quarantine was always short-lived, in response to perceived emergencies, and within the royal prerogative. There was as yet no question of permanent measures or of parliamentary involvement. Below the monarch, the chain of communication was fairly clear. The Privy Council exercised and promulgated the Crown's wishes, although how far quarantine was delegated to the Council's own subsidiary bodies – the fledgling Cabinet and the Committee on Foreign Affairs – is difficult to gauge. The Council gave directions to the Lord High Treasurer, who in turn instructed the farmers of the Customs (later the Customs Commissioners) to enforce the provisions. Neither at this stage nor at any later one, was quarantine more than one of the burdensome distractions of the Customs service, 'not being a Part of the general Business'.[101] In the seventeenth century quarantine was too fitful and localized to cause the service a lasting problem, but in the next century that position was to change. Two other bodies little affected by quarantine at this period were the Navy Board and the Board of Admiralty. The latter were concerned with the disposition of warships, but the number of these ships necessary to meet the quarantine regulations of the seventeenth century was small, so problems were still a decade away.

There were, however, some interesting constitutional aspects to the application of quarantine, especially after the Restoration. It was Charles II who was most closely connected with the risks and indeed the opportunities that quarantine presented. Opportunity sounds a strange word in this context, but Charles was soon to realize that the unwarranted imposition of quarantine was a potent political weapon. It could undermine the concept of free trade by denying pratique to ships of a particular nation. This is exactly what happened in the Mediterranean, to England's disadvantage, in 1662–63.[102] The Spanish, wishing to harass England, claimed there was plague at Tangier where the English were trading. Because of this, English ships were denied pratique in Spain, and then at Toulon. Charles feared that the same might happen, disastrously, at ports like Leghorn and Genoa,

---

100 *APCCS (1680–1720)*, p. 254.

101 J. Lane, *The Reports of the Commissioners appointed to examine, take, and state the Public Accounts of the Kingdom ...* (London, 1787), p. 366.

102 *Calendar of State Papers Venetian* [*CSPV*] (1661–4), p. 199.

and the Venetian ambassador was asked to persuade Italian rulers that Tangier was perfectly healthy.[103] But the least suspicion of infection was enough to rattle the Italian sanitary authorities, and in December 1663 Charles was forced to send an envoy to Leghorn to demand pratique for English ships.[104] Pepys, who had no first-hand knowledge of quarantine, was scathing of the Mediterranean practice 'where a man may buy a bill of health for a piece-of-eight, and my enemy may agree with the *Intendent* ... for ten pieces-of-eight or so, that he shall not give me [one]'.[105] It is against this background that the measures taken against the Dutch in 1663-64 must necessarily be examined. But there is no evidence that the English quarantine precautions, including the banning of ships from Holland for three months, were instituted to any significant degree by a basic dislike of the Dutch. The French had anticipated the English by making an absolute embargo against Dutch ships, and Pepys was a frank-enough diarist to mention any political aspect to the quarantine, had one existed. Moreover, it was in England's interests to receive cargoes from Holland, as the cordage at Yarmouth indicates, whatever the nationality of the ships that carried them.

Among the state papers is an interesting undated memorial referring to the advantages which might accrue in England from a permanent quarantine 'Office'.[106] This document has been endorsed with a suggested date of March 1665. The memorial refers to a petition to the King against 'bringing in the Pest' – a petition which seems not to have survived – advocating the adoption of procedures which existed in 'most other well governed Kingdomes and Republicks professing Christianity'. Thus the new office would have been like a Board of Health. The memorial was not concerned with the medical argument, only the contingent advantages. The case was argued on four grounds: collusion between the farmers of Customs and 'the directors of ... [the] office' would ensure that duties were paid; importers of goods would see their ships liable to equal detention, 'so as hee that first arrives makes not the proffitt alone'; it would be known what ships and cargoes were in detention, which would keep prices moderate; and people coming into the country would be monitored, so bona fide travellers could be distinguished from spies. The memorialist was particularly struck by the second argument, against forestalling, drawing an analogy from Holland where ships could only come and go 'in Fleetes'. But the quarantine arrangements of Holland, unlike its trading practices, were never a model for the European states. In muddying the waters between trade and disease, this mercantilist paper seems to have had no impact on Charles or his advisers. But it is important as the earliest advocacy for a permanent quarantine establishment.

No evidence of political manoeuvring, in the realm of quarantine, is apparent among the royal advisers. The post of Secretary of State had been divided before 1680 between northern and southern divisions (Holland in the former, France in the latter), but at the time of the measures against the Dutch this distinction, if it

103 Ibid.

104 Latham & Matthews (eds), *The Diary of Samuel Pepys*, vol. 4, pp. 417–18.

105 Ibid.

106 NA SP 29/116/122, from which remaining references in this paragraph are taken.

existed at all, was probably weak.[107] It would seem to have been Clarendon, as Chancellor, who formulated quarantine policy at that period (perhaps in Cabinet) but there are no grounds for assuming that quarantine and political ambition were linked, or that any one man made it his speciality. As for the Secretaries of State, interest in their role arises from their relationship not with the Crown but with the Privy Council, which they appear occasionally to have sidelined. This was most noticeable among the 'grace and favour' exemptions cited above from the quarantine restrictions of the 1660s. Of the fourteen instances, seven were sanctioned by the Privy Council, one by Secretary Morice and four by his successor, Bennet.[108] The remaining two were recorded as authorized by licence and warrant respectively, but with no source; as they were not minuted in the Privy Council's register, the authority presumably was Bennet's.[109] Thus the dispensations were shared equally between Privy Council and Secretary of State. Again, in 1692, Secretary Nottingham conveyed Queen Mary's pleasure straight to the Lord High Treasurer, and quarantine against Barbados and the Leeward Islands was in position before the Privy Council had even issued the Order. Of course, the perceived need for immediate action justified a precipitate move in this instance, and it is possible that some committee of Council had sanctioned the Secretary's action whenever he appeared to act by his own initiative, or by a direct route from the Crown.

Another body whose role in quarantine procedures changed after the seventeenth century was the Corporation of London. It has been seen above that the Lord Mayor was consistently canvassed for advice, and even offered executive action. There were three factors at work here. The first was the delicate relationship between the Crown, working from Westminster, and the international merchants working a few miles away in the City of London. As long as the economic affairs of the country were within the royal prerogative, tension with the City was at times inevitable: there was therefore a political reason to consult the City in any issue, such as quarantine, which threatened to disrupt business.[110] The second factor was the body of expertise in the City about the nature of plague, the means of its transmission, and the precautions taken in the Mediterranean to prevent it. Only a Turkey merchant, or a trader to Leghorn or Venice, knew at first hand what quarantine measures were used in the hot spots, and what they meant to the merchant or freighter. The third factor follows closely on the second; only in London were all these people gathered. London was, by a spectacular margin, the most important entrepôt of the country, with four-fifths of the foreign trade.[111] It is

107 For the divisions, see M.A. Thomson, *The Secretaries of State, 1681–1782* (Oxford, 1932), pp. 2–3.

108 The dispensations made by the Secretaries of State were to individuals, with the exception of Sir John Hebdon and the pregnant Mrs Watson who were dealt with by the Privy Council.

109 These were again dispensations to individuals (Cromwell and Lady Davidson).

110 For relations between Crown and City, see C. Wilson, *England's Apprenticeship, 1603–1763*, 2nd edn (London, 1984), pp. 47, 48, 58.

111 E. Lipson, *The Economic History of England. The Age of Mercantilism* (3 vols, London, 1943), vol. 2, pp. 249ff.

unsurprising that nowhere else in the country seemed to matter very much when overseas business was being considered.

The exact nature of the plague, pest or pestilential contagion against which quarantine defended was little discussed. It is doubtful whether the 'plague' reported in Holland and France in 1629, and at Rouen in 1634, was bubonic plague, but when mortality was high the exact diagnosis was of no consequence, and in any event beyond the scope of contemporary medicine.[112] There was no attempt to classify as plague, or as anything else specific, the disease from the West Indies which caused the Queen's panic reaction in 1692. Indeed, this instance is remarkable. It was to be nearly 150 years before disease in the West Indies was again the cause of quarantine in England, although the eighteenth century was to witness more than enough sickness coming into the country from that quarter. Within Britain, however, 'plague' had long existed in various places at different times, and the Privy Council routinely intervened to control the spread of disease, sometimes with significant consequences to local trade. A feature of this early period was the use of quarantine, airing and other controls within the British Isles. This was more than a question of Scotland denying access to people and goods from across the border. It has been shown above that London in 1580 barred ships from Plymouth, and in 1666 all cloth from Colchester to London had to be aired at Stratford before entering the capital.[113] Particularly affected by constraints, some from the Privy Council, others from neighbouring boroughs, was the port of Hull. Ravaged by periodic epidemics, the town's merchants were forbidden to trade in the dire years of 1637–38.[114] The eighteenth-century historians of both Hull and Newcastle refer to eras in their respective towns when business was at a standstill because of plague and grass grew in the streets.[115] In 1645 the corporations of Hull and York took joint action against Leeds, to prevent plague arriving from there in infected cloth.[116]

It has been seen that most impositions of quarantine involved the airing of cargoes. Indeed, in earlier years the airing was the main provision, and the length of detention was whatever time was deemed necessary for the cargo to be aired. There were thus two distinct elements to quarantine – the period of detention for ship and people, and the time needed for fresh air to nullify the contagious elements of the cargo. Ideally these events happened simultaneously, but the lack of airing space was a conspicuous problem and was to become worse in the years ahead. At this period, as later, there is little or no evidence that airing actually took place; for instance, in the measures taken against Holland in 1663–64 the attempt to find space for a lazaretto and airing ground clearly failed, and the emphasis changed

112 J.-N. Biraben, *Les Hommes et la peste en France ...* (2 vols, Paris, 1975–76), vol. 1, Annexe 4.

113 NA PC 2/58/394: the cloth had to be 'well ayred with Brimstone'.

114 NA PC 2/48/226, 227. When the restraint was lifted, the mayor of Hull was warned 'to bee very cautious' still.

115 Hadley, p. 95; J. Brand, *The Histories and Antiquities ... of Newcastle upon Tyne ...* (2 vols, London, 1789), vol. 2, pp. 455–6.

116 L.M. Stanewell (ed.), *Calendar of the Ancient Deeds ... of ... Hull* (Hull, 1951), p. 209.

to quarantine pure and simple. Yet the European perception that some goods were more 'susceptible' to harbouring disease than others was certainly understood in England. Cloth was thought one of the most deadly transmitters: this is why the linen ships from Morlaix were targeted in 1638, and why textiles from Colchester were to be aired at Stratford in 1666. Any fibrous material, including hemp and flax, was reckoned highly contagious, although tar and pitch were thought to form an effective barrier. Thus the cordage at Yarmouth was susceptible, but not when tarred. In the years ahead the division into susceptible and non-susceptible goods was to be a science in itself, with every conceivable import placed in one category or the other, with grades of susceptibility.

Mention of cordage introduces the tricky issue of naval stores. With England almost continually at war with one or more European neighbour, the supply of material for shipbuilding and repair was vital for the efficiency of the navy. The depletion of English forests, the particular suitability of Norwegian pine for masts and spars, and the reliance on the Baltic for hemp and flax (for rope and canvas), combined to make England vulnerable if supplies were disrupted. It was for this reason that the cordage was allowed in at Yarmouth for naval use. As the hemp had been processed in Holland the import was not a breach of the Navigation Act. A wider discussion of this subject will be necessary when the quarantine measures, specifically against the Baltic, are discussed.

If the navy was in need of stores, it was in even greater need of men. There is a large literature on impressment and the history of its use and abuse need not be examined here, although the theme will be recurrent in this work. The seventeenth century saw a significant problem with men being pressed from ships liable to, or even undergoing, quarantine. At this early period some excuse can be found for the navy's actions: for one thing the relative novelty of quarantine made the inviolability little understood. There was the problem of disseminating information to ships' captains, not only that quarantine existed but what it stood for. A captain who had spent the best part of his life capturing enemy merchant ships, regardless of the state of health in the ports his prizes had sailed from, would not hesitate taking men from an idle ship which had a theoretical chance of infection. In 1692 this very much worried the Customs Commissioners, who complained to the Privy Council.[117]

There are many other respects in with the seventeenth-century measures foreshadowed later experience. None of them is particularly significant in itself, but together they form an indication of where the contentions of the future would lie. Shipowners became discouraged from hiring out vessels which would lie for long periods unproductive: the cost of supporting a ship and crew in quarantine was considerable, and the liability sometimes uncertain. Ships could be leaky and seawater might spoil a cargo. Merchants might be called upon to honour bills of exchange against a cargo which had not yet landed. All these issues would develop in the years ahead, but they were questions for individuals and none of them particularly bothered the Privy Council or Secretaries of State. What did trouble the authorities, however, was the widespread evasion of, or deliberate

117 NA PC 2/74/458.

disregard for, quarantine, and the circular letter from the Privy Council of 1664 was evidence of their real concern for this intractable issue. It was one thing to bend the rules for a diplomat or aristocrat who wanted to be rid of the stinking prison which a quarantined ship might become; but quite another to see common seamen sneaking ashore to the local tavern, or even going home. The British never entirely overcame the issue of favouritism, and the problem of deliberate contempt was destined to run and run, embroiling all branches of civil and military administration.

Scotland

Measures against plague in Scotland were being vigorously undertaken while England was still groping for some kind of effective response. This head start was partly born of necessity in that most of the trade, particularly on the eastern seaboard, was conducted with Scandinavia, the Baltic, the Low Countries and France. If exposure to plague were not controlled, the whole population of eastern Scotland, not to mention its economy, could suffer dramatically. Another major difference from the English situation was the plethora of small ports, many of them clustered around the Forth estuary, each with its interest in overseas trade. Whereas in England quarantine measures were aimed at protecting London, while the outports were left largely to their own devices, the system in Scotland had to be workable across a score of harbours, very few of which were large enough to offer quarantine facilities. Another important difference was that, while the enforcement of quarantine in England was handled by the Customs service, in Scotland it was a matter for local government – that is, the burgh councils and magistracy.[118] In both kingdoms, however, it was the Crown acting through the respective Privy Councils (in Scotland initially the 'Secret Council') who formulated policy by a series of Orders and Proclamations. The latter were used more literally than in England: an Order in Scotland was proclaimed at the market cross in burghs and seaports.

The measures themselves were sometimes a simple embargo on trade or landing, and the Scottish Council never flinched from including England among countries on the quarantine blacklist.[119] It was a paradox of the Scottish system that detention periods, whether for ships, crews or airing, were distinctly vague while the process of purification was precisely set out. In July 1564, for instance, merchants trading with Danzig were asked to put in where they could at 'quiet places', rather than the main ports, until further notice.[120] Two months later they were still there, the ships were getting leaky, and the cargoes beginning to spoil. In a decision which predated, quite significantly, the classification later adopted in England of enumerated goods, the Scottish authorities reckoned that only the

118 J. Ritchie, 'Quarantine for plague in Scotland during the sixteenth and seventeenth centuries', *Edinburgh Medical Journal*, 55 (1948), 691.

119 Ritchie, p. 692.

120 *Register of the Privy Council of Scotland* [*RPCS*], vol. 1, p. 279.

flax element in a cargo of naval stores was dangerous.[121] At the expense of the owners, the flax was therefore to be opened and aired on Inchcolm Island in the Firth of Forth, while pitch, tar, iron and timber could stay on board.[122] The ships themselves were to be half scuttled and lie in the water for 'ane or twa tydis' (one or two tides), while the cargoes were washed, cleansed and partly fumigated with burning heather.[123] As well as being precise, these measures were harsh and threatened irreparable damage.

Another characteristic of the Scottish system, again in contrast to the English, was the nominal severity of punishment. In Scotland a Proclamation could carry its own penalties for those in breach, and these were invariably death. This threat might even extend to merchants whose goods, declared 'safe' on arrival, were later believed to have carried a fatal infection.[124] When some crews came ashore in Leith, in breach of the Proclamation of 1564, they were to be seized, and the Proclamation reread at strategic locations to remind people that its provisions were to be enforced 'undir the pane of deid'.[125] Similarly, in 1574, when 'seik and fowll' persons inland presumed to break their isolation for infection, they were to suffer the ultimate fate.[126] In fact, it will be seen that magistrates were lenient with offenders and the cruellest aspect of the Scottish measures lay arguably in the indeterminate duration of quarantine while the 'clengeris', or cleansers, went about their business. In a complicated incident of 1580 (which gave rise to two Proclamations), some seamen and passengers from a Danzig ship spent 115 days in quarantine on Inchcolm.[127]

In the seventeenth century the ferocity of punishment was theoretically maintained, while other measures were introduced to deal with the nature of the risk. A ship which arrived at Dunbar from Norway in 1618, suspected of carrying plague, was summarily ordered back to sea with such provisions as the town would allow.[128] In the summer of that year, the magistrates of Edinburgh were given full power to act as they pleased in relation to quarantine while the lords of the Council dispersed to their respective homes to organize the local harvest.[129] Soon Scotland developed a relatively sophisticated system, whereby ships from suspected places were intercepted before entering port and the master was asked by the local authority to respond to a questionnaire, covering such matters as the port or ports where he had loaded, the 'estate and conditioun' of the area at that time, the health of the people on board, and the nature of the cargo.[130] Satisfactory answers led to a licence to land; if danger was still apprehended, the ship could be sent elsewhere for 'tryall' (detention to see if infection developed) or for

121 *RPCS*, vol. 1, pp. 280–82. The Scottish word for flax was 'lynt'.

122 Ibid.; Ritchie, p. 692.

123 Ibid.

124 Ritchie, p. 692.

125 *RPCS*, vol. 1, pp. 280–82.

126 *RPCS*, vol. 2, p. 415.

127 *RPCS*, vol. 3, pp. 313–14; the full story is in Ritchie, pp. 694–6.

128 *RPCS*, vol. 11, p. 410.

129 *RPCS*, vol. 11, p. 417.

130 *RPCS*, vol. 12, pp. 62–3 (1619).

cleansing.[131] These arrangements were in force, at various times, against arrivals from the East Country, and especially from Denmark and Königsberg.[132] As the Scottish Proclamations invariably claimed the plague in those areas was most violent and infectious, it is all the more curious that England had no quarantine protection against the Baltic until a century later. At times, the Scottish Council could still appear very severe, for instance ordering an Anstruther vessel 'not altogidder voyde and frie of danger' to Inchcolm where the crew had more or less to fend for themselves, as well as unload their cargo for airing.[133] The penalty, of course, was death for infringement at any step of the way.

Despite such precautions, and new measures against Holland, parts of Scotland were attacked by plague in 1624–25, causing court sittings to be cancelled in Edinburgh, and the Privy Council to migrate to Stirling.[134] Plague continued to afflict the Scottish capital, off and on, over the next decade. But as the enthusiasm of the Privy Council for preventive action at the seaports increased (particularly against the Low Countries), there was no inclination by local magistrates to insist on the full penalties of the law. Sailors who left their ships without licence were simply fined, and the offenders were happy to plead guilty.[135] The Council also became aware that provosts and bailies in the seaports were sometimes not doing their duty. In 1629 they summoned the bailies of eight ports between Burntisland and Fife to appear before them and answer for their neglect; the bailies of Leith appeared separately and were asked to keep ships from suspect places routinely out of harbour, for which, and similar measures, they were given a special commission.[136] Similar powers, by specific commission, were later extended to the ports on the northern shore of the Forth, and to Dundee, St Andrews and Montrose, following reports of plague in France, Orkney and Shetland.[137]

An ad hoc commission was appointed in 1635 to examine one William Muddie (or Mudie), master of a ship from the Low Countries, accused of 'most undewtifullie and mischantlie' letting a sick man go ashore.[138] Muddie was not the only skipper to be accused of letting people land, and the Council positively ranted against intercourse with certain Dutch ships, 'being a mater verie suspicious and dangerous and carying with it verie pregnant presumptions of great evill to follow ...'[139] A year later (1636) even ships from English ports, especially London and Newcastle, were subject to special watch.[140] One hapless master of a London ship, arrived at Prestonpans, had the temerity to allow ashore his entire ship's company.[141] For this he was summoned to appear before the Council who, in full

131 Ibid.

132 *RPCS*, vol. 12, pp. 62–3, 322–3.

133 Ibid.

134 *RPCS*, vol. 13, pp. 622, 652, 699, 700.

135 *Extracts from the Burgh Records of Edinburgh* [*EBRB*] (1626–41), pp. 176–84.

136 *RPCS*, 2nd Series, vol. 3, pp. 380–87 *passim*.

137 *RPCS*, 2nd Series, vol. 3, pp. 386, 388–9.

138 *RPCS*, 2nd Series, vol. 6, pp. 119–20.

139 *RPCS*, 2nd Series, vol. 6, p. 126.

140 *RPCS*, 2nd Series, vol. 6, p. 247.

141 *RPCS*, 2nd Series, vol. 6, p. 277.

bluster, announced 'for ... his proud contempt he aucht to be exemplarlie punished to the terror of others to committ the like'.[142] It is by no means clear that he was. Rumours of the plague on the English side of the land border with Scotland in 1637 led, not for the first time, to the total embargo of communications between the kingdoms.[143]

Once Scotland had shaken off the plague, which was not until the late 1640s, a measure of calm allowed the quarantine regulations against Holland to be codified with some precision. In 1655 a Proclamation set out procedures which were well in advance of the English practice, and for the first time allowed the Collector of Customs as well as magistrates to issue a licence to land.[144] A certificate was demanded that the port of loading was not infected, but 20 days' quarantine was still necessary; if the port *were* infected, the quarantine period was 40 days. Any unlawful communication with the shore was to be punished by imprisonment – the death penalty, which had probably never been used, was now discredited and abandoned. Magistrates were responsible for supplying quarantined ships with provisions at reasonable rates. As the Scottish Privy Council were to be made aware of all ships arriving from the United Provinces, the way was paved for each vessel to be monitored and treated on its merits, its discharge being handled by a body which was, save only in name, a Board of Health. In this system lay the roots of the practice which was to overburden the English Privy Council more than 50 years later.

Unfortunately, the 1655 arrangements did not survive the panic which gripped Scotland during the next decade, when plague again ravaged the Low Countries. This outbreak was preceded by other scares from Danzig and Königsberg, leading the Scottish Privy Council to distinguish between black plague in the Baltic and white plague in Holland.[145] To those ships' masters who traded also with England, the almost perpetual fear in Scotland of plague from the Baltic was irrational and unjustified. In 1662 Matheus Janson, master of the *Nicolai* carrying flax and other goods from Pilau, pointed out that not only was the region free of plague, but people and produce could enter London from the Baltic as they pleased.[146] Janson won his point, and soon the Council became so preoccupied with Holland that the Baltic was no longer an issue.

In October 1663, roughly when quarantine against Amsterdam and Hamburg was being introduced in the Thames, the Scottish Privy Council wrote to seaports banning all ships from Holland from entering harbour until they had been visited, after which suspect vessels would 'abyd a tryall'.[147] At the same time a letter was written to Sir William Davidson, Conservator of Privileges in Holland, informing him of this decision and hoping that he would keep the Council informed of ships

142 Ibid.

143 A good summary of the plague worries in Scotland appears in *RPCS*, 2nd Series, vol. 6, pp. xii–xv.

144 Bibliotheca Lindesiana, vol 6: *Ireland and Scotland* (Oxford, 1910), p. 352.

145 *RPCS*, 2nd Series, vol. 8, pp. 83–4.

146 *RPCS*, 2nd Series, vol. 8, p. 135.

147 *RPCS*, 2nd Series, vol. 8, p. 452.

from suspected places.[148] In the following month, the rather vague provision about 'tryall' was superseded by a simple, direct requirement for 40 days' quarantine against arrivals from Amsterdam and Holland, as compared with the 30 days which England had just imposed.[149] One noticeable feature of these decrees was the absence not only of any mention of the death penalty for disobedience, but of any penalty at all. When the inevitable accusations of breach of quarantine ensued, the Council were simply content for ships to complete their time, or leave it to local magistrates to arrive at a suitable punishment, which could include sequestration of goods.[150] Indeed, in February 1664 matters became so relaxed that for certain ships' masters in Bo'ness, the 40 days could be reckoned from the date the ship had set sail.[151] This was in response to information from Davidson that the plague was abating.

By June 1664, however, it was clear that plague in Holland was actually on the increase, and the full 40 days' quarantine was again demanded of all arrivals. This time the instrument was a Proclamation, and in referring to the many breaches which had arisen, it set out the new punishments – confiscation of ship and goods and imprisonment during the Council's pleasure.[152] This led to a coordinated protest on behalf of those masters who arrived daily from Holland without cargo or passengers, but simply to load coal, which meant income to Scotland from Customs dues and the import of specie.[153] An accommodation was reached by which coal could be lightered to vessels waiting offshore, against a bond of the master in £1000 that there would be no other communication with the land.[154] It was clear, however, within a week that many people, including the collier crews, came and went as they pleased.[155] This fact, coupled with even gloomier news from the Low Countries, led to a new Proclamation on 8 July 1664.[156] Past measures were recognized as insufficient, and now all trade with Holland was embargoed from 1 August until 1 November; persons contravening were to lose 'their lyfe, ship and goods, without mercy'. This, then, was a return to the old days, with death as the ultimate sanction. Ships which should arrive in the meanwhile were to stay offshore until magistrates allowed people to land, 'bringing ashore their goods to such houses and places as shall be designed for them and there to handle their goods and commodities daylie be the space of fourty dayes …' This amounted to the provision of lazarettoes, but with an astonishing lack of precision as to how they would actually work and be financed.

Again the measures were largely ignored, probably because they were impracticable, and the Privy Council's resolve was tested to the limit. At Bo'ness several ships, mainly Dutch and apparently colliers, were arriving to load and 'most

148 *RPCS*, 2nd Series, vol. 8, p. 451.
149 *RPCS*, 2nd Series, vol. 8, p. 454.
150 *RPCS*, 2nd Series, vol. 8, pp. 461, 466, 467.
151 *RPCS*, 2nd Series, vol. 8, pp. 492–3.
152 *RPCS*, 2nd Series, vol. 8, p. 534.
153 *RPCS*, 2nd Series, vol. 8, p. 541.
154 Ibid.
155 *RPCS*, 2nd Series, vol. 8, p. 544.
156 *RPCS*, 2nd Series, vol. 8, pp. 561–3.

contumaciously' doing as they liked.[157] The ships were ordered out of harbour, some within 48 hours, others within 24, after which, if they refused, the local bailie was ordered to burn them.[158] In early August some merchants of Edinburgh and Glasgow petitioned for a ship, just arrived at Bo'ness from Holland, to be unloaded, hoping that if they agreed to abide by a period of quarantine they might sidestep the total embargo.[159] But the Privy Council would have none of it; the ship was ordered to leave as soon as weather conditions allowed, with the master under pain of death.[160] Whether or not the threat would have been carried out, news of the tough stance was reported back to Holland by the Dutch ambassador in London.[161] Meanwhile, one of the Dutch ships ordered out of Bo'ness had simply moved to the next port and the crew were going ashore and socializing with the locals, as well as loading coal.[162] In a move which questions the Privy Council's resolve, the previous threat was not carried out, but simply repeated.[163] The only difference now was that those supplying the coal were summoned to appear before the Council.

Faced with continuing petitions from Scottish merchants, the Council blew hot and cold. At least one merchant won a concession from the Council about unloading: Thomas Crawfurd of Glasgow petitioned in mid-August for a ship to unload in the Clyde, where it had lain 26 days after six weeks at sea from Holland.[164] As the cargo was basically iron, and therefore non-susceptible, the Council had no real reason to disagree, although it was still to be cleansed 'at the sight of' local magistrates.[165] This leniency provoked another concerted petition from merchants of Edinburgh and Glasgow for the ship recently ordered out of Bo'ness to land its cargo, as it had arrived before 1 August.[166] But this merely provoked a repetition of the earlier hard line. The next ploy, in November 1664, was to claim that three ships had been forced into Bo'ness 'by the stresse of weather', which caused the Privy Council to ask for a report from a board of local aristocrats.[167] The board made no comment on the circumstances of arrival and generally favoured ways and means of getting the cargo ashore, subject to safeguards at the merchants' expense; as the cargo included iron and barrels of oil, it was recommended that they lie in the sea 'for the space of thrie tydes'.[168] The Privy Council roughly agreed but decided on a somewhat tougher line, ordering

157 *RPCS*, 2nd Series, vol. 8, pp. 567–8.
158 Ibid.
159 *RPCS*, 2nd Series, vol. 8, p. 583.
160 Ibid
161 *CSPD* (1663–64), p. 670.
162 *RPCS*, 2nd Series, vol. 8, p. 584.
163 Ibid.
164 *RPCS*, 2nd Series, vol. 8, p. 591.
165 Ibid.
166 *RPCS*, 2nd Series, vol. 8, p. 594.
167 *RPCS*, 2nd Series, vol. 8, p. 617.
168 *RPCS*, 2nd Series, vol. 8, pp. 621–2.

that any goods which could not be cleansed should be burnt, and that all persons aboard should do 40 days in quarantine.[169]

The same terms were decreed for a ship which had been lying at an exposed mooring off Greenock for the previous 15 days, after a stormy crossing from Holland.[170] The point here was that the ship had been forced out of Holland to avoid being seized. The Laird of Greenock was to provide empty houses in which the cargo might lie during cleansing, and this set a precedent: within a few weeks, the bailie of Bo'ness had to find houses for both goods and people while cleansing and quarantine were performed there.[171] Another ship which claimed to have left Holland in a hurry, to escape seizure, rode outside Burntisland for 40 days; the master then petitioned to land his cargo of 'fyftein barrells of train oyle and certan hogsheids of lint seid'.[172] The Privy Council left it to the local magistrates to make a decision. The minutiae of quarantine work were evidently beginning to pall.

When plague broke out in London in 1665, the Scottish Privy Council were distracted from the position in Holland, although the problems from there did not go away. The new situation was not without irony. However much there was a threat to Scotland from its seaborne trade with London, the excuse to retaliate against its southern neighbour for the perceived injustice of the recent Navigation Act was a big temptation. By the 1662 Act Scotland had been disadvantaged to the same extent as any other foreign nation.[173] Representations to London had had some success, but there were English interests which threatened to undermine it.[174] Against the retaliation argument, however, must be set the fact that embargoes on trade with England, albeit normally across the land border, were nothing new. In any event, a Proclamation against trade with London, and any other English town which might become infected, was issued on 12 July 1665, to be effective until 1 November.[175] Ships already at sea were to be subjected to 40 days' quarantine, and there were restrictions at the land border. Penalties were vague to say the least, and curiously confined to the magistrates themselves, and to others responsible for the execution of the 'act', who if they failed would 'be punished in their persons and goods to the terrour of others'. The Dutch ambassador in London did not fail to let the States General know of this firm stance by their chief trading partner against a virtual enemy of Holland.[176]

As far as can be judged from the many petitions which ensued, it was the Scots themselves who were most inconvenienced by the restriction. A surgeon had his drugs stopped at Berwick-upon-Tweed, and a merchant, sending goods home, saw them stranded in Carlisle.[177] But it was the middle classes and aristocracy who suffered most, struggling to get home from London, Yorkshire or even

169 Ibid.

170 *RPCS*, 2nd Series, vol. 8, pp. 623–4.

171 *RPCS*, 2nd Series, vol. 8, p. 639.

172 *RPCS*, 2nd Series, vol. 8, p. 641.

173 Lipson, vol. 3, pp. 126–7.

174 *EBRB* (1655–65), p. xiv.

175 *RPCS*, 3rd Series, vol. 2, 71–4; *CSPD* (1664–65), 473.

176 *CSPD* (1664–65), p. 488.

177 *RPCS*, 3rd Series, vol. 2, pp. 79–80.

France, and sometimes forced to get a bill of health at Newcastle.[178] The majority of these people were women travelling with servants, all in good health, and in no mood to be put to the expense of exile for the sake of a theoretical risk. The Privy Council, of course, capitulated without condition on every petition, and licences to 'converse at freedom' appeased ladies, merchants and doctors who felt as isolated within Scotland as their compatriots felt outside it.[179]

Despite these concessions, the Scottish Privy Council remained very jittery. In October 1665 two ships in Leith harbour, and one at Prestonpans, were rumoured to carry plague.[180] It was not stated where they had come from. All three were summarily ordered to the island of Inchkeith to air their goods for 40 days.[181] If the masters refused they were to be hanged there and then, and the ships and cargoes burnt.[182] In November the master of one of the ships petitioned that he, his crew and his passengers were virtually dying of exposure.[183] The Privy Council asked the bailies of Leith to establish, as far as they could, whether cleansing had worked; it was then up to the bailies to decide whether the ship could return, 'as they will be answerable'.[184] This encouraged the master of another ship to make a similar, but less dramatic, petition, which was handled the same way.[185] The fate of the third ship is not recorded.

There were two subsequent Proclamations against trading with England, one on 21 December 1665 (continuing the embargo until 1 March), and the other on 2 March 1666, to continue until 1 June.[186] The latter recognized that the plague was abating, but regretted that 'by sad experience it hath bein found that the infection may lurk for a long tyme in merchand wares and commodities, and after handling thereof will break out againe to the great prejudice of the people ...'[187] There appear to have been no petitions arising from either of these later Proclamations, from which the inference must be that they were either very closely respected, or very heartily ignored. Certainly the remainder of the seventeenth century saw very few alarms and incidents at Scottish ports, one brief exception being quarantine for seamen with 'spotted feavers' arriving at Bo'ness from the Low Countries in 1678.[188]

The most interesting aspect of the Scottish measures lies in the insistence that cargoes should be 'cleansed', either by the very radical measure of immersion in sea water for a day or two, or by opening and airing. In this respect the country

178 *RPCS*, 3rd Series, vol. 2, pp. 85, 88.

179 *RPCS*, 3rd Series, vol. 2, p. 87.

180 *RPCS*, 3rd Series, vol. 2, p. 95.

181 Ibid.

182 Ibid.

183 *RPCS*, 3rd Series, vol. 2, p. 100. The island of quarantine is here named as 'Inshcomb'.

184 Ibid.

185 *RPCS*, 3rd Series, vol. 2, p. 102.

186 *RPCS*, 3rd Series, vol. 2, pp. 119–20, 147–8. The latter is referred to in the margin as an 'Act', although there was no Scottish statute to that effect.

187 *RPCS*, 3rd Series, vol. 2, p. 148.

188 *RPCS*, 3rd Series, vol. 5, p. 491.

was nearer to the Continental practice than was England where, for lack of a convenient airing ground in the Thames estuary, and for the insouciance of the Privy Council about what happened in the outports, the focus was on quarantine itself. Admittedly, Scotland had two advantages. The first was the concentration of ports around the estuary of the Firth of Forth, so that one or two airing grounds would suffice for much of the east coast. The second was the location of several small islands in the Forth estuary, of which one or more might at times be suitable.[189] Islands were, in the nature of things, the best places for quarantine and certainly for airing a cargo which was suspected of harbouring infection. The problem which Scotland was soon to face, however, was exactly that which was destined to trouble England – all land, including islands, belonged to somebody and potential plague grounds were not popular with proprietors.

189 cf. Ritchie, p. 692.

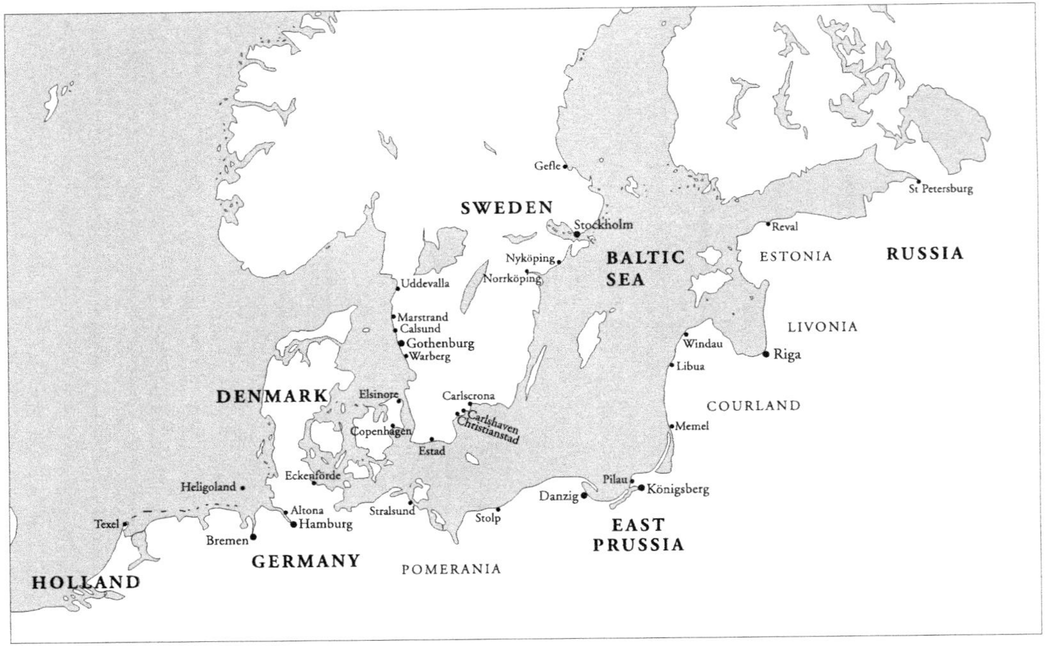

Map 1.1 The Baltic Sea and northern Europe, *c.* 1710. Ports shown with a larger font were those chiefly affected by quarantine in Britain.

Chapter Two

The Baltic Crisis, 1709–1714: Policy and Procedure

Panic measures

In the reign of Queen Anne, England's relationship with the Northern Crowns (as the states around the Baltic Sea were collectively known) reached a peak of complexity. Interest in the region had seriously developed in Elizabethan times, when English cloth gained a strong foothold on the eastern shore, an area known in Britain as the East Country. In 1579, the year when the Hanseatic League lost its privileges in London, English Baltic merchants formed themselves by royal charter into the Eastland Company.[1] This began as a regulated company (in which merchants traded under their individual stock) and it stayed that way, unlike the slightly earlier Russia Company which at times had joint-stock status.[2] Another early regulated company had been the Merchant Adventurers and there was some overlap in boundaries. The Eastland Company shared the German territories bordering the Baltic and parts of Denmark with the Merchant Adventurers and could, in exceptional times, ship goods through Hamburg which was the Merchant Adventurers' staple.[3] But in terms of the Baltic Sea, the Eastland Company was the organization which had most to gain or lose. The Russia Company was later to compete in the Gulf of Finland, but its activities for the time were confined to Archangel.[4]

Politically, the Baltic during the seventeenth century was very much in the grip of Sweden.[5] Finland, plus the area around the Gulf of Finland and the territories to the south (the modern Estonia and Latvia), were already or became under Swedish control. Further south again, Prussia controlled the ports of Memel and Königsberg, while Poland, Germany and Denmark possessed the remaining shoreline. Denmark also controlled Norway, and the southern tip of Sweden, facing its own territory, until 1658. Wars were frequent and vicious, as between Sweden and Denmark from 1675 to 1678, and the whole region became seriously destabilized on the death of Charles XI of Sweden in 1697. Poland, Russia and Denmark combined to catch Sweden wrong-footed, and the Great Northern War erupted. But the extraordinary

1 R.W.K. Hinton, *The Eastland Trade and the Common Weal in the Seventeenth Century* (Cambridge, 1959), p. 5; M. Sellers, *The Acts and Ordinances of the Eastland Company* (London, 1906), p. x.

2 E. Lipson, *The Economic History of England. The Age of Mercantilism* (3 vols, London, 1943), vol. 2, p. 196.

3 Hinton, p. 5; Lipson, vol. 2, p. 318; Sellers, p. xvi.

4 S.-E. Åström, *From Cloth to Iron. Part 1 …* (Helsingfors, 1965), p. 189.

5 J.F. Chance, *George I and the Northern War* (London, 1909), p. 676.

prowess of the boy king, Charles XII, led in the short term to even greater Swedish supremacy. Russia suffered a humiliating defeat at Narva in 1700, but eventually all the Swedish territory on the eastern side of the Baltic was overrun by Russia between 1704 and 1714.

England wanted no part in any of this fighting, and had long adopted a passive foreign policy in the Baltic, while ensuring that its interests were not upstaged by the Dutch.[6] This meant maintaining a balance of power, particularly between Sweden and Denmark, as they glared at each other across the narrow strip of water known as The Sound. With the Great and Little Belts (the alternative channels through the Danish islands) dangerous because of shoals, all shipping out of the Baltic passed through the Sound. There it paid a toll at Elsinore to the King of Denmark, who exacted it, under duress if necessary, at the highest rate he could get away with. England acquiesced in this, as long as Denmark remained relatively weak. But when there was threat of this 'turnstile' being closed, or other interests were threatened, England's policy became suddenly very positive, and between 1658 and 1814 England sent warships to the area nearly 20 times.[7]

The strategic importance of the Baltic to England lay in its provision of naval stores. Through the seventeenth century, exports of cloth to the East Country declined, but the Eastland Company (and interlopers) found good business in the import of hemp, flax and masts from Prussia, and iron, tar and pitch from Sweden.[8] During the Commonwealth the need for naval stores became acute, and they were exempt from the first Navigation Act.[9] Thereafter demand never slackened, and the War of the Spanish Succession, which began in 1697, required a permanently strong fleet against France. Soon a nervous Government sought an alternative supply source from the American colonies but the quality of materials from the Baltic could not be matched.[10]

One of the many problems worrying England was the increasing ability of Sweden to control the market. The Stockholm Tar Company, established in 1689, refused to supply its product except in Swedish ships at its own price, and later through its own factors.[11] Generally, relations between England and Sweden had been good in the seventeenth century, but soured significantly when England, as a guarantor of the Treaty of Travendal of 1700, failed to send troops in support of Charles XII when he urgently needed them.[12] Charles placed retaliatory restrictions on trade with England resulting, for instance, in nine ships with naval stores being prevented from sailing in 1709.[13] In the words of Secretary of State St John, the King of Sweden

---

6 R.G. Albion, *Forests and Sea Power: The Timber Problem of the Royal Navy, 1652–1862* (Cambridge, Mass., 1926), pp. 140, 164ff.

7 Albion, p. 165.

8 Hinton, pp. 22, 37ff., 61, 98–101; Albion, pp. 153ff.

9 Lipson, vol. 3, pp. 122–3.

10 Albion, pp. 148–9, 240, 243.

11 National Archives [NA] CO 388/12, Part 2/71.

12 J.F. Chance, 'England and Sweden in the time of William III and Anne', *English Historical Review*, no. 63, vol. 16 (1901), 684–7.

13 NA SP 104/154/95–6.

was 'neither unwilling nor unable to hurt us.'[14] In another letter, he claimed that the King's interruption of the trade to Riga was 'groundless and intolerable', but at least it affected Holland as well as Britain.[15] To add to the problem, the Baltic was infested with privateers of the various combatant nations, who paid little regard for a ship's nationality if the cargo were from an enemy source.[16]

Statistics of trade with the Baltic reveal the extent of England's dependency, and how much the balance of trade was against her. Between 1697 (when annual figures began) and 1709, England had an average annual trade deficit of nearly £22,000 with the East Country, and almost £138,000 with Sweden.[17] This imbalance offended the mercantilist philosophy of the day and renewed calls for the plantations to produce alternative supplies.[18] An Act of Parliament gave muscle to this movement in 1704, but there was to be no quick fix from across the Atlantic.[19] The Baltic remained vital to British interests and England's policy towards the Northern Crowns did not alter. When Robert Jackson took up his post as English Resident in Sweden in 1710, Anne reminded him first of her concern for the 'Good of Europe by preserving a due Balance in the North'.[20] She went on to state the dire need for ships to get through: 'you are to endeavour to put that matter upon such a foot, That our Navy may be constantly and sufficiently supply'd; and particularly you are to make application to obtain a free Exportation of Masts, and all other naval stores from any Part in Sweden.'[21] As if this messy and dangerous situation, with implications for national security, were not a sufficient trial for Anne, she was already facing an imponderable complication of another kind – the arrival in the Baltic of bubonic plague.

This was far worse than the periodic local epidemics to which western Europe had long been accustomed. The threat now was from a relentless scourge, springing from the Ottoman Empire, rampaging north-west, and killing those who stood in its way. It was as if a new Tartar horde had burst from the eastern fringes of Europe in some devilish, incarnate disguise. Not since the Black Death had the West been faced with such a virulent, invisible enemy. In 1707 Poland was badly attacked and the disease travelled inexorably north to Danzig, which lost up to 25,000 inhabitants, perhaps two-thirds of its population, in 1709.[22] The plague crossed the Baltic to

---

14 G. Parke, *Letters and Correspondence of Lord Bolingbroke* … (4 vols, London, 1798), vol. 1, p. 171.

15 Parke, vol. 1, p. 291; Chance, 'England and Sweden in the time of William III and Anne', 698.

16 Albion, pp. 151, 176.

17 Sir C. Whitworth, *State of the Trade of Great Britain* … (London, 1776), Part 2, pp. 7, 35.

18 Albion, pp. 158–9; Chance, 'England and Sweden in the time of William III and Anne', 678.

19 3 & 4 Anne, c.9, encouraging the import of naval stores from North America.

20 NA SP 104/214/33–8.

21 Ibid.

22 [A. Boyer], *The History of the Reign of Queen Anne, digested into Annals* (11 vols, London, 1710–13), vol. 8, p. 158; D. Panzac, *Quarantaines et lazarets. L'Europe et la peste d'orient (XVIIe–XXe siècles)* (Aix-en-Provence, 1986), pp. 58–9; from which remaining references in this paragraph are taken.

Sweden, killing close to 40,000 people, mainly in Karlskrona and Stockholm in 1710. Denmark was severely affected in the following year, with some 28,000 deaths at Copenhagen. The sickness then spread to Hamburg and Bremen and threatened to move west, ever closer to the British Isles.

There was no sense of alarm in England until the epidemic reached Danzig. This was understandable as plague in the Empire was endemic, and fighting in Poland masked the reality of the threat, as armies were often ravaged by disease. It was only when plague reached the civilian population on the Baltic shore, where English ships collected cargo, that the risk was understood. In the late summer of 1709 Boyer noted that 'besides the Calamities of War, Poland, and the neighbouring Countries were afflicted by a violent Plague, that raged most furiously at Danzick, where for several Months, above 1,500 Persons a Week were swept away'.[23] It was Danzig, also, which featured in the Privy Council's deliberations of 22 August 1709, when ships from that port, and places adjacent, were stopped from coming further up the Thames than The Nore.[24] The navy was to prevent any goods, seamen or passengers from those areas being landed in London or the outports 'untill they be under the Care of the Officers of the Customes who are to take Care ... according to the Intention of this Order'.[25] But what *was* the intention of the Order? Was this quarantine? Evidently there was confusion, as another Order followed quickly on 5 September.[26] This stated that landing could only occur at places 'provided for airing the ... Persons and Goods for 40 Days appointed for performing their Quarantain'; Customs officers were empowered to release the ships after that period.[27]

This second Order was as hasty and ill-considered as the first. The concept of airing appears misunderstood: people were never 'aired', only cargoes, and no open spaces were appointed by the Order where airing could take place. The lessons of the seventeenth century had not been learnt. As regards the Thames, the second Order repeated that The Nore was the closest point to London for suspect ships, unless Customs officers should choose somewhere else after consultation with the Lord Mayor of London. But if the City felt once again that its savoir-faire was in demand, the satisfaction was short-lived. On 14 September there was a third Order which did little more than repeat the second, but with two important differences: the infected area was now designated as the 'Baltick Seas', and the consultation clause was discontinued.[28] The City was never again asked for a view.

As it was, the City had favoured quarantine at Black Stakes, near the mouth of the Medway.[29] Apparently the Queen, and no doubt the City as well, had blocked a proposal that quarantine should be at The Hope, which was judged too near London.[30] The Customs Commissioners, who had been asked to consider an exact site with the

23 Boyer, vol. 8, p. 118.

24 NA PC 2/82/419.

25 Ibid.

26 NA PC 2/82/420.

27 Ibid.

28 NA PC 2/82/427–8.

29 NA PC 2/82/427; *Calendar of Treasury Books* [*CTB*] (1709), p. 360.

30 *CTB* (1709), pp. 357–8.

Navy Board, were hurriedly called in to advise the Lords of the Committee.[31] The Privy Council, on 16 September 1709, appointed the holding ground as Stangate Creek, a remote backwater further up the Medway than Black Stakes.[32] If it became overcrowded, ships were to use nearby Sharfleet Creek, with further capacity, if needed, in the Thames at the Lower Hope.[33] After a quarantine of 40 days (if all was well), passengers could go ashore at the discretion of Customs officers and goods were to be unloaded and aired for a further week.[34] Release was then a formality and the ship could continue to its place of discharge. There were, however, certain goods – linen, Polonia wool, hogs' bristles, spruce-yarn, feathers, hemp and flax – which medical opinion considered highly susceptible to harbouring infection.[35] These items were to be reported to the Privy Council for further instructions. As these 'enumerated' goods contained two vital naval stores, hemp and flax, the problems ahead might well have been imagined.

The continuing Orders testify to something very much like panic in a thoroughly rattled Privy Council. Members were relearning the practicability of procedures which had engaged the minds of past councillors, but the corporate memory had effectively lapsed. On 26 September 1709 it was ordered that the Isle of Grain would be the airing ground for ships bound for London, while Customs officers and magistrates in the outports were to appoint similar places locally.[36] Unfortunately, airing grounds were no easier to establish in this century than they had been in the last. The Isle of Grain had salt pans with a wharf and warehouses, but the owner, Lord Teynham, was in no mind to agree terms with the Customs Commissioners.[37] Through his agent, he demanded £2,000 to compensate for land already settled on his daughters, for the inevitable flight of tenants from their farms, and for the upkeep of sea walls.[38] The Commissioners were unimpressed; their own agent found the wharf in disrepair, most buildings nearly derelict, and the whole claim 'very extravagant'.[39] For a quarter of the cost, he reckoned 'a small stage and a large shed' could be built more conveniently in the Medway creeks, and the Commissioners were empowered to treat.[40]

Meanwhile, even the use of the quarantine creeks was not unopposed. At low tide they were little more than dreary mudflats among inaccessible, featureless marshlands, divided into islands on the western shore. The area was unhealthy and desolate but it provided a livelihood for the free fishermen of Milton or Middleton Hundred, who paid the lord of the manor £100 a year for the right to dredge for

31 NA PC 2/82/427; *CTB* (1709), p. 358.

32 NA PC 2/82/429. The name was subject to many corruptions and variations (Stanlet, Stanley, etc.), and was frequently written Standgate.

33 Ibid. The spelling Sharpfleet (Sharpe Fleet) was equally in usage.

34 Ibid.

35 Ibid.

36 NA PC 2/82/434–6.

37 NA PC 2/82/436; *CTB* (1709), pp. 382, 393.

38 NA PC 2/82/466–9; *CTB* (1709), p. 417.

39 Ibid.

40 Ibid.

oysters.[41] The Customs Commissioners were asked to arrange a buyout, as the trade could no longer be tolerated.[42] That was 6 November 1709, but ships in quarantine had already been there for some weeks: the oysters had long been ruined and the Commissioners did little negotiation. A bigger problem at that time was the site of the proposed airing ground. Attention was focusing on Hoo Fort Island, higher up the Medway. This was controlled by the Board of Ordnance, who already allowed goods to be aired there.[43] But the Privy Council had conflicting advice: the Navy Board, supported by other interests, felt the island 'one of the most improper Places that can be', while the Lord Treasurer, speaking for the Customs Commissioners, stressed its 'great Conveniency'.[44] Up to three ships could unload there at one time, and preparations continued for the reception of cargoes – but only goods from Stockholm or Riga and other places not actually infected with plague. The Privy Council felt this practice should continue; the purpose of the limitation was to allay fears in Rochester and the surrounding towns.[45]

The absurdity therefore existed that goods were being aired against plague despite no perceived risk of infection. The corollary was that goods from infected ports, like Danzig, were not being aired at all. It was probably the policy to develop Hoo Fort Island from small beginnings; in other words, once the locals had become accustomed to the airing ground, the island could be used for ships from higher-risk locations, and indeed for ships which were actually infected. In the meanwhile, even as Hoo Fort Island was receiving ships, £2,100 was being spent in making 'stages and other conveniences' at the quarantine creek.[46] The idea was that goods from infected ports could be offloaded for airing on the deserted islands or Chetney Marshes.

In the event, this was money wasted: the region was uninhabited because it was uninhabitable, unable to support the infrastructure of buildings, population and supply routes which a properly organized airing ground demanded. The provision of landing stages merely brought the problems into focus; it was pointless taking potentially infected goods out of ships' holds unless the airing ground allowed several cargoes at once to be kept distinct, opened, turned, repacked and reloaded. The manpower needed for labouring, supervision and security was immense; and even this set-up would fall short of a full-scale lazaretto, as there would be no facilities for passengers or crew. It is doubtful whether any cargo was ever aired at Stangate Creek, or if the 'stages' were even completed. The Customs Commissioners had no illusions about the unsuitability of the site. In December 1709 they reiterated their concerns to the Treasury: 'opening and airing … will be attended with great difficulty; [some goods] cannot be landed, opened and aired without great damage, and others not without

41 NA PC 2/82/465–6; *CTB* (1709), p. 418.

42 Ibid.

43 NA PC 2/82/486.

44 NA PC 2/82/482, 486; *CTB* (1709), p. 445.

45 NA PC 2/82/486.

46 *CTB* (1709), p. 449.

both and none without danger of infection both to the persons that open them and to the country thereabouts ...'[47]

Opposition to Hoo Fort Island came from the Medway towns, led by Rochester. This was an ancient and populous river port, about three miles away; even closer (within two miles) was the important dockyard town of Chatham, while the smaller community of Gillingham was distant by a matter of yards across the main channel of the Medway. The towns more or less acquiesced in the use of Hoo Fort Island for most of 1710. This can be explained by the work under way in the quarantine creek, at a safer distance from the population, and by the assurance of the Privy Council that only non-infected cargoes would be aired at the island. What caused a new Kentish outcry was the Proclamation of 9 November 1710, the first in England to enforce quarantine since 1635, and followed soon afterwards by an Act of Parliament.[48] In clause five of the Proclamation it was stated that the airing ground for Baltic goods destined for the Thames 'shall be the Island of Stowfort in the River Medway'. There was, of course, a mistake here as Stowfort did not exist, but it was no more than an error of transcription by an engrossing clerk.[49] The intention was now publicly announced: Hoo Fort Island was to be the main airing ground in England for cargoes, regardless of their susceptibility to infection. When the Customs Commissioners were told to build airing sheds, the mayor of Rochester reacted with an angry petition, also on behalf of Strood, Chatham and Gillingham.[50] The very concept of quarantine in the Medway seemed under attack. The mayor was asked what suggestions he had for a better location.[51] He could offer only Stangate Creek as a more suitable airing ground.[52] This answer at least conceded that quarantine in the Medway was acceptable, and in recognition of this, or because the Council genuinely recognized the risk, airing at Hoo Fort Island was scaled down.[53] But with no airing facility elsewhere, quarantine policy was already in disarray.

Encouraged by the resistance of Rochester, it was now the fishermen who returned to the attack. They petitioned in February 1711 that they had received no compensation for the ruined oyster beds, that they were forbidden from entering the creeks, and that 70 families had their livelihood at stake.[54] Again, they were treated cavalierly, with no recompense until March 1712.[55] By then an investigation had revealed that the fishermen were, in some respects, understating their grievance. Some 80 families were found to be at risk, and their losses included £300 worth of oyster stock when the quarantine ships first arrived. There were evidently other

47 *CTB* (1709), p. 460.

48 The text of the Proclamation is in PRO PC 2/83/147–9. For the Act, see below.

49 This error had a remarkable longevity, almost as if Stowfort became the accepted nomenclature even in legislation.

50 NA SP 44/245/211–12; *CTB* (1711), p. 137.

51 *CTB* (1711), p. 164.

52 *CTB* (1711), p. 177.

53 But certainly not abandoned. When plague at Marseilles caused the scare beginning in 1720, the airing sheds were again used.

54 *CTB* (1711), pp. 169, 621.

55 *CTB* (1712), pp. 217–18, from which remaining references in this paragraph are taken.

oyster grounds open to them, but they still paid rent for rights in the banned areas and losses were reckoned at £1,000. The Treasury conceded a payment of £250 for damages to Michaelmas 1711, and £100 annually thereafter for as long as quarantine should continue in Stangate Creek.

One reason for such a delay in settling with the fishermen was the preoccupation with other expensive issues, peripheral to quarantine itself. In February 1711 the Treasury were reminded by Mr Hunt, quarantine officer for the Medway, that no watch had been established in adjoining parishes to prevent illicit communication with the shore.[56] There was now a statutory obligation on local magistrates to provide one, but the expense was not allocated by the Act. The parishes thought the cost should be borne by the hundred, the hundred by the county, and the county by the country.[57] The Attorney-General was asked whether soldiers could be used. He thought they could and as a company of invalids was stationed at Upnor Castle on the Medway, a detachment of an officer, sergeant, corporal and 18 men was sent to patrol Chetney Marshes, on the eastern (or mainland) side of Stangate Creek.[58] But even by the middle of March, their further duty was out of the question. The governor of Upnor Castle reported to his superior: 'the places where they keep guard are two or three miles distant from each other, & as far from any house, & they are forc'd to stand in the open Marshes to do their Duty, which is so deep, that they are up to their knees, so that it is impossible for them to live, unless there be some Guard house made, or Tents provided to keep them from the Severity of the Weather'.[59]

The reality of the situation was now becoming apparent: however useful for quarantine the Medway creeks might be, the adjacent Chetney Marshes were patently unsuitable for any purpose whatsoever. But in a few decades' time the corporate memory would again fail, and the mud would suck down the money as it did a soldier's boot.

Legal framework

The Proclamation of November 1710 began with a preamble lamenting that quarantine was being broken; some people 'have Presumed to come on Shoar, and have Appeared in the Publick Streets, and Mingled Themselves wth Our Subjects', while others had been going aboard and offloading goods.[60] To remedy these evils, the Proclamation sought to integrate the piecemeal measures accomplished by the many Orders of the preceding 14 months. It did not, however, supersede those Orders; the hope was that, now they were brought to people's notice, no one could 'Pretend Ignorance' of their existence. It also embodied policy formulated empirically as procedural questions arrived from north of the border. It was no accident that Scotland, in the aftermath of the Act of Union, should grasp the pertinent issues; Scottish magistrates had long been implementing quarantine laws in their own land and it was probably with some

56 *Calendar of Treasury Papers* [*CTP*] (1708–14), p. 248.

57 Ibid.

58 NA SP 41/3.

59 Ibid.

60 NA PC 2/83/147–9.

smugness that they give the Privy Council something to think about. For instance, it was a Scotsman who asked from what date quarantine should commence.[61] The answer was when the ship came to anchor in the quarantine harbour: no part of the voyage, even if the ship had earlier arrived at some British landfall, would be deducted from the reckoning.[62] Thus the policy of 1692, which must have puzzled and bothered the Scots, was corrected. Likewise, it was the magistrates at Edinburgh who wondered if non-enumerated cargo, at the expiration of quarantine, could be removed from a ship's hold when that hold contained also susceptible goods; and, if so, whether the labourers had to undergo a new quarantine when they had finished.[63] The answer to both parts of that question was yes.

There were nine numbered provisions in the Proclamation. The first clarified when quarantine should begin, as mentioned above, but did not confirm the duration. The second named the quarantine creeks for ships bound to the Thames and Medway; for the outports, quarantine was to be at such places as the Customs officers should appoint. The third forbade persons or goods to leave a ship during quarantine. The fourth provision was more complicated: if, after quarantine had been performed, the Customs officers were satisfied that the ship was healthy and the master had sworn to that effect before a magistrate, then people could come on shore. But the cargo had to be landed, opened and aired for a week; and if the cargo contained the enumerated goods mentioned in the Order of 16 September 1709, it had to stay on board until the Privy Council should decide otherwise. Although this provision did no more than reiterate existing policy, it would have greatly disappointed many merchants and shipowners who, as will be seen, were finding the law unworkable.

The fifth provision has already been dealt with: it clarified the airing ground for the Thames as 'the Island of Stowfort'. The sixth placed under quarantine any ship or person who should receive men or goods from any vessel itself in quarantine. This had already happened in the (probably innocent) context of a man-of-war from Hamburg;[64] more significantly, it seems to have been a warning to the navy not to impress seamen from temptingly inactive merchant ships. The seventh provision imposed quarantine on men who separated iron, tar, pipestaves and timber from susceptible goods, as enumerated in the Order of 16 September, in a ship's hold. The eighth provision enjoined naval captains to prevent goods or people coming ashore before a ship was under the direction of Customs officers; and the ninth urged the Customs officers to do their work diligently. The Proclamation ended as it began, with reference to the lawbreakers: it encouraged people to obey the rules 'upon Pain of being Proceeded against wth the utmost Severity that the Law will Allow ...'

The problem with the Proclamation was that the law entailed no such severity. The breaking of quarantine was not an offence in the statute book, which is why in some ports the rules were still being flouted as they had been in the seventeenth century. Jonathan Swift, for one, was very aware of this. In his *Journal to Stella*, he wrote in December 1710: 'We are terribly afraid of the plague; they say it is

61 *CTB* (1709), p. 416; NA PC 2/82/458.

62 Ibid.

63 NA PC 2/82/540.

64 NA PC 2/82/458.

at Newcastle. I begged Mr. Harley for the love of God to take some care about it, or we are all ruined. There have been orders for all ships from the Baltick to pass their quarantine before they land; but they neglect it.'[65] In fact, the plague was not at Newcastle after all, but as Swift claimed to be 'daily conversant with the persons then in power', his statement is one to be reckoned with.[66] As he was reporting the conversation of a dinner *à trois* at which Robert Harley and Matthew Prior were the other diners, presumably his use of 'We' means the others shared his fear. This has implications for a later discussion on quarantine policy at Cabinet level, but at this stage it serves to confirm that the Orders had not been successful. What Swift must have known, but failed to tell Stella, was that a new way of bringing the country to order was about to be tried. This was an Act of Parliament.

The *Act to oblige Ships coming from Places infected more effectually to perform their Quarentine* had a remarkably rapid progress through Parliament.[67] In an age when Whig and Tory differences reduced most questions to the infighting of party politics, and when the Crown would not expect an issue concerning the royal prerogative to be received by the Commons without opposition, the Quarantine Bill was a model of what could be achieved when the threat to parliamentarians was personal, mortal and indiscriminate. The passage through both Houses took only eight days.[68] On 15 December 1710 leave was given to bring in the Bill; on the 20th William Lowndes, MP for Seaford and Secretary to the Treasury, presented it, and on that same day it received its first and second readings. On the 21st, at 8 o'clock in the morning, it entered committee stage and received 'several' amendments to which the House agreed, although one was itself amended. The following day the engrossed Bill was read the third time, and received a new section (dealing with airing) and some further minor amendments. Later that day the Bill was carried to the Lords who agreed it almost instantly, and without amendment, despite the further requirement for three readings and a committee stage. On 23 December the Bill received royal assent, and was in force from the 25th. Copies of the Act were dispatched over the next three days, mostly by 'Common Post', to all ports in England, Wales and Scotland.[69]

There were a number of advantages in getting parliamentary sanction for quarantine while not disturbing the royal prerogative, which the preamble to the Act expressly protected.[70] Proclamation was to continue as the notifying instrument of the future. But the measures now carried more weight and demonstrated to the public that the Establishment was united. As Parliament was backing the Crown, the situation was manifestly serious; this, in theory, concentrated the minds of those

---

65 J. Swift, *Journal to Stella*, ed. H. Williams (2 vols, Oxford, 1948), vol. 1, pp. 115–16.

66 S. Biddle, *Bolingbroke and Harley* (London, 1975), pp. 4–5, quoting other work by Swift.

67 9 Anne, c.2.

68 *Journal of the House of Commons* [*JHC*], vol. 16, pp. xvi, 436, 439–41, 443–4; *Journal of the House of Lords* [*JHL*], vol. 19, pp. 179, 180; cf. P. Russell, *A Treatise of the Plague* (London, 1791), p. 441.

69 NA SP 44/109.

70 Quarantine was to be 'in such ... places for such time and in such manner as hath been or as shall from time to time be directed ... by Her Majesty or her successors'.

at risk of spreading or receiving infection. Another advantage of parliamentary involvement was that it prepared the way for an estimate of supply if the expenses of quarantine became significant. But most important of all at this worrying juncture, it enabled specific penalties to be introduced 'in a more expeditious manner' to punish those who wilfully neglected or ignored the measures.

To appreciate just how toothless the system of Order and Proclamation had been, it is necessary to revert once again to the seventeenth century. The enforcement of quarantine had been characterized by bluster and threat, disguising an impotence by Crown and Privy Council to take positive and effective action. Whenever possible the consequences of infringement were left to others, or simply ducked. For instance, in the alarm year of 1635 a group of French gentry were allowed ashore in Yarmouth as long as they remained in an appointed house.[71] But somebody gave them 'horses and means', and they reached London.[72] The Corporation was ordered to find out who did it, but any punishment was left to them.[73] In the following year the same Corporation let a man land from Rotterdam, an infected port, and the Privy Council sent a sharp letter stating 'we doe not a little marvell' at the decision.[74] The culprit was ordered to be apprehended, kept in solitary custody for a month, and then to appear before the Privy Council 'according to his Bond'.[75] But nothing further seems to have happened. In May 1664, when a sailor and his family jumped ship at Topsham to escape quarantine, they were roundly accused by the Privy Council of 'insolent obstinancie'.[76] But the infringement itself was not punished; the transgressors had simply to complete their 40 days. In July 1664, also at Topsham, the master of the *Saphir* broke quarantine.[77] This resulted in a letter to the mayor and justices of Exeter, and to the county justices, with another indication of extreme displeasure. But once more, the offender had simply to complete his quarantine, although any house harbouring him was to be shut up, as if with plague.[78]

When the Act of Parliament was mooted, the Attorney-General evidently wished that breaking quarantine should be a capital offence.[79] This, after all, would be nothing more than the penalty required and exacted in the main Mediterranean ports. But the Privy Council backed away, on the grounds that the penalty was so severe that nobody would be prosecuted. They favoured fines for those who could afford them, and a harsh detention for those who could not.[80] This is basically what the Act provided, but it also dabbled in how quarantine was conducted. There were nine sections, the first being also the preamble, setting the scene, and confirming the general constraints which the Orders and Proclamation had set out to establish. The second section allowed for a ship to be forfeited to the Crown if a master allowed

71 NA PC 2/45/287.

72 Ibid.

73 Ibid.; more precisely, they were to 'punish them as they think fit'.

74 NA PC 2/45/401–2.

75 Ibid.

76 NA PC 2/57/104.

77 NA PC 2/57/186.

78 Ibid.

79 *CTP* (1708–14), pp. 230–31.

80 Ibid.

anyone to go ashore, or on any other vessel, during quarantine. The third section allowed for those who jumped ship to be returned to quarantine, after which they would be prosecuted. The maximum fine was £20, with up to one-third going to any informer, or hard labour for no more than a month.

The fourth section targeted those who presumed to go on board and then leave a ship during its quarantine. They were to be forcibly returned for the full 40 days, but curiously no further punishment was exacted. The fifth section punished any Customs officer who wilfully let anyone leave a quarantined ship, by a fine of £100, with up to half going to any informer. It was from this point that the Act interfered in practical issues: the same clause empowered Customs officers to seize a ship's boats. By the sixth section, magistrates were to set up 24-hour watches in the parishes around the quarantine harbours; as noticed above, the costs of that responsibility were not allocated. Arrangements for concluding quarantine were dealt with in section seven: in this respect, unusually, the Act trespassed on a provision already covered by the Proclamation. Quarantine was to be lifted automatically when the time had expired, once a master and two other persons had sworn before a Customs officer or magistrate that the ship was healthy. A certificate would be granted to that effect. Section eight merely allowed the official who heard the oath to charge one shilling, over and above stamp duty. At that point the Act might well have ended but, as already mentioned, a ninth section was formulated during the third reading, when the Bill was already engrossed.[81] This required that goods, after quarantine, should be opened an aired in such places and for such time as required by Proclamation.

The importance of this first quarantine Act is simply that it existed at all. As a piece of legislation it bore all the hallmarks of the panic which engendered it, and its sections suffered from the almost unseemly speed with which it rampaged through the parliamentary process. There was no coherent message as to what the few, brief and diverse provisions were trying to achieve. Certainly, there were now statutory punishments for infringement, but the penalties, when seen in the judicial context of the era, were not such as to strike fear into the mind of a would-be transgressor. Also, the Act tinkered in a minor way with procedural matters best left to the Proclamation. Enabling Customs officers to seize a ship's boats is one minor example; of more significance was section seven, which more or less paraphrased clause four of the Proclamation in the matter of oaths. But it also added that the official who received the oath could issue a certificate, in effect pratique, after which the ship 'shall be liable to no further restraint during that voyage …'. This had not been part of the Proclamation, which it contradicted, effectively removing from Privy Council scrutiny any ship, with whatever susceptible cargo, which happened to have lain in Stangate Creek for 40 days. At the eleventh hour the error was realized, and provision was added by section nine for airing all cargoes according to the Proclamation in force. This implicitly cancelled half of section seven, and the Privy Council was tacitly reintroduced (*pace* the Proclamation) as the controlling authority for pratique. A clumsier piece of legislation could scarcely have been imagined.

81 *Statutes at Large* has a footnote to section 9 stating it was 'annexed to the Original Act in a separate Schedule'; cf. Russell, p. 441.

For better or worse, this mishmash of Orders, Proclamation and Act of Parliament controlled the practice of quarantine for much of 1711. There was not the least hope that the whole messy business could be cancelled. The progress of plague around the Baltic was being monitored with unease. Useful sources of knowledge were Robert Jackson at Stockholm and Daniel Pultency, envoy to Denmark, both in distinctly unhealthy surroundings. As early as 3 October 1710 the Duke of Queensberry, as Secretary of State for Scotland, had given Jackson permission, pending Anne's agreement, to leave the capital if he felt in danger.[82] Jackson stayed on, despite further anxiety in London for his safety, and kept the Queen abreast of developments. In this time of war, all news from Sweden was vital, but the recipients became increasingly jittery about the letters themselves; Jackson was asked to ensure they did not pass through infected hands as 'we have not yet taken any Extraordinary Precaution in airing, or opening, them'.[83] In January 1711, Under Secretary Rowe congratulated Jackson on 'being still in this World' and renewed the request for letters 'thro[ugh] hands that are Sound as well as Safe'.[84] The point about 'Safe' was that Denmark had been interrupting the normal mail route to and from Sweden. Ostensibly this was on health grounds, but of course the war had a lot to do with it. A makeshift postal route out of Sweden had been arranged from Ystad to Stralsund, with a connection to Hamburg for London, but it was a constant source of frustration to Rowe that letters to and from Sweden seemed to miscarry, or were inordinately detained.[85]

By the end of 1710 the plague had reached Stralsund.[86] Its course thereafter was erratic and gave rise to conflicting reports. The Prussian Resident in London, in February 1711, hoped that his country and England could now trade normally as the infection in Prussia was allegedly over.[87] But the Commissioners of Customs felt otherwise and quarantine remained. Later came rumours of the plague having attacked the German North Sea coast. On 1 August, Secretary St John of the Northern Department asked Lord Dartmouth, his colleague of the Southern, to inform the Privy Council that plague was spreading around Hamburg; a regiment marching through Holstein was infected, and precautions should be taken to stop the disease reaching Britain.[88] The result was a new Proclamation of 6 September 1711 extending the quarantine measures to Hamburg and other towns on the estuary of the Elbe, as well as to Bremen on the Weser and Emden on the Ems.[89] This time the Proclamation preceded the Order, which was dated the following day, but it did nothing to change the substance of what had gone before. It was still necessary for all cargoes to be aired for one week after quarantine (at Hoo Fort Island in the case of the Thames and Medway) and for enumerated goods to be reported to the Privy Council. Whereas the restrictions so far had upset only the Eastland Company and merchants trading

82 NA SP 104/154/122–3.
83 NA SP 104/154/132–3.
84 NA SP 104/154/133–4.
85 NA CO 388/13/62; for Rowe's frustration, see SP 104/154/*passim*.
86 *Journal of the Commissioners for Trade and Plantations* [*JCTP*], vol. 2, p. 194.
87 *JCTP*, vol. 2, pp. 238, 242.
88 NA SP 34/16/34/52–3.
89 NA PC 2/83/302–5.

with Sweden, they now threatened the Merchant Adventurers who enjoyed Hamburg as their staple. After some months of frustration, they petitioned for the lifting of quarantine on the grounds that Hamburg and adjacent places 'are not nor have been infected', and that Holland had lifted restrictions.[90] On 3 April 1712 the petition was referred by the Privy Council to the Treasury, the principal Secretaries of State, and the Commissioners of Trade and Plantations.[91]

This was not the first time that the Board of Trade (to use the Commissioners' more convenient title) had been asked for a view. This body, the successor to several committees of the Privy Council, had been established in 1696 to study and review the state of trade, to devise means of making the poor productive, and to familiarize themselves with the governance and business of the plantations.[92] Their role was always advisory, never executive, and in later years the Board became largely nominal. At this period, however, members took their responsibilities (at least, the first and the third) seriously and responded conscientiously to referrals, mainly from the Secretaries of State.[93] In quarantine matters they were being groomed, albeit gradually, as the main source of advice for the Privy Council. This was logical as quarantine was inherently linked to trade, and indeed some members of the Board were merchants and likely to be familiar with procedures abroad. But in response to ad hoc issues, as distinct from general policy, the Board could only seek a view from parties whom they considered to be more knowledgeable than themselves; and if those parties needed to consult others, a substantive reply to the Secretary of State could be delayed by some weeks. When Secretary St John referred to the Board the letter of February 1711 from the Prussian Resident, it was 17 days before he got a reply.[94] In that time alone the plague could have waxed or waned significantly.

In the case of the Merchant Adventurers' petition, the delay was exceptionally long. It will be recalled that the petition was referred by the Privy Council to the Board of Trade on 3 April 1712. The Board eventually asked the Eastland Company for a view, but there were other Baltic matters exercising the latter's judgement, and the Board seemed reluctant to bother them.[95] It was not until 6 May that Thomas Phelp, their Deputy Governor, appeared before the Board to clarify the position.[96] What he said did nothing to inspire in the Board any sense of their own importance. The Eastland Company had already laid before the Customs Commissioners several letters from Elsinore, dated between mid-October 1711 and mid-March 1712, about the prevalence of the plague, and was under the mistaken impression that

90 NA PC 2/83/410.

91 Ibid.

92 A.H. Basye, *The Lords Commissioners of Trade and Plantations Commonly Known as the Board of Trade, 1748–1782* (New Haven & London, 1925), pp. 1–5.

93 C. Wilson, in *England's Apprenticeship, 1603–1763*, 2nd edn (London, 1984), p. 167, regards them as 'a "Third Force" between dynasticism and vested economic interests'.

94 *JCTP*, vol. 2, pp. 238, 239, 242.

95 The Board and the company were engaged in discussing an earlier referral about British ships being taken as prizes by the Danes and Swedes.

96 *JCTP*, vol. 2, p. 361.

the Commissioners had passed them on. In the event, they had forgotten or just not bothered.[97]

While Phelp promised further copies, the Board wrote hurriedly to the Customs Commissioners asking for whatever information they might have specifically relating to Hamburg.[98] On 8 May the Commissioners replied by sending the Board a copy of the material they had already sent their superior, the Lord High Treasurer, in response to a direct referral.[99] To complete the Board's humiliation, the secretary of the Hamburg Company (that is, the Merchant Adventurers) had appeared before them on the previous day and produced a copy of this same report which had thus bypassed the Board completely.[100] The Board had one last chance of recovering some dignity and making a meaningful submission to the Privy Council – by quoting correspondence between Hamburg and London which only the Hamburg Company could produce.[101] As this production would take further time, the Board sent a temporizing reply to the Privy Council.[102] On 9 May 1712 a Mr Van Heymaert appeared before the Board and showed letters which indicated the healthiness of the Prussian Baltic coast, and that this was recognized in Holland.[103] The Board were now in a quandary: should they respond again to the Privy Council? They had already half answered the original referral of 3 April and the new information, although encouraging, was geographically wide of the mark. Eventually, from one source or another, the Council got the gist of the position: on 24 June 1712 quarantine was lifted from places outside The Sound, that is to say outside the Baltic.[104]

The Merchant Adventurers had only a few weeks in which to enjoy the restoration of their trade, which had taken 82 days to achieve. On 28 July 1712, in response to a report of plague at Glückstadt, the quarantine restrictions were summarily reimposed.[105] A committee of the Privy Council had recently been set up to consider the state of health in foreign parts and 'what might be most properly done for Preventing any Infection'.[106] This committee reported on 27 August on the basis of letters received only from the Secretaries of State and the Admiralty.[107] There is no indication that the Customs Commissioners (by way of the Treasury) or the Board of Trade were in any way involved or consulted. As regards the Board of Admiralty, their one letter seems to have been fortuitous; the Board decided to write to Lord Dartmouth on 22 August with information that fishing boats going to Heligoland for lobsters were in constant communication with diseased Glückstadt.[108] This hearsay was relayed to the ad hoc committee, whose report of 27 August was a dismal

97 Ibid.
98 *JCTP*, vol. 2, p. 362.
99 *JCTP*, vol. 2, p. 363.
100 *JCTP*, vol. 2, p. 362.
101 *JCTP*, vol. 2, p. 364.
102 Ibid.
103 *JCTP*, vol. 2, p. 365
104 NA PC 2/83/434–5; *CTB* (1712), p. 338.
105 NA PC 2/83/450–51; *CTB* (1712), p. 387.
106 NA PC 1/2/225; PC 2/83/426; 2/84/7.
107 NA PC 2/84/8.
108 NA ADM 3/27.

litany of infection based on the weakest of evidence. The committee reckoned that Hamburg 'and the whole Circle' were dreadfully worried.[109] Contagion was raging at Glückstadt and on the Danish side of the Elbe; on the German side it was nearing Bremen and had infected two guard posts of soldiers positioned to exclude it.[110] As for Heligoland, the lobster boats communicating with the infected mainland warranted inclusion in a new Proclamation.[111] On 31 August 1712 this, the third Proclamation in England in the subsisting crisis, duly appeared, repeating the measures in force and adding Heligoland to the places from where quarantine was due.[112] In ironic testimony to this haste and confusion, the Council's minuting clerk contrived yet another bizarre variant, 'Stowford', for dysphonic Hoo Fort Island.

The problem with the Heligoland embargo was that the lobster boats were English. In fact, they were owned by interests in London, which threatened the *entente*, so necessary for quarantine to work, between the Crown and the City. The practice was for London boats to stay offshore and collect the lobsters from local fishermen about half a mile from the island's cliffs.[113] Perhaps for seasonal reasons, or because they thought the restrictions would not last, the fishmongers were slow to react. Not until February 1713 did one of them, George Wensley, petition the Privy Council; his case was referred to the Customs Commissioners, who supported him.[114] It was established that Heligoland was unaffected by plague, and indeed that there was no communication allowed with the German mainland. The Council had no difficulty in deciding that Wensley's two boats could be exempt from quarantine whenever they returned to London.[115] The problem with that decision, however, was that it did not offer exemption for all fishing vessels trading with Heligoland, and Wensley was by no means the only practitioner. Later in 1713, at least eight other City parties sought the same favour as had been granted to Wensley, and from the tenor of their petition they found the privilege quite elusive.[116]

While the Hamburg Company, to all appearances, had now resigned themselves to the inevitability of quarantine restrictions, the Eastland Company were less quiescent. They petitioned the Privy Council in June 1713, claiming that Danzig, Königsberg, Riga and Memel had been in perfect health for at least three years, and requesting that quarantine from those ports be lifted.[117] This was clearly a collusive action with certain Members of Parliament for Scotland, whose petition was received the same

109 NA PC 2/84/8.

110 Ibid.

111 Ibid. The Customs Commissioners had been asked to comment on the Admiralty's letter, but there was scarcely time for them to have investigated and responded by 27 August (*CTB* (1712), p. 427).

112 NA PC 2/84/9–12; *CTB* (1712), p. 433. The Order was dated the same day.

113 *CTB* (1713), p. 172.

114 NA PC 2/84/81, 85

115 Ibid.; *CTB* (1713), p. 172.

116 NA SP 34/22/12/23–4. The petition, to 'his Lordship', never arrived at the Privy Council. In October 1713 two lobster vessels, possibly from Heligoland, were made exempt from quarantine but the petitioners, Edward and William Watson, were not among those who signed the petition above (*CTB* (1713), p. 381).

117 NA PC 2/84/193–4.

day, seeking freedom for quarantine on the same grounds for all ships coming to Scotland from Danzig, Riga, Stockholm 'and places within the Baltick'.[118] These petitions were referred to the committee of Council which had been monitoring the situation abroad for at least a year. A letter was immediately sent to the Board of Trade, who responded with equal dispatch, but the substance of their comments was not revealed in their minutes.[119] In any event, the committee were not impressed with the petitioners' case. In fact, Secretary of State Lord Bolingbroke (as Henry St John had now become) was inclined to even harsher measures. On 18 August he wrote to the Queen about his concern for mid-Europe, where plague was still so rife that the King of Prussia had forbidden trade with Austria, Moravia, Bohemia, Silesia and Ratisbon.[120] At Vienna, plague had reportedly reached the Emperor's household. As for Hamburg, Bolingbroke reported 'but too much reason to believe, that this town is at last infected, notwithstanding all the care which has been taken ... to prevent it'.[121] That choice of words amounted to a tacit admission that the Hamburg Company had been right all along.

None of Bolingbroke's information related specifically to the Baltic, but on 23 August 1713, the Privy Council moved to tighten the restrictions by issuing a new Order.[122] The vagueness of the threat was acknowledged in the words chosen to justify their decision: the Queen had 'certain Information that the Plague Encreases and Spreads in many places abroad'. There was not even a pretence that the Baltic was at risk, or that its goods posed a danger to England. Nor was there any attempt to widen the quarantine barrier, perhaps to include countries more directly in line between England and the known areas of infection. The thrust of the new Order was not to increase the restrictions but to insist on the letter of the law. That is to say the requirement laid down by the Proclamation of 31 August 1712, that all goods had to be opened and aired for a week after quarantine was over, was to be strictly adhered to. This requirement had long been nominal. Also, enumerated goods had now to stay on board until further advice as to the health of the place whence they came. The excuse for this decision, which would lead to weeks and weeks of delay beyond the 40 days of quarantine, was a sudden fear (of unexplained origin) that opening and airing might not be enough to remove latent infection.

Such reactionary moves could not be sustained. Whether or not by collusion with merchants, the Customs Commissioners began to adopt new formulae in their reports to Council on ships of the Eastland Company carrying enumerated goods. It was conceded that the ships had come from the Baltic, but claimed that timber had been taken to the place of shipment in rafts, whereby the water automatically cleansed infection.[123] Also, it became usual to state that a ship had not sailed within 30 leagues of Hamburg, or any other German port, or any place known to

118 NA PC 2/84/194.

119 *JCTP*, vol. 2, p. 440.

120 Parke, vol. 4, pp. 237–8.

121 Ibid.

122 NA PC 2/84/227–8; *CTB* (1713), p. 364.

123 NA PC 2/84/191–2, 21 June 1713: 'Wood passes thro' water – by Floots [floats] to Gottenburgh'.

be infected.[124] With some occasional variation (60, even 200 leagues), this formula was presented time after time as a reason why the enumerated goods should not be subject to the extra formalities. And the Privy Council, as if ashamed of their earlier over-reaction, seemed comfortable accepting the Commissioners' recommendations. In such a bizarre situation, the end of all quarantine from the Baltic was already in merchants' sights. The consequence, however, of pinpointing Hamburg as the location of danger was that ships from there could hardly avoid the full rigour of quarantine and airing.

A boost to the Eastland Company's prospects came in February 1714 with a memorial to the Privy Council from Count Gyllenborg, the Swedish minister in London. He claimed there had been no 'contagious distemper' in Sweden for the last year and requested the removal, without specifically mentioning quarantine, of 'any hindrance or Molestation' to trade.[125] The Council, as if relieved to have this excuse to retreat from an uncomfortable position, agreed immediately to lift all quarantine constraints against Sweden.[126] This did not in itself benefit the Eastland Company, whose privileges in Sweden had been lost many years ago, but it encouraged them to seek further testimonies from the eastern shore of the Baltic that all was well, and had been so for years. These facts were presented by petition to the Queen, who was also receiving letters and certificates from Prussia, Hamburg and Bremen.[127] The evidence was incontrovertible that the German and Baltic seaboards had returned to good health. By Order in Council of 21 April 1714, after the best part of five years, all quarantine restrictions were lifted.[128]

Machinery of state

In discussing quarantine under Anne, it is necessary first to determine how far the Queen herself was the source of policy. The traditional view of Anne saw her inhibited by her sex, endowed 'with rather dull wits', and reliant on the judgement and initiative of her Ministers of State, two of whom, Harley (Lord Oxford) and St John (Lord Bolingbroke), were fiercely at loggerheads.[129] This appraisal would suggest that the royal prerogative, under Anne, was manipulated to a greater or lesser degree by her advisers; in other words, that she acquiesced in a quarantine policy which one or more of her ministers took under his wing. Such a conclusion, however, is unlikely to be correct. For one thing, Anne was naturally motivated to take the threat of plague very seriously; and for another it is impossible to bestow on Harley the credit for definitive thinking about quarantine, which his pre-eminence and influence might suggest. Indeed, the lack of a clear policy in this national emergency was a hallmark of the administration.

124 First used NA PC 2/84/239–40, 27 Sept. 1713.

125 NA PC 2/84/332; *CTB* (1714), p. 160.

126 Ibid.

127 NA PC 2/84/356–7; *CTB* (1714), p. 234.

128 Ibid.

129 M.A. Thomson, *The Secretaries of State, 1681–1782* (Oxford, 1932), pp. 12–16.

More recently Anne has been reassessed, and such adjectives as conscientious, deliberate and sensible give scope for assuming that her role over quarantine might actually have been quite positive.[130] Set against 'limited intellectual capacity' was an 'independence of judgment', manifesting itself sometimes as stubbornness, a capacity for hard work, attention to the detail of government and strong religious principles.[131] She was, indeed, heavily reliant on her ministers but ill-health had a lot to do with it. From among her attributes, religious conviction was particularly significant, as defence against the plague, perceived to emanate and be tolerated in the Mohammedan Middle East, was regarded as a Christian duty. More generally, concern for plague sits well with the cautious and responsible aspects of Anne's character, particularly as it impinged upon foreign policy and to some extent the navy, both of which were royal prerogatives.

Set between the Queen and her Privy Council, who to the country at large appeared to control the policy and practice of quarantine, lay the Cabinet and the Lords of the Committee. The identity and function of these bodies has long been the subject of debate, but quarantine has never been identified as an issue for one or the other.[132] Both bodies were composed of an inner circle of privy councillors, with the Lord Chancellor, Lord Treasurer (or First Lord when the Treasury was in commission), President of the Council, Lord Privy Seal, Lord Lieutenant of Ireland, Commander-in-Chief and the principal Secretaries of State entitled to attend.[133] The Cabinet met roughly twice a week at royal palaces, in the Queen's presence, with foreign policy very much on the agenda.[134] The Lords of the Committee met even more frequently at the Cockpit in Whitehall; the Queen was never present although it was usual for other parties to be summoned to give advice or to be questioned on national issues.[135] Broadly speaking, it was the Lords of the Committee who formulated a strategy, which passed to the Cabinet for ratification before the Privy Council took executive action. In the absence of formal minutes of the Cabinet or Lords of the Committee, it is difficult to establish the source of quarantine policy under Anne's style of government.

There do exist, however, informal minutes taken by or on behalf of Lord Dartmouth for meetings of both the Cabinet and the Lords of the Committee.[136] These are very helpful for 1710–12, with some 15 references to quarantine or plague.[137] Only five of these meetings were held at royal palaces and were therefore

130 Biddle, p. 150.

131 Ibid.; cf. J.P. Mackintosh, *The British Cabinet*, 3rd edn (London, 1977), p. 44: 'she had a mind of her own and some capacity …'

132 J.H. Plumb, 'The organization of the Cabinet in the reign of Queen Anne', *Transactions of the Royal Historical Society*, 5th series, vol. 7 (1957), 137–57, recounts and sometimes refutes past contentions.

133 Plumb, 'The organization of the Cabinet in the reign of Queen Anne', 145.

134 Plumb, 'The organization of the Cabinet in the reign of Queen Anne', 142–3, 147.

135 Plumb, 'The organization of the Cabinet in the reign of Queen Anne', 147–8.

136 The Dartmouth Papers in Stafford (now at the County Record Office) are more extensive than Plumb realized.

137 Staffordshire Record Office [SRO] D(W)1778/V/188, D742/U/1/1–139 and D742/U/2/1–77.

meetings of the Cabinet; the others were held at the Cockpit and were therefore meetings of the Lords in Committee. The Cabinet's main involvement concerned the petition of the mayor of Rochester about the unsuitability of Hoo Fort as an airing ground; the Cabinet sent it straight to the Treasury, for the attention of the Customs Commissioners, and later directed that the report of the Commissioners should be considered by the Lords of the Committee – or, as they called them, 'the Committee at the Cockpit'. That is why the referrals have escaped the Privy Council register. The Cabinet also considered questions of quarantine in Ireland and Scotland.

The minutes reveal that the Lords of the Committee dealt with wider issues involving plague abroad, instructions or advice to the Admiralty, and shared an interest in Scotland with the Cabinet.[138] The Privy Council's anti-infection committee has been recently mentioned above; this was set up, certainly by May 1712, to monitor health in Europe and was yet another body where quarantine was discussed. The committee twice received reports of the Customs Commissioners to whom petitions from merchants (for the release of ships) had been referred.[139] In this way it helped free the Privy Council from just a fraction of the relentless minutiae of quarantine business. As every ship was eventually considered, at some meetings of the Privy Council quarantine was the only issue; invariably it comprised most agenda items, although there is no way of knowing how thoroughly the report on each ship was considered.[140] It is perhaps a mark of how seriously quarantine was taken that the scope of the committee was not extended: there was no question, it seems, of systematically delegating the release of quarantined ships to this subordinate body. The committee were, however, asked by the Cabinet to consider the question of Heligoland lobster boats.[141] They reported at the Council Chamber in Whitehall – that is to say, to the Privy Council itself.[142]

If the Cabinet and the Lords of the Committee were the bodies in which quarantine policy was created, it is still tempting to seek within them an individual who made the running. The obvious candidate is Harley, who was close to the Queen and, if not Prime Minister in any formal sense, was certainly *primus inter pares* for much of her reign. It has already been related that Swift made a passionate appeal to Harley to make quarantine more effective, and the latter's selfless, principled and God-fearing public life make him a likely opponent of the plague.[143] On the other hand, Harley has been described as 'culpably negligent', at least when he had been a Secretary of State between 1704 and 1708, and his attendance at meetings of the Cabinet and Lords of the Committee, in the crucial period between October 1710 and June 1711,

138 As regards the risk of infection, the Lords recommended to the Queen that no letters should be received from Holland and Flanders except from Townshend, Marlborough '& so from the respective ministers' (SRO D(W)1778/V/188, 31 Oct. 1710).

139 NA PC 2/83/431; 2/84/7.

140 As early as May 1710 (PC 2/82/588–90), quarantine occupied six out of seven agenda items.

141 SRO D742/U/2/1–77, 24 Aug. 1712.

142 NA PC 2/84/8.

143 Biddle, pp. 15, 20, 25–6.

was not good.[144] On 8 March 1711 he was stabbed by Guiscard (in fact, during a meeting of the Lords of the Committee), which kept him absent from all subsequent meetings of both bodies until 21 May.[145] Another problem with Harley is that when quarantine precautions were first taken he was Chancellor of the Exchequer; this was not a position relevant to the emergency itself, and indeed his Cabinet ranking was unusual.[146] There is a much better case, however, for Harley's involvement following his convalescence, as he returned to public office in the powerful role of Lord Treasurer. This put him in direct supervision of the Customs service.

Lord Dartmouth, whose minutes are mentioned above, was Secretary of State for the Southern Department from June 1710 until August 1714, when he was succeeded by Bolingbroke. It is interesting that he was given an active role in quarantine matters, because the source of the feared infection, the Baltic, was more properly within the remit of his colleague of the Northern Department. The Secretary of State who ran the Northern Department, when the plague crisis loomed, was Henry Boyle. He was followed in September 1710 by St John, who succeeded Dartmouth in the Southern Department in August 1713. The vacancy thus created in the Northern Department was filled by William Bromley, who held office until September 1714, by which time the emergency was over. Boyle has been characterized as 'an unambitious tranquil man' and he was not in office long enough to influence the key Proclamations and statute; as for Bromley, the policymaking was all but over when he arrived in a position of influence.[147]

Dartmouth's unexpected role can be explained to some extent by St John's encroachment into the Southern Department when Harley was stabbed; this came about because the peace negotiations with France which Harley had been conducting needed to continue their momentum while he convalesced, and France fell within the Southern Department.[148] Dartmouth redressed the balance, to some extent, by dealing with northern issues, but his real connection with quarantine arose from his responsibility for dealing with the Admiralty. In October 1710, before Harley's injury had altered the ministerial status quo, Dartmouth recorded at a meeting of the Lords of the Committee 'that I should write to [the] Lds. of the Admiralty to lett them know the Lords [of the Committee] have been informed that there is not sufficient cair taken in the quarantine of the ships and that there is danger from the Pilots going on board and comeing back and how that may be prevented'.[149] This exemplifies the role of Dartmouth, who has been described as 'colourless', as a purveyor of policy rather than an instigator.[150]

In February 1709 a third Secretary of State was appointed; this was the Duke of Queensberry, responsible for Scotland. Queensberry was involved in northern

144 Thomson, p. 19; Plumb, 'The organization of the Cabinet in the reign of Queen Anne', 143.

145 Plumb, 'The organization of the Cabinet in the reign of Queen Anne', 143.

146 Ibid.

147 The quotation is from Thomson, p. 23.

148 Thomson, p. 24.

149 SRO D(W)1778/V/188, 8 Dec. 1710.

150 The description of Dartmouth is from Thomson, p. 20.

European issues, a gesture from his English counterparts with whom he had fractious exchanges.[151] This is interesting as Scotland had a long tradition of managing the plague threat and Queensberry might well have been useful in the early discussions. But he died in July 1711. By elimination, St John would seem to have made the decisive contribution throughout the emergency. He was intellectually brilliant and forthright, and impressed Marlborough by his application to business.[152] On the other hand, he was preoccupied with managing the peace negotiations with France and the tedious procedural detail of quarantine is unlikely to have appealed to him. In brief, no one man seems to have made quarantine his own, and the decisions taken in Committee and in Cabinet were perhaps truly the result of collective thinking. This is consistent with the point, already argued, that quarantine was one of the rare matters in which parliamentary factions, with all the shades of persuasion which they embraced, had little meaning or relevance in the context of a deadly epidemic.

Quarantine and the navy

To the British navy in 1709, the imposition of quarantine was a thorough nuisance. With the country at war with France, much of the fleet which was not engaging the enemy or seizing its shipping was tied up in convoys. While French privateers worked almost in sight of English harbours, it was necessary for merchant ships to muster at convenient locations along the Channel and North Sea coasts to await the arrival of the navy to escort them on the next leg of their voyage. This put serious demands on the availability of warships, which were usually undermanned. Ships' captains were still ruthless and indiscriminate in 'pressing' seamen out of merchant vessels to make up the complement of a man-of-war. In the new emergency, the navy now had the extra tasks of supporting Customs officers in policing the law, and providing guard-ships at quarantine stations; while at the same time a source of its manpower was removed and its own ships were liable to detention. It also faced imponderable delay in the arrival of stores from the Baltic on which the efficiency of the fleet was utterly dependent.

The organization of convoys was a matter for the Admiralty Board, which controlled the administration of the navy and questions of policy, subject always to direction from a Secretary of State or the Privy Council.[153] There were other bodies junior to the Admiralty Board, the chief one being the Navy Board which was responsible for the condition of the fleet. Quarantine affected these boards in different ways. The Admiralty Board delegated quarantine issues, whenever possible, to Sir William Jumper, who had been appointed Captain Resident at Chatham in 1708 and was responsible for the Medway, and with it Stangate Creek.[154] Jumper soon found himself visited with unpleasant and difficult duties, but seems to have sidestepped the most irksome, which was to return a continuously updated account of ships under

151 Thomson, pp. 31–2.

152 Biddle, p. 59.

153 A good summary of the respective spheres of the Admiralty and Navy Boards can be found in D.A. Baugh, *Naval Administration, 1715–1750* (London, 1977), pp. 1–4.

154 For Jumper's career, see *Oxford Dictionary of National Biography.*

quarantine.[155] What he could not avoid, however, was the ambiguous stance of the Admiralty in the matter of impressment, about which instructions were also sent by the Board directly to ships concerned.

The first advice given to Jumper, in December 1709, was that he should spread the word among detained vessels that impressment was 'not intended'.[156] Such a weak form of words, when disseminated among fighting ships, did not prevent the captain of HMS *Deal Castle* at Harwich from boarding an Eastland ship in quarantine there and taking out some of the crew.[157] This action led the Admiralty to put the captain himself into quarantine, and presumably his ship as well, as its new tour of duty was cancelled.[158] But the navy could ill-afford to have a warship lying idle, and about ten days later the *Deal Castle* was sent to Lynn to convoy the 'trade' (as merchants ships were collectively termed) to Newcastle.[159] Just before this, some men from HMS *Fox* in Newcastle went on board a ship under quarantine there; but the captain was only sent a letter of disapproval.[160] The infringements continued, and in January 1710 a letter to the captain of the *Rochester Prize* asked for affidavits from his officers and men that they had not broken the rules.[161] This tougher line did not last: in October the captain of HMS *Jolly*, who had allegedly pressed men from a ship in the Medway, was reprimanded, but the master of the merchant ship was not allowed to reclaim his men, as the *Jolly* was now itself under quarantine.[162] That smacked of a convenient way to keep the men impressed, and in the same month Jumper was no more than 'recommended' to prevent impressment out of quarantine ships for the future.[163] For merchants and shipowners, the uncertain position was yet another headache, as if wars, disease and petitioning for convoys were not problems enough. Sir Randolph Knipe wrote specifically to the Admiralty to request that men from his East Country ships should not be pressed.[164] He won his request, and eventually the Admiralty adopted a stronger line, partly to its own detriment. Warships on convoy duty were forbidden to press crewmen once the ships they were protecting had reached port, on the grounds that men would not then be induced to run ashore.[165] Only a pragmatic reason, not a simple instruction, was likely to deter a naval captain sailing in wartime with 30 men short.

A growing tension developed between the Admiralty and the Customs Commissioners as the former were drawn inexorably, and increasingly, into areas where they had no wish to be. Relations were not helped by the use of the Customs Commissioners, presumably at the Treasury's request, as a medium for conveying complaints against impressment. The guard-ships were another catalyst

155 NA ADM 3/24 [unpag.], 15 Nov. 1709.
156 NA ADM 3/24, 15 Dec. 1709.
157 NA ADM 3/24, 20 Dec. 1709.
158 Ibid.
159 NA ADM 3/24, 30 Dec. 1709.
160 NA ADM 3/24, 24 Dec. 1709.
161 NA ADM 3/24, 17 & 25 Jan. 1710.
162 NA ADM 3/25, 5 Oct. 1710.
163 NA ADM 3/25, 9 Oct. 1710.
164 NA ADM 3/24, 7 Feb. 1710.
165 NA ADM 3/25, 21 Sept. 1711.

for problems, particularly at Stangate Creek. At first, the Collector at Rochester controlled all aspects of shipping in the Medway, but soon a Mr Hunt was appointed with a delegated responsibility for quarantine and its ramifications.[166] From around March 1710, the question of quarantine enforcement in the Thames estuary called for naval supervision, and a brigantine, HMS *Fly*, was dispatched from Harwich to The Nore.[167] The Customs Commissioners upset the Admiralty by asking for naval personnel to board and bring back certain ships which had deliberately sailed passed the quarantine checkpoint.[168] The Admiralty at first acquiesced, but later replied that no men could be spared; the point that this boarding would have made them subject to quarantine themselves was not argued. But it was soon necessary to summon the sloop HMS *Hare* from The Downs to act as a guard ship in Stangate Creek, supported by an additional small boat.[169]

For the next two years, HMS *Hare* was at the centre of repeated allegations by Hunt that she was not doing her duty. The complaints, at first vague, crystallized into a claim that men were breaking quarantine by going on shore to farmhouses, presumably from ships' boats.[170] Jumper was sent to investigate, and the outcome was that boats from vessels liable to quarantine were to be surrendered to the *Hare* on arrival.[171] But still the allegations came of 'Irregularities', presumably connivance, and in February 1711 the boatswain of the *Hare* was dismissed.[172] Meanwhile, the navy got its own back. A letter from Captain Edwards, claiming lax quarantine requirements by Customs officers at Harwich, was sent to the Commissioners for information.[173] A similar letter from another officer was sent some time later, when the Admiralty expressly desired the Commissioners to prevent quarantine abuse from happening.[174] This authoritative line, proper or not, became a hallmark of the Admiralty's position. When Lord Dartmouth asked them to oblige merchant ships off the coast of Scotland to perform quarantine, the Board responded by requesting Dartmouth to ask as much of the Customs Commissioners.[175] And having initiated the scare which caused Heligoland boats to perform quarantine, the Board advised Sir Christopher Musgrave, clerk to the Privy Council, to use the *London Gazette* and not the Admiralty (as he had wished) to warn away shipping.[176]

The Board's tetchiness can be attributed to ever-increasing demands on their material resources while they were still prosecuting the war with France. They were losing ship after ship to quarantine because, like the merchant ships which they escorted from the Baltic, they were subject to the rules which applied to all arrivals

166 Hunt, who was in post throughout the emergency, first appears in the negotiations with Lord Teynham in autumn 1709 (NA PC 2/82/466–9; *CTB* (1709), p. 417).

167 NA ADM 3/24, 27 March 1710.

168 NA ADM 3/24, 24 May & 10 July 1710.

169 NA ADM 3/24, 7 Aug. 1710.

170 NA ADM 3/25, 3 Nov., 13 & 19 Dec. 1710.

171 NA ADM 3/25, 26 Dec. 1710.

172 NA ADM 3/25, 24 Jan. & 7 Feb. 1711.

173 NA ADM 3/25, 16 Dec. 1710.

174 NA ADM 3/26, 16 Aug. 1711.

175 NA ADM 3/26, 6 Sept. 1711.

176 NA ADM 3/27, 28 Aug. 1712.

from places suspected of infection. Some ships, like HMS *Ruby*, did quarantine more than once in a year. For warships this was generally at The Nore, but The Downs were also used, as was The Motherbank in the Solent. At one point matters were so desperate that the *Ruby*, supposedly in quarantine at The Downs, was on standby to escort a merchant ship with naval stores to Spithead, where her quarantine would have continued.[177] In 1712 the position was at its most difficult. No fewer than four warships, each with additional eight-oared boats, were required at The Nore to enforce the Privy Council's requirement for extra precautions, while Sandwich Haven was added to the growing number of quarantine harbours where warships were expected to attend.[178] Soon, at a dozen locations between Plymouth and the Moray Firth, some 15 small naval vessels were dodging in and out of quarantine, passing the baton as guard-ships, and no doubt awaiting with impatience the order to get on with the war.[179]

A lurking problem for the Admiralty was knowing the extent of its powers. Late in 1711 the captain of HMS *Dispatch* asked what should happen next as the merchant ship *Constant* refused to go to a place of quarantine.[180] The Admiralty Board did not know and asked Lord Dartmouth for the Queen's pleasure. The matter was considered by the Lords of the Committee – the only time in which a particular quarantine incident was brought to their attention – and Dartmouth was instructed to reply by sending the Admiralty a copy of the Order in Council of 6 September 1711, 'and lett them know the Queen takes them to be the proper officers to see it put in execution.'[181] This was a feeble response, ignoring the existence of statute and Proclamation, and demonstrating that the Cabinet were equally at a loss. The fact was that the navy's legal responsibility ended once a ship was under the 'direction' of the Customs service, as it was in this instance. Commanders of warships, forts and garrisons had been 'aiding and assisting' Customs officials for more than two years, but this phrase gave no indication of the degree of force which was admissible. Indeed, so far from clarifying the authority of naval guard-ships, the law made no actual provision for their existence. Perhaps unsurprisingly, the *Constant* is not recorded among ships which performed quarantine.

The Navy Board had a quite different outlook on quarantine. Being responsible for the arrival of raw materials in the royal dockyards, they might well have agonized publicly over the way quarantine aggravated an already precarious position. In fact, the Board did all they could to avoid such issues. So far from monitoring the detention of ships carrying naval stores, they resorted to asking the merchants themselves, if necessary, when the quarantine of a ship was likely to end.[182] The Board entered into the fullest discussions with Baltic merchants, particularly about hemp. The procedure was for the merchants to attend the Board, state the prices at which they were prepared to supply the home ports (that is, the Thames dockyards),

177 NA ADM 3/25, 9 Feb. 1711.

178 NA ADM 3/27, 29 Aug., 9 & 11 Oct. 1712.

179 NA ADM 3/27, Aug. 1712 – Apr. 1713.

180 NA ADM 3/26, 14 Dec. 1711.

181 SRO D742/U/1–139, 16 Dec. 1711.

182 National Maritime Museum (NMM) SER/63 [unpag.], 23 Oct. 1710.

plus Portsmouth and Plymouth.[183] The Board then reported to the Admiralty and Treasury, by whom Lord Dartmouth and eventually the Queen were drawn into a view. Eventually the merchants were called to the Board to hear what quantities, in what apportionment per merchant, were acceptable and after further haggling a deal would be struck.

There is no evidence that delay in delivery, caused by quarantine, even entered the bargaining, and the Board must have made it clear at the outset that, as this issue was beyond the control of either side, contracts would be discussed as if quarantine did not exist. So whether or not a ship was detained for 40 days, the contract price would stand. Thus in May 1711, Plymouth yard was instructed to receive pitch and tar at the contract price of the previous year, although the time had overrun.[184] Indeed, as contracts were prepared a year in advance, there was probably a belief that quarantine would have been abolished by the date of delivery. Such thoughts, however, did not prevent individual merchants petitioning for their ships carrying naval stores to be exempt from quarantine detention. The Navy Board would have nothing to do with such questions and referred them to the Admiralty. The attitude of the Admiralty will be seen, once again, to have been ambivalent.

183 The process is well illustrated in NMM SER/64 [unpag.], during February and March.

184 NMM SER/64, 14 May 1711.

Chapter Three

The Baltic Crisis, 1709–1714: Mercantile Worries

Documentary evidence

For the conduct of quarantine against the Baltic, the historian is lucky to have two detailed and complementary sources – one from the Privy Council, the other from the Treasury. They give largely the same information, gathered at different stages, but as neither source is comprehensive or wholly accurate in itself, one tends to correct the other or make up any shortfall. The position will be clearer once the procedures and processes of quarantine are explained. It should be understood that these steps represent the mature system, in the context of a ship not owned or freighted by a contractor to the Navy Board. That consideration does not affect the extent of the evidence (which shows liability to quarantine as well as its performance), but it does mean that some ships, as will be seen, escaped the worst of the rigmarole and expense.

After 40 days had expired, and the master and others had made oath as to the good health of the crew, the merchant petitioned the Queen (or King) in Council for the ship's release.[1] The Privy Council referred the petition to the Treasury, who delegated it to their subordinate body, the Commissioners of Customs. The Commissioners made enquiry and reported back to the Treasury, who referred the report to the Privy Council. Once release was agreed at that level, the Privy Council made an order to the Treasury and the Treasury made an order to the Commissioners. The best evidence comes from the registers of the Privy Council, because that body was involved either side, so to speak, of delegation to the Treasury.[2] But Treasury books and papers are equally important, and for this period the calendars have been published.[3] The advantage of publication is inestimable, and it is doubtful whether quarantine at this early period could be adequately studied without these authoritative, reliable and indexed volumes.

It seems almost churlish to suggest that such scholarship might have a drawback, and indeed set against the totality of the benefit the flaws are minuscule. But

1 The procedure outlined here can be deduced from Privy Council and Treasury records, but is also outlined in *Journal of the Commissioners for Trade and Plantations* [*JCTP*], vol. 2, pp. 194–5.

2 Register books relevant are NA PC 2/82–4. No minute books of the Privy Council (less formal records) survive for this period.

3 Relevant for this period are *Calendar of Treasury Books* [*CTB*], vols 24–8 (1949–69) and *Calendar of Treasury Papers* [*CTP*], vol. 4 (1879).

certain problems do exist. For instance, in August 1711 the phrase 'and deals for Denidge goods' follows iron, pitch and tar as part of a particular cargo.[4] The calendar interprets Denidge as Danish (placed in square brackets after the word); but the supposed adjective is actually a noun, dunnage, meaning material used as packing or protection on the voyage. The point is significant, not only because Denmark had no stake in this particular Swedish cargo, but because the deals, if only dunnage, were a minor part of the cargo and possibly damaged. In another list of cargoes, the unknown word 'oales' is interpreted as '[?oils]', but recourse to the Privy Council register shows the word to be bales.[5] The real mistake there was by a Treasury clerk, and clerical transcription at both Privy Council and Treasury level was sometimes distinctly careless. Difficulty in spelling obscure Baltic ports is understandable; more trying are the problems associated with ships' names. Not only is the spelling at times inconsistent between the two levels of evidence, but there are many problems in deciding if a ship with apparently two linked Christian names (a common practice) is actually two different ships of one name each. For instance, in the Treasury calendars, the *George and John* should be two ships, as should the *Salvator and Prince,* the *Benjamin Hope* and the *John Thorowgood.*[6] This can be proved from the Privy Council registers.[7] Calendaring, of course, makes another opportunity for error. If it was difficult for contemporary clerks to be certain, it was doubly so for the archivists, faced often with an ambiguous text, or evidence of doubt or second thoughts on the part of the scribe. An associated problem was the frequency of certain names, both abstract nouns like *Providence* and *Love* and single female Christian names, such as *Ann(e)* or *Elizabeth*. Even when all the evidence is correct, it can be difficult to differentiate between ships.[8]

In these years before registration, the practice of showing the master's name after that of his vessel was the only way to distinguish between apparently identical ships. Luckily the Privy Council registers do, at times, give masters' names when the Treasury records do not; this means that a *Mary Flower* in one source and a *Mayflower* in the other can be identified as the same ship, and similar comparisons are almost endless.[9] Foreign names were a particular bewilderment for clerks: the Swedish prefix *Hedvig* (as in *Hedvig Sophia* or *Hedvig Eleona*) was sometimes cast as *Headway* or *Headwick*; and *Lady Kerdrant* to a clerk in the Privy Council was *Lady Herdrowt* to his colleague in the Treasury.[10] The Treasury calendars correct

4 *CTB*, vol. 25, part 2, p. 407.

5 *CTB*, vol. 26, part 2, p. 540; National Archives [NA] PC 2/84/54–5.

6 *CTB*, vol. 26, part 2, p. 114; *CTB* vol. 24, part 2, p. 486; *CTB*, vol. 25, part 2, p. 488; *CTB*, vol. 25, part 2, p. 213.

7 NA PC 2/83/360; NA PC 2/83/360, 127–8; NA PC 2/83/360, 321–2; NA PC 2/83/360, 214–15.

8 The number of ships with 'unique' names is very much the minority. Even *Young Tobias* occurred three times in 1712.

9 *CTB*, vol. 27, part 2, p. 126 and NA PC 2/84/80. Sometimes both sources appear in error; the ship named *Gilly Flower* in Privy Council and Treasury was apparently *July Flower* (NA CUST 84/12/43, 47).

10 *Headway* occurs in *CTB*, vol. 25, part 2, p. 221 (and also in the Privy Council); *Hedwick* is in NA PC 2/83/86, 93; *Lady Kerdrant* is in PC 2/83/432; *Lady Herdrowt* in *CTB*,

Ufro to *Juffrouw*.[11] It would be tedious to extend variants and inconsistencies any further, but it is necessary to draw attention to them as another reason why, in the Baltic period, no absolute list of ships subjected or liable to quarantine can be drawn up.

A troubling aspect of the two main sources is the extent to which each is incomplete in itself. It can be expected that in the complexity of Treasury records certain aspects of quarantine were overlooked, or have not survived, but it is not at all clear why the registers of the Privy Council should be so inconsistent in recording both the referral of a particular ship and its eventual discharge. Of the nearly 900 ships mentioned in the registers, only 442 are recorded at both these stages. It is perhaps understandable that petitions for the release of ships were, for reasons of speed, favour, mischance or mistake, referred directly to the Treasury, and missed an initial entry in the Privy Council registers. But it is curious that, on 44 occasions, no discharge was ever registered against ships which *had* been referred in the proper way. The position is complicated by the occasional referral of just 'ships' – that is to say, an undeclared number of unnamed vessels. These vague, block entries which occur in both main sources make another reason why the total number of quarantined ships cannot accurately be known. Rather more ships, in total, are mentioned in the Privy Council registers than in the Treasury calendars, but curiously 40 ships are included in the Treasury records that are omitted altogether (that is at both referral and discharge stages) from the Privy Council registers. No fewer than 32 of those omissions occurred in 1713, the year when quarantine netted by far the greatest number of vessels.

Other sources which mention Baltic quarantine are entry books of the Secretaries of State and records of Customs officers in the English east-coast outports. When quarantine was first introduced, the entry books registered petitions in full (and enlightening) detail, but within a year the sheer volume of them, and no doubt the tedium of repetition, led to increasingly curtailed entries, and finally to no entries at all.[12] As for local Customs records, these mainly consist – where they exist at all – of letters from the Board in London to the local collector.[13] While these do contain instructions for the discharge of named ships, much of the material concerns notices and circulars for information. An important survival, however, are the records of Harwich outport, being copies of letters from the collector to the Board.[14] At no other local port in the Baltic period can quarantine be glimpsed from this angle. While none of the ships reported from Harwich escaped the Privy Council registers, the information on port of departure, cargo, and place of quarantine confirms and often amplifies the evidence from other sources. Another unique glimpse at quarantine

vol. 26, part 2, p. 305.

11 *CTB*, vol. 26, part 2, p. 316.

12 NA SP 44/245 has 27 petitions between July 1710 and November 1711.

13 The most useful series are Board to Collector, Yarmouth (NA CUST 97/74A), and ditto, Newcastle (CUST 84/122).

14 NA CUST 99/1.

from the local standpoint comes from the water bailiffs' records at Hull.[15] These are not Customs records per se, neither are they in any way complete; but the fragments which survive from 1709–11 show many ships which could not have escaped quarantine, and yet are unmentioned by name in the Privy Council registers. These are some of the 'lost' ships comprised in the block entries mentioned above.

By piecing together these large and small pockets of evidence, more than a thousand merchant ships over less than five years can be positively identified as caught up in the quarantine restrictions against Baltic and north German ports. The 'lost' ships – those in the block entries – might add another 10 per cent to that total.

The quarantine ports

Despite the massive supremacy of London as the entrepôt of British seaborne trade, many of the naval stores imported from the Baltic were destined for the dockyards of the Thames estuary, Chatham, Portsmouth and Plymouth. Other naval stores (naval meaning maritime rather than military) were destined for Hull and Newcastle; as well as hemp, flax, pitch, tar, masts and spars, these supplies included large amounts of bar iron which were converted into nails in the Tyne valley.[16] These nails were then dispatched by sea to London and the southern dockyards, which thus required the manufactured product of Baltic goods as well as the raw materials. Other supplies, notably fir, came from Norway.[17] The demand for naval stores was therefore spread along the south and east coasts of England – but particularly the east coast. As Stangate Creek was placed roughly halfway along that total coastline, it might appear convenient for it to have acted as a quarantine clearing station for ships heading west and north, as well as to London and the Medway. Unfortunately, war and the winter weather conspired to make Stangate Creek less useful than it should have been.

If a ship were making for London she did not necessarily sail direct, particularly in time of war. Harwich was well placed geographically to receive and dispatch convoys: not only was the North Sea journey relatively short, but the Thames was within easy reach, and coastwise convoys could escort northbound ships to Hull, Newcastle and intermediate ports. Whether this gave Harwich the edge over Stangate Creek as England's busiest quarantine port is an interesting proposition, and there is evidence to suggest that it did.

Taken from the various sources already discussed, Table 3.1 has been prepared.

---

15 Hull City Archives [HCA] WB 8, 9. The file of 'account sheets' includes also ships from Norway, Holland and Germany.

16 By Sir Ambrose Crowley.

17 H.S.K. Kent, 'The Anglo-Norwegian timber trade in the eighteenth century', *Economic History Review*, 2nd series, 8 (1955–56), 62–6.

Table 3.1 Ships at quarantine stations in England and Scotland, 1709–1714

Q. Station	Ships	Ships shared with other stations	Total
England			
Harwich	149	5 with Newcastle; 8 with Hull; 24 with Stangate Creek	**186**
Stangate Creek	77	1 with Hull; 24 with Harwich	**102**
Newcastle	66	5 with Harwich	**71**
Hull	17	1 with Stangate Creek; 8 with Harwich	**26**
Portsmouth/ Solent	2		**2**
Exeter	2		**2**
Cowes	1		**1**
Studland Bay	1		**1**
Scotland			
Inverkeithing Road	5		**5**
Inverness/ Cromarty	3		**3**
Dumfries	1		**1**
Kirkudbright	1		**1**
Leith Road	1		**1**
'Scotland'	3		**3**

Note: These are known ships at known quarantine stations, not definitive totals.

Source: Privy Council registers and Treasury calendars

Before Harwich is awarded the accolade, it must be conceded that for many ships the place of detention was not stated in the Privy Council registers, or elsewhere. The Harwich total is also slightly inflated by the inclusion of 11 ships in spring 1714 which the collector reported as quarantine detainees, but which were released soon afterwards when the system was abolished.[18] When the quarantine port is not stated, and if the petitioners are known to have been London merchants, there must be a presumption in favour of Stangate Creek. As the total number of ships in the above table is 405, or only some 40 per cent of the number which quarantine affected, there is clearly scope for Stangate Creek to take the honours. But there are also good reasons to suggest that the supremacy of Harwich could be correct. There were evidently flat-spots in the Creek's business: when the detachment from Upnor Castle pleaded to return from Stangate Marshes early in 1711, their trump-card argument was that there were no ships doing quarantine at that time.[19] Even more telling was the complaint by the superintendent at Stangate Creek, early in 1714, that ships were choosing to go to Harwich because 'a greater liberty is given them' there.[20] This, of course, was vigorously denied by the Harwich controller (who thought the opposite was the case), but the evidence, such as it is, supports the balance of business as being at the Essex port.

The above table indicates that some ships were placed in quarantine on their arrival at one place, but allowed to continue their journey to another to complete the 40 days. The two known ships at Exeter (there were probably more) and the one in Dorset represent the trade from the German North Sea ports, rather than from the Baltic. It is interesting that much of this trade also did quarantine at Harwich, although few of the cargoes could be characterized as naval stores. The procedure at Harwich was straightforward, and representative of the wider system: when a ship arrived from a port suspected of infection, she was immediately put under quarantine. The collector, every day if necessary, wrote to the Board in London with a list of arrivals; he gave ships' and masters' names, and brief details of cargo and provenance. He wrote again when the period of 40 days had elapsed, confirming that the master and others had gone ashore to make their sworn declarations, and that crewmen were free of infection. Thus when the Commissioners in London needed to report to the Treasury (for the Privy Council) following the referral of a petition for discharge, they should already have had confirmation that quarantine was completed. That was all very well in the case of Harwich, only 70 miles from London, but it will be seen that for ships in Scotland the system was perfectly dreadful.

Dozens of ships, especially those from Germany, chose to do quarantine at the island of Texel in Holland before reaching England.[21] There is no evidence that this diminished the quarantine period in Britain, although this was probably a hope. There were no onshore airing facilities at Texel, and the British outports were similarly disadvantaged, despite the Order in Council that a site be agreed between

18 NA CUST 99/1 [unpag.].

19 NA SP 41/3.

20 NA CUST 99/1, 23 Feb. 1714.

21 As well as receiving individual ships, Texel welcomed them in convoys of 9, 12 and even 24, bound for England (NA PC 2/83/336, 384–5, 422–3).

local Customs and magistracy. However inadequate and controversial were the airing grounds in the Medway, they did at least exist. At Harwich, ships simply lay with their hatches open, weather permitting.[22] At Hull, quarantine was performed in Whitebooth Roads in the Humber. There is evidence of 'Airy Sheds' existing on land by January 1710, but perhaps not for much longer.[23] At Newcastle, airing was the subject of an early and deep division between collector and corporation which led to Privy Council intervention.[24] The collector was given the last word, but there is no reason to believe that an airing ground was ever established: the Privy Council later asked in vain what facilities existed there.[25] One aspect of quarantine in the outports is that local corporations, despite the sensitivity of airing-ground selection, did not deal with these matters in formal council. At both Newcastle and Hull, the borough records are silent.[26] This is especially curious at Newcastle, which was comfortable sending representations to London on matters including plague and maritime trade, yet in the town's Common Council Order Book there is no hint of controversy with the local collector about his chosen site.[27]

In Scotland, the position was muddled. A Scottish Board of Customs had been set up following the Act of Union in 1707, and early in 1710 the magistrates in Edinburgh joined forces with the Commissioners to put a number of quarantine issues to the Privy Council in London.[28] One question concerned an airing ground. It would be convenient to use Inchcolm (which had proved useful in the seventeenth century) but the Earl of Murray would not agree.[29] What should happen now? The reply was weak, evasive and irrelevant: the question was simply not deemed 'requisite' as enumerated goods were prevented from landing anywhere until the Privy Council had given orders for their disposal. This attitude was in marked contrast to the Council's robust stance in England, where local Customs officers had the power to appoint airing grounds in defiance of objections, at least from magistrates.

Ports of departure

Table 3.2 seeks to give an idea – and little more than that – of the foreign ports whose trade was most affected by British quarantine.

---

22 For example NA PC 2/84/296, where the master complained of 'no conveniency' for airing ashore at Harwich.

23 NA PC 2/82/568.

24 NA PC 2/82/459; *CTB*, vol. 23, part 2, p. 411; NA CUST 84/122/34.

25 NA PC 2/83/322–3. There is no reference to this question in CUST 84/122.

26 At Hull, the 'Bench Book', 1682–1741 (HCA BRB 6), is scarcely interested in any harbour matters, although the town's main merchants were successively elected mayors.

27 Tyne and Wear Archives [TWA] MD/NC/2/3.

28 NA PC 2/82/540.

29 Ibid.

Table 3.2 Ports of departure of ships affected by British quarantine, 1709–1714

Port of departure, with no. of ships sailing direct		Ships calling also at one other port	Ships possibly from this port (i.e. in composite lists, with other ports as shown below)	Total
Sweden (Western Baltic)				
Calsund	1			**1**
Carlscrona	1			**1**
Carlshaven	1			**1**
Christianstad	2			**2**
Gefle	10		4 with Gothenburg, Nyköping; 4 with Nyköping, Gothenburg, Hamburg; 9 with Stockholm, Königsberg	**<27**
Gothenburg	133	45 (29 from Stockholm)	4 with Gefle, Nyköping; 4 with Gefle, Nyköping, Hamburg; 5 with Stockholm, Riga, Königsberg; 6 with Hamburg, Bremen; 14 with Stockholm, Riga, Königsberg, Danzig, Hamburg	**<211**
'Long Sound'		1		**1**
Norrköping	1			**1**
Norrköping	1			**1**
Nyköping	2	2	4 with Gefle, Gothenburg; 4 with Gefle, Gothenburg, Hamburg	**<12**
'Pewsterswick'	1			**1**
Stockholm	127	47	5 with Gothenburg, Königsberg, Riga; 9 with Gefle, Königsberg; 14 with Gothenburg, Riga, Königsberg, Danzig, Hamburg	**<202**
Warberg	1			**1**

Unspecified	56			**56**
Eastern Baltic				
Danzig	66	15	14 with Gothenburg, Riga, Königsberg, Stockholm, Hamburg	**<95**
Eckenförde	2	1		**3**
Königsberg/ Pilau	58	21	5 with Hamburg; 5 with Gothenburg, Stockholm, Riga; 9 with Gefle, Stockholm; 14 with Danzig, Gothenburg, Riga, Stockholm, Hamburg	**<112**
Libau	1			**1**
Memel	4	6		**10**
Petersburg	1	4		**5**
Reval	1			**1**
Riga	17	22	5 with Stockholm, Königsberg, Gothenburg; 14 with Danzig, Gothenburg, Riga, Stockholm, Hamburg	**<58**
Stolp	1			**1**
Windau	1			**1**
Unspecified	12			**12**
Denmark				
Copenhagen	1			**1**
Germany				
Altona		1	36 with Bremen, Hamburg	**<37**
Bremen	38	17	6 with Gothenburg, Hamburg; 36 with Altona, Hamburg; 24 with Hamburg;	**<121**

Hamburg	70	18	4 with Stockholm; 4 with Gefle Nyköping, Gothenburg; 5 with Königsberg ; 6 with Gothenburg, Bremen; 14 with Danzig, Gothenburg, Königsberg, Riga, Stockholm; 24 with Bremen; 36 with Altona, Bremen	**<181**

Totals:

Sweden (Western Baltic):	<517
Germany:	<339
Eastern Baltic:	<299
Denmark:	1

Note: The symbol < in the Total column means up to the number indicated.

Sources: NA PC 2/82–4; Calendar of Treasury Books, vols 24–8; NA SP 44/245 and CUST 99/1; Hull City Archives WB 8, 9

There were only a few ships whose port of departure was unrecorded in one source or another, so the evidence of this table can be regarded as fairly complete. The information, however, is only as good as the accuracy of contemporary clerks. It might well have been normal for them to précis the knowledge at their disposal, to save time and page space, and so omit the names of ports which they could neither spell nor pronounce. With that reservation, the information is useful, but the table as a whole needs explanation.

The second column lists ships which appear to have loaded and sailed direct from the port named in column one. The third column lists ships which are known to have called at one other port before or after arriving at the port in question; that one other port also lists that ship. For instance, the one vessel recorded against 'Long Sound' called also at Gothenburg, and is included among the 45 ships under Gothenburg in column three. Purely in the interests of clarity, it has not been possible to state in column three (except in the Stockholm–Gothenburg relationship) which other port was involved. Column four has tried to make useful, as far as possible, the composite lists which appear quite often in both Privy Council and Treasury records. These lists, submitted in petitions for discharge, gave maybe a dozen ships' names followed by the ports from which all or any lesser number might have sailed. For instance, an order of discharge in January 1712 lists 14 ships of Henry Lyell, summarized as from Hamburg, Altona and Bremen. It is impossible to tell which ships came from where. These 14, therefore, are included in column four, under *each* of the three ports, among the total of ships occurring in such circumstances. If there are ships in column four, then column five almost certainly shows too high a figure. The symbol indicates that the true figure is up to the number shown; it is impossible to know for any one port how near to the truth that number might be. The combined effect, of course, is to give a grand total of ships which exceeds the number believed to have been quarantined. There is, nevertheless, some merit in column four as it gives an idea of trade patterns, showing, for instance, that some ships which set out from the German North Sea ports for Britain had sailed originally from the Baltic, perhaps calling at more than one port there. This fact shows why so many petitioners in 1713–14 (when the Baltic was supposed to be clear of plague, while the German ports were not) had been keen to demonstrate that their ships had not sailed within so many leagues of Hamburg.[30]

Another strength of the table is that it shows the relative amount of business between the Baltic ports and Britain. Gothenburg and Stockholm (iron and deal) clearly had the strongest links, while Danzig and Königsberg (hemp and flax) were still the major ports of the eastern seaboard. The position of Gothenburg, however, needs some comment. After loading higher in the Baltic, a ship would sometimes spend the winter at Gothenburg or at nearby Masterland (the modern Marstrand), before braving the North Sea gales, or waiting for a convoy with naval escort. While more cargo might have been taken aboard, many of the 45 ships in column three, against Gothenburg, would not have opened their hatches.

An interesting aspect of the table is that it shows how relatively strong was the import trade from the German North Sea coast. The number of ships from there exceeded those from the Eastern Baltic, although the quarantine restrictions began two years later. Of course, numbers mean little by themselves, and only when allied to tons burthen and relative cargo values does the real picture become meaningful. Unfortunately, these wider statistics are difficult to find. As regards size, such little evidence as there is would suggest that ships could be as small as 30 tons burthen from Hamburg, and as large as 400 tons burthen (but more generally 250 or even 150 tons) from the Baltic.[31]

It is worth noting that only one ship in ballast was affected by quarantine, testimony that trade from the Baltic and German North Sea coast was very much in one direction, a point made clear by merchants in a submission to the Board of Trade.[32]

Commodities

Table 3.3 indicates the relative incidence of commodities, distinguishing whether, and how often, they were part of a larger cargo.

30 See Chapter 2: petitions stated that ships had not been within 30 or even 200 leagues of Hamburg or any other infected German port.

31 The number of crew (men and boys) varied between five and twelve.

32 This ship was the *S*[ta] *Brigitta* which arrived at Newcastle from Danzig (NA PC 2/82/496). For Swedish merchants' submission, see *JCTP*, vol. 2, p. 119: 'our ships [now] going out in ballast and taking in their loading in the Baltick'.

Table 3.3 Commodities in quarantined ships, 1709–1714

Commodity per ship[1, 2]	Sole cargo	+ 1 other	+ 2 others	+ 3 others	+ 4 others	+ > 4 others	Total
Iron (g)	15	139	92	108	63	83	**500**
Deals	2	110	41	96	53	62	**364**
Tar (g)		2	52	89	37	41	**221**
Pitch	1	6	29	92	33	26	**187**
Flax	8	25	25	28	18	82	**186**
Staves[3] (G)	12	24	3	33	42	40	**154**
Hemp	1	9	14	28	13	75	**140**
Potash (g)		4	9	22	28	68	**131**
Linen (g)		6	4	19	12	79	**120**
Piece goods (G)	8	12	1	26	32	19	**98**
Clapboards (g)	1	14	8	29	33	12	**97**
Bale goods (G)	17	14	3	1	3	22	**60**
Lampblack (G)		15	1	25	26	7	**74**
Wooden wares	3	20	26	9	1	12	**71**
(Spruce) yarn (g)		1	2		9	53	**65**
Plank (G)	21	11	1	4	2	13	**52**
Hogs' Bristles (g)		1		5	1	41	**48**
Sturgeon (g)		1		8		38	**47**
Masts	1	6	14		7	11	**39**
Spars			2		24	1	**27**
Spruce beer				2		23	**25**
Baulks (g)			1		1	19	**21**
(Fir) 'Timber'	4	1	7	5		4	**21**
Feathers						14	**14**
Copper				4		8	**12**

Tinplate (G)				1	1	9	**11**
Mum (G)	1	2	2			5	**10**
Amber						9	**9**
Hartshorn[4] (g)				1	1	6	**8**
Linseed			2	1	1	4	**8**
Wire						8	**8**
Latten (g)						7	**7**
Polonia wool						6	**6**
'Naval stores'	4						**4**
Match				4			**4**
Trunnills			1			3	**4**
Scoops					1	3	**4**
Firewood						3	**3**
Spars					1	2	**3**
Silk (G)				1		1	**2**
Skins (G)				1		1	**2**
Smalt (G)				1	1		**2**
Whalebone (G)			2				**2**
Antimony				1			**1**
Beeswax				1			**1**
Cucumbers					1		**1**
Knappel					1		**1**
'Knapwood'				1			**1**
Oars					1		**1**
Paving stones (G)						1	**1**
Rhenish wine (G)						1	**1**
Rye	1						**1**

Notes:

(1) Items italicized were 'enumerated' as particularly liable to convey infection (see Chapter 2).

(2) (G) means the product was imported from the German North Sea ports; (g) means the product was essentially from the Baltic, but also imported from Germany.

(3) The term 'staves' includes hogshead, barrel and pipe-staves.

(4) Hartshorn includes buckhorn.

Sources: NA PC 2/82–4; Calendar of Treasury Books, vols 24–8; NA SP 44/245 and CUST 99/1; Hull City Archives WB 8, 9

The usual caveat applies: that the information is only as good as the details which were entered in contemporary records. One ship might carry as many as eight commodities, some in very small measure. It was usual for Privy Council and Treasury clerks to round up a cargo to its main components; this can be proved by comparison with the few petitions mentioned in the entry books of the Secretary of State, where details are much fuller. Another problem is that of the composite entries, already discussed. If this practice led to some ambiguity in the context of ports of departure, it also means that some details of cargoes may not be applicable to all ships in a given list. There are also two other points which concern cargoes of iron and deals. It has been mentioned that the latter were sometimes used as dunnage (packing) to protect the main cargo and indeed the ship from damage during the journey. Subsequently, the deals were of little or no commercial value. Iron, on the other hand, was sometimes loaded primarily as ballast, but it could still be used for manufacturing. This wide application is well illustrated by the table, where the two products top the list of commodities and feature strongly as both main and auxiliary freight. Although some iron was shipped, or trans-shipped, from Hamburg, by far the greatest supply came from Sweden.

The so-called enumerated cargoes affected chiefly the Baltic ports but, as 'Piece goods' comprised textiles, deemed particularly susceptible to infection, it can be understood why the later focus of quarantine restrictions was on the German North Sea coast. One of the strengths of the table is that it shows the variety of products caught in the quarantine net. The term 'bale goods' was ambiguous, as it could refer to any cargo not classified as 'case' goods, but there was much more at stake than naval stores. Potash was used by soap-makers. Deals had a market in the building trade, and staves, although very much in demand for shipboard barrels, had a wide sale among coopers. Clapboards, although sometimes used also for barrels, were the material for wainscoting. Lampblack, or blacking, was used to make ink. Mum was a German beer. Smalt was a blue glass crushed to make pigments. But the temporary absence of such minor commodities would not have sent ripples through Government, as did the threat to naval stores. It is worth noting that one cargo of rye (imported to Newcastle) is the only significant foodstuff in the list, although the Danish prize *Helena*, forced to do quarantine in Stangate Creek, carried a cargo of corn which the prize agent was anxious to sell.[33]

33 The rye was from Danzig (NA PC 2/84/297). The *Helena*, not freighted for Britain, is excluded from the table.

In summary, the table quantifies the extent to which Britain relied on the Baltic to keep her navy and merchant marine supplied with the key raw materials of iron, deals, tar, pitch, flax, staves and hemp.[34]

The petitioners

The first year of quarantine was chaotic and it was the Swedes as much as the British who found most cause for worry or complaint. The main problems were the definition of enumerated goods, the mixture of enumerated and non-enumerated items in one shipment, the impracticability of airing cargoes, indecision by the Privy Council and consequent delays, and even the definition of the Baltic.[35] Solutions to most of these problems were slow, painful and empirical. The Swedish envoy Leijoncrona made the early running with Secretary Sunderland, but most diplomatic intervention was by his successor, Count Gyllenborg, who regularly harassed the Duke of Queensberry for leniency towards Swedish vessels and tolerance for the mistakes of crewmen who were simply ignorant of the rules.[36] While he had some progress in establishing that the port of Uddevalla was outside both the Baltic and The Sound, and should therefore be exempt like Norway from quarantine, Gyllenborg had little success over individual ships.[37] He became exasperated by prevaricating referrals to Treasury and Admiralty, and sought to attach quarantine to a wider diplomatic agenda. Referring to the spirit of the trade treaties between Britain and Sweden, Gyllenborg found it inconsistent that England should have an open trade with one enemy, that is, Spain, and allow the Dutch to pursue their business with France, while friendly Sweden found its ships stopped 'upon all sorts of frivolous pretences', with owners put to great expense and crews being 'ill nay Barbarously used'.[38]

As quarantine slowly established its rhythm, Gyllenborg became a less frequent correspondent, sometimes writing on behalf of the Duke of Holstein, who had no minister in London, or to ensure his own countrymen were not disadvantaged.[39] He still championed the cause of those who erred by mistake or misdemeanour. In spring 1711, for instance, he forwarded the petition of a Swedish master who had gone ashore from his quarantined ship in the Humber, allegedly 'destituted of necessaries', and was prevented by the weather from returning the same night.[40] When opportunity presented, Gyllenborg continued to battle for Sweden's total

34 For tables comparing volumes of naval goods (pitch, tar, masts and hemp) imported from the East Country and Sweden relative to elsewhere, see NA CO 388/17/95.

35 The Scottish Customs Commissioners agreed a tight definition of the Baltic with the magistrates of Edinburgh: it was to begin 'at the point of Ulekkerin or Ledgsons over against Jutland and so comprehend all the seas within the north point of Jutland and the aforesaid point …' (West Register Office, Edinburgh CE 14/1 [unpag.], 20 Nov. 1710).

36 NA SP 100/61/31, 53, 59 etc.

37 NA SP 100/61/53, 55, 59.

38 NA SP 100/61/61, 17 Aug. 1710.

39 NA SP 100/61/65/72, 76, 78.

40 NA SP 100/61/118/128.

exemption from all quarantine restrictions, but his efforts generally wrung few concessions from London.

Most petitioners to the Privy Council were owners and/or freighters of ships, professing to act 'for themselves and others'. That formula reflected the complexity of shipowning, when one or two active merchants usually managed affairs for many other 'sleeping' partners.[41] Occasionally two merchants petitioned separately for the same ship, or series of ships, but mostly they petitioned together, or sometimes in larger groups. Ships' masters might also petition, but not often, in support of merchants or on their own account. When a master was sole petitioner, he might also have been owner, or co-owner, of the vessel. A revealing feature of the Hull water-bailiffs' records, haphazard as their survival has been, is that masters trading from the Baltic invariably carried a small quantity of goods, sometimes different in kind from the main cargo, under their own name.[42]

The merchants who petitioned are named in Appendix 3. The list cannot be complete, as some petitioners were referred to impersonally in the Privy Council as 'divers merchants', but it shows the main players, and the variety of combinations and shared interests. The merchants form two main groups – those trading with the East Country, and those trading with Sweden. The former were members of the Eastland Company, and could if necessary speak by that corporate voice. The latter had no formal, regulated existence but could nevertheless petition Government as a group and were recognized as a coherent entity by the Board of Trade.[43] The Swedish merchants were, in fact, an offshoot of the Eastland Company, formed when its privileges were curtailed in 1673, and some maintained an interest in the eastern Baltic, or in other regulated and joint-stock companies. Although the appendix is in many respects a roll-call of the most prominent London and east-coast merchants, some notable names, such as Heathcote and Gould, are absent.[44] They may, of course, have had an interest in cargoes for which others petitioned. Within these broad groupings were specialist importers, particularly of naval stores, and invariably with a Government contract. But before their quarantine experience is examined, it is necessary to look at the wider fortunes of merchants as a whole.

The first petition for an individual ship was submitted by Jacob Jacobsen and referred by the Privy Council to the Treasury on 24 October 1709.[45] By that date, three cornerstones of policy had been laid: all affected ships had to perform 40 days' quarantine; their cargoes had to be aired for one week after quarantine had expired; and enumerated goods (that is, those listed as most risky) could not be released unless and until the Privy Council made an order to that effect. Jacobsen's ship, the *Ashfat*, could hardly have been a more taxing initiation for all parties. The vessel had

41 R. Davis, *The Rise of the English Shipping Industry* (London, 1962), p. 82.

42 HCA WB 8, 9.

43 There are petitions of merchants trading to Sweden in, for example, NA CO 388/12(2)/65, 78. For Board of Trade, see, for example, *JCTP*, vol. 2, p. 125: 'Mr. Wordsworth and 20 other Swedish merchants attending ...' (10 Feb. 1710).

44 cf. S.-E. Åström, *From Cloth to Iron. Part 1. The Growth, Structure and Organization of the Trade* (Helsingfors, 1963), pp. 162ff.

45 NA PC 2/82/454.

arrived in the Thames from Danzig, the port most feared at that time, but Jacobsen argued that her departure had predated the plague.[46] The *Ashfat*'s main cargo was iron, deals, hemp, flax and potash. On 13 November the ship was authorized to proceed to her place of discharge without further restraint, despite the hemp and flax being enumerated items.[47] But Customs officers, discovering small amounts of wool and feathers, took it upon themselves to suspend the unloading and report the existence of these further enumerated goods to the Treasury.[48]

When this news reached the Privy Council on 15 December, members were discussing another Swedish vessel, the *Ufro Christiana* from Riga, with a similar cargo of hemp, flax, iron and deals.[49] This ship had already been discharged after 40 days' quarantine, but again Customs officers were uncomfortable: while airing should apply to all cargoes, in practice not even enumerated goods were being aired, let alone detained until the Council had taken stock of the risk. The Privy Council's grasp of their own decisions was being put to the test: the flax and hemp were being 'stayed' by the Commissioners of Customs until the Council should give proper orders for their disposal. With tacit admission that the issues were beyond them, Council asked the Commissioners to 'do therein, as they shall judge most safe.'[50] As for the *Ashfat*, the Council decided to mull things over. By 8 January 1710 all the cargo had been unloaded except the feathers and wool, which were the subject of another petition.[51] The Council, of course, referred it to the Commissioners. On the strength of their report, the *Ashfat* was ordered to 'carry back' the wool and feathers 'wch are soe lyable to Infection and Coming imediately from Dantzick which hath been soe Grievously afflicted with the Plague'.[52] Customs asked the merchants to give security that the goods would not be landed. When the Council got to hear of the merchants' refusal, Customs were asked to 'take speciall Care that the said Wooll & Feathers be not upon any account whatsoever landed in any part of this Kingdom'.[53] Jacobsen was joined by Cornellisen, who owned the 10 bags of Polonia wool and was at his wit's end. Why not just throw the wool in the river?[54] To the Privy Council that seemed a practicable solution, and on 9 March they ordered the wool to stay under water for 6 days.[55] After that, no doubt, it was ruined, but the impasse was broken and 15 months after loading at Danzig the *Ashfat* was rid of its cargo. The ship, and possibly the crew, had suffered a quarantine of 166 days.

The significance of the *Ashfat* and *Ufro Christiana* cases was that the Privy Council, which had ordered the fate of enumerated goods to be referred back to themselves for an ultimate decision, discovered they had no constructive suggestions as to what that fate should be. In London and the outports, cargoes of hemp and flax were arriving

---

46 Ibid.
47 NA PC 2/82/469–70; *CTB*, vol. 23, part 2, p. 425.
48 NA PC 2/82/488; *CTB*, vol. 23, part 2, p. 459.
49 NA PC 2/82/481, 490; *CTB*, vol. 23, part 2, pp. 436–7, 461.
50 Ibid. The PC reference (490) is clearer than the one in *CTB*, p. 461.
51 NA PC 2/82/509; *CTB*, vol. 24, part 2, p. 127.
52 NA PC 2/82/529. Paraphrased in *CTB*, vol. 24, part 2, p. 157.
53 NA PC 2/82/537–8; *CTB*, vol. 24, part 2, p. 178.
54 NA PC 2/82/543; *CTB*, vol. 24, part. 2, p. 191.
55 NA PC 2/82/549.

daily, vital for the war effort, and yet incapable of being used. The Eastland Company petitioned in December 1709 for the release of seven ships from Danzig, Königsberg and Memel, which between them carried every enumerated product, particularly hemp and flax.[56] These were vital cargoes for the home dockyards. What was the Privy Council to do? Meanwhile a chorus of voices from Newcastle, petitioning for the discharge of two flax ships which had sailed from Königsberg in 1708, insisted that their goods would be 'much damnifyed & diminshed' by opening and airing.[57] And then Hull joined the battle.[58] To the beleaguered Privy Council, there seemed only one way out: they would shelter behind the oath required of every master, after quarantine, that his ship and crew were healthy, and on that basis the Eastland ships were conditionally released.[59] Unfortunately the Customs Commissioners would have none of it.

Following a presentment by the Commissioners to the Treasury, the Privy Council learnt in February 1710 that feathers and nine 'fats' of undeclared hogs' bristles had been found among the cargoes of the seven Eastland ships.[60] In exasperation, the Council ordered these items to be carried out to sea.[61] The merchants were now incensed. The enumerated goods were owned by Phill, Bullock and Thomas Coutts, who had paid import duty when the ships were initially released.[62] Now they were being told that the feathers and bristles were to be dumped at sea – but they had already been discharged into lighters. Could they, please, get on and deliver the goods or be paid their value?[63] Meanwhile the Privy Council's attitude had caused confusion in Scotland. The *George* of Elie had arrived at Leith from Danzig with hemp and flax worth £400, loaded during the plague, as well as other non-enumerated goods.[64] After quarantine had been performed, she was ordered to carry back the hemp and flax, although five weeks earlier the *James* of Dumfries, also from Danzig, had been allowed to unload flax with her iron.[65] For merchants at Hull, the Privy Council's instructions were equally baffling. The *Vine* from Königsberg had performed quarantine and very properly delivered her flax into airing sheds.[66] But on 26 March 1710 her freighters were given a choice: the flax could either remain indefinitely in the sheds 'in such manner that no Person be permitted to come at it', or it could be carried out to sea and presumably dumped.[67] This was too much for

56 NA PC 2/82/485; *CTB*, vol. 23, part 2, p. 441. Full details of the ships and their cargoes emerges only later.

57 NA PC 2/82/493.

58 Petition of Philip Wilkinson for release of *Catherine* with flax from Memel (NA PC 2/82/501).

59 NA PC 2/82/503. On 21 December 1709 the Privy Council had originally decided that only ships carrying wood, iron and potash should unload (NA PC 2/82/494).

60 NA PC 2/82/537.

61 Ibid.; *CTB*, vol. 24, part 2, p. 179.

62 NA PC 2/82/556; *CTB*, vol. 24, part 2, p. 222.

63 Ibid.

64 NA PC 2/82/540; *CTB*, vol. 24, part 2, p. 178.

65 Ibid.; NA PC 2/82/503; *CTB*, vol. 24, part 2, p. 118.

66 NA PC 2/82/543; *CTB*, vol. 24, part 2, p. 203.

67 NA PC 2/82/558.

Sir William St Quentin and William Maister, the most powerful merchants in Hull, who pointed out that the *Vine* had been discharged from quarantine on 17 December 1709, and the flax had been in airing sheds since around 11 January.[68] The position was ridiculous. On 2 April the Privy Council met solely to reconsider their recent decision and allow the flax to be delivered.[69]

With policy now in tatters, the Council were saved from further humiliation by, ironically, another petition of thinly veiled frustration. In April 1710, John Gordon and Thomas Coutts complained of the great loss and inconvenience caused by the detention of ships in Scotland long after quarantine had been completed.[70] They were particularly concerned for three cargoes of flax, hemp, iron and copper which had arrived from the Baltic five months earlier.[71] Gordon and Coutts put forward their own suggestions: as long as wool, feathers or hogs' bristles (popularly deemed to be the items most susceptible to harbouring infection) were not on board, and provided proper affidavits that quarantine had been completed and crews remained healthy were accepted by local Customs officers, may ships be immediately released?[72] The Privy Council were against anything which smacked of automatic discharge, but they did allow the flax and hemp to be unloaded at the same time as the iron and copper.[73]

The wider benefit of this decision was that flax and hemp were now generally to be regarded as non-enumerated goods, despite being classified to the contrary. Merchants could now petition for a standard objective, which was that their goods (unless they included wool, feathers or hogs' bristles) should be summarily discharged once the 40 days of quarantine were over. In other words, they were petitioning for goods to be released without airing. It will be remembered that airing, strictly speaking, applied to *all* cargoes anyway; but with so much trouble over enumerated goods, the prospect of infection from other commodities was no longer an issue. But even now, in terms of enumerated products, the Privy Council might have an aberration. In September 1710 they allowed cargoes to be discharged from two ships at Newcastle, except the flax 'which is to remain There untill further Order'.[74] This decision, of course, was reversed under protest, and the Council were equally capable of an aberration in the other direction, as testified by an earlier order to release hogs' bristles and linen without airing.[75]

For the remainder of the quarantine years, policy remained far from consistent. From the merchants' point of view, it was helpful to arrive at a petition which was near standard in wording as well as in purpose. In winter it was useful to stress the hazards of the season, particularly if a ship had a coastwise voyage after quarantine to

68 NA PC 2/82/568; *CTB*, vol. 24, part 2, p. 233.

69 Ibid.

70 NA PC 2/82/569; *CTB*, vol. 24, part 2, p. 242.

71 Ibid.

72 Ibid.

73 NA PC 2/82/577; *CTB*, vol. 24, part 2, p. 293.

74 NA PC 2/83/96; *CTB*, vol. 24, part 2, p. 456.

75 NA PC 2/83/108–9; 2/83/86, 94; *CTB*, vol. 24, part 2, pp. 430, 444. The ships had, however, performed a very long quarantine – a punishment on the masters for having come up the Thames illegally.

arrive at the port of discharge.[76] Seasonal considerations aside, a routine formula was now appearing: the port of departure had been healthy, the crew had been and still were in perfect health, and the goods were not, by nature, liable to retain infection. Once Customs had confirmed these points, discharge by the Privy Council was a formality. Even enumerated goods, for the most part, were released without airing. But the position was soon to change. Following the Quarantine Act and Proclamation, late in 1710, it was hardly possible for the less 'risky' enumerated cargoes, such as flax and hemp, to continue to be released on the nod. Again, it was the Customs Commissioners who made all the running; it was their practice to remind the Privy Council, whenever they reported back on a ship with enumerated goods, that these should be aired.[77] In April 1711 coordinated petitions from masters and merchants forced the Council, once again, to back down, and even the Commissioners were forced to agree the impracticability of reloading a cargo once it had been aired (for taking on to the port of discharge), and the likelihood of it having been spoiled in the airing.[78]

By the autumn of 1711 the Commissioners were again emboldened to press the Privy Council for tighter restrictions. The catalyst was the Proclamation of 6 September which extended quarantine restrictions to the German North Sea coast, and repeated the necessity for airing all cargoes, whether or not they were enumerated. In a landmark case of 1 October, the Commissioners reported, on referral, that eight ships from various Baltic ports were carrying iron, potash, amber, sturgeon, linen, hemp, flax, spruce beer and wooden wares.[79] Their quarantine had been completed 'but the Comm^{rs}. Submitt to Her Ma.^{ty} whether they are to be Discharged, some of the said Ships being Loaden with Goods that are by the Act of Parliament and Her Ma.^{ts} Proclamation not only to be aired a Week but to remain there till her Ma.^{ts} Pleasure is further Signifyed.'[80] This time, however, they were wasting their ink. The Privy Council, in a defiant, irrational stand of questionable legality, released all the ships instantly without airing.[81] And so it went on for month after month. The Commissioners went through the motions of reminding the Council of the law, and the Council declined to obey it. In the end, the Commissioners weakened. In March 1712, possibly for the first time, they raised no objection to a ship, the *Margaret* from Danzig, discharging her flax without airing.[82] The reason, apparently, was that the master and crew had weighed and packed the flax themselves, and overseen the loading.[83] By September 1712 the Commissioners were raising no objections to anything – even hogs' bristles.[84] During 1713, especially in the autumn, there was evidence of a return to airing, especially for baled products from Hamburg, now

76 For example NA PC 2/83/151.
77 For example NA PC 2/83/207–9.
78 NA PC 2/83/232.
79 NA PC 2/83/320–21.
80 Ibid.
81 Ibid.
82 NA PC 2/83/383.
83 Ibid.
84 NA PC 2/84/23–4.

being described as 'Exceptionable Goods'.[85] But basically the battles were over. In December 1713 a group of masters from Hamburg railed at the impossibility of airing 'at the distant Ports where they lye, where there is no Conveniency', and the Privy Council, in conciliatory mood, allowed the ships to be released if the masters had done all they could.[86] Within a few more months, quarantine was over.

The experiences quoted above applied to most merchants and owners, but within both the Swedish and Eastland camps were individuals who fared better, sometimes much better, than their colleagues. These were the merchants, like John Taylor, who had contracted with the Navy Board to import supplies for the royal dockyards, but the group included Sir Ambrose Crowley (succeeded by his son John) who imported iron on his own account for manufacture into nails.[87] Crowley's nails travelled coastwise from his factories in the Tyne valley to a depôt in London, and then on to the south-coast dockyards. For these petitioners (who won the envy of general importers) the aim was not release without airing, but total exemption from quarantine.[88] Although neither the Navy Board nor the Admiralty Board championed individual petitions, Taylor (who also imported naval stores from North America) won the early backing of Josiah Burchett, secretary to the Admiralty. In November 1709 letters from Burchett and Taylor induced the Privy Council to allow the ship *Purveyor*, with plank for the navy, to unload without airing (but probably after quarantine).[89] In January 1710 Taylor successfully petitioned for three ships from Riga to be released during quarantine itself, on the strength of the masters' oaths as to the health of the crew.[90] It now became almost normal for Burchett to intervene, and in May 1710, when a petition from Crowley was still in the balance, he succeeded in getting total exemption for two ships arrived in Newcastle.[91]

In September 1710 Burchett again joined Crowley, this time in seeking exemption for several ships 'that are Coming' from Sweden.[92] As the vessels had not arrived, and so their state of health could not be known, it is unlikely that this was conceded. But exemption upon arrival (if the crews were demonstrably healthy) was now not unusual for either Taylor or Crowley: in August 1711, Crowley won this concession for a dozen ships at once.[93] Later, the exemption was less automatic. The Privy Council, who had usually been coming to their own decisions about contractors' vessels, sometimes referred the petition to the Treasury, and thereby the Customs Commissioners, for a report. A new formula was gradually arrived at: ships would be exempt only if, after strict examination by Customs, the various statements and

85 NA PC 2/84/262–3.

86 NA PC 2/84/282.

87 The business of the Crowley dynasty has been fully set out in M.W. Flinn, *Men of Iron: The Crowleys in the Early Iron Industry* (Edinburgh, 1962).

88 The 'envy' point is well illustrated in NA SP 44/245/131–2, where Alexander Mitchell complains that his three ships which arrived in the same convoy are still at Harwich, whereas the latter's ships had been released a month earlier.

89 NA PC 2/82/464; *CTB*, vol. 23, part 2, p. 417.

90 NA PC 2/82/513; *CTB*, vol. 24, part 2, p. 143.

91 NA PC 2/82/588; *CTB*, vol. 24, part 2, p. 312.

92 NA PC 2/83/109; *CTB*, vol. 24, part 2, p. 467.

93 NA PC 2/83/285; *CTB*, vol. 25, part 2, p. 407.

allegations were found to be true. The Crowleys were always wary of the Privy Council's attitude, looking around for arguments to strengthen their case. They had long used the ploy that ships were leaky or unsafe, but that was a common complaint among merchants.[94] The new and irrefutable argument, used also by Taylor, was that Her Majesty had 'immediate occasion' for the iron, and John Crowley eventually succeeded where his father had probably failed – that is, in achieving exemption for ships even before they had arrived.[95] Lesser merchants were not so fortunate: Ralph Robinson and George Morley, contracted to supply iron, pitch and tar to the navy, found their petition of October 1713 referred to the discretion of the Treasury.[96]

Petitioners who were furthest from London suffered the most, mainly because letters to and from the capital took such a long time on the road. When quarantine was first imposed, William Crowle of Hull organized his London correspondents, Abraham Crop and William Skinner, into petitioning on his behalf.[97] That, however, was an isolated example. More common was the practice of petitioning a few days before quarantine was over; by the time the petition had reached the Privy Council and been referred, it was hoped that news would have reached the Customs Commissioners from the quarantine station, that the 40 days had been completed.[98] Such nicety of timing was unavailable to the Scottish, who were severely disadvantaged by the Privy Council's London address. Without the Scottish Customs Commissioners meeting in Edinburgh, the situation would have been wholly unworkable, with every message between outports and Customs, and vice versa, travelling the length of the Great North Road. But the Scottish Board still needed to correspond with the Treasury in London, so delays in Scotland were at least double those which obtained in England. The *Concord* of Leith was placed in quarantine at Inverness on 6 November 1710 and discharged on 9 February 1711; two ships quarantined in the Cromarty Firth on 5 November 1710 were still there three months later, with referral to the Treasury only just beginning.[99] Some delays seem explicable only by misplacement of papers: the *George* of Montrose, with iron and flax from Königsberg, did quarantine in Inverkeithing Road, and then moved to Montrose river on 10 September 1710, where it was boarded by a physician.[100] With all crewmen well, the routine for release was duly followed, but the report of 13 October from the Scottish Customs Commissioners was not heard by the Privy Council until 13 December.[101] In the case of the *William* of Greenock, it was confessed that papers had miscarried. The ship arrived in Scotland in November 1713, but release was not possible until March

94 For leaky ships, see NA PC 2/83/84, 232–3; PC 2/84/273, 326; SP 44/245/64–5, 91–2.

95 NA PC 2/84/229; for 'immediate occasion', see also 2/84/204, 283–4 etc.

96 NA PC 2/84/263–4.

97 NA PC 2/82/463.

98 For confirmation that merchants petitioned before quarantine had been completed, see *JCTP*, vol. 2, p. 195.

99 NA PC 2/83/188.

100 NA PC 2/83/338.

101 Ibid.

1714.[102] For the *Jean* of Kirkcaldy, quarantine expired on 26 June 1713, but she was released only on 18 October, following a petition that the cargo (hemp and flax) was 'become Damnifyed by lying so long'.[103]

Costs

In analysing the financial hardship caused by quarantine against the Baltic, a division must be made between the costs of the quarantine process and losses by damage and delay. The former can be dealt with comprehensively, thanks to Josias Wordsworth. The circumstances of his revelation were unusual. In November 1710 the Board of Trade were considering a number of issues affecting the Baltic, especially the interruption by the King of Denmark of letters to Sweden. In their normal way, the Board asked for comments from the Swedish merchants. The reply came from Wordsworth, a favoured correspondent of the Board, who took the unsolicited opportunity to air his complaints about quarantine.[104] The 40 days per se did not worry him unduly, but the costs were a different matter. Referral of a petition from the Privy Council to the Treasury cost £3, 2s, 6d; the referral from the Treasury to the Commissioners of Customs cost another 15s. The report from the Commissioners to the Treasury was also 5s, while the order for discharge from the Privy Council was £2, 12s, 6d, with 30s more for a duplicate to the Admiralty. Another 30s was payable to the Treasury for relaying to the Commissioners the order of Council, while the Commissioners themselves wanted 15s as a discharge fee. The total cost, therefore, of releasing a ship, 'though never so small or her cargo inconsiderable', was £11. Wordsworth, in full flow, went on to list the less obvious expenses, such as 'money to clerks and doorkeepers for dispatches and coach hire, and great loss of time in attendance.' All this, added to 40 days' victuals and wages for seamen 'is very severe & no way helps to prevent the Evil we would avoid'. To Wordsworth, the rigmarole for discharge was costly nonsense: after 40 days 'can it be imagined they [the goods] are infected? Or that this Attendance so troublesome to the Queen, her Council & Officers as well as so Expensive to the Merchts. does any way help to prevent it?'

The Board of Trade were clearly taken aback; 'finding that some matters in the … letter wanted explanation', the Board summoned Wordsworth before them on the following morning.[105] He attended with Messrs Joy, Thomlinson and Green. This was the first and only occasion when a far-reaching, general complaint was raised or heard during the Baltic crisis. In solidarity, the four merchants outlined the system. Men from the guard-ship at the quarantine station monitored the crew of a detained ship for each of the 40 days. When the time had elapsed, a Customs officer went on board, and oaths were made ashore as to the health of all involved. Then the visitors made certain allegations: seamen were 'frequently permitted to come on

102 NA PC 2/84/346. The miscarriage was during dispatch of the referral from the Treasury in London to the Customs Board in Edinburgh.

103 NA PC 2/84/260.

104 NA CO 388/13/63, from which all references in this paragraph are taken.

105 *JCTP*, vol. 2, pp. 194–5, from which all references in this paragraph are taken unless otherwise stated.

shore' before quarantine was over, and ships arriving from Sweden at Lynn and Plymouth performed no quarantine anyway. The merchants had a practical solution to streamline procedure: if quarantine had to be, then let local Customs officers, once the 40 days were over and the oaths administered, have authority to make the discharge. The Board of Trade, as was usual in this era, conscientiously forwarded the comments to the Duke of Queensberry. Five days later, on 14 November 1710, the Board were informed that the Lords of the Committee, predictably, thought no changes should be made to procedure.[106] The matter was never registered in the Privy Council's proceedings, and the merchants had achieved nothing but a vent of their feelings.

Wordsworth's figure, when multiplied by the number of ships known to have been quarantined, indicates that merchants and owners spent more than £11,000 in fees to Government and its agencies. It is difficult, however, to feel *too* sorry for Wordsworth. Clearly the rigmarole for release was most vexatious, but fees would often have been subdivided: most merchants petitioned in association with colleagues, and £11 when set against a cargo valued at several hundred pounds would not really have bothered the better-off. The other expenses, however, were a different matter, especially when the cost of keeping crew paid and victualled ran considerably longer than 40 days. In unusual circumstances, for instance if the ship were a prize, the Privy Council would ask Customs to provide victuals at public expense.[107] Generally, ships were allowed to provision at their own charge (passed on to merchants) and by the use of their own boats, which rode unmanned at the length of their hawsers, while provisions were dropped within.[108] Exceptionally, boats could fetch food which had been placed on a nearby beach.[109] A large ship might have twenty-three men and boys, although some had as few as five.[110] In considering these aspect, however, it should be remembered that journeys from the Baltic, quarantine aside, were often extraordinarily long. The practice of overwintering around Gothenburg meant a voyage from say Königsberg to England which could, in the summer, take only eight weeks, might well last a year.[111] An overall journey of six months was normal, although the leg from Gothenburg to Newcastle might take as little as ten days.[112] There were, of course, ships which plied regularly to and fro, but for most a further delay of six or so weeks is unlikely to have made the difference between profit and loss.

Damage to commodities during quarantine, typically from a leaky hull, was an expensive risk for the master; he was responsible for the cargo while it remained on

---

106 *JCTP*, vol. 2, p. 196.

107 NA PC 2/82/470 (*CTB*, vol. 23, part 2, p. 424) in the case of the Danish prize *Helena*, whose provisions were allegedly taken by the capturing warship.

108 This instruction was issued to local Customs by way of a circular letter; see NA CUST 84/122/32v for an example of such a letter being received.

109 NA CUST/97/74A/343.

110 NA SP 44/245/91–2, 104–05.

111 NA PC 2/82/493; it was possible to take nine months even from Bremen, when a stop was made in Holland en route (PC 2/84/38).

112 The *Henrietta* pink left Gothenburg for London 16 July 1710; reached Newcastle 25 July and lay there ten days; reached Harwich 8 August and stayed there four days; and arrived London (very leaky) on 14 August (NA SP 44/245/64–5).

his ship. There were several petitions by masters that testify to their concern.[113] The concept of insurance at this era was too embryonic to offer comfort or redress.[114] Also, a master, by mischance or misdemeanour, could seriously embarrass his merchant by risking the seizure of the vessel. When William Astell learnt with alarm that his ship *Young Dick* had been arrested at Newcastle (because the master and two men had been found drinking at an alehouse during quarantine), he petitioned not to suffer for another's mistake.[115] It is surprising such pleas were not more frequent, as the evidence for men going illegally ashore is plentiful (in this respect Wordsworth was right), and the Privy Council insisted on prosecution.[116]

Delay in getting the cargo to market was, perhaps, the merchants' overriding concern. Payments were by bills of exchange which criss-crossed between countries; one cargo could be covered by as many bills as there were merchants who drew them.[117] Bills were often drawn on correspondents in Hamburg and Amsterdam, but some British importers had bank accounts in Sweden.[118] In the summer of 1711 the *Richard & Joseph* loaded iron and tar at Stockholm for London; the ownership of the cargo was divided between two independent merchants (of whom one was in partnership with a third), who paid by bills 'partly remitted from London to Stockholm and partly drawn from Stockholm on Hamburg'.[119] Given generous maturity dates, bills could probably be honoured even after a cargo had been several weeks in quarantine, although the system was not geared for such imponderable delays. An examination of protested bills might well indicate the merchants and agents, some in mainland Europe, who were the financial casualties of British quarantine.

Many of the merchants engaged in the Baltic and North German trades were substantial traders with varied interests. Some were knighted, forming part of the London mercantile élite, rich and influential, which had arisen in the seventeenth century.[120] Sir Ambrose Crowley and Sir Randolph Knipe were City aldermen; Astell, Crowley, Jacobsen and Charles Joy were directors of the South Sea Company; some had accounts with the Bank of England (Knipe was a director), and trading connections in India and the plantations; Jacobsen ran the Hanseatic steelyard in

113 For example NA PC 2/84/282, 325–6.

114 V. Barbour, 'Marine risks and insurance in the seventeenth century', *Journal of Economic and Business History*, 1 (1928–29), 591, comments with regard to the late seventeenth century: 'But, even in these leading commercial cities [London, Amsterdam, Paris], insurance continued in the hands of merchants, who were by turns too timid or too rash'. The war years of the early eighteenth century saw few developments in the management of risk.

115 NA PC 2/84/81.

116 For example NA PC 2/84/190, 262–3. The best glimpse of the problem at local level is in the Harwich letter-book, collector to Board (NA CUST 99/1), towards the end of 1713.

117 Åström, pp. 91ff., discusses most aspects of payment by bills of exchange in the context of Sweden and the Baltic.

118 Åström, pp. 96, 113.

119 NA CO 388/14/94.

120 J.H. Plumb, 'The mercantile interest: the rise of the British merchant after 1689', *History Today*, 5 (1955), 762–7, sets the background.

London.[121] For these men and their like, quarantine was never more than an irritation. Similarly the main merchants at Hull, among them Crowle, Maister and Mowld, and at Newcastle, especially Ridley, were perfectly good for their obligations while cargoes were detained.[122] At Dumfries, it was a similar picture: John Crosby ranted at Customs over the detention of the *James* from Danzig, but he was the rich provost of the burgh making money from the import of tobacco.[123] Quarantine was not going to break him.

The parties most at risk were merchants importing in a small and speculative way, and, ironically, the lesser contractors to the Navy Board. The practice was to remunerate them with bills from the Navy Office paid in a queue, usually years overdue, known as 'the course'.[124] The bills could be discounted, but at significant loss. By the time of Baltic quarantine, complaints against this system had been long-standing and heated. It is interesting that in September 1709, exactly when quarantine began, the Navy Board were directed to pay interest on bills which became due, but could not be honoured.[125] This can be seen, perhaps, as a realization that delays and expenses of quarantine might have driven some contractors out of business. Of course, this was no more than a sop, and within three years, when the Navy debt stood at around £6 million, there came about the South Sea Company to fund the Government's liabilities. In any event, the big men like Crowley and Taylor would have comfortably survived, although Crowley was, and had been for a dozen years, the heavyweight petitioner for a better system of payment.

Conclusion

If the Baltic plague did not reach Britain, how far was this due to quarantine? The answer, of course, is imponderable, but as no seamen were ever reported to be sick in quarantined ships, it could be argued that the system was never tested. The traditional belief that goods, as much as people, were conveyors of infection, and evidence that quarantine was often taken lightly by crews and by the navy, impart no confidence that the defences would have held. As procedures were deliberately broken for the war effort, in a confused vision of what was ultimately in the national interests, it was perhaps just as well that the epidemic stopped where it did. The Privy Council had shown themselves incapable of pursuing a consistent policy.

Equally imponderable is the damage which quarantine did to the economy. Ship after ship in a very small fleet – indeed the only ship for a master–owner – was kept out of harbour for weeks on end, with deadlines being missed for unloading

121 A.B. Beaven, *The Aldermen of the City of London* (2 vols, London, 1908–13), vol. 2, pp. 122–4; J. Carswell, *The South Sea Bubble* (Stroud, 1993), pp. 245, 247, 250, 251; Flinn, *passim*.

122 G. Jackson, *Hull in the Eighteenth Century: A Study in Economic and Social History* (Oxford, 1972), pp. 96ff. (for Hull). The Ridley family were also bankers.

123 WRO CE 51/1/1 [unpag.], esp. 24 Dec. 1711.

124 Flinn, pp. 154ff.; Carswell, pp. 41ff.; B.W. Hill, *Robert Harley. Speaker, Secretary of State and Premier Minister* (New Haven & London, 1988), p. 135.

125 Flinn, p. 157.

and return. But even before the introduction of quarantine, British merchants doing business with Sweden and the East Country had faced increasing problems. The difficulty is in knowing to what extent quarantine made a bad situation worse. That the situation *was* already bad can be readily established. In 1709 the Board of Trade reported to the Privy Council that trade with the Baltic 'is much Decreased Since the Year 1700 when the Warr broke out between the Sweeds & Muscovites'.[126] Official statistics of trade for England and Wales begin only in 1697 and therefore give little perspective to the slump. For the early eighteenth century, however, figures have been quoted by Schumpeter in five-year average values, giving the following breakdown (in £ thousand):[127]

Imports from East Country: *1701–5*: 154; *1706–10*: 126; *1711–15*: 125; *1716–20*: 130

Imports from Sweden: *1701–5*: 195; *1706–10*: 182; *1711–15*: 176; *1716–20*, 87

There are slight grounds here for believing that the quarantine era of 1709 to 1714 was slightly worse for trade than the years which had preceded it, but the poor total against Sweden for 1716–20 indicates that imports were even weaker when quarantine was no longer a factor. An obvious drawback with Schumpeter is that the periods straddle the years when quarantine was in force. Luckily the figures can be amplified by recourse to Whitworth's eighteenth-century analysis, giving totals for individual years (rounded here to nearest £ thousand):[128]

Table 3.4 Annual value of imports from the Baltic, 1700–1715, to nearest £ thousand

From East Country		From Sweden	
1700	135	*1700*	199
1701	167	*1701*	191
1702	100	*1702*	143
1703	211	*1703*	236
1704	195	*1704*	202
1705	96	*1705*	206
1706	143	*1706*	209
1707	148	*1707*	171
1708	157	*1708*	210
1709	65	*1709*	145
1710	115	*1710*	174
1711	98	*1711*	148
1712	123	*1712*	168
1713	169	*1713*	160
1714	140	*1714*	237
1715	95	*1715*	166

Source: Sir C. Whitworth, State of the Trade of Great Britain ... (London, 1776), part 2, pp. 7, 35

126 NA PC 2/82/423–5; *CTB*, vol. 23, part 2, p. 364.

127 E.B. Schumpeter, *English Overseas Trade Statistics, 1697–1808* (Oxford, 1960), p. 18.

128 For problems with the strict accuracy of these figures, see G.N. Clark, *Guide to English Commercial Statistics, 1696–1782* (London, 1938), pp. 35–6.

From Table 3.4, the position is clearer, but still not definitive. The year 1709 was indeed bad for trade, but there are problems in making quarantine too decisive a factor. For one thing, restrictions were introduced only late in the year. Also, British merchants and shipowners were struggling to match an advantage enjoyed by Holland in dealing with the Danes. Eventually, they acquired certificates of lading (which the Dutch had been using for some time) to speed the progress of ships through customs at Elsinore. But trade suffered during months of confusion and frustration while passes and certificates were being drafted.[129] In 1710 imports were certainly weak from the East Country, but reasonably strong from Sweden. The main reason for the low figures from the East Country in 1710–11, was the commercial blockade imposed by Charles XII on the ports he had recently lost.[130] It might also be argued that quarantine was beginning to bite. But in 1712, when more ships were detained in British ports, trade totals somewhat recovered; and in 1713, when quarantine was strictly enforced, imports from the East Country showed a paradoxical rise. Figures for 1714 were influenced only slightly by quarantine, which was discontinued in the spring, while the weak figure for 1715 is another warning that the complexities of Baltic history, independent of plague and its prevention, must never be overlooked.

To disentangle the impact of quarantine from other factors which contributed to the downturn in trade, the need is for a statistic which offers insight into the movement of shipping, and therefore of freight. If British ships were being detained in quarantine ports, then there was a greater opportunity for Swedish ships (or others in conformity with the Navigation Acts) to take a greater share in the export of iron and deals from the Baltic. Statistics, therefore, of total imports (or indeed statistics of the import of particular commodities), might be disguising the damage done to mercantile interests which were essentially British. Fortunately, there is one source which enables such a supposition to be tested, as the multitude of published tables analysing the Danish Sound tolls include a breakdown, as follows, of voyages made by ships' masters.

---

129 *JCTP*, vol. 2, pp. 176, 274, 284, 310; NA PC 2/82/423–5, 552–6; SP 34/11/70; SP 34/34/43A.

130 J.F. Chance, 'England and Sweden in the time of William III and Anne', *English Historical Review*, 16/63 (1901), 677, quantifies the loss to the Eastland Company.

Table 3.5 Statistics of ships' masters on the return leg of a round trip, passing through The Sound (between Denmark and Sweden)

Year	English (Scottish) masters: number of round trips in stated year					
	1	2	3	4	5	6
1690	9 (3)	70 (14)	0 (1)	2 (1)	0 (0)	0 (0)
1700	14 (14)	177 (53)	6 (2)	36 (6)	0 (0)	1 (0)
1710	5 (16)	81 (26)	1 (0)	0 (0)	0 (0)	0 (0)
1720	24 (14)	187 (69)	2 (0)	11 (3)	0 (0)	0 (0)
1730	16 (12)	263 (37)	1 (2)	50 (1)	1 (0)	1 (0)

Note: These statistics are only available at ten-year intervals.

Source: N.E. Bang & K. Korst, Tabeller over Skibsfart og Varetransport gennem Øresund, 1661–1783 ... (Copenhagen and Leipzig, 1930)

Table 3.5 indicates that virtually no British masters, and therefore no British ships, made more than two return journeys to the Baltic in 1710, the first full year of quarantine, and the only year during those restrictions for which statistics are available. This is a striking contrast from 1700, when 42 masters made as many as four return journeys. Also, the total number of English (Scottish) ships in 1700 was 234 (67) compared with only 87 (42) in 1710. This is strong encouragement for believing that quarantine played a part in disrupting procedure, because ships were detained which would otherwise have made more journeys. The discrepancies are far greater than the relative decline in imports. They are also more than can be attributed to the war; the need for convoys certainly delayed ships which would otherwise have sailed, but the war had been interrupting commerce for a decade, while the years of quarantine showed (albeit inconsistently) a further deterioration in trade. The conclusion, therefore, is that Swedish ships, many freighted by British merchants, compensated for British tonnage which was detained in the quarantine ports. These ships, of course, would also have been quarantined on arrival, but a larger total of vessels in transit would have kept imports at a reasonable level. Although there are many cases where the records of quarantine indicate that a ship was Swedish (perhaps through the involvement of the Swedish minister, or simply by the master's name), sources do not give nationality as a matter of course. This situation precludes a proper analysis of the proportion of Swedish ships which were quarantined and, when coupled with the absence of Sound toll statistics for the other quarantine years, means any inference as to the impact on Swedish shipping can only be tentative. Despite this, the argument can be sustained from other figures.

If the number of return trips fell, then it would be logical for the volume of exports to the Baltic to have dropped correspondingly. This is exactly what happened, as the following figures indicate (rounded to nearest £ thousand):[131]

Table 3.6 Annual value of exports to the Baltic, 1705–1715, to nearest £ thousand

To East Country		To Sweden	
1705	100	*1705*	47
1706	110	*1706*	62
1707	147	*1707*	93
1708	134	*1708*	59
1709	57	*1709*	22
1710	30	*1710*	28
1711	47	*1711*	24
1712	71	*1712*	65
1713	81	*1713*	42
1714	88	*1714*	27
1715	51	*1715*	166

Source: Sir C. Whitworth, State of the Trade of Great Britain ... (London, 1776), part 2, pp. 7, 35

Table 3.6 shows a decline in the quarantine years consistent with the reduction in British shipping through The Sound. Although Swedish ships might have imported goods from Sweden into Britain, the Navigation Acts restricted them in relation to return cargoes. With fewer British ships available, exports to the Baltic could only have suffered. The usual caveats apply, of course, as to other factors which might have caused the decline. With so many unpalatable ingredients in the pudding of Baltic trade, it is impossible to say how far quarantine caused a uniquely nasty taste. But an enforced inactivity of at least 40 days, once or twice a year, could only have exacerbated the difficulties of merchants, and more especially shipowners, struggling against a conspiracy of natural and man-made misfortunes. Without the availability of Swedish ships, quarantine might have cost Britain its naval stores, and ultimately its war with France.

131 The same warning applies as in footnote 128.

The chief losers, in effect, were not the dockyards, the merchants, the shipowners, the masters, or even the seamen confined to six weeks of stultifying boredom; they were the two Boards of Customs, in England and Scotland, and their subordinate officers in the outports, for whom the dreary, thankless business of quarantine had just begun in earnest. It was destined to become ever more troublesome.

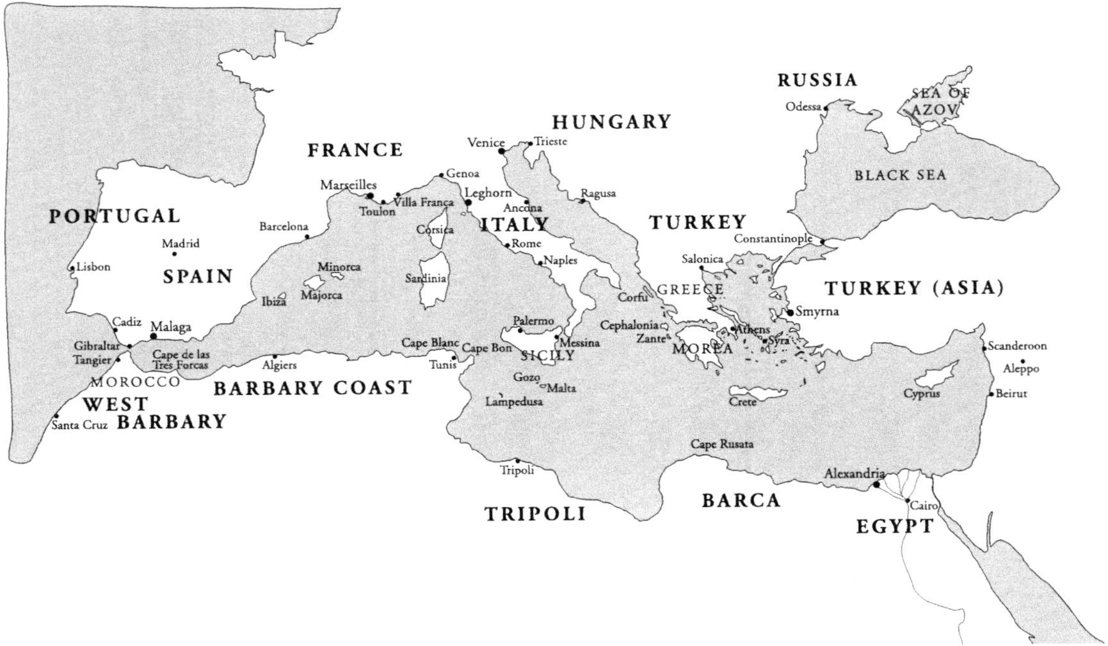

Map 3.1 **The Mediterranean Sea in the eighteenth century.**

Chapter Four

The Marseilles Crisis, 1720–1723

Plague at Marseilles

In 1720, six years after Britain had abandoned quarantine restrictions against the Baltic, Marseilles was decimated by one of the deadliest outbreaks of bubonic plague ever to strike terror into post-medieval Christendom.[1] Nearly half the population of 100,000 was wiped out, with the same ratio dying in many nearby towns, including Toulon. Frantic attempts were made to control the epidemic by cordons sanitaires. Western Europe, especially the maritime nations of Britain and Holland, reacted with panic and disbelief; Marseilles was one of the Mediterranean ports where quarantine procedures were supposedly a model for dealing with disease from the East.

Marseilles had not been the first port to institute permanent quarantine regulations – that honour is generally awarded to Venice – but they became a necessary concomitant to the free-port status which the port was granted by Colbert in 1669.[2] The experience of Leghorn, which had built its first lazaretto in the late sixteenth century, demonstrated to the French that a successful free port could only hope to deal with commerce from Turkey and the Levant if its merchants and inhabitants were protected from the threat of plague.[3] As early as 1622 sanitary arrangements in Marseilles had been the subject of a decree of the parliament at Aix, and over the next 60 years edicts from the same body ensured that merchant ships from the Levant, bound for France, could perform quarantine nowhere else.[4] There was a lazaretto at Toulon, but only for the navy.[5] The first royal ordinance affecting quarantine, under the title of precautions to be taken for preventing the introduction of plague,

---

1 For the history of the Marseilles plague, see C. Carrière et al., *Marseille ville morte. La Peste de 1720* (Marseilles, 1968); also J.–N. Biraben, *Les Hommes et la peste en France et dans les pays européens et mediterranéens* (2 vols, Paris, 1975–6), vol. 1, pp. 245–51. There were many contemporary tracts.

2 Venice is sometimes thought to have instituted quarantine in 1348 (W.F. Bynum & R. Porter (eds), *Companion Encyclopaedia of the History of Medicine* (2 vols, London & New York, 1993), vol. 2, p. 1232), but other authorities (J. Davy, *Notes and Observations on the Ionian Islands and Malta* … (2 vols, London, 1842), vol. 2, p. 325, and D. Panzac, *Quarantaines et lazarets. L'Europe et la peste d'orient (XVIIe–XXe siècles)* (Aix-en-Provence, 1986), p. 198) argue for a real beginning in 1423, when a lazaretto was established.

3 For Leghorn lazaretto, see Panzac, p. 34.

4 Panzac, p. 33; R. Paris, *Histoire du commerce de Marseille* … (5 vols, Paris, 1949–57), vol. 5, p. 23.

5 Panzac, p. 193. For instructions from Colbert about quarantine at Toulon, see P. Clément, *Lettres, instructions et mémoires de Colbert* (9 vols, Paris, 1864), vol. 3, pp. 167–9, 250–51.

was in 1683, laying out very specific procedures to be adopted at both Toulon and Marseilles.[6] That was the culmination of Colbert's energetic attention to maritime matters since he had become chief financial minister to Louis XIV in 1661. The monopoly of Marseilles for mercantile quarantine soon grew into a monopoly for commerce with the Levant.[7] Within the port, quarantine was run by the Health Office (*bureau de la santé*), consisting of 16 officials (*intendants*) appointed from merchants and sea captains, working under the direction of the Chamber of Commerce.[8] Rules were nominally approved at Aix and Paris, but as time passed the authorities in Marseilles were left largely to their own devices.

When the Conseil de Commerce was founded in 1700, akin to the British Board of Trade, the monopoly of Marseilles was immediately under attack. Toulon still had mercantile aspirations, the Languedoc wanted commercial independence, and even ports opening to the Bay of Biscay wanted a share of the Levantine trade.[9] But gradually Marseilles developed as the quarantine port for all France, a status recognized by royal ordinance in 1709.[10] That, of course, was the year when plague reached the Prussian seaboard. The Baltic crisis left France initially unruffled, as she had little direct trade with the Northern Crowns, but when the epidemic reached the German North Sea ports there was some alarm. In January 1712 de Pontchartrain, Minister of the Marine, raised the matter with the Conseil, and four ships from Hamburg were soon in quarantine at Rouen.[11] There was talk of making a lazaretto at the mouth of the Seine and of banning all commerce with the areas around Hamburg, Bremen and Lübeck.[12] An embargo on the importation of certain suspected goods, including flax and hemp, was not lifted until 1718.[13] By comparison with Britain, however, the French response was on a small scale, and the protest from Dunkirk, as late as December 1714, that English and Dutch ships were conveying northern goods to France without quarantine, suggests a view of the Baltic crisis prompted more by mercantile jealousy than public health.[14]

The loss of quarantine monopoly during the Baltic epidemic had no deleterious effect on Marseilles, which continued to dominate commercial relations with the Levant. In 1716 precise instructions were printed about the functions of the *intendants* of both the Health Office and the lazaretto, and the duties of guardians and others responsible for the management and supervision of ships, crews, passengers and cargoes.[15] These described the actual practice of quarantine, giving periods

6 [A.J.L. Jourdan], *Receuil général des anciennes lois françaises* (28 vols, Paris, 1822–30), vol. 19, pp. 431–4.

7 Paris, vol. 5, pp. 23–4.

8 Paris, vol. 5, p. 139; P. Masson, *Histoire du commerce français dans le Levant au XVIIIe siècle* (Paris, 1911), p. 53.

9 Paris, vol. 5, pp. 24–5.

10 Paris, vol. 5, p. 24.

11 P. Bonnassieux (ed.), *Conseil de commerce et Bureau du commerce 1700–1791 …* (Paris, 1900), p. 64.

12 Bonnassieux, pp. 69, 74.

13 Bonnassieux, p. 94.

14 Bonnassieux, p. 75.

15 Reproduced in Panzac, pp. 127–39.

of minimum detention (which depended on the bill of health), and the process of purification. Such procedures were tested day after day without the least cause for alarm. But then, on 25 May 1720, arrived the local ship *Grand Saint-Antoine*.[16] She was back from the Levant, having embarked several passengers at Tripoli in Syria, where a clean bill of health was issued. On the return leg to Cyprus one of the passengers died and the rest left the ship. More cargo was loaded, and the vessel cleared for France on 18 April, again with a clean bill of health. Within a few days of sailing two sailors had fallen ill, and before long five men were dead, including the surgeon, and another three were sick. Partly for this reason, but also for fresh stores, Captain Chataud deviated to Leghorn. Arriving on 14 May, he was ordered by the Health Office to stay out of harbour. In strict quarantine, the ship was guarded day and night, and the three sick crewmen died. When their bodies had been landed, the medical diagnosis was a malignant, pestilential fever; this was actually some comfort to the crew, who had feared bubonic plague. The authorities at Leghorn endorsed the bills of health with the events of the ship's detention, the diagnosis of the disease, and a general warning to take every precaution. On that basis the ship left for Marseilles with a new surgeon.

The *Grand Saint-Antoine* dropped anchor at the island of Pomègues, about three miles from Marseilles, the holding-ground for all ships from the Levant and Barbary.[17] By now another man was ill. Captain Chataud reported to the Health Office, who ordered that his cargo be transferred to the lazaretto, known as Les Infirmeries, for purification under the strictest regime, as if the bill of health had been foul. The cotton wool was initially destined for cleansing at the relatively distant island of Jarre, but the bureau changed its mind on 3 June, and all the cargo arrived at Les Infirmeries. On 14 June those aboard the ship were allowed to land after various rituals, and the ship itself was fumigated at Pomègues. It was a bad omen that, only the day before, one of the guards keeping an eye on the ship had died; the diagnosis was old age and cholera morbus. Ten days later the cabin boy fell ill, then died, and events gathered a grisly momentum. In vain did the Health Office send the ship to Jarre for a further fumigation. Six porters who had handled the cargo, a priest who had delivered the last rites, and the surgeon of the lazaretto quickly succumbed. The Health Office were at first dilatory in realizing the seriousness of the position, and the diagnoses were equivocal. The chaos which ensued shocked sensitivities even a hundred years later. The *Quarterly Review* found it too painful to:

> represent in detail the early doubts and obstinate denials that the disease was the plague; the fears of the magistrates to alarm the people; the unwillingness of the people to believe; their terror at its first announcement, and, after a short and deceptive calm, their drunken joy and mad confidence; the contests between the physicians and the magistrates; the insults offered by the populace to the former; the scarcity of food; the bodies collected in the houses and in the streets, for want of persons to remove them; the fires lighted in the squares and market–places, and before the doors of every house, for the purpose of

---

16 The following account is taken mainly from Carrière et al., but *Quarterly Review*, vol. 33 (1825–26), 222–5, is also useful.

17 The use of islands off Marseilles for quarantine purposes is described in Masson, pp. 225–7; see also Paris, vol. 5, p. 140, and Panzac, pp. 180–82, for Les Infirmeries.

> burning out the contagion, till the whole city was a blaze; the flight of the people from the town; the immense graves; cart–loads of bodies tumbled into them in the utmost disorder; the shops and public places closed, and the streets deserted … [18]

Alarm in the Privy Council

News of the epidemic was published in the London press on 10 August 1720, quoting a letter from Genoa dated 27 July.[19] Morale in the capital was already low by the failure of the South Sea scheme. Details of the illness were necessarily sketchy, and the Privy Council were slow to take cognizance of the threat. As George I was in Hanover, it was for the Lords Justices to preside at Council. On 23 August, presumably following new and alarming information received via James Craggs, Secretary of State for the Southern Department, they were galvanized into a rapid and worried discussion.[20] Customs were asked to give the 'Proper Directions' to their officers at the outports to prevent any landings from anywhere within the Mediterranean until further notice.[21] That was impossibly severe but it bought time in which the Attorney-General could draft a Proclamation. Meanwhile the Council took the unusual step of appointing a committee to meet that same evening to consider further measures, with Customs Commissioners in attendance. The main task was to consult the archives of ten years earlier to establish a form of words for an Order in Council which would also, of course, be the basis for the Proclamation.[22]

Two days later the Lords Justices issued an Order which was a virtual resurrection of the texts used in the Baltic crisis, even repeating the aberration of 'Stowfort' Island as the airing ground for Thames-bound goods.[23] The Order continued the troublesome requirement for all goods to be aired for a week before a ship left for its place of discharge, but it varied and enlarged the enumerated goods which (as before) could not be discharged at all until the Privy Council had given ad hoc permission. These goods were now defined as hemp and flax; paper and books; raw, thrown or wrought silk; linen, cotton wool, cotton in yarn or manufactured; wool raw or in any way wrought; feathers; grogram or mohair yarn; human hair; goats' hair; Carmenia wool, carpets, cambletts, burdetts or other manufactures of silk and cotton; kid skins; and skins in the wool or hair.[24] Hemp and flax were essentially Baltic naval stores, but supplies were occasionally brought from the Mediterranean. Also on 25 August appeared the Proclamation, issued 'that no Person … may Pretend Ignorance of Our

---

18 *Quarterly Review*, vol. 33 (1825–26), 223–4.

19 J.W. Joyce, *Daniel Defoe and the Plague in Marseilles (1720–1722)* (Leeds, 1957), p. 2.

20 NA PC 2/86/472.

21 Ibid.

22 NA PC 2/86/475.

23 NA PC 2/86/476–7.

24 Many of these items of cotton, silk and wool are difficult to interpret in modern terms. The large *Oxford English Dictionary* simply defines burdetts (burdet) as 'some kind of cotton fabric'. The word cambletts, better known as camlets, covers a number of fabrics from silk to linen. Carmenia wool (not in the *OED*) must have taken its name from Carmania, a province of Persia.

Command', repeating (and numbering) the points in the Order, and ending with a warning that offenders would be punished 'with the utmost Severity'.[25]

In fairness to the Council, they could have done little else in their rush to bring out some temporizing measure than reverse the polarity of the restrictions imposed under Anne. That is to say, they had learnt from Customs the main products imported from the Levant, directly or via the Mediterranean free ports, and enumerated those which were deemed particularly susceptible to conveying infection. But there was one important difference from the Council's position of ten years earlier – they had openly sought medical advice. Although quarantine measures in 1664 had followed the recommendations of the College of Physicians, the regulations drawn up in the Baltic crisis were apparently arrived out without formal consultation with that body or its representative.[26] In 1720, however, the Lords Justices asked Richard Mead, the leading physician of the day, to assemble his thoughts on pestilential contagion and the methods used to prevent it. Those words are virtually the extended title of the 'Short Discourse', which Mead set about producing, having 'most readily' undertaken his task, 'though upon short Warning, and with little Leisure'.[27] The book bears a dedication to James Craggs dated 25 November, explaining that the commission had come from the Lords Justices; without that statement it would be difficult to make any connection between Mead and the Privy Council. As no mention is made of him in the Council register, he would seem not to have attended the committee meeting on the evening of 25 August. The conclusion must be that Mead's involvement had been more a matter for the Cabinet than the Privy Council.

It is also unclear why the Lords Justices wanted Mead to publish his thoughts and recommendations, rather than keeping his advice to themselves.[28] The advantage of publication was that those whom quarantine was likely to affect would now see the medical basis for their expense and inconvenience; it was also an exercise in transparent government in an age when daily newspapers, one run by the influential Daniel Defoe, might well have disseminated their own wild thoughts in the absence of a government line.[29] But there were also disadvantages; the obvious one was that the same mania to publish might spawn a host of other medical views, some not in agreement. The other danger was that Mead himself might have opinions which were in conflict with accepted practice and beliefs, at home and abroad, and undermine the credibility of measures which had traditionally satisfied the Customs Commissioners, the Privy Council's other advisers. Both these drawbacks were realized.

Mead believed in the role of the disposition (or constitution) of the air, which doctors as far back as Galen had thought preceded and even occasioned an outbreak

25 NA PC 2/86/478–80.

26 P. Russell, *A Treatise of the Plague* (London, 1791), p. 323, states that the College of Physicians was recommending quarantine 'according to the custom of Italy' as early as the beginning of the seventeenth century.

27 R. Mead, *A Short Discourse concerning Pestilential Contagion* ... (London, 1720), title-page.

28 It is possible that the Lords Justices, at the outset, had not intended Mead to publish his advice, but felt they could not do otherwise than acquiesce in his wish.

29 For Defoe, see Joyce, pp. 2–3.

of plague.[30] But the epidemic also depended, in Mead's view, on the release of noxious matter from infected persons, which was carried on the wind.[31] This was contagionism, but not in the most literal sense. But as far as goods were concerned, Mead was orthodox. He held that an infected body produced 'an active Substance, perhaps in the Nature of a Salt'.[32] He made analogy with pervasive animal scents, like civet, and deduced that animal products were likely to have the same potential to retain the noxious exhalations from a human being.[33] Thus furs, feather, silk, hair, wool and skins were particularly dangerous, and any bale of fibrous material, such as cotton, hemp or flax, posed a similar risk. So did clothes. These opinions led Mead to a rather unusual view of quarantine. He saw little use in confining men on their ship as infection in wearing apparel might outlast the detention, especially if further sickness occurred on board.[34] He was very much in favour of lazarettos, preferably on islands, for people and goods.[35] If the ship were infected, all the men should be landed, the well being separated from the sick.[36] Both groups would have their clothes burnt and undergo a quarantine of 30–40 days.[37] If the ship were healthy, Mead saw no reason for quarantine at all, provided the men were washed and their clothes aired for a week.[38]

The lazaretto for goods, according to Mead, should be separate, and all susceptible materials, including paper and books, should be aired in warehouses for 40 days.[39] 'This may perhaps seem too long; but as we don't know how much Time precisely is necessary to purge the Interstices of Spongy Substances from Infectious Matter by fresh Air, the Caution cannot be too great ...'[40] Cotton from Turkey was deemed the most dangerous conveyor of infection. If a ship came from a place where plague was more virulent than usual, Mead felt the goods should be burnt, and even the ship.[41] He followed up this with a passionate diatribe against smuggling, which he thought more liable than anything else to import the epidemic from France.[42] Generally, he was in favour of severe punishment for transgressors. But once plague had erupted, Mead was again controversial. Treatment should be 'Compassionate Care' rather than 'Discipline' and 'Punishment'.[43] Shutting up houses, he thought, creates 'Seminaries of Contagion'.[44] He was comfortable with the idea of cordons sanitaires, but not so as to restrict all egress, as in France, 'which is an unnecessary

30 Mead, pp. 2–3.
31 Mead, pp. 14–15.
32 Mead, p. 17.
33 Ibid.
34 Mead, pp. 21–2.
35 Mead, p. 21.
36 Mead, p. 23.
37 Ibid.
38 Mead, p. 24.
39 Mead, pp. 24–5.
40 Mead, p. 25.
41 Mead, p. 27.
42 Mead, p. 30.
43 Mead, p. 32.
44 Mead, pp. 34–5.

Severity, not to call it a Cruelty'.[45] Mead's view was that people should leave, if they wished, after a quarantine of 20 days.[46]

The popularity of Mead's *Discourse* was demonstrated by the printing of seven editions within a year and an eighth, with additions, in 1722.[47] But that is not to say he 'was effectual in allaying the public alarm', as claimed by one biographer; and his ideas were far from 'universally approved', as was suggested nearly 50 years later.[48] Patrick Russell, at the turn of the eighteenth century, largely agreed with Mead (but found him too critical of plague restrictions in London instituted by James I);[49] Gavin Milroy, writing in 1861, had scarcely a good one word to say for him, pointing out that Mead had no experience of the plague, or even of a lazaretto, and was basing his medical views on hearsay, on reading and on the diseases of the metropolis.[50] At the time, opposition to Mead was forceful. He had opened a public debate on contagion and the plague, which was to rumble and roar for the next century and a half. Defoe suddenly recollected the events of the Great Plague of London and issued, anonymously, his *Due Preparation* for body and soul.[51] George Pye, on the other hand, set out systematically to refute all that Mead had written. Part of Pye's attack was that plague could not be propagated by goods, a point in which 'Explainer', having referred to Mead's 'Conceits and Contradictions', concurred.[52]

These attacks (and there were others) were published too late to affect Privy Council policy for the first year of the crisis. They were, however, to be most important in the long run as the wisdom and effectiveness of quarantine, cornerstone of plague defence, was now under attack. This is not the place to rehearse the elaborated arguments of the anti-contagionists, but two points stand out: the first was that Mead had weakened his own position by insisting that air, not contact alone, was responsible for the spread of plague; and secondly that Britain had been importing cotton and other goods for many years from Turkey and the Levant. If cotton was so dangerous, why had the disease not reached England already? There were, of course, those who claimed on 'irrefrigable Authority', that the Great Plague had been started by a bale of Turkish cotton or silk, imported via Holland, but that did not explain England's immunity in direct trade.[53] Quarantine was dismissed by the anti-contagionists as useless, an incentive to the running of contraband, and 'a very great Injury to a trading Nation'.[54]

---

45 Mead, pp. 53–5.

46 Ibid.

47 See *Oxford Dictionary of National Biography* [*ODNB*]

48 *ODNB*; *The Immediate Necessity of Building a Lazzaretto for a Regular Quarantine* ... (London, 1768), p. 24.

49 Russell, preface [unpag.].

50 *British Parliamentary Papers* [*BPP*], vol. 58 (1861), p. 265.

51 For full title, see Bibliography.

52 G. Pye, *A Discourse of the Plague* ... (London, 1721), pp. 36–43; 'Explainer', *Distinct Notions of the Plague, with the Rise and Fall of Pestilential Contagion* (London, 1722), pp. 3, 97–131.

53 The quotation is from N. Hodges, *Loimologia* ... (London, 1720) p. 30.

54 Pye, p. 43. He also argued (p. 50) that quarantines 'propagate and keep up Fears and Frights amongst the People'.

The Levant Company

If quarantine under Queen Anne had risked friction between Government and vested interests in the Baltic, especially the Eastland Company, the crisis under her successor threatened the monopolists trading with Turkey.[55] English trade with the Mediterranean had been insignificant until the sixteenth century. A small number of London merchants obtained a charter from Elizabeth, in 1581, to trade exclusively with Turkey for seven years, on a joint-stock footing.[56] Parallel concessions had been granted to others for trade with Venice and the Levant, and in 1592 these interests were merged with those of the Turkey merchants by the creation of a new Company.[57] The charter allowed for over 50 members, but with an indistinct division between joint-stock and regulated status. The Company was definitively set on a regulated base when a new charter, more than doubling the membership, was granted in 1605.[58] Despite the 'free trade' aspirations in which this latest charter was conceived, entry to the Company retained some exclusivity; indeed, under Charles II, freedom of the City became a further prerequisite for would-be members living within 20 miles of London, unless they were aristocracy or 'gentlemen of quality'.[59] Most new entrants were qualified by patrimony or apprenticeship, and in 1720 the Company had around 200 members.[60] An important constitutional aspect of the Levant Company was that it had the right (at times contested by the Crown) to appoint the ambassador at Constantinople, while maintaining consuls and vice-consuls at strategic Turkish ports.[61] Stationed at these ports were factors, nominally under Company control, who organized the purchase and dispatch of goods.[62] These people were also, of course, very knowledgeable about the risks of the indigenous plague.

Trade with Turkey and the Levant was essentially an exchange of English woollens, dyed and dressed, against the raw materials of silk and cotton and their many associated fabrics, some of Persian origin. Additional exports from England were lead and tin, while other imports included currants, galls and spices. The intention was that the value of these goods should roughly equate, but in practice an excess by value of imports was normal, and the Company had sometimes to send

55 The standard histories of the Levant Company are by M. Epstein, *The Early History of the Levant Company* (London, 1908) (to 1640) and A.C. Wood, *A History of the Levant Company* (Oxford, 1935).

56 E. Lipson, *The Economic History of England. The Age of Mercantilism* (3 vols, London, 1943), vol. 2, p. 337; Epstein, p. 16; Wood, p. 11.

57 Lipson, vol. 2, pp. 337–8; Epstein, pp. 20–24, 36; Wood, p. 20.

58 Lipson, vol. 2, pp. 340–41; Wood, pp. 39–41; Epstein (pp. 153–212) transcribes the charter.

59 Lipson, vol. 2, p. 341.

60 D. Macpherson, *Annals of Commerce, Manufactures, Fisheries, and Navigation …* (4 vols, London, 1805), vol. 3, p. 115; Wood, p. 151.

61 Lipson, vol. 2, pp. 342–3; Epstein, pp. 74–99; Wood, pp. 250–53, lists all the ambassadors and consuls.

62 Wood, p. 216, points to the Company's difficulty in exercising 'any effective control … over the factors'.

specie to redress the balance.[63] In 1720 goods worth nearly £400,000 were imported from Turkey, while exports were valued at nearly £360,000.[64] Goods at this period travelled in large, well-armed, merchantmen (known as 'general' ships), chartered several times a year, in which members rented space.[65] The voyage, which might take two months in each direction, was dangerous, with ships very liable to attack from Barbary corsairs and sometimes Spanish warships.[66]

Despite the high value of return cargoes, and the importance to English manufacturers of the annual export of 20,000 broadcloths, the role of the Levant Company in the national economy was relatively slight.[67] In 1720 the value of trade with Turkey amounted to only some 4 per cent of the total value of English trade, although business with the Mediterranean in general was much stronger; at that date, the combined value of English trade to Spain, the Straits and the Mediterranean, including the Levant, was around 20 per cent of the national total.[68] This was partly because many goods, both inward and outward to Turkey, travelled via the entrepôt of Leghorn. This trans-shipment was much to the chagrin of the Levant Company, who sought the prohibition of raw silk imports from Leghorn, although their own ships traded at times with the Italian ports.[69] Equally significant for the Company was the increasing threat from the French, now that a native woollen industry was developing; it worried them that Marseilles was fast developing as a free port with a monopolistic claim to Levantine trade, by virtue of its lazaretto. At first sight, and from a purely commercial standpoint, the Levant Company might have seen the outbreak of plague in its main competitor as a proverbial ill wind. If they did, the viewpoint was not to last.

Tightening control

The autumn of 1720 brought increasingly harrowing accounts of the devastation in Marseilles and its hinterland. Writing in *Applebee's Journal*, Defoe was graphic in his description and found the state of the town 'scarce credible'.[70] Reports reaching the Privy Council from diplomatic sources were just as worrying. Via Holland and Genoa, there was nothing but bad news.[71] A further complication was the nature of trade within France itself. With the plague escaping beyond the confines of Marseilles, danger was perceived from the kid skins of Languedoc, brought for export to Bordeaux and other ports of the Atlantic seaboard. The result, in mid-

63 Lipson, vol. 2, p. 345.

64 Sir C. Whitworth, *State of the Trade of Great Britain* … (London, 1776), part 2, p. 37.

65 R. Davis, *The Rise of the English Shipping Industry* (London, 1962), pp. 251–2.

66 Ibid.

67 The number of broadcloths is from Lipson, vol. 2, p. 344.

68 S. Conn, *Gibraltar in British Diplomacy in the Eighteenth Century* (New Haven, 1942), p. 267.

69 Davis, p. 252; Lipson, vol. 2, p. 347.

70 Joyce, p. 2.

71 NA PC 2/87/26.

October, was the summary extension of quarantine to arrivals from ports in the Bay of Biscay.[72]

This latest move, added to the quarantine regulations introduced in August, brought about a situation quite impracticable for shipowners and masters. With no naval stores to worry about, the Lords Justices felt entitled to follow a policy of monumental exclusion. Absolutely every ship reaching Britain from anywhere in the Mediterranean, and from the Bay of Biscay, whatever the cargo, was now liable to detention. But for every general ship of the Levant Company bound for London, there were 20 smaller vessels, locally owned, beating up the western approaches from Spain and beyond. Few of these ships were heading for London, and many 'broke bulk' in the south-west of England, or ran goods into fishing boats when nearing land. Merchants and masters trading lawfully out of ports farthest from London were particularly disadvantaged. Quarantine in Stangate Creek was a ridiculous concept for the master and part-owner of a Penzance vessel, sailing to Leghorn with pilchards, to return via Malaga with wine, fruit and currants for south-west England.[73] The Customs Commissioners recommended, therefore, that ships should have the option of quarantine at London or Bristol, and the intervening ports of Falmouth, Plymouth and Portsmouth.[74] The Privy Council were evidently reluctant and asked the Admiralty to comment; in the meanwhile they set about risking another rumpus with Rochester by building airing sheds on Hoo Fort Island.[75] For those in Whitehall, still the only port that mattered was London.

Unhappily for English shipowners, a rumour that the plague was now at St Malo reached the Lords Justices via the Admiralty.[76] Thoroughly rattled by what seemed the epidemic's inexorable progress, the Council rushed out a new Order and Proclamation within 48 hours.[77] Thus on 27 October 1720, for the first time ever, quarantine was demanded at the mainland against ships from the Channel Islands and the Isle of Man. It might seem strange to have included the latter as there was no quarantine imposed against arrivals from Ireland. Ironically, the Isle of Man was the subject of a plague scare in the following month, but in October health was a secondary issue. The island was a large, illicit entrepôt and the idea was to inhibit 'running'. The Privy Council conceded that the quarantine ports were now London, Portsmouth, Plymouth, Falmouth and Bristol, and airing grounds were to be summarily appointed by local Customs. Animal skins and human hair were now deemed the imports most likely to retain infection, and as they might arrive as re-exports they were to be detained at the Privy Council's pleasure, even in ships not otherwise liable to detention. Among minor clauses, pilots were not to go on board (unless prepared to undergo quarantine) and were to operate from a small boat to

72 NA PC 2/87/15–7.

73 Some ships quarantined on their return to England had originally carried fish to Leghorn from Newfoundland.

74 NA PC 2/87/24–5. This was also presented as an anti-smuggling move. If ships could be grouped at strategic ports, it would mean fewer arrivals at the smaller ports where Customs officers were too thin on the ground to prevent running.

75 NA PC 2/87/25.

76 NA PC 2/87/26.

77 NA PC 2/87/27–35, from which all references in this paragraph are taken.

windward. Finally there was a clause mentioning the 'most pernicious Trade' of smuggling, and enjoining the agencies of the Crown to enforce the law 'with utmost rigour'. No one was to assist smugglers on pain of incurring the King's 'Highest Displeasure', and severe penalties. Thus the Manxmen were given their rationale.

The situation was now reached, as it had been in 1710, that parliamentary muscle was needed to make these penalties meaningful and specific, and demonstrate that the Crown was acting with the approval of the people's representatives. It would also have been recognized that public money might be necessary to relieve the King from expenditure over and above his normal allowance. Nothing was done, however, for some weeks and it was widely accepted that Dr Mead's *Short Discourse*, not published till late autumn, was a model for the Bill which soon followed.[78] In so far as the provisions departed from precedent and included elements of Mead's advice, this seems a logical deduction, but there are reasons for questioning the closeness of the link. The first is that Mead's dedication was, as noticed above, dated 25 November 1720, while leave to bring in a Bill was granted on 17 December.[79] Given the time necessary for the book's production, the interval appears too short. Of course, Craggs was probably aware of what Mead was going to write, but if the aim of the latter's commission was to make people aware of the reasons for such drastic action, it was pointless to anticipate the publication of his book by parliamentary proceedings. It may be countered that the Bill did not get going until the following year (the first reading was 10 January), but that delay was for another reason: 60 members of the Lords had been asked on 21 December to inspect and consider the legislation already in force.[80] It was their rejection of the Act passed under Anne, mingled with Mead's advice, which coloured the Bill now in hand.

In a mark of political neutrality, the Bill was introduced by the Attorney-General and Solicitor General, who were instructed to include provision for the repeal of the quarantine Act of 9 Anne, Chapter 2.[81] The Committee stage, which was chaired by Craggs, lasted a week, delayed by a petition of the Levant Company who feared the total cessation of their trade.[82] The Commons were uneasy and further amendments were made on report.[83] But passage through the Lords was uneventful, and the Bill received royal assent on 25 January 1721.[84] The resulting Act (7 Geo. I, c.3) was a faithful expression of the mood, not far removed from terror, which the situation in southern France had brought about in England. The preamble stated that 9 Anne, Chapter 2 had been found 'by experience' to be 'defective and insufficient', and the penalties inadequate. It is unclear whether this experience had been gained in the Baltic crisis, or just in the few months since August, but there was no doubting the determination of Parliament to control and coerce, albeit through the Crown.

78 For example Gavin Milroy in *BPP*, vol. 58 (1861), p. 265.

79 *Journal of the House of Commons* [*JHC*], vol. 19, p. 389.

80 *Journal of the House of Lords* [*JHL*], vol. 21, pp. 383–4.

81 *JHC*, vol. 19, p. 395.

82 *JHC*, vol. 19, pp. 400–401, 403.

83 *JHC*, vol. 19, p. 403. As well as discussing amendments in Committee, the House introduced new ones.

84 *JHL*, vol. 21, pp. 404, 407; *JHC*, vol. 19, p. 411.

The Act began by acknowledging the royal prerogative of managing the performance of quarantine by Proclamation. What followed was virtually a list of penalties: a master who concealed plague on his ship was to be guilty of felony; one who dissembled in his answers was to be fined £200; one who allowed egress from on board, or would not sail to his quarantine port, was not only to be fined but to forfeit his ship. Those who had left the ship were to be forcibly returned and suffer six months in prison as well as a £200 fine. If England became infected, the penalties would be stiffened. The King might then, through the Privy Council, authorize the purchase of wasteland for the provision of lazarettos and airing grounds. Infected persons were to be obliged to go there 'by any kind of violence'. For downright refusal, or escape, the penalty was to be death. The same punishment was ordained for any uninfected person who boarded a diseased ship, refused to undergo the same quarantine as the crew, and sought to escape. The King could also cause 'lines' to be 'cast up' around infected places. Again, death was ordained for those who would cross the lines without licence. It was to be the responsibility of neighbouring parishes, acting under the supervision of two justices, to ensure the lines were patrolled day and night. Parishioners who refused or neglected their duties were subject to fines and imprisonment. The King could also enumerate goods for special precautions. He could even cause a ship from an infected port, or carrying goods from that port, or with infected crew, to be burnt. Under normal circumstances, however, a ship would be released from quarantine against an oath (of the master) and certificate (from Customs), the goods having been opened and aired as the King directed; these were the only clauses which echoed the system under Anne. Again in times of infection, the King could prohibit vessels under 20 tons burthen from sailing out of any port in Great Britain, until the master had given £500 security against going to any country mentioned in the Proclamation. The Act was to commence on 10 February 1721 (from which date the Act 9 Anne, Chapter 2 would stand repealed) and continue in force for three years.

Continuing legislation

Such Draconian procedures, garbling the edict of James I, the lessons of the Great Plague and the cordons sanitaires of southern France, shocked the English sensibility. There was scarcely a clause which did not provoke questions of civil liberty, mercantile freedom and the unwelcome resurgence of royal authority. For Government, one advantage of the Act was the opportunity it presented, from the most specious of excuses, to crack down on smuggling and the losses it represented to the revenue. This was the point of singling out vessels of under 20 tons burthen; if these could be deterred from criss-crossing the Channel, then many fewer goods would be run ashore in the creeks and coves of southern England. One of the problems with smuggling was that many members of the public, who were beneficiaries of contraband in one way or another, were prepared to condone it. Ineffectual statutes already existed by which vessels below a certain burthen were forbidden to import spirits.[85] Running parallel to the laws of quarantine, and justified by the mantra of public health, there was soon to arise a long series of statutes to prevent the clandestine running of goods and the consequent danger of infection. Invariably such provision formed part of a composite measure and was unrelated, sometimes quite strikingly, to the rest of the enactment.[86]

The first attempt to strengthen the link between quarantine and smuggling occurred within a few months of the main Act, just described, but ran into difficulty. On 4 July 1721 leave was given to bring in a Bill to prevent the introduction of infection by clandestine running, but it was soon opposed by wine and spirit merchants based in London.[87] The intention of Government once again was to ban all imports of spirits in vessels below a certain tonnage, or else the ship and its cargo would be forfeited; other clauses were designed to ensure that unloading took place only in the presence of Customs officers, who were to have powers to stop and search at night, and demand a certificate of duty paid. The merchants argued that such measures would discourage recruits to their lawful trade.[88] The Commons made several amendments but too few to appease the merchants, who repeated their opposition when the Bill was in the Lords.[89] By the end of July the Bill had been rejected.

When Parliament reassembled in the autumn, George I was back in London.[90] The plague in Provence had largely ceased, the immediate cross-Channel threat was over, but preventive measures were still much in evidence. The King's speech ended with a reference to the 'unspeakable misery and desolation' which the plague had caused in Europe [*sic*] and the need to continue precautions.[91] 'And as all other provisions will be altogether vain and fruitless, if the abominable practice of running of goods be not, at once, totally suppressed, I most earnestly recommend to you, to let no other consideration stand in competition with a due care of preserving so many thousand lives.'[92] Evidently ministers still felt the occasion to batter smuggling was too good to miss. In December 1721 a new Bill was introduced, and this time it passed; the penalties were distinctly savage – transgressing ships might be burnt and their tackle sold – but the minimum size of vessel was now raised to 40 tons burthen.[93] An interesting feature of this Act, which dealt also with the disparate topic of copper ore produced in British plantations, was that it remedied an oversight in the recent quarantine enactment. Masters were not refusing to go to the appointed quarantine

85 Earlier Acts are summarized in the preamble to 8 Geo. 1, c.18. See also N. Williams, *Contraband Cargoes: Seven Centuries of Smuggling* (London, 1959), p. 108, and his chapter 4 generally.

86 8 Geo. 1, c.18 involved also the regulation of copper ore in the Plantations. Perhaps the most involved composite Act was 28 Geo. 3, c.23 (1788) which again concerned Plantations, seeking to prevent the seducing of workers in the iron and steel trades to work overseas.

87 *JHC*, vol. 19, pp. 624, 636. In the early eighteenth century the volume of French wines smuggled into Britain was around a third of the legal trade.

88 *JHC*, vol. 19, p. 636.

89 *JHL*, vol. 21, p. 582.

90 The King had been presiding in the Privy Council since 15 November 1720.

91 *Parliamentary History of England* [*PHE*], vol. 7, p. 914.

92 Ibid.

93 8 Geo. 1, c.18.

ports, but some were leaving them immediately without authority, claiming they were bound elsewhere, even overseas. In future they would forfeit their ship and be fined £200.[94]

It was remarkable that in this sitting of Parliament two more enactments ensued resulting indirectly from the Marseilles plague. Their stories are intertwined. Both Bills received the royal assent on 12 February 1722, and therefore overtook the anti-smuggling measure just discussed, which did not become law until 7 March.[95] The earlier Bill was introduced 8 November 1721 with the aim of allowing the King to prohibit commerce for one year with any country infected by plague.[96] This was not the death knell to trade or the constitutional aberration which the title suggested, as the King's powers were to be circumscribed by the present emergency. It was not the intention to establish a contingency measure, to be taken from a shelf and dusted off whenever infection might threaten in the future. Any proclamation had to be issued before 12 December 1722 and would form an ultimate defence against the crisis in France, should the plague regain its vigour. Amendments in the Bill's passage were relatively few. A lobby of the Levant Company, led by Sir Gilbert Heathcote and Nathaniel Gould, argued that their ships should be exempt from the more severe penalties, or else their trade would in effect be prohibited.[97] But other members felt the penalties were best left to the King and his ministers. Thomas Broderick was afraid 'the king would be too merciful, rather than too severe', and the Levant Company got nowhere.[98]

It was realized by now, ironically, that the declining death toll in France allowed the duration of the main quarantine Act to be reduced. During its passage through the Lords, therefore, the above Bill attracted a rider. This was that the Act 7 George I, Chapter 3 would not be in force after 25 March 1723; in other words, it would cease nearly a year earlier than originally decreed.[99] The second Bill was to become a more direct attack on the severity of the main Act.[100] This time trenchant divisions of opinion revealed the seriousness of constitutional issues which the passing of the Act had served only to highlight. It was a complicated matter, which ruffled the equanimity of the Lords. The origins of the new Bill were distinctly oblique. On 6 December 1721 the Corporation of London petitioned the Upper Chamber, under the slight misapprehension that their lordships were considering an amendment to 7 George I, Chapter 3.[101] In fact, the Lords were still discussing the Bill allowing the King to prohibit commerce with infected countries for one year, and the only aspect of the main quarantine Act being debated was the date it should terminate. The City was worried that 'not only the rights, privileges, and immunities, but the trade, safety, and prosperity' of its people were under threat.[102] The Lords as a whole

94 8 Geo. 1, c.18, s.14.

95 *JHC*, vol. 19, p. 743; Russell, p. 443.

96 *JHC*, vol. 19, p. 664. Enacted as 8 Geo. 1, c.8.

97 *PHE*, vol. 7, p. 929.

98 Ibid.

99 8 Geo. 1, c.8, s.6.

100 Enacted as 8 Geo. 1, c.10.

101 *JHL*, vol. 21, pp. 622–3.

102 Ibid.

felt the petition was inappropriate and it was rejected. But this prompted 18 peers, led by Lord Bristol, to dissent.[103] There were several grounds for this dissension: the liberty of petitioning was 'the birth-right of the free people of this realm'; the petition itself was proper in form and content; the right to petition had never in the past been denied to even 'the meanest corporation' and, even it had, the City of London by its importance, prestige and susceptibility to the plague was surely a special case.[104] The dissenting lords particularly felt that relief against quarantine was appropriate for the City in view of recent losses by the South Sea debacle. They also felt that if a petition from the City were rejected it would discourage other petitions from elsewhere, to the general detriment of the parliamentary process. They argued that if the City's petition had been accepted it would have caused no conceivable harm, no significant interruption to business, and no increase in the disaffection with Government which was generally being felt. Finally, the lords challenged the two specific reasons for the rejection: that a general Act should not be attacked by a sectional interest; and that acceptance in this instance might lead to other and 'tumultuous petitions'. In the view of Lord Bristol and his associates, such tumultuous petitions were more likely from the rejection.[105]

A few days later, on 11 December 1721, the Upper Chamber was again ruffled by what the record called 'a very warm debate'.[106] The subject now was the 'lines' around infected areas which had been sanctioned by the quarantine Act. Lord Cowper moved that London and Westminster be excepted; Lord Harcourt thought this pointless as even 200,000 soldiers would be insufficient to enforce any cordon and such an army did not exist.[107] The motion was defeated by 45 votes to 20. It should be remembered that this further debate was still in the context of the relatively uncontroversial Bill to allow the King to prohibit trade with an infected country for one year. But there was a groundswell of opinion in the Commons, now that the French epidemic was in check, that the main quarantine Act had been far too coercive, and the Bill gave an opportunity, or at least an excuse, for these points to be raised. The aim of the Lords' debate, therefore, was to rehearse the arguments before an ad hoc Bill to repeal aspects of the quarantine Act could be brought before the Commons. The latter found encouragement from the views expressed by the 18 dissentients mentioned above, by the 20 who had backed Lord Cowper's motion, and by a new group who attacked the whole concept of cordons sanitaires.

This latest group were backing a new motion by Lord Cowper debated on 13 December. With the Lords in grand committee, Cowper moved that a Bill be brought in to repeal powers under the main quarantine Act to force people into lazarettos, and create lines around infected places. In other words, he was extending his cause beyond the metropolis to include the country as a whole. This motion was also

103 Ibid.

104 There are three versions of the arguments of the dissenting peers: *JHL*, vol. 21, p. 3; *PHE*, vol. 7, pp. 930–31; and a printed paper in the British Library, shelf mark 622–1881. a.5.(1).

105 Ibid.

106 *PHE*, vol. 7, p. 931.

107 Ibid.

rejected, but by the narrower margin of 39 votes to 20. Cowper's supporters were headed by the Archbishop of York and they wished their dissentient views to be on record.[108] They felt it to be wrong that well-to-do people living alone, and therefore no risk to others, could be forced into common lazarettos. At the first prospect of the creation of cordons, the rich would disperse to the country while the poor starved and trade was discontinued. In principle, the powers were thought unconstitutional and repugnant, even tougher than the measures under James I and relying more on military force than the civil magistracy. France was considered a poor precedent for the British to follow, as the Government there was 'conducted by Arbitrary Power, and supported by Standing Armies'. In any event, they argued, even without the cordons the Great Plague of 1665 had not spread to remoter parts of the country. If this exceptionable part of the Act were repealed, the Crown still had ample authority to deal with a crisis. The admission that the powers would probably never be used was a reason in itself why the powers should not be available in the first place. They may be a mark of confidence in the King's 'wisdom and goodness', but at the risk of making 'him [more] terrible than amiable to his subjects.'

With such encouragement from the Lords, a motion was debated in the Commons on 15 January 1722 for a Bill to repeal those clauses in the quarantine Act that gave power to remove persons from their habitations, or to make lines about places infected.[109] It passed by 115 votes to 75.[110] With only minor amendments, the Bill raced through both Houses, and the Lords, influenced by the minds of their outspoken minority, raised no objection. On 12 February 1722 the Bill had the royal assent, and each House had assuaged its collective conscience.[111]

More tough measures

While the quarantine Act had been passing through Parliament, the Privy Council continued to tighten their control. Two warships, accompanied by armed sloops, were put at the disposal of the Customs Commissioners, guards were placed on coasts, and the governor of Upnor Castle was to 'watch' the sheds being erected on Hoo Fort Island.[112] With so much attention to the south of England, it was ironic that the first maritime scare, discussed by the Privy Council on 14 November 1720, came from Newcastle. The ship was the *Lambton Anne* which had delivered corn to Marseilles, and was returning with brandy for Rotterdam.[113] The master 'presumed' to enter the Tyne to do quarantine; the ship was expelled immediately and barred from all other British ports.[114] Customs officers were to examine 'by what Neglect' the ship had

108 There are again three versions: *JHL*, vol. 21, pp. 629–30; *PHE*, vol. 7, pp. 933–5, and the paper in the British Library. Most of the references below are taken from *PHE*.

109 *JHC*, vol. 19, p. 712.

110 Ibid.

111 *JHC*, vol. 19, p. 743.

112 NA PC 2/87/35–6.

113 NA PC 2/87/49.

114 Ibid.

been admitted at all.[115] The Privy Council were in no mood to be distracted from the danger they perceived to London. On 15 November 1720 they wrote to the Lord Mayor to 'recommend' him to appoint 'knowing' persons to open, air and repack goods after quarantine.[116] These men were to act under the supervision of Customs with such 'allowances' as the Corporation should think reasonable to be paid by the proprietors of the goods.[117] Similar letters were then sent to the outports, where they were probably received with dismay.[118] By what yardstick could local authorities impose an equitable charge?

Early in 1721 the Privy Council (with the King now presiding) received several petitions and gave short shrift to most of them. Not unexpectedly, Jersey and Guernsey complained about being in quarantine from the mainland.[119] The merchants of Jersey were the more upset. If they took all precautions themselves, sent ships to England carrying only the produce of the island, and confined their imports to Southampton, could the quarantine be lifted?[120] The request was referred to the Treasury, and thence to the Customs Commissioners; the matter was ultimately handled by a Privy Council committee, who stalled for more time to consider reports from the French coast.[121] This same committee was presented soon afterwards with a petition from the Isle of Man, submitted by Lord Derby, complaining that quarantine 'obstructs their little Trade'.[122] But nothing was conceded. The Merchant Adventurers of Bristol, backed up by merchants from elsewhere, all trading to and from Italy, wanted ships with non-enumerated goods, to discharge immediately after quarantine.[123] The Privy Council referred this to the Treasury as usual, but the Customs report was favourable and the Bristolians, at least, won their day.[124] Finally, a petition came from the free fishermen of Milton Hundred who had restocked their oyster beds around Stangate Creek 'at great expense', following the cessation of quarantine in 1714.[125] They had been told not only that the creek was again out of bounds but that, if people died on board ship during quarantine, 'the Dead Bodys are to be put into a Chest and flung over into the said oyster Grounds'.[126] They wanted this ruling overturned and renewed access to their fishing, or compensation in lieu. The Customs Commissioners, via the

---

115 Ibid.

116 NA PC 2/87/55.

117 Ibid.

118 Ibid.

119 NA PC 2/87/98.

120 NA PC 2/87/113. The Jersey petitioners were represented by counsel.

121 NA PC 2/87/165.

122 NA PC 2/87/162. One argument of the Manxmen was that small ships could not ride out quarantine in winter gales. In June 1721 Lord Derby petitioned that the Lieutenant-Governor of Man might be allowed to visit his lordship on the mainland without quarantine. The Privy Council's fatuous response was to ask the Treasury to report back with accounts they had received about the health of the island (NA PC 2/87/247).

123 NA PC 2/87/98.

124 NA PC 2/87/191.

125 NA PC 2/87/121.

126 Ibid.

Treasury, were visited with this problem as well.[127] For the servants of the Crown, the traditional complications of quarantine were coming home to roost.

The Order and Proclamation which followed the quarantine Act were both dated 5 February 1721.[128] They stated that Marseilles was still infected, and that kid skins, silk, cotton, human hair and other susceptible goods were regularly brought from Languedoc to Bordeaux and the Biscay ports. Ships from these areas, it was claimed, touched frequently at the Channel Islands and Isle of Man, so that all arrivals from the stated French areas and British offshore islands would be subject to 40 days' quarantine. Again Bristol, Falmouth, Plymouth, Portsmouth and London were declared quarantine ports, with ships to proceed to the one nearest their destination. In the offshore islands, a quarantine location was to be appointed by the Governor, Deputy Governor or Commander-in-Chief. Then followed the established clauses to prevent unlawful communication to and from ships, to ensure pilots stayed to windward, and to allow release of ships under normal circumstances against oath and certificate. The cargo, however, would now be opened and aired for a week unless the King in Council prescribed otherwise. That contentious measure harked back to the Baltic crisis and had already caused the petition of the merchants trading with Italy. But with regard to enumerated goods, which were the same as those listed in the Order of 25 August, a change was made; these were to stay on board ship for such time as the Customs Commissioners, not the King in Council, should appoint. The Privy Council were passing the buck.

Within two days of the quarantine Act becoming law on 25 January 1721, the Levant Company, in consternation, dispatched a transcript to their ambassador in Constantinople, with copies for him to forward to Smyrna, Aleppo and Cyprus.[129] The consuls at those ports were also written to directly.[130] The aim was to prevent the general ships loading any return cargoes for England before the Company had applied to the King in Council to establish some relief.[131] A meeting of the factory was to be convened at Aleppo, and special measures recommended for the ships *Chandos* and *Wentworth* which were believed to be sailing from Scanderoon to Tripoli and back again, where they would probably now need to unload. Masters generally were to be allowed demurrage and, on any rumour of plague at Cyprus (a normal port of call), ships were to bypass the island and sail straight back to England. The fear of problems at Cyprus was explained by events then devolving in London, although on 27 January, when the Levant Company was writing, the really bad news had not been broken. The Company could hardly have guessed that within a few months two of their finest general ships would be deliberately destroyed.

127 In a report to the Privy Council, the Customs Commissioners recommended, *inter alia*, that bodies should be taken ashore to the salt marsh and buried there. This was approved (NA PC 2/87/157–8).

128 NA PC 2/87/122–6 (Order), 126–31 (Proclamation), from which all references in this paragraph are taken.

129 NA SP 105/116 [unpag.], 27 Jan. 1721.

130 Ibid. The letter to Consul Cooke at Smyrna is also in NA SP 105/332/100–101.

131 NA SP 105/116 [unpag.], 27 Jan. 1721, from which all references in this paragraph are taken.

Burning the boats

The strange truth about this dramatic precedent is that it had no intrinsic connection with the plague at Marseilles. The two ships involved were the *Bristol Merchant*, which arrived from Scanderoon and Cyprus late in 1720, and the *Turkey Merchant*, which arrived from Alexandria, Acre and Cyprus early in 1721.[132] Both were general ships, carrying cotton wool and other enumerated, and non-enumerated, goods. Unfortunately, they had foul bills of health from Cyprus as plague had been in the island when or just before they called. Indeed two or three men who had been loading the *Turkey Merchant* subsequently died. According to the British consul at Genoa, the ships had been chased out of Messina by gunfire, although they were able to touch briefly at Leghorn where foul bills were a little less unwelcome.

A few months earlier, plague in Cyprus or the Levant would have been a matter of indifference to the Privy Council. If quarantine restrictions against the Mediterranean as a whole had not been introduced, both ships would have docked at London and no one would have been any the wiser about the potential risk. As it was, Britain was now locked into the methods and attitudes which had long subsisted in the Mediterranean. The more the voyages were probed, the greater became the alarm and confusion. The Privy Council asked the Customs Commissioners to consider 'with the utmost Care and Circumspection' whether the holds could even be opened without danger and the non-enumerated goods separated from the rest.[133] It is interesting that this was still considered a matter for regulatory officers as opposed to physicians. A committee of Council was formed at which the law officers, Customs Commissioners, merchants and owners worried and haggled about what to do.[134] The fear of the Council, infection aside, was that if stern action were not seen to be taken, certain Mediterranean countries might prohibit trade with Britain 'inasmuch as Publick Notice was sent to all Parts to have a Strict Eye on these Ships'.[135] This was the historic first expression of a deep worry which was to underpin quarantine policy in Britain until the very end of the nineteenth century.

The committee saw no solution but the destruction of both ships and their cargoes. Owners would need to be compensated at public charge 'for preventing any Discouragement to the Turkey Trade'.[136] The King approved this radical step on 5 March 1721, but the Customs Commissioners struggled to value and apportion the losses, and it was many months before the matter could be settled.[137] It was not only the owners who felt themselves entitled to compensation. Masters petitioned for extraordinary expenses, wages, and provisions while their ships and crews lay idle in Stangate Creek.[138] They also wanted 'some regard' for clothes and cabin furniture,

132 NA PC 2/87/60, 64, 109, 35, 140–41, from which all references in this paragraph are taken.

133 NA PC 2/87/64.

134 NA PC 2/87/140–41.

135 Ibid.

136 Ibid.

137 NA PC 2/87/157, 239.

138 NA PC 2/87/178.

'besides their Private Adventures and Loss of … Employments'.[139] Seamen wanted compensation for chests, apparel and personal effects, if these could not be released from the holds.[140] William Farrington, British consul at Cairo, had dispatched his books and papers on the *Turkey Merchant*, along with two cases of 'Curiositys and odd things'.[141] Luckily for Farrington, his goods had been nailed up in crates at Cairo in his own presence, and then stored in the ship's gunroom and not in the hold. They were allowed ashore.[142]

Not before 16 June 1721 was the whole matter before the Commons.[143] There was now a distinct sense of urgency and little dissent. A sombre House agreed on 22 June to a supply of £23,935 for the King to make satisfaction to the owners, freighters, masters and other interested parties.[144] But still it dragged on. On 9 July the masters petitioned for a 'Speedy relief' to their virtual imprisonment in the fetid creek.[145] Not until 28 July, on receipt of yet another petition, this time from owners and merchants, did the Privy Council make the fateful resolution.[146] The ships were to be taken to a prescribed spot, holes were to be bored in their decks, and flaming tar was to be poured on the cargoes; two vessels from the Customs and two from the Admiralty were to witness the total destruction of what would have been considered, less than a year before, to be two magnificent and 'healthy' merchantmen.[147]

The worst fear for both Government and traders was that this hideous and costly burning would need to be repeated. In this context must be seen the appeal of Sir Gilbert Heathcote in the Commons, later in 1721, arguing that the Turkey trade should be exempt from the ultimate power (burning of ships) being granted to the Crown as part of the measure to prohibit trade with an infected country for one year.[148] It will be recalled that he argued in vain. But this protest was only part of a wider campaign by the Levant Company which had been going on for months. Just after the Company had written to their ambassador and consuls in the Levant, they petitioned the Privy Council on 31 January 1721, pointing out that 140 years of trading with Turkey had been carried on 'without any ill consequences', despite the absence of quarantine.[149] As Turkey was a vast country, never entirely free of the plague, the Company hoped that ships might be exempt from quarantine if they had

139 Ibid.

140 Ibid.

141 NA PC 2/87/154–5.

142 NA PC 2/87/154–5, 170–71.

143 *JHC*, vol. 19, p. 593. The need was for the Commons to approve the valuations, which they considered while meeting as a committee to discuss a treaty with Sweden.

144 *JHC*, vol. 19, p. 606.

145 NA PC 2/87/260.

146 NA PC 2/87/267–8.

147 Ibid. Destruction was to take place at 'the Red Sand' or 'the Mouse'.

148 *PHE*, vol. 7, p. 929.

149 NA PC 2/87/135. C. Maclean, *Remarks on the British Quarantine laws and the so-called Sanitary Laws of the Continental Nations of Europe, especially those of Spain* (London, 1823), pp. 8–9, has much of the text of the Levant Company's petition, of which there is no detail in the Privy Council register. Indeed, it was 5 February before the petition was considered.

sailed from ports certified as uninfected at the time of departure and had remained healthy during the four or so months of the voyage.[150] It was far from the Privy Council's intention to alienate any lobby from the City of London, but this idea was too radical; a committee was set up to liaise with the merchants directly. On 4 March 1721 the Company submitted, at the committee's request, a memorial proposing the system of quarantine reckoned least detrimental to their trade.[151] It is not clear what they suggested but the committee asked Customs to comment. On 14 April the full Council pondered the Customs Commissioners' report, but sent it straight back again 'to consider what Orders His Majesty may fitly give'.[152] This meant the Council disliked the recommendations but felt unable to amend them themselves. In early June another meeting of the committee was held with the Customs Commissioners and Levant Company in attendance; this was also inconclusive.[153]

Making no progress with the Privy Council, the Levant Company continued their parliamentary pressure and sent unhappy letters on 12 July 1721 to Abraham Stanyan, the ambassador they had appointed at Constantinople, and to their main consuls.[154] Ships at Smyrna were to stay another 50 days in port, leave only if they could bring a clean bill of health, and then sail directly for England, calling at Gibraltar for any messages.[155] At Scanderoon, the port for Aleppo, ships were to load over 60 days and then return under the same conditions.[156] New forms were sent for bills of health, in the hope they 'will be better esteemed of here'.[157] But on 21 July further letters were hastily drafted in part rescinding the earlier orders; news had again reached England of plague in Cyprus where two general ships, the *Sea Horse* and the *Duke of Cambridge*, had called for cargo on their outward leg from London.[158] It was imperative that these goods did not stay on board until the ships re-sailed for England. They were to be offloaded at Scanderoon and deposited in rented warehouses for opening and airing.[159] Anything less would expose the ships to burning when they arrived in England. Letters from merchants to their correspondents in Aleppo were sent to Phillip Wheake (soon to be appointed consul at Cairo) who was in Paris; Wheake was to send them by express to the southern French port of Sète, where he was to ask the master of the first ship for Scanderoon to take them, whatever the cost.[160] If no ship were due to sail, members of the Company authorized one to be hired, as the letters 'are of that consequence to their Trade as to need the

150 Maclean, *Remarks on the British Quarantine laws*, p. 8.

151 NA PC 2/87/154.

152 NA PC 2/87/175. The King was not present.

153 NA PC 2/87/227.

154 NA SP 105/116 [unpag.], at date.

155 Ibid.

156 Ibid.

157 Ibid.

158 Ibid.; for the detention of these ships when they arrived in England, see NA PC 2/87/154/553, 557.

159 NA SP 105/116 [unpag.], at date.

160 Ibid.

utmost Dispatch'.[161] This was the measure of the seriousness of quarantine to the Levant Company.[162]

The London headquarters of the Company were surprised by a strong memorial from Stanyan to Lord Carteret, who had recently succeeded Craggs as Secretary of State for the Southern Department.[163] In a letter to Stanyan of 6 December, markedly more deferential than the ones which had preceded it, the London members thanked him for using his influence, apparently unsolicited, in arguing the Company's cause. But Stanyan, unfortunately, had stated that little or no damage would occur to wool, silk and cotton in the process of airing. The members wanted him to write once again to Carteret and correct himself. They pointed out that the facilities for opening and airing in England were primitive. There were no lazarettos to compare with Italy and elsewhere, 'but only open Boarded Sheds on a small Island, in ye River Medway, a great distance from home, which have been twice overflown by the Tides'. Silk, they insisted, would lose its gum or gloss and become 'Fuzzy' if exposed to wetness or even air, and the importers' marks on the bales would become confused after opening. They also feared embezzlement, with no person accountable for losses during airing, unlike the practice abroad. They worried, too, about cotton, which dropped in price by a penny per pound simply after repacking and without other damage.

On 20 December 1721 the General Court of the Levant Company, taking into account 'the great hazard their Estates may be lyable to' because of quarantine, tried again to regulate their general ships.[164] The intention was to bypass Cyprus until there had been no infection there for 40 days; when ships did call, they were to load only silk and drugs, not cotton. If any factor, even at Aleppo, allowed Cyprus cotton on to a general ship he would suffer a 'broke' of 20 per cent of the value. Other cotton being loaded was to be certified as to place of growth. If plague broke at Smyrna, Aleppo or Scanderoon before the ships arrived, they would not be loaded; the Company would no longer allow demurrage to masters but consuls would release them from their charter party if their wished. If plague broke out during loading, the consuls were to 'adjust' with the masters for their loss of time and expense. Two ships were specifically prevented from loading any goods at Constantinople, again under a penalty of 20 per cent *ad valorem* to be paid by the factor. In July 1722, and again in December 1723, the General Court made similar rulings, adjusting to the latest intelligence and planning for contingencies.[165] For instance, if plague broke out among crewmen, ships could not load until 60 days after they were free of infection. And at Smyrna, no cotton, mohair yarn or other enumerated goods could be loaded without a certificate showing the goods had been opened and repacked under supervision at least 20 days after plague had ceased. Some Company members

161 Ibid.

162 Yet quarantine at this period is not mentioned in Wood's history of the Levant Company.

163 NA SP 105/116 [unpag.], 6 Dec. 1721, from which all references in this paragraph are taken.

164 NA SP 105/332/103; also in SP 105/210/34–7, from which references in this paragraph are taken, until indicated otherwise.

165 NA SP 105/332/106–7, 109–10 (cf. SP 105/210/43–6), from which remaining references in this paragraph are taken.

shipped goods via Leghorn, in the hope that its pedigree as a quarantine port might alleviate some of the difficulties in England.

The case of the *Peckar* will illustrate the problem from the Privy Council's point of view. This was a large vessel of the Levant Company which had arrived at Smyrna in May 1721.[166] Two months later she set sail for Leghorn, where the goods she had loaded at Smyrna were put into the lazaretto for quarantine. When this was finished, she reloaded, took on other cargo, and set off for Malaga and Alicante to complete her lading. In June 1722 she was back at Stangate Creek after a passage of 65 days from Leghorn. Apart from thirty-two crew, including a surgeon, the ship had seven passengers. An infant had died on the journey, 'Strangled in drinking Brandy'. The bill of lading stated wine, raisins, oil, silk, anchovies, rhubarb, capers, drugs, carpets, brimstone, clothes, soap, argol, kid skins and a horse. Customs also found stone images, vitriol and books. The Privy Council had to decide whether this ship should be treated as from Smyrna or from Leghorn. The silk had come from Smyrna (as had the horse) and much of the cargo was enumerated. The ship had no bill of health from Smyrna as this had been given in at Leghorn. On the other hand, the most susceptible cargo (silk) had already done quarantine in the lazaretto at Leghorn. But arrivals from that port were not exempt from the restrictions in England. Another practical complication was that enumerated items were sometimes at the bottom of a ship's hold, with less susceptible cargoes loaded above. The decision of the Privy Council had to match principle with feasibility. It was decided that the *Peckar* might unload her wine, fruit and oil, but that the ship and the rest of the cargo, including passengers, had to perform full quarantine, during which bedding and apparel were to be aired on deck for one week. There was no provision for passengers to perform their quarantine ashore. At this era, most travellers of social distinction would have returned to England from Leghorn overland, but here can be glimpsed the beginning of a problem which was to become dominant as the century progressed. The long-suffering horse was no doubt released to quarantine in a field.[167]

Coming to terms

It had been a feature of the Baltic emergency that the Privy Council gradually relaxed the harshness of their decisions – often to the annoyance of the Customs Commissioners – despite the letter of the law, most of which was of their own making. In the context of the Marseilles crisis, severity was also to soften, but not before the Levant Company had been thoroughly upset and restrictions widened further against France. On 27 September 1721 the Council sat, without the King, solely to instruct the Attorney-General to prepare an Order obliging all persons arriving in this country from the French coast north of Biscay, to bring a bill of health

166 NA PC 2/87/47, 70, from which all references in this paragraph are taken.

167 It was by no means unusual for general ships to carry horses and their immediate release was sometimes the subject of a specific petition, in case the animal be 'spoyled' (e.g. NA PC 2/87/477, 484, 532). The Privy Council were amenable as long as the owner(s) paid duty.

or be subject to quarantine.[168] On 2 October, with the King then present, an Order and Proclamation were duly issued on those lines.[169] Bills or certificates were to be signed by magistrates at the port of departure. All persons on packet boats 'of what Condition or Quality soever they be' were to produce their bill to the master before sailing, or the whole ship would be quarantined.[170] The immediate result was that the smuggling communities of Jersey and Guernsey did a good trade in blank bills acquired illegally in ports like St Malo.[171] The summary effect of the rulings now in force was that Britain had placed all ships arriving from the French Mediterranean and Atlantic coasts under quarantine, and all persons crossing the Channel under the necessity to prove that they, and their port of departure, were healthy. The point where the Atlantic (Biscay) coast ceased and the Channel coast began was not defined in law. Ships from the French Channel ports were not subject to quarantine, nor were their cargoes unless they comprised skins and hair.

Common sense would suggest that the requirement for bills of health from France was abused and evaded. It certainly caused a problem for the navy. A sloop accosted two French boats ostensibly fishing off Beachy Head.[172] Normally the captain would have boarded them, being convinced they were smuggling, but the Frenchmen told him they had no bills of health. If, therefore, the captain had boarded them and then returned to his sloop, he would have been legally obliged to perform quarantine, because he had no bill of health for himself when he left a vessel originally from France. This absurd dilemma was delegated from the Privy Council to a committee, which got rid of it to the Customs Commissioners.[173] It was more than three months later, in May 1722, before legal minds clicked into gear and naval officers were allowed a dispensation to board suspected vessels without risk of quarantine on return to base.[174] In the interval, no doubt, smuggling with impunity had been rampant.

Masters and shipowners engaged in the Mediterranean trade endured the same rigmarole of petitioning which had overburdened their colleagues trading to the Baltic some ten years earlier. Initially, responses from the Privy Council were far from helpful. The first two petitions for release from quarantine, in the autumn of 1720, were summarily dismissed.[175] But persistence mellowed the mind; the Council came to accept that north Italy and Spain were not a direct threat, and too many petitions would swamp their own business. On 8 November 1720, for instance, the Council heard 13 petitions, and on some days the number reached 20.[176] Of course, it had not been unusual in the Baltic crisis to consider as many ships as that at one meeting, but then they were often contained in just two or three petitions. Now there could be almost as many petitioners as ships. Certainly, the names of several merchants recur

168 NA PC 2/87/313.

169 NA PC 2/87/314–17.

170 Ibid.

171 NA PC 2/87/334.

172 NA PC 2/87/466.

173 NA PC 2/87/466, 531.

174 NA PC 2/87/569–70.

175 NA PC 2/87/6, 13.

176 The record was probably 14 April 1721 when the Council heard 21 (NA PC 2/87/178–81).

throughout the lifespan of the quarantine Act, but this time there were no arrivals by convoy, and no one importing on the scale of a Brander or a Norris.

The object of petitioning, which was only necessary by law for the release of enumerated goods, was to allow cargoes to be discharged after quarantine without airing. There was a general resignation in the early months that 40 days' detention was unavoidable, but no importer wanted fruit or wine to stay on board for one day longer than necessary. Merchants understood that the Privy Council merely referred petitions to the Treasury, which sent them straight on to the Customs Commissioners. It might, therefore, take six days before the Privy Council made an order for discharge, and for this reason most petitions arrived before the ship had completed quarantine. By early November 1720 the Council were conceding that a ship with, say, currants from Zante, or lemons and wine from Malaga, or prunes from Bordeaux, could discharge without airing, although for some weeks all cordage and linen packing had to be destroyed.[177] In the case of larger ships with more complex cargoes, merchants petitioned for the non-enumerated goods to be discharged without airing, and the enumerated goods to be aired so as not to be damaged.

The vulnerability of silk was a particular concern, whether the product were imported from Italy or the Levant. Raw silk of Turkish origin rarely escaped airing (and almost certain damage), but the Privy Council were soon persuaded that raw or wrought silk should not be aired if suitably certified as the growth or manufacture of Italy and Sicily.[178] This concession was even extended to silk of the growth of Barbary, although the African countries were widely reckoned to be hotspots of the plague.[179] One ship with Barbary silk, imported via Venice and Leghorn, was excused airing because the master claimed to have sailed with the hatches open.[180] Another ship, the *Rumney*, was allowed to land grogram yarn and other susceptible goods from Smyrna, of all places, without airing on the strength of a particularly eloquent bill of health from the consul, who reported 'not so much as the least Apprehension of any Infectious Distemper'.[181] But at other times the Privy Council could still be difficult. Cotton and goats' wool from Turkey might still need airing, despite quarantine being done at Leghorn.[182] Yet at other times three bales of goats' wool might slip through without it.[183]

For the Levant Company, inconsistencies of policy were yet another grievance. Sir John Williams brought the matter to head over the *Mary* from Smyrna, which arrived at Stangate Creek in April 1721, carrying raisins, coffee, cotton, carpets and

177 For example in the case of the *Eaton* frigate with 571 boxes of lemons from Genoa (NA PC 2/87/37–8, 46–7).

178 This concession first occurred in January 1721 (NA PC 2/87/106). No raw silk or mohair yarn from Asia could be trans-shipped to Britain through Italian ports after 29 September 1720 (by virtue of 6 Geo. 1, c.14), so in theory the risk of infection via Leghorn or Genoa was much diminished.

179 NA PC 2/87/106.

180 NA PC 2/87/111, 134.

181 NA PC 2/87/155, 166.

182 NA PC 2/87/135, 161.

183 NA PC 2/87/179, 219. For some reason the interval between referral and the Customs' report in this case was around six weeks – that is, more than three times longer then usual.

galls.[184] She had a clean bill of health and the Customs Commissioners, to whom her petition had as usual been referred, were disposed to allow her to discharge after quarantine without airing. But the Privy Council suffered one of their fits of the jitters and asked the Commissioners to reconsider.[185] This prompted Williams to point out that the Turkey ships *Clapham* and *Rumney* had already been allowed to deliver their cotton without airing.[186] In the face of intransigence, Williams resorted to technicalities; the cotton could not be infected as it grew two days' camel journey from Smyrna and was carried there 'some times in the Nutt itself, and pick't out there' and repacked for shipping.[187] His final plea, in some desperation, was that his ship be allowed to sail as close as possible to the airing ground, presumably on Hoo Fort Island, and air the cargo on its own decks.[188] The Customs Commissioners had reservations about the practicability, but this became a precedent for Turkish cotton, some ships airing their cargo while staying in Stangate Creek.[189]

The place of growth or manufacture developed into the guiding criterion for Privy Council policy. If any substance could be certified as 'local', that is not from the Levant, it was excused airing after quarantine as a matter of course. This proved vital for items of intrinsic fragility, such as books, prints and paintings, which formed a small but important part of many cargoes from Italy, as the diplomats and Grand Tourists sent home their trophies of travel. The ruling was also beneficial for cordivants (Cordovan leather goods) loaded at Gibraltar, and eventually for cork.[190] With its air-containing cells, cork was viewed initially as susceptible to conveying infection. But when it was shown that cork imported from Bordeaux had already been five years, or longer, in a warehouse, restrictions were lifted.[191] This was important as cork was often used as dunnage, or protective packing, for larger cargoes and it would have been unfortunate to delay a cargo for a further week for the sake of airing its cushion.

Distinctions in 'growth' called for meticulous paperwork to satisfy both Customs and the Privy Council. Bills of lading, bills of health, letters of advice, invoices and business correspondence could all be produced to rid a cargo from the dreaded obligation of airing. When such documentary proof was unavailable, goods were immediately dispatched to Hoo Fort Island, or to a warehouse at Deptford primarily used for airing skins and hair. This building was called the Red House, one of a collection of warehouses on Crown-held land from which the large Victualling Office developed in the eighteenth century.[192] The relative proximity to London of

184 NA PC 2/87/188.

185 NA PC 2/87/217.

186 NA PC 2/87/228. For the *Rumney*, see above.

187 Ibid.

188 Ibid.

189 Ibid., in the case of the *Hind.*

190 The precedent for cordivants was the *Neptune* (NA PC 2/87/179, 186).

191 NA PC 2/87/147, 151, 166, referring to *Lady Ann.* Even nine years in a warehouse was possible.

192 For the Red House, see E. Hasted, *The History and Topographical Survey of the County of Kent* (4 vols, Canterbury, 1778–99), vol. 1, p. 8; N. Dews, *The History of Deptford* ..., 2nd edn (London & Deptford, 1884), pp. 267–8; A.J. Dunkin, *History of the County of Kent*

the Red House, and the space and shelter of its large interior, encouraged the Privy Council to use it for airing items which needed delicate handling in more ways than one. For instance, when a ship arrived with bales of silk from Genoa, they were sent to the Red House along with a case of pictures for the Duke of Chandos and a parcel for Lord Carteret's office, neither of which could be proved as the 'growth' of Italy.[193] It would have been very unwise to send such items, or books and prints, to swampy Hoo Fort Island.

Ships from the Channel Islands fared particularly badly. They were invariably asked to do full quarantine on arrival, usually at Portsmouth, although the criteria of local 'growth' or 'produce' spared them the need for airing. Exports to the mainland were typically stockings, oil, wine, cider and pebbles. Why a small ship carrying 20 tons of pebbles and 30 hogsheads of cider needed to perform full quarantine is difficult to explain, unless part of a wider deterrent against smuggling.[194] Only one ship from the Isle of Man ever petitioned for release; her macabre cargo of tombstones earned her an immediate discharge.[195] Later in the crisis, when quarantine regulations for ships from the Mediterranean began to be relaxed, the off-islands enjoyed no corresponding respite in the severity of their treatment.

In the early months of the crisis, the only commodities to be favoured with total exemption from quarantine, as well as from airing, were specie from Iberia and wine from Bordeaux.[196] The latter, destined for the Prince of Wales, constituted whole shipments, twice in April 1721 and twice in March 1722.[197] The petitioners were the Board of Green Cloth, who argued that immediate discharge 'will be for the preservation of the Wines'.[198] The Privy Council agreed. Exemption of another kind was afforded to warships. This was not automatic and ships were generally quarantined on arrival. But chests and apparel were allowed ashore without airing, to avoid keeping crew longer in quarantine, and therefore in pay, than was necessary.[199] By the same token, detention might be curtailed on the grounds of 'easing the Publick Charge'.[200] One warship which had done a token quarantine at Lisbon was given an immediate discharge for paying off and laying up.[201]

Before long, meaningful concessions were extended to the mercantile sector, and the beginning of this process can be accurately traced. On 27 May 1721 the *Cadiz Merchant* arrived at Stangate Creek from Genoa, loaded with lemons.[202] The master

... *Deptford* (London, 1854), p. 580; E. Walford & W. Thornbury, *Old and New London* ... (6 vols, London, 1873–78), vol. 6, p. 158.

193 NA PC 2/87/240, 264, referring to the *Levant*.

194 The example is from NA PC 2/87/201, 208, referring to the *Jersey Sloop*.

195 NA PC 2/87/321, 325.

196 Bullion (both gold and silver) was imported by merchants from Lisbon and Cadiz in British warships (NA PC 2/87/71, 77, 350, 354).

197 NA PC 2/87/178, 181, 184, 529, 532–4. The ships themselves were not exempt from quarantine.

198 NA PC 2/87/178.

199 NA PC 2/87/40–41.

200 NA PC 2/87/168.

201 NA PC 2/87/230.

202 NA PC 2/87/229.

petitioned a week later for the immediate discharge of his 'suffering' cargo, and the Privy Council agreed.[203] This was a significant departure from policy and probably took merchants by surprise. As in the Baltic crisis, there was discussion and collusion among petitioners, resulting in uniformity of argument and presentation. But whereas most petitioners before had been merchants in a large way of business, nearly half in the present crisis were masters and co-owners concerned with individual ships; it was therefore more difficult to formulate strategy. There were only two standard ploys: the first was to begin petitioning for discharge long before quarantine was due to end; the second was to tell the Privy Council as little as possible about the totality of a cargo. Thus a petition would stress the non-enumerated goods, especially if these were the bulk of the lading, and omit the silk or the cork or the paper.[204] Of course, the extra items would come to light in the Customs report, but there was always the hope that whole cargoes might be discharged early in a fit of benevolence, or out of carelessness, or simply by mistake. In the case of the *Cadiz Merchant*, it is interesting that the petitioner was the master; it was the man on the spot, witnessing his cargo perishing, who finally made the breakthrough. It was now up to the wider community of merchants to press home the advantage, which they were slow to do.

The 'Gang of Five'

It seemed for a few weeks as if the episode of the *Cadiz Merchant* had been an aberration. But then in late June and early July 1721, three more ships were treated with unusual leniency. The first had sailed in ballast from Civita Vecchia to Lisbon, where she loaded wine and fruit; the second was carrying pipe-staves and iron hoops from Port Mahon; and the third had loaded wine and lees at Bordeaux.[205] All were allowed to discharge immediately, although this had not been requested. As ten or so days elapsed between the referral of each petition and the Privy Council's decision (which then had to be relayed to Stangate Creek), it is very probable that the ships were already out of quarantine by the time they had the news. But the point was that they could be released even if the 40 days had not been completed. In a sense, none of these concessions was remarkable: the first ship had allegedly done quarantine in Lisbon; the second was carrying naval stores; and the third was enjoying a privilege which had already been afforded to the Board of Green Cloth. But the concessions came roughly together, and the merchants were emboldened.

The lead was taken by Joseph Chitty & Co., shipowners and freighters of London, and experienced petitioners. In July 1721 the firm had two ships doing quarantine at Stangate Creek, both from Malaga with wine, oil and fruit. Despite the small quantities of cork and leather also on board, Josiah Chitty (probably brother of the principal) petitioned for immediate discharge, as opposed to discharge

203 Ibid.

204 By way of example might be cited the *Mercury* from Genoa; the petition mentioned non-enumerated goods but the Customs reported silk and paper, which had to be aired (NA PC 2/87/70, 95).

205 NA PC 2/87/250, 257–8, 261, 266. The ships were the *Restoration*, *Ann & Mary* and *Robert*.

after quarantine without airing.[206] This was granted on condition that the cork and leather could be certified as local growth.[207] Soon other shipowners and masters began petitioning for the same privilege, and invariably an immediate discharge was granted (unless the cargo consisted basically of silk), even when the petitioner had not asked for it. Now Chitty was tempted to go a stage further. On 2 October 1721 he asked whether the *George*, in transit from Malaga with wine and fruit, might be discharged as soon as she arrived at Stangate Creek.[208] In other words, could she be spared quarantine altogether? The Privy Council referred this question, as usual, to the Customs Commissioners, who took unusually long (16 days) to reach a decision.[209] In that interval they had been visited with four other similar petitions for the same liberty. The first was from Joseph Chitty, the second was from Thomas Downs, also a shipowner and freighter, and the other two from ships' masters, in one case supported by his freighter.[210] All these ships were from Malaga, carrying basically fruit, so there had been collusion.

The report from Customs, which the Privy Council accepted, was not ill-disposed towards the fruit, but expressed concerns about the bedding and apparel on board, in the belief they could harbour infection.[211] Quarantine was still necessary, therefore, for the ships and crewmen, if not for the cargoes. At this stage, the interested parties evidently conferred again. They submitted a joint petition asking whether the cargoes of all five ships might be immediately discharged into lighters.[212] The Privy Council agreed, but insisted that the bedding and apparel should be aired on deck during the last week of the ships' quarantine.[213] The petitioners realized this was the best they could expect, and the concessions granted to these five ships became the benchmark for the rest of the crisis. Shipowners, freighters and masters usually asked for perishable cargoes to be discharged immediately, not so much into lighters as into small sailing vessels called hoys. Although these craft were normally associated with the Thames estuary, and therefore with detention in Stangate Creek, hoys were also mentioned at quarantine ports elsewhere, as far away as Plymouth.[214]

Towards the end of the period that quarantine had to run, merchants began routinely to petition for ships to be released after ten days of detention. This first occurred in August 1722 and was occasioned by reciprocity with Spain.[215] In May 1722 the Privy Council learnt that the Spanish King had reduced a political quarantine

206 NA PC 2/87/269.

207 NA PC 2/87/274.

208 NA PC 2/87/321.

209 NA PC 2/87/333.

210 NA PC 2/87/326–7. The other freighter was Richard Merry. All the petitions were heard in the Privy Council on 11 October.

211 NA PC 2/87/332–3.

212 NA PC 2/87/343. Inverkeithing, it would seem, harboured the only vessel to have done quarantine in Scotland. This lack of ships is not surprising given the virtual exclusion of any reference to Scotland in the Orders and Proclamations, but cargoes which had passed through quarantine may have been trans-shipped in London on to coastal vessels.

213 Ibid.

214 NA PC 2/87/348, 355.

215 Ibid.

against England to ten days, and was urged by merchants to make the same reduction against Spain.[216] The concession for soft fruit to be unloaded immediately into hoys did not free the ship itself from the delay and expense of 40 days' quarantine. Now, ships, passengers and other cargoes (if non-enumerated) could be released after only ten days, although during that time the bedding and apparel of the crew had still to be aired for one week. The Privy Council heard its last six petitions on 15 February 1723.[217] Within a few more weeks the irksome machinery of quarantine ended overnight, when the Act had run its course.

Synopsis

Although Treasury papers are calendared for the 1720s, there are no lists of ships in quarantine, as there had been during the Baltic crisis. There is, therefore, no printed source to compare with the Privy Council registers and consequently no easy way of knowing how far the latter included every vessel. There is, however, a likelihood that the registers are comprehensive, subject to certain caveats mentioned below in relation to the islands. Ships were not arriving in large convoys, so there was less chance of one being omitted accidentally from lengthy lists submitted by just a few petitioners. Also, by the Navigation Acts, ships were British owned and crewed, so there was no misunderstanding of names, as there had been with Swedish vessels trading from the Baltic. Furthermore, it was a shorter period of quarantine, with fewer ships to elude the clerks in the Privy Council's scriptorium.

Table 4.1 summarizes the ports of departure, the numbers of ships from each (with other main ports of call), and the main cargoes.

Table 4.1 Voyage statistics of ships quarantined from the Mediterranean, 1720–1723

Port(s) of Departure	*Ships*	*Main Cargoes*
Scanderoon	5	Silk, galls, goats wool, grogram yarn
Smyrna	8	Cotton wool, carpets, coffee, fruit
Smyrna, Zante, Messina, Leghorn	1	Silk, carpets, cotton wool, hemp
Smyrna, Zante, Leghorn	1	Silk, carpets, cotton wool, hemp
Smyrna, Leghorn, Malaga, Alicante	1	Wine, oil, fruit, silk, carpets, drugs
Smyrna, Gibraltar	1	Grogram yarn

216 NA PC 1/3/106; PC 2/87/595, 600–601.

217 NA PC 2/88/199.

Alexandria	1	Wine, coffee, elephants' teeth
Alexandria, Candia, Tunis	1	Senna, drugs, oil, coffee
Cephalonia	2	Currants, fustic
Cephalonia, Messina	1	Currants, silk
Nathalico, Zante	1	Currants, wine, vine-plants
Zante	8	Currants, fustic, bugles, silk
Zante, Leghorn	1	Fruit, silk, currants, wine, straw hats
Zante, Venice, Gibraltar	1	Currants, silk, cordivants
Zante, Gibraltar	1	Currants, fustic, oil, cordivants
Venice, Zante	6	Currants, fustic, silk, wine, books
Venice, Zante, Cephalonia	5	Currants, fustic, beads, books, drugs
Venice, Zante, Cephalonia, Gibraltar	1	Currants, beads, drugs, wine
Venice, Zante, Messina	3	Wine, fruit, beads, drugs, silk, oil
Venice, Cephalonia, Messina	1	Drugs, bugles, currants, fustic, silk
Venice, Cephalonia	2	Currants, fustic, beads, soap
Venice, Ithaca	1	Wine, currants, galls, pictures
Venice, Leghorn, Port Mahon	1	Argol, brimstone, wine
Cesenatico, Ancona, Gibraltar	1	Argol, hemp, wine [Cesenacho]
Gallipoli [Apulia]	8	Oil, soap, books
Gallipoli, Naples	1	Oil, catlings
Cirella	1	Raisins
Belvedere	3	Raisins, oil, wine, anchovies, hats
Naples	3	Fruit, wine, oil, raisins, argol
Naples, Leghorn	1	Fruit, wine, silk, marble, books, prints
Naples, Leghorn, Malaga	1	Silk, cotton yarn, wine, oil, fruit
Naples, Belvedere, Gallipoli	1	Wine, fruit, oil
Naples, Gallipoli, Messina, Leghorn	1	Wine, oil, silk, catlings
Civita Vecchia, (ballast to) Lisbon	1	Wine, fruit (ex-Lisbon)

Genoa	11	Silk, fruit, hemp, paper, capers, stone
Genoa, Leghorn	3	Silk, hemp, goats wool, fruit, oil
Genoa, Leghorn, San Remo	1	Lemons, oil, anchovies
Genoa, Leghorn, Gibraltar	1	Silk, lemons, paper, books
Genoa, Naples, Belvedere, Syracuse	1	Wine, raisins, argol
Genoa, Majorca, Alicante, Benicarlo	1	Wine, oil, brooms
Genoa, Alicante	1	Marble, hemp, oil, wine, cork
Genoa, Alicante, Denia	1	Marble, wine, argol, fruit, oil
Leghorn	36	Silk, wool, oil, fruit, wine, marble
Leghorn, Genoa	5	Oil, wine, silk, books, cloth, kid skins
Leghorn, San Remo	1	Marble
Leghorn, Gallipoli	1	Wine, currants, cork, oil
Leghorn, Crete	2	Oil
Leghorn, Cagliari	1	Wine, oil, fruit, cork, anchovies, salt
Leghorn, Naples, Corella	1	Fruit, capers, wine, oil, anchovies
Leghorn, Naples, Messina	1	Silk, kid skins, books, prints
Leghorn, Messina, Lipari	1	Wine, fruit
Leghorn, Port Mahon, Gibraltar	1	?
Leghorn, Palamos, Benicarlo	1	Wine, currants, cork
Leghorn, Alicante	1	Fruit, oil, anchovies, wine
Leghorn, Alicante, Malaga	1	Wine, oil, marble, straw hats
Leghorn, Gibraltar	1	Silk
Sicily, Leghorn	1	Silk, wine, oil, fruit, anchovies
Lipari	2	Fruit, wine, oil, brimstone
Lipari, Messina	4	Fruit, wine, pumice stones, silk, oil
Messina, Lipari, Naples	1	Raisins, currants, silk, argol, catlings
Messina, Leghorn	2	Silk, hemp, wine, oil, marble, argol

Messina, Leghorn, Gibraltar	1	Oil, wine, marble, drugs, cordivants
Messina, Leghorn, Genoa	1	Silk, paper
Messina, Saragossa [sic]	1	Argol, wine, reeds, brooms
Cagliari	1	Salt
Port Mahon	4	Naval stores
Port Mahon, Gibraltar	1	Naval stores, wine, wool, skins
Tripoli, Tunis (bound Portugal)	1	Rice
Barcelona	3	Wine, cork
Barcelona, Benicarlo	1	Cork, wine
Barcelona, Benicarlo, Alicante, Gib.	1	Cork, wine, fruit, almonds
Barcelona, Salou, Denia	1	Fruit, nuts, wine
Barcelona, Salou, Alicante, Cadiz	1	Wine, nuts, cochineal, cork, silver
Barcelona, Alicante, Carthagena	1	Wine, cork, capers, barilla, wool
Barcelona, Malaga, Cadiz	1	Wine, raisins, cochineal, cork, bullion
Barcelona, Majorca	1	Oil, cork
Salou	2	Wine, nuts, fruit, cork, whisks
Vinaros	1	Wine, nuts, cork
Benicarlo	4	Wine, lemons
Benicarlo, Alicante	3	Wine
Benicarlo, Alicante, Cadiz	1	Wine, fruit, barilla, cochineal, cork
Benicarlo, Denia, Malaga	1	Wine, fruit
Denia	15	Raisins, fruit, wine, almonds, cork
Denia, Malaga	1	Fruit, wine
Alicante	26	Wine, fruit, raisins, cork, barilla, oil
Alicante, Denia	2	Raisins
Alicante, Valencia	1	Wine, oil, soap
Alicante, Malaga	3	Wine, fruit, oil, cork, barilla, salt
Malaga	81	Wine, fruit, marble, whisks, oil, cork

Malaga, Gibraltar	7	Wine, fruit, potatoes, cordivants
Malaga, Cadiz	3	Wine, fruit, cochineal, bullion
Carthagena	1	Barilla, wine, cork
Gibraltar	3	Fruit, salt, wine, skins, naval stores
Cadiz	3	Wine, oranges, lemons, silver, cork
Bordeaux	33	Prunes, wine, brandy, kid skins, cork
Bordeaux, St-Martin	1	Wine, salt, brandy
La Rochelle	3	Prunes, brandy, kid skins, nuts, pears
St-Martin (Ile de Ré)	3	Salt, rosin
Le Croisic	12	Salt
Alberoon [?Ile d'Oléron]	2	Salt
Jersey	28	Pebbles, cider, stockings, wine
Guernsey	14	Stockings, pebbles, wine, cider, hides
Isle of Man	1	Tombstones

Note: The table does not indicate when ships called at other ports, typically Gibraltar, for water or provisions, without loading new cargo. Also, it does not cater for warships, and excludes one ship arriving at Bristol in ballast. No other ships in ballast are mentioned. The sources are Privy Council registers (NA PC 2/86–8) for the duration of the crisis.

This table has a corollary value as an accurate snapshot of British maritime trade with the Mediterranean for the two and a half years when quarantine subsisted. A total of 435 ships were detained, of which 392 were from abroad (that is, not from the Channel Islands or Isle of Man). When arrivals from west of Gibraltar are deducted, only 335 ships from the Mediterranean and the Straits were quarantined. Malaga is revealed as the port sending by far the most ships to England (roughly a quarter of all arrivals from the Mediterranean), with Leghorn well down in second place, even after the composite ports are added to its total. The incidence of only one ship from the Isle of Man is absurd, and to some extent the low number of arrivals from Guernsey gives grounds for suspicion. Was quarantine against the islands effectively ignored in certain mainland ports? Were cargoes simply smuggled to the mainland? Did other patterns of trade materialize, for example shipment via Ireland? The position would repay a separate, detailed study.

It will be recalled that ships had a choice of ports along the south coast, as well as London and Bristol, where they might pass their quarantine. The Privy Council registers reveal only rarely which port was chosen. It can be assumed that most cargoes were destined for London, and therefore quarantined in Stangate Creek, but from the 10 per cent of cases where an outport is known, it would appear that Plymouth and Portsmouth, with 16 and 13 ships respectively, were the most popular harbours. In the case of Plymouth, bad weather in the Channel might have accounted for some arrivals, yet there is little evidence of quarantine at Falmouth, an equally safe haven. Inverkeithing, it would seem, harboured the only vessel to have done quarantine in Scotland.[218] This lack of ships is not surprising given the virtual exclusion of any reference to Scotland in the regulations, but cargoes which had passed through quarantine may have been trans-shipped in London on to coastal vessels sailing north. The extent to which Scotland was untouched by the Marseilles crisis is one of the defining differences between that emergency and those from the Baltic.

It must be stressed that information as to quarantine ports in the registers is occasional and haphazard, and may give the wrong impression. Only two ships, for example, were noted as quarantined in Bristol, whereas the real number would have been second only to London. If Bristol's trade had not been so significant, the city's Merchant Adventurers would not have petitioned for favours, as mentioned above. Furthermore, the names of Bristol merchants – Thomas Freke, Nathaniel Wraxall, John Angier, Stephen Perry, William Hart, Joseph Silvester and Jacob Elton – featured strongly in the early months of the crisis. These men were concerned with the fruit trade, and a few other merchants from the south-west can be similarly identified. Thus Robert Tristram and Nicholas Dennys imported to Barnstaple, William Hill to Falmouth, and Philip Pentyre to Plymouth. Also at Plymouth was Samuel Wallis, who imported salt from Brittany. The main merchants, however, were based in London. Of these the most frequent petitioners (13 times each) were Claude Jamineau, who imported currants from Venice, Zante and Cephalonia, and Francis (and James) Porteen, whose activities stretched to Smyrna. Next came Joseph (and Josiah) Chitty, who imported fruit from Malaga and Denia, and Richard Merry, who was in much the same line of business and traded also with Leghorn. These men had 12 petitions each. Gideon Leglize (six petitions) imported prunes from Bordeaux and oil from Gallipoli, and many other men had several petitions to their name, including George Hammond, Thomas Downs and Sir John Williams. The last-named was a member of the Levant Company as were, undoubtedly, Jamineau and Porteen and an unknown number of the others. Some merchants petitioned on behalf of, or jointly with, others (as had been noticed in the Baltic crisis), reflecting the various interests in one cargo.[219]

Skin and hair

It remains to consider one more aspect of quarantine in the Marseilles emergency, which was the airing of kid and hare skins, and human hair. This was an issue to which the Privy Council paid close attention, as medical opinion held that skin and

218 This was one of the ships from 'Alberoon'.

219 The above comments are a synthesis of information in the Privy Council registers, NA PC 2/86–8.

hair were especially prone to harbour infection.[220] Skins were sometimes imported in ships which were liable to quarantine anyway, but in the great majority of cases they formed part of a cargo in vessels from the near Continent, especially Hamburg, Amsterdam and Rotterdam. As these ships were not themselves detained, they do not form part of the statistics of quarantine and are excluded from the above table. Most of the skin and hair went to the Red House at Deptford, which has already been discussed. Skins were imported in vast quantities for the leather trade; as many as 28,000 in one consignment, sometimes spread between two ships, and packed in bales, casks or 'fatts'.[221] Other skins were imported through Ireland, which did not exempt them from the quarantine restrictions. Human hair for the wig and peruke makers was imported generally in quantities of 50 to 70 lbs, packed into bags or barrels, although 500-lb cargoes were not unknown.[222]

The overriding concern for Customs and the Privy Council was not the port of departure of the ship but the place of 'growth' of the product. A ship from Holland might have kid skins from, say, Bayonne, in which case the bales would need to be opened and aired after 40 days of quarantine. More often, however, skins imported via Holland could be proved as the growth of Germany, in which case the Privy Council were more relaxed, and the cargo was released without airing. The same was true of Irish skins, if it could be shown they were Irish in origin. Human hair was treated similarly, with the same bizarre form of words. Thus a consignment from Hamburg would be released if it could be proved 'of the Groweth [*sic*] of Germany'.[223] Hair of the growth of Spain was equally acceptable.

Most of the problems with skins and hair were caused by the growth of France. A frequent route of importation was the packet from Dieppe to Rye, where Thomas Grebell & Sons had a warehouse. This building was accepted by the Privy Council as equal to the Red House at Deptford for the purposes of airing. The Council had to make a fine judgement as to the 'safety' of the hair arriving in Rye, depending on the area of France from which it originated. Thus hair from Rouen or Caen would not be aired; but hair of the growth of Bordeaux or even Tours would be aired for one week. Petitions from Grebell & Sons were submitted on their behalf by Alexander Valière, a London merchant. This happened six times. The total number of petitions over skin and hair was 79 – the highest individual number, nine, coming from Matthew Boehm of London, sometimes in association with John William Lutkins.[224]

And so ended the second great episode of British statutory quarantine. Although the machinery of control was identical to that of the Baltic crisis, the Privy Council had shown a better grasp of what to do. Despite brief periods of near panic, and agonizing over the ships of the Levant Company, there was none of the utter chaos in

---

220 In the Privy Council registers, petitions over skin and hair are indexed separately. This can be taken as a mark of their significance in relation to petitions of other kinds.

221 NA PC 2/87/422, 456; PC 1/3/101.

222 The 500 lbs of brown human hair were from Normandy, imported from Dieppe to Rye (NA PC 2/87/534, 541).

223 NA PC 2/87/100, 134.

224 The above comments are a synthesis of information in the Privy Council registers, NA PC 2/86–8.

decision making which had marred the previous episode. Relations with the Customs Commissioners were not strained; the mercantile lobby was more resigned than indignant; and the Council had made the bold move of consulting, very publicly, with the best medical opinion. But this had been a less complicated crisis. Naval stores were not at stake, there were no volatile Northern Crowns to offend, Scotland was hardly implicated, and Britain was not at war. If the Privy Council had handled it any worse, there might have been moves to deny to the King the sweeping powers with which Parliament were still prepared to entrust him. One body noticeably absent from any involvement in this episode was the Board of Trade, whose influence over quarantine was so feeble that even the Levant Company did not bother to enlist them. The Board's next contribution to policy was nearly half a century away.

If anything positive came out of the Marseilles crisis, then it was the recognition of the true value to the country of its Customs officers. In December 1722 the Treasury granted the service an additional allowance of £200 for 'a very great Addition of Business … no way relat^g to your Duty as Managers of the Custo^s'.[225] It was a very inadequate gesture.

---

225 E.E. Hoon, *The Organization of the English Customs System, 1696–1786* (Newton Abbot, 1968), p. 41.

Chapter Five

Gibraltar and Minorca, 1720–1814

Gibraltar unexploited

When Britain faced up to the Marseilles crisis, she already had two possessions in the Mediterranean, namely Gibraltar and Minorca. The measures against infection adopted in 1720–22 necessarily interfered with arrivals from both places, but not to the same extent. The few vessels sailing from Minorca were warships or merchantmen carrying only naval stores, so enumerated goods were not a problem. By contrast, arrivals from Gibraltar were frequent, and many ships carried commercial cargoes, often of high value and originating in the suspect Levant. Although some vessels called at Gibraltar to load cordivants and imports from Morocco, most dropped in only for water or provisions and, in the case of the Levant Company's ships, to receive intelligence.[1] It is difficult to be precise as to the number of ships entering quarantine in Britain which had called at Gibraltar on the way, as the information was not systematically recorded.

The vagueness attaching to arrivals from Gibraltar was matched by the slapdash analysis of shipping movements within the colony itself. When Lieutenant-Governor Kane received a request from the Board of Trade in 1728 for an annual total of visiting ships and their nationalities, he could only reply that the numbers were unknown, but large, and British ships outnumbered other nations put together.[2] This lame response was symptomatic of an absence of ideas on the part of Government as to what Britain expected from Gibraltar, or indeed if it wanted the Rock at all. Gibraltar had been taken by Admiral Rooke on his own responsibility in July 1704, during the War of the Spanish Succession. By the Treaty of Utrecht, 1713, which marked the end of the war, Spain recognized British control. Despite this concession and Gibraltar's obvious strategic importance, it is notorious that British Governments, by 1783, had made six grovelling attempts to return the Rock to Spanish rule.[3] Only public opinion, and a Spanish foreign policy as inept and erratic as the British, ensured that Gibraltar developed as a Crown colony. Britain had no political agenda for the Mediterranean. Tangier, to the south-west of Gibraltar, had already been acquired

1 Cordivants were products of Cordovan leather (for an example of export from Gibraltar, see National Archives (NA) PC 2/87179, 186). A. Anderson, *An Historical and Chronological Deduction of the Origin of Commerce* (2 vols, London, 1764), vol. 2, p. 242, mentions Gibraltar as 'a refreshing place' for merchant ships and warships. For the Levant Company and its intelligence, see NA SP 105/116, letter 12 July 1721.

2 S. Conn, *Gibraltar in British Diplomacy in the Eighteenth Century* (New Haven, 1942), p. 133.

3 Recounted succinctly in W.F. Lord, *England and France in the Mediterranean, 1660–1830* (London, 1901), pp. 3–20.

and squandered.[4] It was to take Napoleon, nearly a century later, to indicate the Mediterranean's potential as a short route to India, via Egypt.

There was a dichotomy between the military and commercial possibilities which Gibraltar offered. The former are not within the scope of this study, but there were geographical factors that influenced both aspects alike. The Rock, for instance, was just that – an enormous barren boulder, wonderful as an observation post, but useless for providing sustenance for its garrison and civilian population. The connection to the Spanish mainland was by a sandy isthmus, only a few feet above sea level, and in wartime too exposed to the enemy to be used for crops or storage. This meant that the necessities of life had to be imported by ship, often from North Africa. But the axis of the Rock was north–south, so access was only from the west through Gibraltar Bay. This route exposed shipping to privateers working out of the Spanish town of Algeciras, across the bay itself, and in an unfavourable wind a vessel might stray within range of the shore batteries.[5] Another problem was the constant strong current from the Atlantic Ocean which, when combined with a westerly gale, could make it impossible for a ship to round Europa Point.

If Britain had adopted an active policy for bottling-up the Mediterranean from her pivotal Rock, it would have occurred to Government, as it later occurred to John Galt, that a toll could be instituted as profitable for the Crown as were The Sound tolls at Elsinore for the King of Denmark. Had Britain owned Gibraltar and Tangier at the same time, the mechanics of enforcement would have been that much more efficient. Showing 'the Herculean energies of the British nation, with a more frank and masterly arrogance,' wrote Galt, '... the possession [Gibraltar] will become less the sentinel of a pass, than the guardian of a rich Hesperides.'[6] Practicability aside, it was never part of the British mentality, or official policy, to cause any obstruction, especially one of doubtful legality, to international trade. 'While England is in Possession of Gibraltar', wrote Joshua Gee, 'the Trade of the Mediterranean will be open to all the Nations of Europe'.[7] In fact, Britain had made Gibraltar a limited free port as soon as the Rock was captured. The limitation meant that only British and Dutch ships (the Dutch having assisted in the capture) saw any benefit; when, in 1711, the Emperor of Morocco suggested that Gibraltar should also be a free port for his trading ships and cruisers, the Board of Trade were unimpressed.[8]

Although Gibraltar was to evolve as a free port in a more catholic sense (to the eventual envy of Malta), for most of the eighteenth century it fell far short of the Mediterranean model. Joshua Gee, writing in 1738, even argued that a free port should be created there, apparently unaware that one of a sort existed.[9] But the

4 Acquired in 1662 as the dowry of Catherine of Braganza and abandoned in 1683 as too expensive in relation to its use.

5 For first-hand experience of the dangers of shore batteries and privateers, see T. Walsh, *Journal of the late Campaign in Egypt* ... (London, 1803), pp. 10–11.

6 J. Galt, *Voyages and Travels, in the Years 1809, 1810, and 1811* ... (London, 1812), p. 403.

7 J. Gee, *The Trade and Navigation of Great-Britain Considered* ... (London, 1738), p. 167.

8 *Journal of the Commissioners for Trade and Plantations* [*JCTP*], vol. 2, p. 276.

9 Gee, p. 160.

concept at Gibraltar was hugely removed from the paradigm of Leghorn, where the principles and procedures of free-port status were the envy of other Italian states, and more especially the French. What Gee wanted at Gibraltar (and for that matter at Minorca) was another Leghorn, where duty-free trade would be complemented by a civil administration, independent of the Governor, backed up by a court of merchants. Trade, wrote Gee, has never flourished anywhere under a military governor, and 'a general Liberty of Conscience' was vital in a free port to encourage merchants escaping from religious or political persecution to settle there.[10] This was the key to Leghorn's superiority, its trade 'not being carried on so much by the Subjects of the Grand Duke, as by the Merchants of divers Nations who correspond there; so that this Port is at it were a great Warehouse, where Merchants may lay up their Goods at a small Charge, to be ready for Transportation up and down the Mediterranean, as Markets may demand'.[11]

Unfortunately, Gee's argument overlooked three vital and practical advantages that Leghorn possessed and Gibraltar lacked. The first was a hinterland open to the reception of imported produce (and the supply of goods for export); the second was wharf space and warehousing able to accommodate a huge tonnage of commodities in transit; and the third was a stern Board of Health operating an efficient lazaretto and an inflexible system of quarantine. True, the problems of space were mitigated to some extent by a new mole and other engineering; but the Rock was always cramped. As for trade with the hinterland, this was impossible even in peace, because from 1728 Spain maintained the colony under constant quarantine, on the excuse that its trade with Morocco, especially Tangier, risked the introduction of plague.[12] The threat of epidemic disease from North Africa was indeed real, and underlines why Gibraltar without a lazaretto could never be taken seriously as a free port. But successive British Governments in the early eighteenth century had no experience of lazarettos and what opinion of them they possessed was soon coloured by the horrific events at Marseilles where the public-health system had demonstrably failed.

When the lack of any political will to be more deeply involved in Mediterranean commerce is added to the equation, the prospect of Gibraltar as a quarantine station, complete with lazaretto, seems more suited to the dreams of the Levant Company than those of the Privy Council or Board of Trade. Yet the Levant Company never, at any period of their existence, hoped to see Gibraltar as a quarantine station; for them it was just a convenient harbour where ships might take on water, receive news and wait for a convoy to sail east or west under naval protection. Before the Marseilles crisis, the Levant Company had not the least interest in raising the disruption of quarantine as a matter for national debate; after the crisis, the Company wanted the very name of quarantine to drop from ministers' vocabulary. And when the word would not go away, and the menace of disease became overwhelming, Gibraltar was always too small and too exposed to offer any kind of solution.

Yet Gibraltar had some value to Britain in questions of health, as it was an early warning station for outbreaks of plague to the east or south. Excluded from the

10 Gee, pp. 161–2.

11 Gee, p. 165.

12 Conn, pp. 125–6.

privileged circulation of Mediterranean consular letters – the eyes and ears of the Boards of Health – Britain traditionally relied on messages from her own envoys, often in northern Italy, or friendly governments; such information was inevitably second-hand, usually unreliable, and invariably out of date. Now, however, rumours were received more quickly and had greater credibility. An early example of Gibraltar's potential occurred in 1735, when the Privy Council pondered letters from Governor Sabine to the Duke of Newcastle.[13] Masters of ships from Barbary, the Morea, the Archipelago and Gulf of Venice had spoken of plague at Smyrna and Alexandria and nearby places. As quarantine had been imposed in Tunis, Sabine had thought it right to order quarantine against Turkey [*sic*] for ships entering the Bay of Gibraltar.[14] There was, of course, nothing very startling in such news, as plague in the Levant was endemic, but the Privy Council referred the matter to a committee who were to consider and report.[15] There is no evidence of any outcome. The likelihood is that the committee were less concerned with the news of plague than with the impropriety of a governor imposing quarantine on his own authority. Such constitutional issues were, all too often, a negative contribution to Britain's laboured defence against imported disease.

Relations with Marseilles

The powerful Boards of Health in the maritime centres of the western Mediterranean formed a clique, dictating quarantine policy against the Levant, constantly revising and reviewing their procedures, and exchanging every scrap of information, even the weakest rumour, garnered from the letters of consuls abroad and the statements of masters newly arrived from the East. The system relied wholly on the honesty of its members, and was to a large extent free of governmental or royal interference, despite the political stance often adopted against enemies of the state. If a ship arrived in, say, Leghorn with evidence or suspicion of plague, a circular was immediately sent to the other ports in the clique with frank and full information, and no offence was taken at Leghorn when quarantine was imposed or increased against its ships arriving in the other harbours. With plague endemic in the Levant, temporary scares were more or less constant, so the continual imposition and relaxation of quarantine, reminiscent of swings and roundabouts, governed the tempo of trade from east to west and between the colluding ports in the West itself. Within the clique, the ports of Marseilles and Leghorn were pre-eminent, with Genoa and Venice a short step behind. At a rather lower level, as their trade was smaller, came Messina, Malta and Ancona. At this period (mid-eighteenth century) the port of Trieste, destined to have a famous lazaretto, was not yet fully developed.[16] The accepted language of communication

13 NA PC 2/93/216.

14 Ibid.

15 Ibid.

16 The first lazaretto at Trieste, opened in around 1730, was followed by a much larger structure built in 1765–69 (Daniel Panzac, *Quarantaines et lazarets. L'Europe et la peste d'orient (XVIIe–XXe siècles)* (Aix-en-Provence, 1986), pp. 35, 195–6). Only then did Trieste join the lower ranks of the clique.

was Italian, a decision with which Marseilles was never uncomfortable. Scores of minor ports along the Christian shores of the Mediterranean modelled their sanitary regulations on those of Marseilles and Leghorn. Any failure to toe the line meant retribution in the form of an arbitrary quarantine against their shipping. It was a system without compassion, without favour and without appeal.

For much of the eighteenth century, Gibraltar neither gave nor sought information about the plague in its limited relations with Continental Europe. The frequency of war, and the fact that no Spanish port was a member of the health clique, made it inappropriate or unnecessary to get involved.[17] The change of mood was brought about by Governor Eliott. It happened after his successful resistance to the siege of the Rock and coincided with peace with France after the War of American Independence. It had not been Eliott's intention to begin a rapport with Marseilles, nor vice versa. What put the two sides in communication, fortuitously, was a particularly severe plague at Tunis, which began in 1784. In July, Eliott wrote to all British consuls around the Mediterranean informing them he was putting into quarantine (for an undisclosed period) every ship arriving from the Mediterranean and the coast of Barbary. In the archives of the Marseilles Board of Health is a copy of that circular together with a French translation.[18] For whatever reason, the British consul at Marseilles must have thought it appropriate to let the Board know of Eliott's intention. The mortality of the plague in North Africa was certainly causing consternation in Marseilles, where quarantine for arrivals from Tunis was increased to 50 days.[19]

The Board at Marseilles wrote to Eliott on 30 August 1784. What they explained to him can only be inferred from Eliott's answer of 16 September, as the Board's copies of their outgoing correspondence have not survived. Evidently there had been mention of a plague-ridden Ragusan ship, and Eliott's reply, regarding this or some other vessel, was critical of a decision to remove cargo from a lazaretto, presumably the one at Marseilles.[20] The Board would have been astonished at this impertinence from an interloper, as their main reason for writing had been to protest at the inconvenience to French ships which called at Gibraltar. It would also have annoyed them that Eliott replied in English (which he continued to do). Retaliation was swift. In his next letter to the Board, dated 6 December, Eliott deigned to justify his policy, but expressed himself most ill-content that arrivals from Gibraltar had been placed under 12 days' quarantine at Marseilles, whereas arrivals from southern Spain were not detained at all. In the British soldier-governor, the arrogance of the Board had met its match. According to what principle, demanded Eliott, is this 12 days' quarantine imposed? Would it not be equally consistent for him, when he took quarantine off other Mediterranean ports, to subject ships from Marseilles to the

17 Spain had no lazaretto until one was built at Valencia in 1721, following the plague in Marseilles (Panzac, p. 35).

18 Archives départementales des Bouches-du-Rhône, Marseilles [ADBR], 200 E 441, 26 July 1784. The first item on the Gibraltar file is a long jotting in Spanish dated 1753.

19 J.P. Papon, *De la peste, ou Epoques mémorables de ce fléau, et les moyens de s'en préserver* (2 vols, Paris, 1800), vol. 1, p. 216. He mentions 400 people a day dying in Tunis.

20 ADBR 200 E 441, 16 Sept. 1784, from which the remaining references in this paragraph are taken.

same delay? Pre-empting the excuse that intercourse with Tangier was the cause of Gibraltar's harsh treatment, he pointed out that his garrison had 'not had so much as an Egg from Barbary these four months, whilst Spain, we are told, imports supplies continually …' Eliott ended by asking the Board what quarantine was performed at Marseilles from the different ports of Africa.

From this inauspicious beginning, the correspondence mellowed. Eliott was clearly more comfortable with the tone from Marseilles, despite being called upon to clarify the definition of 'garrison', by which he had meant all the inhabitants of Gibraltar.[21] Both sides sought uncontentious ground. There were pious exchanges as to the theoretical infallibility of bills of health and the unfortunate way they were impaired by events in the voyage. The Board pumped Eliott for a better understanding of Privy Council policy, and the extent to which he could alter it in the context of Gibraltar. Eliott's frank answer is probably the only explanation of this important point. After a lukewarm endorsement of the 40 days' quarantine demanded in Britain against arrivals from the Mediterranean, he confessed he was bound by the same Order 'using, but most cautiously, a discretionary power of abatement or prolongation … according to particular circumstances …'[22] He went on to imply that they should not expect too much from him; once London had imposed 40 days' quarantine on arrivals from within the Straits, he had little option but to follow suit. Eliott was experiencing one of the basics facts about quarantine: it was easier to impose than remove it.

By the spring of 1785, Eliott was on such good terms with Marseilles that information, warmly acknowledged (certainly by Eliott), was exchanged by return of post. Gibraltar had not entered the clique, because it did not correspond with the other members, but there was now a cooperation between two traditional enemies in the interests of public health. Marseilles had a lot to gain from Eliott, poised as he was on the fringes of Barbary. Information from merchants and consuls about 'malignant' fever in Algiers and Tripoli was relayed from Eliott to the Board, who no doubt compared it with facts or rumours from their established contacts. In return, the Board confessed to Eliott, as fully and regularly as they would have done to Leghorn or Genoa, the state of health in their lazaretto, with good news or bad. Eliott was effusive in reply, with platitudes about the blessing of God and compliments – perhaps more patronizing than the Board might have wished – about their judicious precautions. On one occasion, Eliott can be accused of a touch of political manoeuvring. In July 1785 he wrote: 'It may not be improper to acquaint you that since the Spanish truce with Algiers, several of their Cruizers have been off the Western Capes, taken portuguese prizes and boarded their ships indiscriminately'.[23] But in most respects the correspondence was remarkably objective. At each end quarantine was regulated or at least influenced by what the other party wrote. The earlier acrimony over tit-for-tat detentions was over, but for Eliott, at least, there was always an apprehension that the Rock might be treated differently from mainland Spain. For instance, he was happy to tell the Board, in October 1786, that 'the perfect

21 ADBR 200 E 441, 10 Feb. 1785.

22 Ibid.

23 ADBR 200 E 441, 25 July 1785.

state of salubrity' to which their lazaretto had returned enabled him to admit ships from Marseilles without quarantine.[24] In the same letter, he noted a like exemption at Marseilles for arrivals from Spain, but the Board had omitted to mention whether or not Gibraltar was included.

Eliott queried this point, but it is unclear how or indeed whether the Board responded. At this stage there is a hiatus in the archives at Marseilles, and the next letter on file is one from Major-General Charles O'Hara, dated June 1787, which began with the news that Eliott had departed for England.[25] There are two other letters on file from O'Hara at Gibraltar to the Board, one in July 1787 and the other in October. It would appear that Eliott had briefed O'Hara as to the nature and advantages of the liaison, as the latter slid easily into the rhythm of correspondence. If anything, O'Hara's style was even more deferential, and a touch more flowery, than Eliott's. The 'Old Cock of the Rock', so called for his colourful attire, lived up to his description when addressing the Board.[26] How far the *intendants* of health at Marseilles appreciated sentences in English beginning 'Permit me, Gentlemen, to say how sensible I am of your attention in communicating intelligence of such importance to humanity' cannot be known, but there was more to O'Hara than a purple passage.[27] He sought information from Marseilles as to how they punished escapees from the lazaretto and played his part in reporting public health in Morocco and Algiers.[28] He also made it clear to the Board how he used their information; he imposed quarantine against Barbary on the basis of their news and relayed all letters to the British navy in Gibraltar Bay.[29] Perhaps with that last admission, O'Hara had gone too far. He wanted the correspondence to continue, but there is no evidence that it did beyond October. It was one of the understandings within the clique that intelligence was for the benefit of trade. Even corresponding with soldiers would have made Marseilles uncomfortable; when the news was being directed, however innocently, to other areas of the military it was time to call a halt.

At Marseilles, there is only one other letter from Gibraltar on file which antedates the abdication of Napoleon. This was written by Governor Boyd, again in English, on 9 February 1792.[30] It was brief and wholly businesslike. He had not been honoured or favoured by their news: two letters from the Board had simply 'been duly received'. But they had nonetheless been useful, inducing Boyd to follow the lead of Marseilles in imposing a precautionary quarantine against Corsica while removing another against ports of the Emperor in the northern Adriatic. Then came a surprising announcement from Boyd: he had no doubt 'that the neighboring Commander in Spain, to whom I impart all advices receiv'd from your Office, will concur in the same measures'. In this rare interval of peace between the Rock and its hinterland, a

24 ADBR 200 E 441, 30 Oct. 1786

25 ADBR 200 E 441, 7 June 1787. The total number of letters from Eliott at Marseilles is 18.

26 For the nickname, see *Oxford Dictionary of National Biography.*

27 ADBR 200 E 441, 7 June 1787.

28 ADBR 200 E 441, 7 June, 9 July & 29 Oct. 1787.

29 ADBR 200 E 441, 7 June 1787.

30 ADBR 200 E 441, 9 Feb. 1792, from which remaining references in this paragraph are taken.

joint stance against plague could transcend nationalistic divisions. But it could not, of course, transcend the reality of war, and Gibraltar and Marseilles, for the next 22 years, kept all information to themselves.

Initiation in Minorca

The island of Minorca had been another trophy for Britain from the War of the Spanish Succession. Captured in 1708, the island was also ceded to Britain by the Treaty of Utrecht. In 1756 it was recaptured by the French (leading to the infamous execution of Admiral Byng), but restored to Britain in 1763 by the Treaty of Paris. A combined force of French and Spaniards regained the island in 1782, although the British recaptured it 16 years later. In 1802 Minorca passed to Spain by the Treaty of Amiens, and the British had no more to do with it. Despite these complications, the island was in British hands for some 71 years out of 94 and managing the island's commercial interests, given its strategic location and proximity to Marseilles, was to exercise and exasperate the Privy Council for most of that time. Minorca also gave Britain its first painful insight into quarantine as practised in the Mediterranean, and witnessed its first fumbling attempts to build and maintain a lazaretto.

The rationale for seizing Minorca was, of course, military. The fine natural harbour at Port Mahon provided a safe winter anchorage for the Mediterranean fleet, and a base between Toulon and the Straits for harassing the French navy. Public opinion in Britain was very much for the island's retention, as it was for keeping Gibraltar. The two colonies, however, offered widely different opportunities, and indeed obligations, from the standpoint of trade. Whereas Gibraltar was a small, rocky peninsula, sparsely inhabited, Minorca was a significant island, 30 miles long, 10–13 miles wide, and supporting a population of around 25,000. Administratively, the island was divided into four districts called terminos, each with a council known as a university (not in any academic sense); the chief universities were Mahon at the south end and Ciudadela at the north. Within the universities were magistrates known as jurats. The islanders grew vines, olives, cotton, capers, fruit and vegetables, and imported corn from North Africa. They spoke Spanish and were proudly Roman Catholic.

Even before its capture, Minorca seemed to some people to offer commercial possibilities. A tract in 1707 urged possession of Mahon to spoil the prosperity of Marseilles and advance British trade.[31] In the following year Lord Raby argued that the island could 'be better than Tangier ever could have been to serve our Turkey trade'.[32] Both sentiments were vague, and the former was largely negative, but the idea grew that Minorca had some kind of potential beyond its military convenience. Late in 1712 Queen Anne appointed John Campbell, 2nd Duke of Argyle, to be Governor and Henry Neale to be the island surveyor. The latter's brief included an assessment of the island's potential as a free port and the means of making it a

31 [G. Penn], *The Policy and Interest of Great Britain, with Respect to Malta, Summarily Considered* (London, 1805), pp. 12–13, quoting a tract of 1707 entitled *An Enquiry into the Causes of our Naval Miscarriages.*

32 British Library Add. MS 22198, fol. 99.

'magazine' of trade in the Mediterranean.[33] Argyle decreed Mahon a free port on 5 December 1712.[34] This status was once again beneath the notice of Joshua Gee, who argued (although less loudly than at Gibraltar) for a proper free port with all the political and religious connotations which existed at Leghorn.[35] In fact, Argyle had sought to encourage immigrants for the promotion of trade, but the Minorcans proved unwilling to accept them.[36]

Before the British arrived, quarantine in Minorca had been a matter for the jurats. Argyle was inexperienced in questions of health and was soon reminded of the traditional rules and the need for them to continue.[37] The Minorcans had also established an admiralty jurisdiction.[38] In 1718 a Vice-Admiralty Court, whose main function was to dispose of prizes, was established along British lines, but there was a reluctance to deprive the islanders of their control over health.[39] In 1724 Lieutenant-Governor Kane (who has been noticed above in a temporary move to Gibraltar) established two new taxes with the jurats' approval. These were the estanque and anchorage duties.[40] The former was a tax on the sale of brandy and its application was to be equally divided between support for the universities and the funding of public works. The latter was to be used only to maintain quarantine procedures, including the building and upkeep of a lazaretto, under the control of the university of Mahon. Although Kane upset the Minorcans in some areas, notably religious tolerance, he can be credited with the fiscal framework from which quarantine was to benefit. He had already erected a pratique house, and a lazaretto was the obvious next step.[41]

These enlightened provisions of one soldier-governor were put at risk, if the jurats are believed, by the rapacity or incompetence of his soldier successors. The first to earn the islanders' wrath was Lieutenant-Governor Anstruther, whom they accused of oppression and the embezzlement of public money. Even before these serious allegations, Anstruther had run foul of the jurats who controlled the pratique house and who applied in vain for his support in applying the rules. Early in 1733 they claimed a British warship had taken on board a boat and three sailors out of a ship from Messina; this vessel had been refused entry, as a health risk, at Leghorn, Marseilles and finally Mahon.[42] And there was a wider problem: the jurats told Anstruther they were generally abused and maltreated by naval officers, who did

33 NA CO 174/15/55.

34 NA CO 174/19/53.

35 Gee, pp. 160, 163.

36 D. Gregory, *Minorca, the Illusory Prize ...* (London & Toronto, 1990), p. 31.

37 I. Lameire, *Les Occupations militaires de l'Ile de Minorque pendant les guerres de l'ancien droit* (Paris, 1908), p. 105.

38 NA CO 174/1/52–64.

39 Ibid.

40 Ibid. For background, see Gregory, p. 59.

41 Gregory, p. 115; J. Armstrong, *The History of the Island of Minorca* (London, 1752), p. 20: 'The eastern Part of the Wharf [below Mahon] is taken up by the Merchants, near which is the *Practica*-House, where Ships newly come into Port must apply, and shew a clean Bill of Health, before they are admitted to break Bulk'.

42 NA CO 174/16/45.

what they liked in quarantine matters.[43] This was a familiar and chronic problem; 70 years later, Customs' officers at Portsmouth would be making similar complaints.

Following wide-ranging allegations to the Privy Council, Anstruther was recalled, examined before the House of Lords, and replaced in 1747 by Lieutenant-Governor Blakeney, a more tolerant and conciliatory man who at first earned the jurats' respect.[44] In matters of quarantine, Blakeney upheld their views, even to his own discomfort. From 1743 the Privy Council distributed all new regulations affecting quarantine in Britain to Ireland, Gibraltar and Minorca, expecting them to follow suit.[45] Thus the two Mediterranean possessions were to conform to policy weeks out of date by the time it had arrived, and not necessarily relevant. For Minorca, there was a further fundamental anomaly: the jurats were responsible for health but the Privy Council were making quarantine policy and sending it to the Lieutenant-Governor for the jurats' information. Thus Blakeney, in September 1749, acknowledged the Order-in-Council of 28 June for laying new quarantine restrictions against Barbary.[46] The jurats went along with that, although their trade with Algiers was important. The discomfort arose in 1752 when Blakeney received an Order-in-Council of 28 May lifting quarantine restrictions on ships from Smyrna with clean bills of health, and limiting quarantine against ships from other parts of the Levant to 20 days.[47] When he informed the local health office, the jurats responded with a 'Remonstrance' suggesting that London could not be aware of the facts.[48] Plague, to their certain knowledge, was in Algiers and it was dangerous to allow free pratique for ships from Smyrna (something Minorca had never done) which was much closer to them than to England.[49] As it was, ships from Minorca were forced to perform quarantine in all ports of the Mediterranean, and if this Order were followed the detentions would be far greater.[50] Blakeney confessed to London that he had suspended the Order.[51]

This incident raises several points. The Privy Council had only lifted the quarantine against Smyrna after a well-argued petition from the Levant Company, followed by their own enquiries abroad.[52] They had been right in those circumstances to make the Order and the jurats, for their part, had been right to resist it. Minorcan ships would certainly have suffered even more delay in neighbouring countries. The problem was the lack of perception in London as to how quarantine was administered in the Mediterranean, and more especially the extent to which it was augmented for

43 Ibid.

44 For Anstruther's recall, see *The Examination of Major-General Anstruther before the House of Lords January 28 1741* (London, 1741).

45 NA PC 2/97/482, 497.

46 NA CO 174/2/150.

47 NA CO 174/2/236. The Order reached Blakeney on 20 June.

48 NA CO 174/2/238, 240.

49 Ibid. It was not spelled out why plague in Algiers should affect ships from Smyrna. The connection lay only in their common exposure to Ottoman rule.

50 Ibid.

51 NA CO 174/2/236. Blakeney had also barred entry to all ships from Algiers, even with clean bills.

52 NA PC 2/103/98–101. The Privy Council had been following the lead of Amsterdam (see Chapter 6).

semi-political reasons. For the merchants at Marseilles, who composed the Board of Health, what better excuse than quarantine incaution at Mahon to get their own back on the British who had settled in Minorca. Let their ships lie idle for another ten days at the island of Pomègues. And as the Boards of Health swapped their gossip, so Leghorn, Genoa and Messina would probably have followed suit. But the historian should not be *too* cynical in applying unworthy motives. The Marseilles plague had taught all Boards – none more than Marseilles – to be ruthless in their measures of prevention and a long detention was simply in keeping with the medical wisdom of the day. Lessons were learnt slowly in London from Blakeney's dilemma, but not before he had received the next Order about quarantine, which was, thankfully for him, an extension of the rules.[53] Gradually a system evolved whereby Minorca received copies of Orders made in London only when they affected ships which might sail from the island to Britain.

But for a bizarre development in London, Blakeney and the jurats might well have continued in reasonable harmony. The problem was that the conscience of the Establishment had reasserted itself. The Lords of the Committee chose to resurrect, in 1752, the report they had made four years earlier when the allegations against Anstruther were being examined.[54] In this report, the Lords had decided to make general regulations 'for the better guidance and conduct' of the island's administrators. Had that been done immediately, when all parties were available, something useful might have been achieved. It is unclear whether the Lords forgot to instruct the Law Officers of the Crown until 1752 (the likely explanation), or whether the latter had been four years in deliberation. In any event, the Law Officers eventually reported to the Committee of Council for Plantation Affairs that they had come to some recommendations, although 'it was impossible for want of further information to ... form a judgment as to the necessity or expediency of all the several regulations proposed'. The Lords of the Committee acquiesced, with some qualms, in this cautious conclusion, and on 28 May 1752 the full Privy Council, meeting under the Lords Justices, read and approved the flawed report.[55] For the administration of the island, not least in respect of quarantine, disaster was in the making.

Rules and unruliness

The regulations of 1752 affected Minorca in both its civil and military administration. The three military clauses, and four of the six in the civil branch, do not concern this study. The two which are important were the third civil regulation, affecting anchorage duty and, less directly, the fifth concerning the estanque. As regards the former, it was decreed 'That the Anchorage Duty Laid by Governor Kane to Build a Lazeretto [*sic*] be received and imployed by the University of Mahon for the Building and keeping in repair the Lazeretto and the Pratique Haven and be actually employed

53 NA CO 174/2/250.

54 NA PC 2/103/62–4, from which remaining references in this paragraph are taken unless otherwise stated.

55 NA PC 2/103/106–8.

for those services only and not Diverted to any Private use whatsoever'.[56] Similarly the estanque duty instituted by Kane for public works, such as town gaols and water cisterns, was to be received and applied by the four universities.[57]

Within weeks Blakeney was complaining loudly to London about the arrogance of the universities. The regulations were a charter for the jurats to shake off the control of the Lieutenant-Governor. Blakeney alleged profiteering, dishonesty and abuse in most of their responsibilities; these included quarantine, where charges had been raised for bills of health.[58] He sent Lord Holderness, Secretary of State for the Southern Department, a memorial from Protestant merchants warning of 'the Arbitrary Powers' with which the jurats of Mahon felt themselves now invested.[59] In February 1753 the Privy Council formed a committee to consider the many letters which Holderness had received from Blakeney.[60] The committee reported on 8 August that the jurats had 'misapprehended' the regulations, which had been intended to redress earlier complaints, not by divesting the Lieutenant-Governor of his proper power 'but by establishing a check and control'.[61] They recommended changes. The proposed new regulation for the anchorage duty was particularly significant:

> the application ... should continue as ... directed solely and strictly to the Building a Lazeretto [*sic*] and to the keeping it when built as also to the Repairs of the Pratique Haven, And ... the Governor ... [should] cause a Plan of the said Lazaretto to be forthwith prepared and laid before him – And ... the building thereof [should] be immediately proceeded upon, and in such part of the Island as will best Answer the design and Intent thereof, and as the Governor shall think proper to direct.[62]

As for the estanque duty, this was not to be demanded from any parties other than those mentioned in the original ordinance. For both the anchorage and estanque duties, as well as the land tax, the Governor was to appoint collectors; they would keep accounts for his inspection, with a copy for the Secretary of State to lay before the Privy Council.[63] These recommendations, with the wider restatement of rules, amounted to a commission to the Governor (or Lieutenant-Governor) to form a civil administration.[64] All the proposals, which reversed the thrust of the previous Order, were accepted by the Privy Council on 10 August 1753; some of them needed implementation by Letters Patent under the Great Seal, the rest less formally by royal signature.[65]

No sooner had materials been collected for the lazaretto, at a site on Quarantine Island in Mahon harbour, than Minorca was again at war. Capture by France in

56 NA PC 2/103/62–4.
57 Ibid.
58 Gregory, pp. 69–70.
59 NA PC 2/103/270–71.
60 NA PC 2/103/313.
61 NA PC 2/103/467.
62 NA PC 2/103/467–78.
63 Ibid.
64 NA CO 174/1/52–64; cf. Gregory, p. 69.
65 NA PC 2/103/480–81.

1756, during the Seven Years War, forestalled the full anger of the islanders towards the new regulations from London. The French noted, perhaps unfairly, that health matters had been almost entirely neglected on the island before they took control, and by royal ordinance '*une chambre ou bureau de santé*' [Chamber or Board of Health] was installed under the aegis of Count de Lannion, the new Governor-General.[66] Ships and goods liable to quarantine were not to be received in the island, but dispatched to Marseilles. The new Board was composed of five *intendants*, supported by a secretary and a messenger. One *intendant*, who ranked above the others, was appointed and paid for by the Marseilles Board of Health. Of the other four, two were from Mahon and two from Ciudadela. The elder man from Mahon was Treasurer, collecting fees for bills of health against a tariff set by the university and approved by the Governor. The Secretary was to be a local man, fluent in French, Catalan and Spanish, chosen by the Board, again with the Governor's approval. The Secretary received 600 livres a year, the jurats 200 a year, and the messenger 30 livres a month.

The work of the new Board was modelled on the rules which had been set for Marseilles in 1730; there was to be a meeting on the first of each month with minutes being sent to Marseilles for information.[67] As the Governor was to be briefed by one of the *intendants*, he was not a participating member of the Board, let alone its president. All procedural matters which were not directly regulated by the ordinance were to conform to the practice at Marseilles.[68] Of course, the Board had few teeth because quarantine in the island was discontinued, but this was very much a Board of Health with at least nominal independence from Government along established Mediterranean lines. It was also not unacceptable to the Minorcans, whose status in health matters had been respected, albeit in emasculated form. The Board was, however, short-lived. Minorca was restored to Britain in 1763 and the French infrastructure was disbanded. Confused responsibilities returned, and acrimony between the jurats and the British administration, both locally and in London, could only worsen.

When Colonel Hamilton Lambert repossessed the island for Britain, he ordered the expulsion of all French inhabitants who had settled there since the capture by France.[69] This was at the instigation of the British merchants, who complained the French were engrossing the trade.[70] France protested that this contravened the Treaty of Utrecht, but Lambert was supported by a petition of the merchants who objected to restrictions against themselves at Marseilles, despite its claim to be a free port.[71] Lambert lost his argument and was soon superseded by the next Lieutenant-Governor. He was James Johnston, a volatile, self-opinionated despot, under whom relations with the jurats reached their nadir. In October 1763, Johnston wrote to

66 Lameire, pp. 135–7, from which remaining references in this paragraph are taken. The ordinance was dated 17 October 1757.

67 Lameire, p. 137.

68 Ibid.

69 NA CO 174/1/52–64; 174/3/28–9.

70 NA CO 174/1/52–64.

71 NA CO 174/3/28–9.

Lord Halifax, the new Secretary of State for the Southern Department, setting out his own erratic vision of Minorca's commercial potential. He did not support the expulsion of the French and dismissed the so-called British merchants as 'second hand Traders' from Gibraltar; they were newly-arrived opportunists, 'only Tavern, and Wine-house keepers' and 'travelling Merchants'.[72] He wanted trade open to all, dropping the name of Lord Egremont who had confided in Johnston his wish for a free port to rival Leghorn.[73] A wiser man than Johnston would have realized that a free port without a lazaretto would be ridiculous. The jurats pressed him to restart the building work. Johnston's response was that a lazaretto was 'not only useless but dangerous': it would lead to the landing of infected goods and put the health of the island at risk.[74]

Any comment on this attitude in London was precluded by Johnston's greater misdemeanour, which was to insult the whole populace of Minorca. He did this by telling them that their religious and civil privileges granted by the Treaty of Utrecht had not been ratified by the recent Treaty of Paris, and therefore their continuation depended on the islanders' good behaviour.[75] Johnston was ordered by Halifax to retract this, but the outrage already caused led to his temporary removal to London in the summer of 1764; the barrage of complaints which Johnston had to answer included allegations of the misuse of the estanque and anchorage duties.[76] In his absence, the jurats had ideas for two lazarettos, one at Port Mahon and the other at Ciudadela.[77] The island, during the interregnum, was under the direction of Lieutenant-Colonel Wren, the senior officer remaining; his responsibilities lasted longer than he might have wished, because the officer designated to stand in for Johnston died soon after his arrival.[78] Wren wrote a guarded letter to London, in August 1764, reporting he had taken 'the necessary precautions' against a bad epidemic in Naples.[79] Perhaps, in reality, it was the jurats who had taken the decisions.

In January 1765 Wren was relieved by Colonel Thomas Townshend, an active and able administrator. Within weeks, the island's merchants had sensed a receptive mind and Townshend received an eight-point petition.[80] Three of these points were quarantine issues. The merchants' first complaint was that ships used to arrive for intelligence of the markets, but now they came only when bound there. They attributed this change to rising and exorbitant port charges, including those of quarantine. Secondly, there was no place to air cargoes, because the lazaretto scheme on Quarantine Island, for which materials had been collected, was abandoned by the French. Nothing had been done since the recapture, although anchorage duty was still being levied. Thirdly, their own ships were being forced to do quarantine, even with clean bills of health, on their return to the island from such neighbouring places

72 NA CO 174/3/38–41.

73 Ibid.

74 NA CO 174/3/52–3; 174/19/9; cf. Gregory, p. 78.

75 NA CO 174/1/52–64; 174/19/9.

76 NA CO 174/3/96.

77 NA CO 174/3/98–102; 174/19/17.

78 This was Colonel John Crauford.

79 NA CO 174/3/142.

80 NA CO 174/3/175–6, from which remaining references in this paragraph are taken.

as Majorca and Gibraltar which were then infection-free. Most of these complaints were levelled against the Health Office.

Townshend was wary, at such a delicate juncture, of causing further ill-feeling among the jurats. He therefore sidestepped quarantine and gave his full attention to less contentious and wider issues. The estanque fund was used to make public roads, and work began on building new barracks.[81] The economy of the island was also much on his mind, and he found a fortuitous ally in Lord Hope, who spent a few days on the island to recover his health. While Townshend tried to import corn from Barbary, Hope promised to speak to Lord Halifax about better trading conditions for the merchants.[82] But, almost immediately, Halifax was replaced as Secretary of State by Henry Seymour Conway. In July 1765 Thomas Hope, a relative of his lordship, had a discussion with Conway, which was followed by a memorial arguing several changes to make the island of commercial advantage to Britain, rather than a liability.[83] Although quarantine was not mentioned, many of these points would have repercussions in that area. For instance, the plan was very much anti-French and confrontational. The free port of Mahon and the island's other harbours would be put on the same footing as regards the French as the free port of Marseilles was to the British; in other words, the French would be as much hindered in Minorca as the British were inconvenienced at Marseilles. It was remembered, or alleged, that in the recent war the town of Marseilles had advanced huge sums to prosecute the expedition against Minorca.[84] Endless opportunities were now looming for disruptive, retaliatory quarantine.

While Thomas Hope tackled Conway, Townshend wrote to Sir Richard Lyttelton, the island's absentee Governor, with upbeat ideas for the island's economy. He felt that Minorca 'in Point of Situation for Trade ... has the Advantage of every other Port of the Mediterranean' and 'might become the General Magazine of Commerce'.[85] He had imported two hundredweight of cotton from Malta and about 80,000 young mulberry trees to diversify the island's economy.[86] In July 1765 Townshend was appointed one of two commissioners to enquire into the complaints against Johnston, and he passed the autumn of 1765 at the peak of his achievements.[87] But before the end of the year, Johnston was back in the island as Lieutenant-Governor. The allegations against him were still being examined, but his presence in London was no longer necessary. The most turbulent episode in the island's administration was about to begin.

81 NA CO 174/3/177–8.

82 NA CO 174/3/203, 209–11.

83 NA CO 174/3/175, 223–4. Other proposals included a Custom House and a Court of Merchants to settle differences among themselves.

84 Ibid.; NA CO 174/19/50.

85 NA CO 174/3/232–3.

86 Ibid.

87 NA CO 174/3/259. It was not all good news for Townshend. He was sent a severe reprimand for continuing the barracks project without authority from London.

Johnston versus the jurats

His sojourn in London had worked to Johnston's advantage; his integrity was intact and he made influential contacts. He probably returned to Minorca with a hint and a nod that the accusations of personal misconduct against him would be dismissed – as they eventually were. His first move was to turn against Townshend, whose stint in the island was at an end. In a letter to the Marquess of Rockingham, head of the coalition ministry in London, Johnston dismissed Townshend as 'a casual Commandant' who had begun the barracks without authority.[88] Johnston stopped all work on the grounds of lack of money. It ruffled him that Townshend had been given investigative powers in the matter of the jurats' complaints, and elsewhere Johnston accused him of conducting more of an inquisition than a free and open enquiry.[89]

But Johnston was experiencing a change of heart. While still brash and arrogant towards the jurats, he realized that the proposals to improve the island's trade were gaining favour in London. The initiative had passed from Conway to Rockingham, and it was in Johnston's interests to go along with it. He now accepted the case for commercial revival and the full apparatus of quarantine which supported it. His first constructive move, in December 1765, was to send London a proposal for an island Chamber of Health.[90] From the most reactionary of soldier-governors there now appeared an idea of some wisdom, showing a grasp in principle of what was needed if the island were ever to meet the standards and requirements of other Mediterranean free ports. But the detail was flawed and in the presentation of his case Johnston reverted to type. Before insulting the jurats, he accused his own predecessors of neglecting to argue for a Chamber which would have obviated the 'irregularities and abuses' of the present magistrates, who claimed a prescriptive right to manage health. They ordain quarantines, wrote Johnston, 'without proper Reflection, and give Prattick in a very arbitrary manner'. Worse, they regarded themselves as gentlemen and would not submit to Governors' wishes, although it was the latter who received Orders from the Privy Council as to how quarantine should be laid. This, of course, was the crux of the problem.

Johnston went on to attack the three jurats of health as 'ignorant and illiterate ... Viz^{t}. The first a Burgess, the second a Farmer, & the third a Mechanic.' There were also two subaltern jurats who could 'neither write nor read'. Here, Johnston played a curious card, claiming that it was the arbitrary behaviour of the jurats which occasioned the rigid quarantine against Minorca in nearby ports. This argument made him appear almost a Francophile, and his knowledge was inaccurate. Did not the French, claimed Johnston, immediately institute a Chamber of Health run by the Governor and *intendants*, to take such matters out of the hands of the jurats? But the jurats had been the *intendants*, to the exclusion of the Governor. And did not this lead to Minorca being in free pratique with the neighbouring ports? With Marseilles handling quarantine, it could hardly have been otherwise. When the French were

88 NA CO 174/3/264.

89 NA CO 174/3/257.

90 NA CO 174/3/256–8, from which all references in the next three paragraphs are taken.

removed, continued Johnston, the jurats resumed control of health 'in their old wrong-headed way' and the quarantines were re-imposed. The only way, argued Johnston, to avoid the complaints of the merchants, to maintain good relations with other ports, and to keep the plague at bay, was to establish a Chamber of Health on the lines he went on to describe.

The Chamber was to be established in Mahon, composed of four *intendants* (Johnston was keen to keep the French term), a secretary, a physician and a surgeon; this body would be chaired by the Commander-in-Chief, who was also the Lieutenant-Governor, as president of the Board. The latter would choose (Johnston used the verb 'elect') the *intendants*, three of whom would be inhabitants of Mahon, one an English merchant, the second a Minorcan merchant, and the third a Mahon burgess. These men, with the Commander-in-Chief, would effectively form the Chamber. The fourth *intendant* would live at Ciudadela and be subordinate in all respects to his colleagues. Every year one *intendant* would stand down, his replacement being elected (this time the verb was correct) by the others and approved by the Commander-in-Chief. 'And as this Employment ... cannot be very laborious, ... the Emoluments to be received shall be the same as they are at present, which they shall divide as the Commander in Chief shall direct, who shall diminish or increase them, as future Exigencies may require.'

This was hopelessly woolly and paid only lip-service to the systems in Marseilles and Leghorn. No mention was made of a lazaretto, a concomitant institution to any Board of Health. The French had relied on the one at Marseilles, but this was not now an option. The Chamber would be no more than a device to wrest control of quarantine from the jurats. Power would now lie with the Lieutenant-Governor and for that reason alone the neighbouring ports would have maintained, or even increased, their restrictions. Johnston had the argument back to front. It was not the jurats in charge of policy who would have bothered the French and the Italians; it was the representative of the Crown. If the jurats knew little in these matters, the British knew less. Furthermore, Johnston had no suggestions in his paper as to whether quarantine policy should originate in London or Minorca. No doubt he suspected that London would interfere, even if he were allowed to set limits for vessels' detention. For Marseilles and Leghorn, where the Boards thought for themselves, any smack of British involvement, any suspicion that policy might be arranged for reasons other than the prevention of plague, would have doomed ships from Minorca to inordinate delays. Gibraltar had been tolerated by the Board at Marseilles because they had something to gain. But there was no benefit from Minorca for the Mediterranean clique. Novice dabblers were far from welcome.

These proposals found no favour in London and in March 1766 the Privy Council resolved to restore the 'full and free' management of health to the magistrates of Mahon on the footing which had existed before the brief reoccupation by France.[91] But as this matter touched upon the allegations of the jurats against Johnston, and as the other complaints were still being examined, the decision was not relayed to Minorca at that time. Meanwhile, the Rockingham administration were concerned with improving the island's economy on the initiative which had started with Townshend.

91 NA CO 174/4/15.

In July 1766 'Hints relative to the Improvement of Minorca' were assembled by Edmund Burke, Rockingham's private secretary, for general discussion.[92] The motive was partly retaliatory. For instance, a 15-per-cent levy was suggested on all foreign goods brought into Minorca to match the same duty imposed on British goods carried to Spain. A kind of Board of Trade was mooted for the island, with a salaried president, 'as His Majesty has not such a Spot of Ground besides [that is, elsewhere], situate among so many different Powers, and therefore admitting of such variety of Connections and Commerce, and [so] suited to be a place … of Business in the Mediterranean'.[93] One aspect of this business was the Turkey trade, and a proper lazaretto was suggested for returning ships; if they went to Minorca the island would receive the income from quarantine which was currently enjoyed elsewhere.[94]

As the argument for a lazaretto was now on the agenda in London, Johnston found himself in the uncomfortable position of supporting a measure which he had previously dismissed as useless and dangerous. Another incentive to Johnston to conform was that his alleged misapplication of the anchorage duty would grow increasingly insignificant if the money were now directed to its proper use. The Privy Council, never enamoured of its inquisitorial role, were only too happy to file anchorage duty under 'Points which do not seem to press'.[95]

Towards a lazaretto

In April 1767 Johnston sent Lord Shelburne, the new Secretary of State for the Southern Department, a plan of Quarantine Island.[96] This indicated progress already made in building a lazaretto, the additions he proposed when enough money had been raised, and accounts of the anchorage duty. From these facts, 'your Lordship may see, that it never was my Intention to pocket that Produce, notwithstanding all that has been most maliciously hinted … I have laid out, and done more in the short Time I have [commanded] … out of that Fund, than all my Predecessors, and all the Jurats, that have had the handling of it since it was originally establish'd'.[97] That boast was true, but only because Johnston was the first Lieutenant-Governor in a position to implement the proposals accepted by the Privy Council in 1753, before the occupation by France had intervened.

Events now progressed slowly, but Johnston was not wholly to blame. For one thing, receipts from the anchorage duty were modest. A total of some 90 dollars (of which 22 had been raised under Townshend) had to meet the expenses of the Inspector of Public Works, who employed bricklayers and labourers on the new lazaretto and struggled to find money for the doors, windows and grates.[98] A second factor was that Johnston was seriously busy in other directions. The same strategic

92 NA CO 174/4/43–5.

93 Ibid.

94 Ibid.

95 NA CO 174/1/49–51.

96 NA CO 174/4/128–30.

97 Ibid.

98 NA CO 174/4/133–4.

location which made Minorca so attractive for military purposes introduced less welcome diplomatic issues. A Venetian squadron arrived from Algiers, with the two countries suddenly at war.[99] As Algiers supplied Minorca with corn, what should be done if the Venetians wanted the island as a base? Then the Corsicans wanted to cruise against the French. Could they use Minorca as a refuge and a port to bring in prizes?[100] Johnston showed himself level-headed and made the Privy Council even less disposed to sacrifice him for the sake of the jurats. Confrontations with the islanders diminished somewhat, and Johnston applied himself to meet the recommendations approved 14 years earlier by the Privy Council. In some respects he met them rather loosely, 'borrowing' money from the estanque fund to finance the fabric of the lazaretto.[101] Even then funds were tight. The conflated figures for estanque and anchorage duties for the year to April 1769 amounted to only the equivalent in sterling of £340.[102]

While Johnston reported his slow progress in completing the lazaretto, he was rewarded in July 1769 by a clear hint from Lord Weymouth, who had succeeded Shelburne, that many of the complaints against him had been found frivolous and vexatious.[103] At that point, an emboldened Johnston appears to have resurrected the question of an island Chamber of Health. He wrote to Weymouth reiterating the rationale for his proposal, which was free of any self-interest.[104] He had never interfered, he claimed, with 'the Business of the Health'; all he wanted was

> a proper Set of People, who may form a regular Chamber of Health as in other Places: and who, from their Permanency, a better Education, a more extensive knowledge of Trade, and a little Geography, may, by keeping up a Correspondence with the other Chambers of Health in the Mediterranean and the Levant, make themselves Masters of their Business, and bring their own Chamber into some Repute, which cannot be expected upon the Footing it now is, from the annual Change and Ignorance of the Jurats.[105]

There was a new suggestion here: that of participating in the network of correspondence between health boards. There had been nothing in the gaunt outline of his earlier proposal which had recommended this fundamental step. But as there were no Chambers of Health in the Levant, Johnston was still displaying a less than full grasp of the Mediterranean scene. He went on to hope that the lazaretto in Minorca would be finished that autumn, and looked forward to poaching trade from Leghorn.[106]

Within a month, Johnston was back on the attack. He was now less reluctant to criticize the jurats. In early September 1769 he wrote to Weymouth, complaining

99 NA CO 174/4/196.

100 NA CO 174/5/93.

101 NA CO 174/5/106–7. The amount borrowed was some 747 dollars.

102 Ibid. That was the conversion of nearly 4,700 dollars.

103 NA CO 174/5/114.

104 NA CO 174/5/124–5.

105 Ibid.

106 Ibid.

of the contraband trade in tobacco to Spain.[107] If the management of health was left in the hands of the jurats, he warned, 'for their own Profit they will not fail to wink at Breaches of the Quarantine Laws, of which at present I have daily Proofs.'[108] In October he wanted the smugglers to carry bills of health, which he claimed would induce Spain to lift its quarantine against Minorca.[109] This would help the island's export trade, as it shipped large amounts of corn to Spain from Barbary, Sicily and Sardinia. But the jurats, he alleged, would not insist that bills were issued. He now envisaged a Chamber where the members (none of them jurats) were salaried to a modest degree from the fees for quarantine and bills of health.[110] Income from these sources was now more than £100 a year and expected to increase when the lazaretto was finished. He would not object to any surplus being distributed among the jurats, as the perquisites from the health office were their only motive, he claimed, for wanting its management.[111]

In March 1770 Weymouth wrote to Johnston that the many charges against him had at last been heard and dismissed, and the Privy Council had confidence in his 'Moderation, Affability & Gentleness'.[112] These were not qualities with which Johnston was conspicuously favoured. In the matter of a Chamber of Health, Weymouth apologized for his silence. His predecessor had ignored a letter written by Johnston on 11 July 1767, on the grounds it might prejudice the general enquiry into matters of health.[113] In fact, on this topic Johnston had not been wholly vindicated, and Weymouth sent him a new Order in Council which reaffirmed that the jurats were to manage health without his interference.[114] With surprising frankness, Weymouth explained that he had distanced himself from this collective decision. He had laid the plan for a Chamber before the King, arguing that 'the important Concern' of quarantine should be vested in Johnston.[115] Even more surprising, therefore, was Johnston's retort to Weymouth, on 21 April 1770, that he wanted nothing to do personally with any Chamber of Health as it would lead to 'numberless Disputes and Coolness' with the captains of warships.[116] Johnston was now a wiser man, having dealt with the Venetians and Corsicans. The good news for Weymouth was that Johnston had now finished the lazaretto according to the plan sent to Shelburne in April 1767. Only two landing stages remained to be built.[117]

It is impossible to know the scale or style of the completed lazaretto. It is not even clear whether the 'plan' sent to London had included an elevation. For reasons which will be discussed elsewhere in this study, the layout of Johnston's building has not survived among the many plans relating to Minorca in the National Archives. Perhaps

107 NA CO 174/5/128. The route was from Ciudadela via Majorca.

108 Ibid.

109 NA CO 174/5/130.

110 Ibid.

111 Ibid.

112 NA CO 174/6/5–11.

113 Ibid.

114 Ibid.

115 Ibid.

116 NA CO 174/6/34–6.

117 Ibid.

even the name lazaretto was too grand, and it seems very doubtful that features or facilities were specifically modelled on any of the Mediterranean exemplars. The island's nineteenth-century historian referred to only ten warehouses for goods, although that may not be right, as Johnston announced proudly to Weymouth that the building was perfectly convenient for both goods and passengers.[118] The construction of the lazaretto was in the hands of Joseph Soler, Inspector of Public Works.[119] His experience in quarantine is unknown. That the lazaretto cost relatively little is certain, but the accounting processes for estanque and anchorage duties make it difficult to arrive at a final figure: the books were kept in dollars, reals and doubloons; the accounting year ended in April before changing in the early 1770s to 31 December; and the amounts transferred from the estanque tax to the much smaller anchorage duty were not always apparent. Only one thing is clear – the most the lazaretto could have cost was several hundred pounds, and on that scale of expenditure it was no more than a makeshift structure of limited use.

International distractions

To Johnston's dismay, quarantine in Minorca became embroiled in another round of political and diplomatic issues. This time it was the Russian fleet, returning in July 1770 with wounded seamen from war against Turkey.[120] In the same month, Johnston put into quarantine a large Danish fleet which had bombarded Algiers.[121] At first it was the Russians who worried him more. The sick and wounded continually arrived in ships from the Levant with no bills of health; whether or not the Minorcans were at risk from this, Spain lost no time in putting ships from the island under 40 days' quarantine.[122] Then it was the turn of the Danes to exercise Johnston's patience. They had claimed only 30 or 40 sailors unwell on board, but when given pratique after the usual interval for warships, they put ashore 600 sick men.[123] At no stage in his correspondence with London did Johnston allude to the usefulness or even the existence of his new lazaretto, in the context of these troublesome allies.

Early in 1771 Johnston was promoted to Major-General and put in command of the 9th Regiment of Dragoons in Ireland.[124] But he was not destined to return to a military arena. Lieutenant-General Mostyn, appointed Governor of Minorca in his place, disliked the island and was soon too sick to do his duties.[125] Although ill himself, in London, Johnston agreed to go back to Minorca.[126] Before he arrived, the island was under the command of Lieutenant-Colonel John Barlow, who was immediately exercised by a further problem with the Russians. As there was the

118 Gregory, p. 143, quoting D. Pedro Riudavets y Tudury.
119 NA CO 174/6/38–9.
120 NA CO 174/6/68–9.
121 NA CO 174/6/77–8.
122 NA CO 174/6/80, 89, 143.
123 NA CO 174/6/89.
124 NA CO 174/7/5.
125 NA CO 174/7/137.
126 NA CO 174/7/163.

prospect of peace between Russia and the Turkish Porte, Barlow wondered whether the quarantine restrictions against Russian ships should not be made tougher. He wrote, in August 1772, that the Chamber of Health planned to impose 40 days' quarantine, or even not let the Russians land if there was any sickness amongst them. Did this have approval in London?[127] The answer to Barlow was a typical example of Privy Council evasion: the Russian warships were to be treated no differently from merchant ships, in conformity with Privy Council Orders of which Barlow was aware.[128] It was true that the Privy Council sent copies of Orders to Minorca which affected the quarantine of ships arriving in Britain from the Mediterranean.[129] This was useful, as some of those ships sailed from Minorca. But not for some years had the Privy Council suggested that restrictions thought necessary for London would be equally appropriate at Mahon.

The other point to arise from Barlow's letter was his reference to the Chamber of Health as if this was actually in existence. He must have been dignifying the jurats with an unofficial title, because the Chamber was never created. Mostyn had shown no interest in the topic, and any feelings which Barlow might have expressed were forestalled by the re-arrival of Johnston before the end of 1772. These were not good years for quarantine in Minorca. The impetus to improve trade and commerce had been lost and the island was embroiled in international politics. As if the Russians in themselves were not problem enough, the Dey of Algiers was stopping all corn exports to Christian countries on the grounds that the Russian consul at Mahon, who was also Captain of the Port, had given corn to the Russians under the pretext of supplying the garrison.[130] Furthermore, Johnston came back a disgruntled man. He had long coveted, and been denied, personal terms which were granted to others. In particular, the title of Vice-Admiral of Minorca, important in the context of the eponymous prize court, had been withheld from Johnston but was given to Mostyn.[131] It was far from Johnston's intention to be constructive; he made no more overtures for a Chamber of Health.

Maintenance of the lazaretto was an ongoing but minor expense from the anchorage duty. In 1773 the duty realized nearly 240 dollars but only some 24 dollars were required for the 'repair' of the lazaretto and pratique house.[132] The larger sum of 45 dollars was granted to the Keeper of Quarantine Island as his salary.[133] In 1774 income had fallen to 208 dollars, but was augmented by a 'House Rent' of 7 dollars from Quarantine Island.[134] Outgoings on the lazaretto stayed much the same. What is interesting is that no income was apparently received from the institutions

127 NA CO 174/7/222–3.

128 NA CO 174/7/226.

129 The most recent had been Orders in Council of 5 and 19 October 1770, acknowledged by Johnston on 20 November (NA CO 174/6/143).

130 NA CO 174/7/3. The news reached London from 'Consul Fraser', not from Minorca.

131 NA CO 174/7/17. Johnston was later to complain also that his successor, Murray, had come on terms which he (Johnston) had always been denied (NA CO 174/9/5).

132 NA CO 174/8/55–6.

133 Ibid.

134 NA CO 174/9/7–8.

of quarantine, including the lazaretto, to help balance the books. These revenues seem to have continued, doubtless to Johnston's chagrin, as perquisites of office for the jurats.

The 1774 accounts were the last ones to bear Johnston's signature. In the following January he was succeeded by Lieutenant-General Murray who was soon preoccupied with military considerations. But even these impinged upon quarantine, especially when France entered the War of American Independence in 1778. Now that French shipping was fair game for British privateers, and given that Minorca had a Vice-Admiralty Court, the island was well placed to provide ships under letters of marque to plunder the trade of Marseilles.[135] When the Spaniards and then the Dutch joined the war against Britain, the Minorcan privateers had very rich pickings. It is reported that Murray built a second lazaretto at Fornells to cater for the large number of ships captured from the Levant, but that must be too grand a name for another collection of huts.[136] It seems unlikely that Murray took more than token precautions against the import of plague. There was, however, a significant health risk, according to the perceptions of the period, in allowing ships from the Levant to dock and unload without stringent measures for airing their cargoes. London was fully aware of the situation in Minorca because Murray returned lists of prizes. One of these for example, dated January 1779, lists five ships bound for Marseilles, of which two were from Smyrna and one from Alexandria, with cotton or cotton wool.[137] All these highly susceptible cargoes were taken to Mahon. But the Privy Council did not express the least concern over this, let alone offer guidance or instructions to Murray as to how cotton should be 'cleansed'.

When Minorca was recaptured by the Spanish and French in 1782, the former attempted to make quarantine more conformable with Mediterranean practice. As the Spaniards had been strangely remiss in providing proper quarantine facilities on their own mainland, the move can be interpreted as a telling indictment of how bad the British lazaretto had become. In 1785 facilities for passengers were either added or improved, but the site was too cramped for expansion.[138] A decision was therefore taken, in 1793, to build a new lazaretto on the peninsula (now an island) to the east of the existing site.[139] Before it was finished, the British had begun their third and final occupation of Minorca, beginning in 1798. In this brief four-year period, the island was first governed by Lieutenant-General the Hon. Sir Charles Stuart, who reconfirmed the traditional responsibilities of the jurats, including their control of public health. He was succeeded in 1801 by Lieutenant-General Henry Fox, who had served under Stuart as Lieutenant-Governor in the previous year.

Fox ran into immediate trouble with the jurats in matters of quarantine. Despite Stuart reaffirming the spheres of authority, he was accused of having taken control

135 Gregory, p. 155.

136 Ibid.

137 NA CO 174/12/27.

138 Gregory, p. 143; B. Velimirovic, 'The quarantine stations at Mahon, Menorca', *Pratique*, 17/3–4 (1992), 80.

139 Gregory, pp. 93, 143; Panzac, p. 248.

of public health and imposing his absolute will.[140] There were also many complaints against the attitude of British naval commanders.[141] Fox recognized his mistake and was soon the most responsible of British administrators in all aspects of quarantine. Unfortunately he had less than two years in which to make his mark. He informed London in 1800 that only a quarter of the new lazaretto begun by the Spaniards had been finished, and he resurrected the arguments for a Board of Health.[142] In doing so he was necessarily critical of the jurats, and there were echoes of Johnston in his accusations of their incompetence. For him, it was their inattention to duty which put the navy at risk, rather than the navy endangering the safety of the island.[143] But there was still no understanding of the kind of Board which would have been acceptable in the main ports where the Minorcans were accustomed to trade. Fox could only conceive of a Board under the presidency of the Governor, and any such body would have run into the difficulties which, less than 30 years later, were to infuriate the British from their base in Malta. So the jurats won the day, and the British conceded Minorca with the worst possible record of quarantine mismanagement. Their Mediterranean neighbours would not forget.

Complications

When they resumed control of the island, the determination of the Spaniards to provide Minorca with a larger lazaretto did not diminish. For many years there were two lazarettos, as the site on Quarantine Island was not vacated until 1817.[144] A plan of Mahon harbour showing, *inter alia*, Quarantine Island was published in 1803 by Thomas Walsh (Illustration 5.1), showing an L-shaped ground plan for the buildings.[145] How far that represented the footprint of the British lazaretto is impossible to know, as the Spanish had enlarged and altered it. Earlier maps do not inspire confidence. A 'Sketch map' of 1772, including Quarantine Island, shows a large building in the middle of it, virtually a rectangle, while a map of 1781 shows no building at all.[146] The handsome elevation shown in an engraving of 1814 in the *Naval Chronicle* (Illustration 5.2) was presumably part of the Spanish enlargement. The accompanying text mentioned 'apartments for the accommodation of persons coming from places liable to the plague, or other contagious diseases, and warehouses to receive goods'.[147]

140 Lameire, p. 713.

141 Lameire, pp. 713–14.

142 Gregory, p. 143.

143 Ibid.

144 Panzac, p. 248; Velimirovic, p. 80.

145 The large naval hospital on another nearby island had been built in 1711 to replace an earlier one (Armstrong, p. 20).

146 BL Maps K. Top. 74–14; there is faint evidence of an open area within the rectangle approached from the side of the building facing George Town. The 1781 map was by John Armstrong (BL Maps 188.o.2 (20)).

147 *Naval Chronicle*, vol. 23 (1814, Part 2), p. 136.

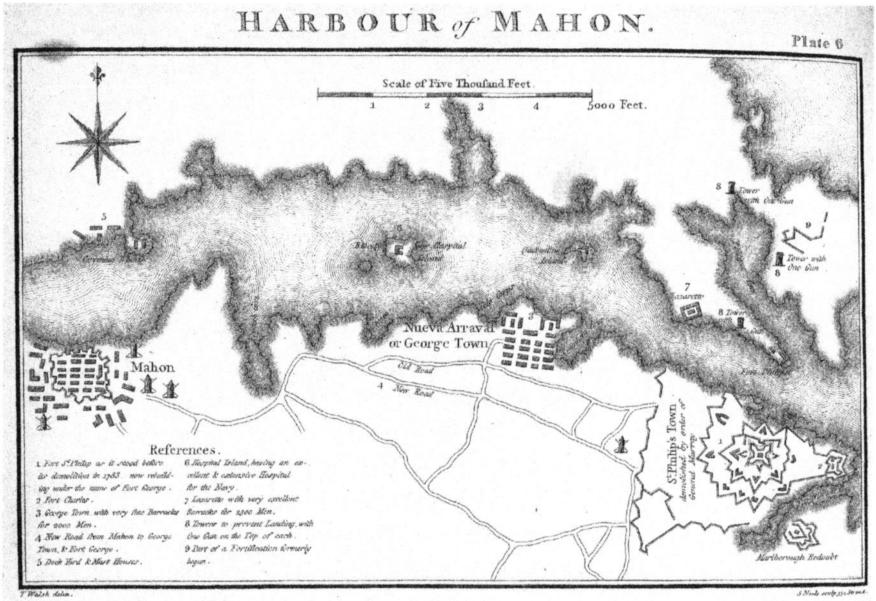

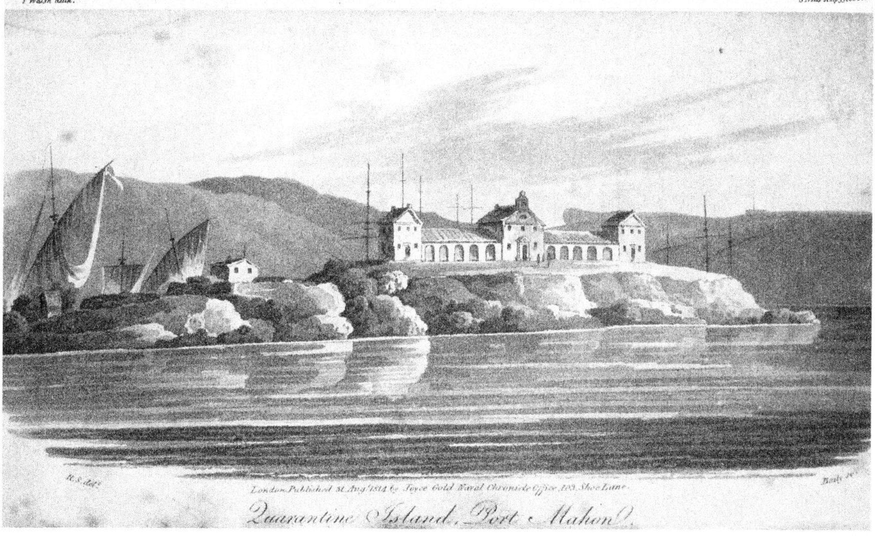

Illustration 5.1 & 5.2 **Map including Quarantine Island near Port Mahon, 1803, plus elevation of its enlarged lazaretto, 1814. The land lazaretto (no. 7 on the map) was virtually a barracks.**

Ralph Green, an army doctor, referred to merchandise being received in 'pavilions … built of wood and jalousied, where a current of air passes through and over every thing; within, the goods are piled on platforms perfectly defended from wet, but fully exposed to the atmospheric air'.[148] Green thought the lazaretto was excellent, and the Royal Navy were equally impressed. In 1812, when Port Mahon was open to British warships, the lazaretto was deemed 'very capacious' and in 1813 it accommodated the 44th Foot.[149] But Green's words, and the experiences of the military, call into question which of the lazarettos they meant. The navy, in 1813, anchored 'in the Quarantine Harbour, Cala Taulena as it was called – a cove over which the Lazaretto was situated'.[150] (This was called Philipet Cove on Walsh's map.) That must, then, be a reference to the second lazaretto, although historians believe it was not finished until 1817, the year when the first lazaretto was abandoned.[151] But this is at variance with Walsh, who visited Minorca in 1800. Walsh wrote that 'nearly opposite to Fort George [built on the ruins of St Philip's], is the Lazaretto, encompassed with high walls, and containing excellent barracks for two thousand five hundred men. There is a second lazaretto built in a small island in the harbour, which is appropriated to the performance of quarantine'.[152] The first sentence conflicts not only with the historians but with the comment of Fox in 1800 (mentioned above) that the new lazaretto was only a quarter built. Walsh would appear to be supported by Sir Lucas Pepys who cited 'the excellent Lazaretto on the island of Minorca ... having double walls of thirty feet high', as a model for Britain.[153] That recommendation was also made in 1800, but unfortunately Pepys is misleading. He had no personal knowledge of the island and had simply been looking at Johnston's plan for a lazaretto, sent to London in 1767, which may or may not have conformed with the building eventually erected on Quarantine Island.

A solution to part of the problem may lie in the definition of a lazaretto. Walsh maintained that only the subsidiary lazaretto on the island was intended for quarantine. Indeed, he implied that the main one was no more than a barracks. There may have come a point (around 1817) when a facility originally intended for military purposes, including military quarantine, acquired a largely civilian use, at which time the older site was superseded.[154] But that does not explain the curious comment by Fox in 1800, about the new lazaretto being so far from completion. Only one thing is clear – whatever the date of the second lazaretto, there is no reason to credit the British with any meaningful hand in its completion.

---

148 *British Parliamentary Papers* [*BPP*], vol. 6 (1824), pp. 165ff. Green was stationed in Malta in 1813 and his experience of Minorca was probably at around that date.

149 M.A. Lewis (ed.), *A Narrative of My Professional Adventures (1790–1839) by Sir William Henry Dillon* (2 vols, Navy Records Society, 1953–56), vol. 2, pp. 201, 251ff.

150 Lewis, p. 251.

151 Panzac, p. 248; Velimirovic, p. 80

152 T. Walsh, *Journal of the late Campaign in Egypt* ... 2nd edn (London, 1803), p. 16.

153 C. Maclean, *Remarks on the British Quarantine laws* ... (London, 1823), p. 18.

154 This civilian use came about slowly. Velimirovic, p. 80, states the 'New Lazaretto' was occupied by English soldiers in 1800, by coastguards in 1803 and by Catalan troops in 1809.

Postscript

Minorca was not developed by Britain for quarantine purposes because politicians never made up their mind why the island was needed. This was an echo of the problem at Gibraltar. There was an initial military requirement for a safe harbour in winter and a base to intercept a French fleet sailing from Toulon to the Straits. But once Malta had been taken, that island became 'infinitely preferable' in the eyes of Alexander Ball (despite Nelson's reservations) to Minorca.[155] In the intervening years, the potential of Minorca was always promised and never realized. James Lind made the famous comment that Minorca had all the advantages of Gibraltar, and in a much higher degree, and none of its disadvantages.[156] As Lind had served in Minorca as a naval surgeon, he knew the island was impossible to defend, unlike Gibraltar, against a determined enemy; it is therefore difficult to understand the nature of the benefits which Lind, and so many other people, envisaged.

The idea that Minorca might be useful for the commercial aspirations of Britain assumed that London had some strategic purpose in the Mediterranean. To the very end, even after the acquisition of Malta, there was a school of thought that Minorca might yet prove its value. John Jackson, writing in 1804, argued for the possession of both islands. 'The Minorkeens are a trading people, have a great number of shipping, and through them England would have enjoyed the greatest part of the Barbary trade, as the Minorkeens have always been accustomed to it'.[157] But the British had no interest in engrossing the trade with North Africa. Neither had they intention of developing Minorca for the Levant trade, although some sectors of the public thought otherwise. The view of Lord Raby, in 1708, has already been mentioned. When the island fell to the French in 1756, it was as if the Levant trade had suffered a fatal wound. A satirical pamphleteer lamented the effect in London: 'many Turkey Merchants, who us'd to have twenty Fires blazing at once … now are forced to do their Business at Coffee-Houses, for Want of Money to buy Coals at Home. Their Wives call aloud for no Coaches, though their own are laid down, their Maid-Servants … sift their own Cinders …'[158]

Such feelings can be well understood. Minorca offered a safe harbour, not too distant from the main sea-lane to Gibraltar. In the mid-eighteenth century, when Britain-bound ships with foul bills of health were obliged by statute to perform quarantine in one of the established (and named) Mediterranean lazarettos, it made sense for the British to have a facility of their own creation.[159] But the idea for that, buried away in a discussion paper of Edmund Burke, called for a conviction that the island could be defended against attack, and a massive endorsement from the Levant Company that their ships would agree to go there. The first criterion was

155 NA CO 158/8/1–4.

156 Quoted in Conn, p. 264.

157 J. Jackson, *Reflections on the Commerce of the Mediterranean* … (London, 1804), p. 8.

158 *Two Very Singular Addresses to the People of England: Faithfully printed from the Originals, 'after performing a Quarantine of more than Forty Days.'* (London, 1757), pp. 5–6.

159 The statute was 26 Geo. II, c.18 (s.12).

impossible and the second did not really happen. Minorca had no place in the Levant Company's strategic planning. A military historian, in 1752, referred to 'the frequent touching of our homeward-bound Levanters here ...', but that situation (if it were true) would have ended a year later with the statute mentioned above.[160] The Levant Company used the established lazarettos at Leghorn and Malta, not simply because of the Act, but from convenience. Malta was exactly on the sailing route, and while Leghorn was a considerable deviation, the Company had many business contacts there, as well as the opportunity to load more cargo. The position changed somewhat when the Mediterranean lazarettos were closed to British shipping in the French Wars, but as Minorca had failed as a free port, so it missed out as an entrepôt. The island offered few cargoes of value for London to supplement the cotton already on the ship.

The Levant Company would also have been aware that any lazaretto at Minorca could not have survived only off the income from the Company's own ships. They were just too infrequent. Therefore, the British Government would have asked the Company to subsidize the upkeep, which they would have been most reluctant to agree to, or the lazaretto would have touted for a more general trade. But as the British would never have agreed to a Board of Health independent of the Lieutenant-Governor, the integrity of a lazaretto would always have been compromised in the eyes of the French and Italians who made all the running about quarantine in the Mediterranean. For the Levant Company, Minorca, in terms of quarantine, was no more suitable than Gibraltar, and it was a matter of commercial indifference to them when possession of the island was lost. As long as Britain held the Rock, convoys could be protected against the Barbary corsairs.

160 Armstrong, p. 22.

Chapter Six

The Messina Crisis, and Legislation, 1728–1754

False alarm

It will come as no surprise that Britain, without a strategic policy for the Mediterranean, had no standing regulations in the early eighteenth century for dealing with infection from the countries which bordered it. When the Marseilles crisis was deemed at an end, the Privy Council sighed with relief and removed quarantine from their agenda. Ships of the Levant Company slipped into London with little formality and the Commissioners of Customs reverted to orthodox business. True, the *Discourse* of Richard Mead continued to appear in new editions, but the public could now view the prospect of plague with philosophical detachment because it had failed to cross the Channel. Whether the national defences deserved all the credit for keeping it at bay was not the point. What mattered was that another Great Plague had somehow been averted, and the defences could be reintroduced if danger threatened again.

For no very good reason, complacency ended in 1728. Russell attributed this to 'the plague being in foreign parts', but as there were foreign parts where the plague was more or less permanent, this vagueness is not enlightening.[1] The Privy Council, it would appear, were startled by information, accurate or otherwise, that the Ionian Islands and the Morea were badly infected, and this region was the source of currants, one of the nation's favourite ingredients. On 4 May 1728 an Order was issued for all ships from those places, especially Zante and Corfu, to perform 40 days' quarantine.[2] Within five days a Bill was before the Commons. Despite a few doubts at Committee stage, the Bill was propelled through all the stages; the Lords made no amendments and before the end of the month (on 28 May) it had gained royal assent, and Parliament was then prorogued.[3]

Given the tight timescale, and the muddle of Acts which had accompanied the scare from Marseilles, it was to be expected that the new statute would be less than perfect.[4] The main surprise was that it omitted to spell out the prerogative of George II (then in his first regnal year) to make Orders for the control of quarantine. But the Act reintroduced the King's power to prohibit commerce with infected countries

1 P. Russell, *A Treatise of the Plague* ... (London, 1791), p. 444.

2 National Archives [NA] PC 2/90/303.

3 *Journal of the House of Commons* [*JHC*], vol. 21, pp. 157, 166–9, 172, 177–9, 181–2; Russell, p. 444.

4 The Act was 1 Geo. II, c.13, from which all references in this paragraph are taken unless otherwise stated.

for one year, provided that any Proclamation to that effect was issued before 24 June 1729, and allowed him to bar entry to individuals. There was no continuation, however, of the royal power to have ships burnt and not a hint of reintroducing the measures for compulsory removal of people, and setting up lines, which had been repealed after the earlier Act. But if Britain should become infected, the King could prevent boats of less than 20 tons burthen from leaving port without security; the opportunity to hit smuggling was, once again, too good to miss. As Russell noticed, this was the last Act to insist on goods being opened and aired *after* the period of quarantine, and it was within the competence of the Customs Commissioners to discharge cargoes when airing had been done.[5] There was no mention of enumerated goods. Penalties under the Act included death as a felon for a master who failed to disclose plague in his ship, for a person refusing to go to, or escaping from, a lazaretto, and for an incompetent or corrupt official who let persons or goods depart without licence. Fines for various misdemeanours ranged from £200 to £500, and ships and goods could be forfeited if the rules of a Proclamation were broken.[6] The Act was to be in force for two years, beginning 1 June 1728.[7]

At this stage, there is evidence of Viscount Townshend, Secretary of State for the Northern Department, influencing policy. This long-serving minister had once been a diplomat in the Netherlands, and he laid before the Lords of the Committee, on 29 June, the translation of a placard issued only two days earlier, extending quarantine in Holland.[8] It is possible that Dutch alarm had inspired the British reaction in the first place; the placard certainly influenced the Privy Council into widening the area affected. On 4 July 1728 the Proclamation and a new Order were issued together, laying 40 days' quarantine against the Levant, especially Smyrna, and the islands of the Archipelago, as well as the Morea and the Ionian Islands.[9] This was to take effect immediately on the mainland, and four days later in the Channel Islands and Isle of Man. The ports of quarantine were once again London, Portsmouth, Plymouth, Falmouth and Bristol, and at such places in the off-islands as their Governors should direct. Release from quarantine could be effected by certificates from Customs officers or magistrates. Then came the troublesome clause: goods should be aired for one week after quarantine unless the King in Council declared otherwise. The usual list of enumerated goods followed; these had to remain on board, or at a place of airing, until released by the Customs Commissioners (or the Governors or military commanders in the off-islands). That was very much a repetition of the provisions in the Marseilles crisis, and the other clauses in both Order and Proclamation followed the established line.

This was the first time the term Levant had been used in quarantine regulations and the Customs Commissioners asked for a definition. The Privy Council, having

---

5 Russell, p. 445, considered airing after quarantine 'productive of very unnecessary delay, not to mention other inconveniences ...'

6 cf. Russell, p. 445.

7 *Calendar of Treasury Books and Papers* [*CTBP*] (1731–34), p. 146, alludes to an opinion by the Attorney-General as to when the Act expired.

8 NA PC 2/90/322.

9 NA PC 2/90/323–7, from which remaining references in this paragraph are taken.

set up a committee, decided it meant anywhere east of a line from Corfu to Cape Rusata (also called Cape Rozat) on the coast of Barca, and this was the subject of a new Proclamation.[10] The Commissioners also wanted quarantine ports to be designated further north than Bristol and London. The Privy Council obliged with Liverpool and Hull.[11]

It was soon clear that the Council had no stomach for a confrontation with the merchants. The spirit of compromise which had softened the regulations a few years earlier was now evident from the outset. Again, both the length of quarantine and the necessity to air cargoes after its completion generated petitions for relief, mainly from London and Bristol.[12] Forty days' detention for currants, a non-enumerated foodstuff, was clearly nonsense, and airing would have ruined them. The Privy Council quickly realized that the airing clause had run its course; or rather, that if airing was necessary it had to be coterminous with quarantine, and probably on board the ship. This was also the view of the Customs Commissioners who, within days of the Order and Proclamation, warned that airing sheds were expensive and seldom used.[13] Soon the petitions produced a pattern of response: ships could discharge without airing after only 20 days.[14] This applied not only to currants at Bristol but to enumerated goods from Turkey at Stangate Creek.[15] The airing of clothes and bedding for one week on deck, a customary requirement of the Marseilles crisis, was seldom demanded.[16] Two Levant ships, the *Asia* and *Dolphin*, were exempt from quarantine altogether as they had clean bills of health from Smyrna.[17]

Before the end of 1729, it was realized that this was a phoney alarm and merchants lost patience with the cost and inconvenience. But the arguments had to be tactically presented as ministers were unlikely to admit to an overreaction. The first attack was on quarantine against Zante; merchants trading to Venice and the Currant Islands claimed, in a petition of 19 November, that there had been no disease at Zante for the last 18 months.[18] A committee of the Privy Council established that quarantine against Venice and Zante had been discontinued some time ago in Holland and at Hamburg, and so Britain followed suit on 11 December.[19] This was just what the Levant Company hoped to hear, and they petitioned on 22 January 1730 for quarantine to be abandoned altogether for ships with clean bills of health, so trade 'may be upon as easy terms as that of our Neighbours', that is, the Dutch.[20] The

10 NA PC 2/90/327, 338, 341. The alternative 'Rozat' appeared, for instance, in PC 2/92/170.

11 NA PC 2/90/342.

12 *CTBP* (1729–30), pp. 183, 185, 188.

13 NA PC 2/90/342.

14 For example *CTBP* (1729–30), pp. 183, 185, 191, 193 etc.

15 *CTBP* (1729–30), p. 191.

16 One instance, however, is recorded at *CTBP* (1729–30), p. 191.

17 *CTBP* (1729–30), p. 91.

18 NA PC 2/91/84; *CTBP* (1729–30), p. 231 (where the interval without disease is given as 'upwards of a year').

19 NA PC 2/91/103,105; *CTBP* (1729–30), p. 169 (where the Order of Council is given as 8 December, which was the date of the committee's report).

20 NA PC 2/91/138.

committee of the Privy Council were again in agreement and recommended that ships should be assessed at The Hope; if the bill 'should not prove Satisfactory', ships should proceed to Stangate Creek.[21] That was evidently deemed too elaborate by the full Council, as Customs were simply empowered, on 2 February 1730, to discharge from quarantine all ships with clean bills.[22] For another 18 months, the Privy Council dismissed quarantine from their mind, and the merchants went about their business.[23]

Bills of health

The Privy Council Order of 2 February 1730 was the first legal instrument in England to mention the concept of a ship's bill of health in relation to quarantine. This was not just a new departure for Orders and Proclamations: none of the quarantine statutes before 1730 had referred to bills of health and it was to be another 23 years before they were mentioned for the first time in an Act. Yet it was vital for the credibility of Britain that the Privy Council recognized bills as prima facie evidence of health at the start of a voyage. Only when the importance of bills was understood, and confidence placed in their validity, could the British claim to operate a system of quarantine which conformed with best practice in the Mediterranean. If that conformity did not exist, British ships visiting Spanish and Mediterranean ports would suffer extra delay as a mark of disapprobation, no matter what evidence they produced that Britain was free of disease.

This is not say that bills of health (often called patents) had played no earlier role in British commerce. Merchants and indeed travellers had experienced them from the late sixteenth century, when a clean bill acted as a kind of passport to enter or leave a city, either in Europe or the Middle East.[24] The idea of a personal bill of health was enduring. Russell claimed that, before 1754, Customs officers in England paid more attention to the patents of passengers than that of the ship.[25] There is certainly far more early evidence of ships leaving Britain with bills of health than arriving with them. Although they were not necessary for voyages to, say, the Baltic, a clean bill was indispensable for trade with southern Europe. The best record of the issue of bills in the early seventeenth century is in the archives of the Burgh of Edinburgh, where the Council supplied them to ships sailing mainly from Leith to Cadiz with woollens, linen, timber and wax.[26] These bills, apparently in English, recorded not only the good health of the port of departure but also the number of persons on board, usually a mixture of merchants and mariners.

21 NA PC 2/91/147.

22 NA PC 2/91/156; *CTBP* (1729–30), p. 505.

23 The Privy Council register which followed this decision (PC 2/92) is remarkable for having no index entry for ships discharged from quarantine.

24 C. Maclean, *Remarks on the British Quarantine laws …* (London, 1823), p. 5.

25 Russell, p. 414.

26 *Extracts from the Burgh Records of Edinburgh* (Edinburgh, 1927–50): 1626–41, pp. 151, 168–9, 196, 248–9; 1642–45, pp. xlviii, 31–2, 50, 52–4, 60, 101, 130, 133–4, 262, 348.

In England the issue of bills of health was a matter for the Customs service, and a manual of 1732 made it clear that no one could land in Portugal, Spain or any Christian shore of the Mediterranean without one, unless he was prepared to undergo quarantine.[27] The English bill was in a standard form, using Latin as a lingua franca. The document began with the classic salutation of a medieval charter and gave the name of the ship and its master, the port of departure, the country (not the port) of destination, and the number of the crew.[28] A flowery final clause testified (in translation) that 'in this port there currently exists neither pestilence, plague, nor any other dangerous or contagious disease'.[29] The same manual made not the least mention of incoming bills, and how they should be acted upon, which bears out Russell's allegation that they were largely ignored. Abroad, bills of health were issued by the consuls of the Levant Company for British ships sailing direct to England and to Mediterranean ports, such as Leghorn.[30] The form was always the same. The text was in English and gave rather more detail than the bills issued in England. There was emphasis on the British nationality of the ship, its crew and its owners, to meet the requirements of the Navigation Act, while the length of time the port and its region had been healthy was stated with some precision. This accuracy was for the benefit of the Mediterranean Boards of Health. It appears that patents for individual passengers were couched in Italian, the normal language for quarantine and matters of health.[31] Russell pointed out that all English bills of health went further than was necessary, by declaring the place of departure to be free not only of plague but of any other contagious disorder.[32] That view certainly accords with the text quoted above.

In the early 1730s the idea of a ship arriving at a British port with a bill of health which was other than clean was not seriously considered. The Levant Company, still priding itself on keeping England free of plague, prevented its ships from loading enumerated goods for London in Cyprus, Turkey or Egypt at a time of infection.[33] If plague broke out when ships were still loading, masters were to take in non-enumerated goods to make up their cargo and leave the port within 12 days.[34] No guidance was given at this early date as to how soon the loading of enumerated goods could resume once the plague had ceased. But for both the Privy Council and the Levant Company, the agonizing over such difficult details, and the problem of foul bills of health, lay just around the corner.

27 H. Crouch, *A Complete View of the British Customs* … (London, 1724), p. 89.

28 Ibid.

29 Ibid.

30 An example is given in Russell, p. 366.

31 Ibid.

32 Ibid.

33 NA SP 105/210/62–3 (General Court resolution, 29 Feb. 1732).

34 Ibid.

Sicilian scourge

When the Messina crisis broke in 1743, Britain had enjoyed some 13 years in which quarantine had faded to a memory. Only briefly in 1733 had measures been reintroduced following reports of plague in Tripoli: unusually, the Lords Justices in Ireland had been the first to take action. In December 1732 they imposed quarantine against ships arriving from places between Cape de las Tres Forcas in Morocco and Cape Rusata in Barca.[35] As if with reluctance, the machinery in England ground into gear and an Order and Proclamation to the same effect were issued by the Privy Council in the following June.[36] It must be doubtful whether a more skimpy and useless Order had ever been issued. Quarantine for the Thames and Medway was to be at Stangate Creek, and for elsewhere as Customs should appoint. That was an archaic form of words, making no mention of the recent quarantine ports between London and Bristol, let alone of Liverpool and Hull. The remaining provisions were almost trite. Nothing was to be landed during quarantine, and any ship or person receiving goods in that period was to be detained for a like duration. Captains of warships were to prevent landings until the Customs took over; Customs were enjoined to be vigilant; and military commanders were to be aiding and assisting. And that was it. The Order, such as it was, formed a random selection of weak clauses resurrected from the time of the Baltic crisis.

There was, however, a new Act.[37] The Bill galloped through Parliament in nine days, receiving the royal assent on 13 June 1733.[38] Its main purpose was to continue for another two years the provisions of the quarantine Act of 1728, which had expired. It also specifically empowered the King, by Proclamation before 24 June 1734, to prohibit contact with an infected place. This, of course, echoed a similar provision in the 1728 Act, and was the last time the King was vested with such authority.[39] In summary, the 1733 measures showed the Walpole administration going through the motions of quarantine without enthusiasm or understanding. Perhaps this was a measure of Robert Walpole's dislike of Townshend, who had influenced the procedures in 1728.[40] In any event, the Prime Minister who did so much for free trade was not interested in impeding commerce with the shackles of quarantine,

35 Bibliotheca Lindesiana, vol. 6: *A Bibliography of Royal Proclamations of the Tudor and Stuart Sovereigns and of Others Published under Authority 1485–1714. Ireland and Scotland* (Oxford, 1910).

36 NA PC 2/92/170, 4 June 1733, from which remaining references in this paragraph are taken. For the Order, see also *The London Magazine*, vol. 2, p. 302, where the quarantine period is given as 50 days.

37 6 Geo.II, c.34.

38 *Journal of the House of Commons* [*JHC*], vol. 22, pp. 171–2, 202–3; Russell, *Treatise of the Plague*, p. 445.

39 This authority was never used. It was the subject of comment in a memorandum among the Chatham papers, dated around 1800, when it was believed that the Privy Council had not thought it right for the King to act (NA PRO 30/8/259, fols 340, 343). Only the Acts of 1721 and 1733 (i.e. not the 1728 Act) were mentioned.

40 For differences between Townshend and Walpole, see *Oxford Dictionary of National Biography*.

which ceased entirely for nine years. Walpole resigned his governmental positions in 1742, shortly before the panic at Messina could test his unconcern.

Unlike at Marseilles, the plague at Messina was not caused by any laxity in the system of quarantine, beyond the venality of a health guard. On 20 March 1743 there arrived a Genoese ship under Neapolitan colours, carrying wool, wheat, tobacco and linen, all loaded in the Morea which had been visited with plague.[41] Consequently the ship sailed with a foul bill of health, but the master made for nearby Missolonghi whence he contrived to depart with a clean one. During the voyage to Sicily, a sailor died of plague. On arrival at Messina, the master produced his clean bill, said nothing of having called at the Morea, declared only wool and wheat as his cargo, and claimed the missing crewman had fallen overboard. The Health Office acted properly and sent the ship to the lazaretto where the cargo would be aired. But during the night before it arrived there, the master, with the connivance of a health guard, sent the tobacco and linen ashore via a local fisherman. It was at this fisherman's house that the plague first made its appearance.

As the outbreak erupted, the anxiety felt in Italy and soon in London, was chronicled in the correspondence between Horace Mann, the British envoy in Florence, and Horace Walpole. As Mann was writing in new-style dating and Walpole in old-style, it will be confusing to give other than a broad outline of chronology.[42] It is clear, however, that by the end of June 1743, Italy was 'in the greatest consternation'; Sicily was cut off from any communication with the mainland, where troops patrolled the seaboard to prevent clandestine landings.[43] Already the death toll in Messina was around 16,000, with the epidemic out of all control and spreading beyond the town boundary.[44] Galley slaves and condemned criminals carried the dead off the streets to burial.[45] Sixteen of the afflicted sailed as best they could for Leghorn, hoping for refuge or treatment in its famed lazaretto.[46] But entry was denied and the weak and the dying were towed to Corsica and abandoned.[47] The Corsicans, outraged, set fire to the boat and no one survived the ill-starred voyage.[48] This was just one incident out of many; the Tyrrhenian Sea was dotted with grisly small ships carrying moribund crew. A month later, Mann wrote that the death toll in Messina was around 30,000 and the plague was still rampant: 'They have no other hopes of its being extinct but from the want of inhabitants …'.[49] Many who survived the disease died of hunger, as

41 Russell, pp. 327–8, from which remaining references in this paragraph are taken. Russell's source was a letter 'from a gentleman who resided in Messina in … 1743'.

42 Until 1752 Britain retained the old-style Julian calendar, which meant dates were ten days behind those of western Europe which had already adopted the new-style Gregorian calendar.

43 W.S. Lewis (ed.), *The Yale Edition of Horace Walpole's Correspondence* (52 vols, Oxford, 1937–83), vol. 18, p. 252.

44 Lewis, vol. 18, pp. 252, 261.

45 Lewis, vol. 18, p. 262.

46 Ibid.

47 Ibid.

48 Ibid.

49 Lewis, vol. 18, p. 269.

the town was isolated from its hinterland and larder by cordons sanitaires.[50] During August the plague abated as it ran short of victims.

In London, Walpole had more than one reason to be alarmed. He had paintings arriving from the Mediterranean on HMS *Pembroke*, which warship, although not from Sicily, was caught up in the quarantine which Messina had brought about. 'I tremble for the pictures', he wrote, 'for they are to be aired at the rough discretion of a master of a hoy, for nobody I could send, would be suffered to go aboard'.[51] In the same letter to Mann, he revealed his wider fears. 'The Regency are so temporising and timid, especially in this inter-ministerium, that I am in great apprehensions of our having the plague: an island, so many ports, no power absolute or active enough to establish the necessary precautions, and all are necessary! 'Tis terrible!'[52] Walpole's greater fear was for the safety of his correspondent, as there were rumours that plague had reached Calabria. He ended 'Adieu! Write me minutely the history of the plague: if it makes any progress towards you, I shall be a most unhappy man: I am far from easy on our own account here'.[53]

For Britain, the prospect of plague had fallen at the worst possible juncture. The last Act of Parliament to underpin the King's authority in matters of quarantine had expired eight years previously. Also, the King was abroad, which caused the Lords of the Regency to think hard before they acted definitively on his behalf. A worse problem was the hiatus in government – what Walpole called the inter-ministerium. The administration of Lord Wilmington had ended at his death on 2 July, and that of his successor, Henry Pelham, did not begin until 27 August. But if the Regency proved indecisive in managing the conduct of quarantine, they had not dithered too badly in the imposition.

Difficult decisions

On 7 July 1743 the Lords Justices, chairing the Privy Council in the King's absence, ordered quarantine of 40 days on all arrivals from Sicily, and 14 days from elsewhere in the Mediterranean.[54] A week later came the Proclamation.[55] Although 7 July was 18 July (by new-style dating) in Italy, that was not a particularly slow response to the developing crisis. Not a year would have passed without gossip of plague in one or more region of the Mediterranean seaboard, and some time was necessary to put the Messina catastrophe in perspective. Another overreaction was to be avoided. The Regency would have been mindful that after a decade without restrictions, the re-imposition of quarantine would have severely upset commercial interests.

50 Lewis, vol. 18, p. 262. Mann wrote (27 July NS): 'It's terrible to think as many have died by hunger as by the illness'.

51 Lewis, vol. 18, p. 282.

52 Ibid.

53 Lewis, vol. 18, p. 284.

54 NA PC 2/97/476; this Order was sent to the Customs Commissioners 'tho' only signed by two of the Lords of the Treasury' (*CTBP* (1742–5), p. 295) – a mark of the urgency.

55 NA PC 2/97/478–9; Lewis, vol. 18, pp. 275–6; *The London Magazine*, vol. 12, p. 358; *The Gentleman's Magazine*, 14 July 1743.

Walpole referred to consternation in the City of London, implicitly at the prospect of quarantine, as for 'merchants there is no plague so dreadful as a stoppage of their trade'.[56]

But the marks of haste and inexperience were stamped all over the Regency's rules. The broad understanding of shipping routes, especially the role of the outports, which had characterized the Orders of 1721 and 1728, were nowhere in evidence. It was the measures of 1733, which had been a feeble reversion to the Baltic crisis, which were now reintroduced, but without statutory backing. This lack of parliamentary support cannot easily be explained. The last two scares had seen Bills precipitated through both Houses, but the Acts had become irrelevant even before their powers had naturally lapsed. It was as though Parliament, in this gap between ministries, could not face a third rushed Bill in case this scare too came to nothing.

Russell took the view that, in default of other legislation, the Act of 1710 was now 'the sole quarantine law remaining in force'.[57] Certainly, an Act of that antiquity was not out of keeping with the tenor of the Order and Proclamation just introduced. There are, however, difficulties with Russell's interpretation, and it was not shared by the Law Officers of the Crown.[58] Russell accepted that the 1710 Act had been specifically repealed by the next quarantine statute in 1721, but pointed out that the latter Act was of finite duration. The question, therefore, was whether the earlier Act revived when the 1721 Act expired. If it did, then the relationship of that Act with the two later short-lived statutes, in 1728 and 1733, was equally problematical. But did Acts really matter anyway? Now that the Crown had issued so many Orders and Proclamations over quarantine, the royal prerogative in that area was no longer exceptionable. But it was still the question of punishment which made the statutory background so important, because Privy Council Orders were meaningless without parliamentary sanction, and when laws expired, so did the penalties. When the *St George* from Gibraltar left The Motherbank without permission to sail to Southampton, the Treasury could only advise the Customs Commissioners to prosecute the master 'and see how it was done last time'.[59] If the 1710 Act were somehow still in force, then the penalties under that Act were also current. But it will be recalled that the penalties under that Act had been distinctly mild – certainly nothing approaching the opportunities for the death sentence which had arisen under the short-term Act of 1728.

It will be wearisome to take the debate any further, except to illustrate a serious anomaly which the legal confusion brought about. In September 1743 the clerk to the *Scipio*, a naval fireship, was sentenced to six months in gaol by a court martial for not performing quarantine according to the directions of the Lords Justices.[60] At the same court martial, the ship's boatswain was convicted of the same offence, aggravated by his leaving the ship, and sentenced to death.[61] Russell, writing nearly

56 Lewis, vol. 18, p. 282.

57 Russell, p. 446.

58 NA PC 2/103/128 (1752), when all quarantine Acts were said to have expired.

59 *CTBP* (1742–45), p. 445.

60 *The London Magazine*, vol. 12, p. 463; Russell, p. 446.

61 Ibid.

50 years later, expressed some misgivings about the latter sentence, and in this instance he must have been right.[62] There was certainly no penalty of death anywhere in the Act of Queen Anne, and the later statutes under which such a penalty might have arisen had long expired. The unfortunate boatswain of the *Scipio* should have lost £20 and not his life.[63]

After this diversion, it is necessary to return to the Lords Justices, who were still struggling to cope. Even the basic structure of quarantine was eluding them. They ordered precedents to be sought in the files for extending quarantine to the Channel Islands and Isle of Man, to say nothing of Gibraltar and Minorca.[64] They even asked the Customs Commissioners whether ships from the Mediterranean ought not to be airing their cargoes.[65] This should have been a requirement of the Order and Proclamation, together with the definition of enumerated goods, a subject which the Privy Council had yet to address. On 21 July 1743, with the benefit of advice from Customs, a new Order was issued.[66] This broke free of the Baltic shackles and reintroduced measures of the 1720s. For instance, pilots were to stay to windward in a separate boat, and goods and bedding were to be aired for one week, but *after* quarantine. It was noticed above that the last statutory insistence on airing after, rather than during, quarantine had been in 1728, but the requirement had been continued by the Privy Council. The new regulations also defined enumerated goods, very much in line with those of the Marseilles crisis, down to straw hats, brushes, matting and artificial flowers. These were to remain on board, even after airing, until the Privy Council had authorized their release.

To facilitate airing, the Lords Justices asked the Lord Mayor of London and magistrates at the outports to appoint proper persons to open and air goods under the supervision of Customs officials, but at the owner's expense.[67] This went down badly, especially in London, and there was confusion in the Treasury as to whether or not a similar request had been made in 1720.[68] The three men approved for airing goods on a special hoy wanted protection against press gangs, and the Corporation were unhappy that owners should pay for labour costs.[69] The Lords Justices agreed to protection for the labourers and promised to refer the second point to the King's 'Grace and Favour'.[70] Meanwhile, on 29 September 1743, they approved the expenditure of £1,672, 11s on airing sheds or lazarets, with houses and sentinel boxes for the workers.[71] These buildings were presumably for land near Stangate Creek, which

62 Russell, p. 446.

63 It is possible that he was reprieved, but the anomaly lay in the sentence.

64 NA PC 2/97/478, 482.

65 NA PC 2/97/483.

66 NA PC 2/97/493; cf. *CTBP* (1742–45), p. 300.

67 NA PC 2/97/516–17; *CTBP* (1742–45), p. 305, where it is clear that the idea came from the Customs Commissioners. See also *CTBP* (1742–45), p. 308.

68 NA PC 2/97/551; *CTBP* (1742–45), p. 307.

69 NA PC 2/97/552; for the approval of the men, see also *CTBP* (1742–45), pp. 314, 373.

70 NA PC 2/97/540, 552. There is no evidence of royal compliance.

71 NA PC 2/97/568; *CTBP* (1742–45), pp. 317, 319. The Treasury added a memorandum: 'Care to be taken if a lease shall be taken ... that at the expiration of the term all the materials,

was now to be the only quarantine harbour for the Thames and Medway as Sharfleet Creek and The Hope had been found unsuitable.[72] The work was not carried out, and it will be seen below that the episode became the focus of parliamentary attention in 1752. The decision to concentrate all quarantine ships in Stangate Creek led to the predictable claim from local fisherman seeking compensation for damage to the oyster beds.[73]

The circular to the outports prompted a complaint from Bridgwater that there were too few Customs officers to compel ships to obey the rules.[74] The Privy Council responded with an order to the Commissioners to report what places had been appointed for quarantine, and what personnel were necessary to enforce it.[75] The only reply which has survived came, on 1 September 1743, from Scotland, which now re-emerged in the quarantine scene after some 30 years in which activity had been virtually confined to the south of England. There were now six quarantine stations in Scotland, as follows:[76]

1. Inverkeithing Bay: for ships bound to Leith, Bo'ness, Alloa, Dunbar, Kirkcaldy, Anstruther and Prestonpans
2. River Tay, opposite Broughty Castle: for Dundee, Perth, Montrose and Aberdeen
3. Cromarty Firth: for Inverness, Shetland, Orkney, Caithness and Lewis
4. Tail-of-the-Bank (Greenock): for Port Glasgow, Greenock, Irvine and Campbeltown
5. Lochryan: for Ayr, Stranraer, Portpatrick and Wigtown
6. Carsethorn: for Dumfries and Kirkcudbright.

The Customs Commissioners in Scotland wanted two companies of soldiers quartered near each place. That was asking too much, and the Privy Council could only instruct General Guest, Commander-in-Chief in North Britain, to provide as many as he thought necessary and could spare.[77] There is no evidence to suggest that any of the above quarantine harbours was widely used, at least for the next few decades.

While Scotland had been organizing its shoreline, the Privy Council in England were facing one of the most difficult decisions which quarantine could ever demand. The ship *Mermaid* had arrived in Stangate Creek from Gallipoli, Leghorn and Sicily. Part of her cargo was silk – an enumerated product – loaded at Messina after the plague had broken out. Then came the *Duke of Lorraine* from Milazzo in Sicily.[78] Fearing the grim necessity of destroying ships and goods, the Privy Council asked

---

&c., used in the … buildings do return to the public.'

72 *CTBP* (1742–45), p. 308: 'the Hope is not a proper place … [for quarantine] in regard great numbers of foreign ships, coasters, fishing vessels, &c. are constantly passing and repassing, insomuch that it is very difficult or hardly possible to prevent their having communication with the ships and people there'.

73 *CTBP* (1742–45), p. 667. This was referred by the Treasury to the Customs Commissioners; the Privy Council seem not to have been involved.

74 NA PC 2/97/518; *CTBP* (1742–45), p. 305.

75 NA PC 2/97/518; *CTBP* (1742–45), p. 308.

76 NA PC 2/97/539–41; *CTBP* (1742–45), p. 371 (but with no list of places).

77 NA PC 2/97/539–41

78 Often spelled *Duke of Lorain* or *Loraine*.

the Customs Commissioners, on 11 August 1743, what steps should now be taken.[79] Being advised that the silk should be burnt, the Council sought a medical opinion on the safety of unloading, which was supplied by Richard Mead and Matthew Lee.[80] The doctors were dogmatic and thoroughly pessimistic: 'We think it will not be absolutely Safe to Open the Hold of a Ship in which there are Goods infected'.[81] They thought there might even be danger in airing them. Some merchants had suggested boiling goods as a means of cleansing them, but the doctors considered that 'very dangerous ... and a very likely way to Spread Infection'.[82] In short, they foresaw only way one to deal with an infected ship and goods: 'Sink them out at Sea in Deep Water'.[83]

That was not what the Privy Council wanted to hear and they had the courage to disregard the advice. The cargoes and not the vessels would be sacrificed. The massive compensation for the burning of the Turkey ships in 1721 could not be countenanced again, especially as other suspect arrivals were possible. Indeed, one Dutch ship from Messina, rumoured to have plague aboard, had already been forced out of Plymouth Sound by gunfire and told not to call elsewhere in Britain.[84] In September 1743, therefore, the Privy Council allowed the non-enumerated goods to be offloaded, but ordered the silk and velvet (some of which had come from Genoa) from both ships to be piled on a sloop of the Customs service and taken out to sea.[85] A warship was appointed in October as an escort and the goods, covered in sheet lead, were dumped overboard.[86] There had been seven bales of silk in the *Mermaid*, while the *Duke of Lorraine* had three bales of silk, one box of silk and velvet, and another box of just velvet.[87]

The question now arose of compensation. The Customs Commissioners reported on the value, and George II was asked whether he wished the estimate to go before the Commons, as it had in 1721 when the Turkey ships were burnt.[88] The King evidently did not, as the Privy Council ordered £1,940, 5s, 6d for the prime cost and freight to be paid out of the Old Subsidy 'in like manner as the Charges of former Quarantine have been paid.'[89] Unfortunately, that was not quite the end of the matter. The *Mermaid* belonged to Joseph Chitty, who now wanted compensation for the long detention of his ship while the Privy Council had made up their mind. It did not augur well for Chitty that the Council had, in October, summoned the secretary to the Customs Commissioners before them and asked him to consider a number of matters relating to quarantine; these included the building of sheds for airing and,

79 NA PC 2/97/518, 549.

80 NA PC 2/97/558; PRO PC 1/13/101; *CTBP* (1742–45), p. 312.

81 NA PC 2/97/558–60.

82 Ibid.

83 Ibid.

84 NA PC 2/97/547. The ship was the *De Resolute* of 400 tons burthen.

85 NA PC 2/97/560, 569; *CTBP* (1742–45), pp. 314, 373 (which indicates that sausages, hats and wine among the cargo of the *Mermaid* were also to be destroyed).

86 NA PC 2/98/3; *CTBP* (1742–45), pp. 375–6.

87 NA PC 2/98/116.

88 Ibid.; *CTBP* (1742–45), pp. 445, 453.

89 NA PC 2/98/248; *CTBP* (1742–45), p. 453.

more pertinently, the opportunity for fraud by people claiming more for a destroyed cargo than it was actually worth.[90] The mood was clear: all claims for compensation would be treated with suspicion. Certainly there was to be no public money for the owners of the *Success*, accidentally burnt when under quarantine at The Hope, but in November 1745 a merchant was allowed £318 'by particular directions' for losses in quarantine incurred by the *Friendship*.[91]

Chitty's initial approach had been to the Treasury, in January 1744, but the lords felt they had no standing in the matter.[92] That did not deter Chitty from trying again in April, hoping that the Treasury would recommend him 'to Parliament for some recompence for accidental loss from enforced quarantine'.[93] That was a dangerous prospect, as a payout would open the possibility of compensation for all detainees. The Treasury called in the Customs Commissioners who reminded their superiors that 'it has been the constant practice to pay for no goods but what have been directed to be actually destroyed'.[94] This further rejection merely encouraged Chitty, in June, to apply to the Privy Council, but they relegated his petition to the Treasury, who got rid of it to the Customs service.[95] In September 1744 Chitty played his last card; he petitioned the King with annexed accounts of his losses, but these papers were buried in a filing room of the Treasury.[96] Chitty had lost.

No relaxation

If the Privy Council were mainly alarmed about Messina, they were also looking warily at other seats of the plague. Reaction to rumour was now immediate. In October 1743 a 40-day quarantine was introduced against Smyrna, and in July 1744 against West Barbary (that is, the Barbary coast which flanked the Atlantic).[97] By that time the detention from Smyrna had been reduced to 14 days, which was the subsisting restriction against all shipping from the Mediterranean, introduced in parallel with the longer quarantine against Messina.[98] By the spring of 1745, the merchant lobby was becoming irritated, as usual, by expense and delay, and the tactic adopted was to argue for relief by reference to the policy in Holland. If that policy had once (in 1728) influenced the imposition of quarantine in England, it could surely now influence its removal, as dangers were receding. In late May there was a petition to the Lords Justices in Council from the merchants of London who 'by repeated and undoubted Advices for several Months past from their Correspondents abroad are

90 NA PC 2/98/14.

91 *CTBP* (1742–45), pp. 482, 831.

92 *CTBP* (1742–45), p. 448: 'My Lords can do nothing in this'.

93 *CTBP* (1742–5), p. 472.

94 Ibid.

95 NA PC 2/98/362, 381; *CTBP* (1742–45), p. 570.

96 *CTBP* (1742–45), p. 582.

97 Smyrna: NA PC 2/98/362; *CTBP* (1742–45), p. 324. West Barbary: NA PC 2/98/433; *CTBP* (1742–45), pp. 504, 576.

98 NA PC 2/98/115, 150; *CTBP* (1742–45), pp. 444, 548.

well informed that the Plague had entirely ceased in Sicily and Calabria'.[99] This, they conceded, was not the time to remove quarantine altogether from those two places, but they wanted it abolished from other Mediterranean ports. This had already happened in Holland, by the placard of 19 January 1745.[100]

The response of the Privy Council was to refer this to a committee of their own members. Although it would be normal for Privy Council committees to seek an opinion from the Customs Commissioners via the Treasury, it was a mark of the Council's growing expertise in quarantine that they were increasingly reliant on their own judgement. Another advantage of a committee was the opportunity it afforded for deliberate indecision, when the way forward was still fraught with risk. With nothing resolved, the merchants renewed their attack in December 1745, claiming that quarantine was a heavy burden on their trade.[101] Messina was now in free pratique with the rest of Sicily; was this not time to lift quarantine altogether? This petition was also referred to the committee, who sought help from the Treasury and purposely took their time in preparing a full and detailed report. Their recommendation, relying heavily once more on the practice in Holland, was that quarantine should be lifted entirely from West Barbary, Sicily and all other places within the Mediterranean, which included the Levant.[102] On 20 March 1746 this was accepted by the full Council and quarantine duly ceased.[103]

The main reason to be dilatory was that with significant rumours of plague being now so common, a quarantine removed on one day might need to be reimposed virtually on the next. It was an administrative nightmare to rush through Orders and Proclamations with all the delays and possible mishaps which dissemination to the outports entailed. If the merchants would only tolerate the inconvenience and costs, a system of permanent quarantine against suspect places – which is what existed in some ports bordering the northern Mediterranean – was far and away the most practicable solution for the Privy Council. It was also, of course, the system most likely to keep Britain free of plague. But in a democracy with its wealth rooted deeply in trade, permanent quarantine was still politically unacceptable. The time to have introduced it, if at all, was in the wake of the Messina crisis. Now that was over, and an illusion of normality had returned, the long-term future for quarantine could hold nothing but endless ad hoc orders followed by endless ad hoc protests.

It would have surprised no one, therefore, that in June 1747 a quarantine of 40 days was reintroduced against all arrivals from West Barbary.[104] The only remarkable aspect was that another two years passed before that quarantine was extended to the ports of Barbary between the Straits of Gibraltar and Cape de las Tres Forcas.[105] Such an interval without quarantine in Britain against some part of the Mediterranean seaboard would not happen again in the eighteenth century. The main importance

99 NA PC 2/99/100; PC 1/13/103.

100 Ibid.

101 NA PC 2/99/278; *CTBP* (1742–45), pp. 744–5.

102 NA PC 2/99/376–8; PC 1/13/103.

103 NA PC 2/99/409.

104 NA PC 2/100/293–6.

105 NA PC 2/101/281.

of 1749, however, in quarantine history, lies not in new quarantine Orders but in the problems posed by ships from the Levant arriving with foul bills of health when no Orders for quarantine against Turkey subsisted. In October the *Venice* and *Samuel & Elizabeth*, both from Smyrna, sailed into Stangate Creek.[106] The *Venice* was owned by Jacob Chitty, one of the family so well known to the Privy Council for persistent and awkward petitions. The ship had left Smyrna on 10 June 1749 when plague was still active or recent. As the Levant Company did not allow ships to sail directly for London with foul bills, the ship was destined for Hamburg, which she reached on 15 September, only to be turned away.[107] London was then the only option. The *Samuel & Elizabeth*, also with a foul bill, seems to have made for London out of solidarity with the *Venice*. Also from Smyrna, she carried wool, carpets, yarn, hair and other enumerated goods, as well as 'Antique Stones'.[108] When Chitty petitioned, in early November, for the *Venice* to be discharged, a shocked Privy Council asked the Customs Commissioners whether the ship's hold should even be opened.[109]

It was another mark of the Privy Council's growing confidence in quarantine matters that they did not seek a medical opinion, as they had in 1743. It was no doubt expected that the doctors would preach overcaution, and the Council had no more wish to offend them by ignoring their advice for a second time, than they had to upset the City by the interruption to its trade. But this was a risky tactic as there were reports in London that seamen had died on the voyage, and it was a short step from there to rumours of plague.[110] In early December the Customs Commissioners were summoned to the Privy Council to discuss their reports on both vessels, and a decision was taken that the cargoes should simply be aired.[111] This prompted a petition from the Levant Company in January 1750, claiming that mohair yarn aired on an open hoy for 14 days would be ruined.[112] Could they not air it between the decks of a warship? The Privy Council could not disagree with the logic, and the Admiralty were asked to provide a 40 or 50-gun warship from those laid up at Sheerness.[113] The Admiralty obliged with HMS *Hampshire*, which was in position in Stangate Creek in the middle of February.[114] On 13 March 1750 the mohair yarn was duly discharged after airing and the warship, supported by another, was then ordered to attend the opening and airing of the rest of the cargoes.[115] This extra ship was HMS *Looe*, which loaded 258 sacks from the *Venice*, all of which were discharged, along with the cargo of the *Samuel & Elizabeth*, on 21 April.[116] It was thus six months before the merchants realized the value of their cargoes, but this time there were no claims

106 NA PC 2/101/324.

107 Ibid.

108 Ibid.

109 NA PC 2/101/324, 326.

110 *The Gentleman's Magazine*, 19 Dec. 1749.

111 NA PC 2/101/376.

112 NA PC 2/101/443, 447.

113 NA PC 2/101/453.

114 Ibid.

115 NA PC 2/101/482–3, 501.

116 NA PC 2/101/551–2. Customs had been told on 16 March not to destroy the packaging of the goods as this would have made it impossible to determine ownership (PC 2/101/502).

for compensation arising from the delay. Chitty would have been only too thankful that his enumerated goods had not been destroyed.

Even before the Privy Council had reached a decision on the two Turkey ships, another vessel had arrived in Stangate Creek with a foul bill of health, this time from Santa Cruz in West Barbary.[117] The cargo included almonds, as well as beeswax, feathers and leather. The owners wanted the almonds removed without airing, and a compromise was reached with the Privy Council: almonds in casks would be left where they were, while their containers were swabbed with salt water and vinegar; but those in sacks would be rebagged and aired for 14 days.[118] In one important respect this ship was easier to deal with, because there was an Order in force for quarantine against arrivals from Barbary. If anything went wrong, for instance if the master were disobedient, then the sanctions of the law – such as they were without the umbrella of an Act of Parliament – could be called into play. The fact that the bill was foul, in the context of Barbary, was irrelevant because the Privy Council had reverted to the traditional stance of making no distinction between them. But for the Levant, the situation was different. It will be remembered that an Order of 1730 had removed quarantine entirely for ships from the Mediterranean with clean bills; had that been still in force, then quarantine measures would have automatically applied for Turkey ships with bills which were foul. But the world had moved on, and the situation by 1750 was that ships from the Levant with any bill type of bill, even foul, were not automatically subject to quarantine, so there were no grounds for destroying their cargoes. This position arose because no Act, Order or Proclamation governed quarantine from the Levant at that date. In the imposition of quarantine and airing, the King was exercising the royal prerogative only on the basis of custom.

The other lesson from this episode was the importance of airing all enumerated goods, an indispensable practice according to medical opinion. But this raised its own problems. Turkey ships were large and their holds carried more bales than could be aired on even a collection of hoys. With no airing sheds to speak of on dry land, the only expedient was to utilize warships of the reserve fleet. If the Admiralty thought that the two ships they supplied in 1750 were a temporary expedient, they were soon to be proved wrong. Questions of availability, suitability and cost were already in the pipeline. When the issue of naval involvement was joined to the uncertainty of royal authority, the ramifications of quarantine were clearly ripe for the attention of Parliament.

Need for a lazaret

It took more than another year before Parliament could steel itself to tackle quarantine in all its aspects. For the rest of 1750, the Privy Council were preoccupied with Barbary, organizing the airing of cargoes on HMS *Looe*, frightened by stories that a plague ship at Safi in Morocco had unloaded its infected goods on to other ships unknown.[119] But Turkey could not be ignored for long, and in April 1751, following

117 NA PC 2/101/352. This ship was the *Neptune*.

118 NA PC 2/101/403, 450, 455, 500.

119 NA PC 2/102/47, 80, 83, 85, 92.

nothing worse than routine rumours of plague at Constantinople, a 40-day quarantine was imposed against the Levant, the extent being defined exactly as it had been in 1728.[120] It was this decision that began to focus parliamentary minds. There was now the prospect of more Turkey ships arriving with foul bills – in preparation for which event another large warship was requested for Stangate Creek – and the problem of airing cargoes was the catalyst for serious discussion.[121]

On 13 February 1752 the Commons resolved to form itself into a committee a week later 'to consider of the most proper and effectual manner of performing Quarantine'.[122] Among those asked to attend the committee were the Master Attendant of the royal dockyard at Deptford and the Assistant to the Master Shipwright at the same place. The other co-opted members were Robert Forster, Daniel Goatly and a Mr Watley. The immediate brief was to discuss a memorial from the Customs Commissioners to the Treasury, dated as far back as 27 September 1743, proposing the building of sheds or lazarets to air goods under quarantine in Stangate Creek. This expense, as has been noticed above, was approved by the Privy Council but nothing had come of it. In anticipation of the Commons' resolution, the Admiralty had already, in January 1752, sent officers from Deptford and Chatham to Stangate Creek to find the best site.[123] With this information before them, the committee met and re-met before reaching three conclusions. The first was that the present mode of airing goods on hoys and ships was 'not well calculated to prevent the Infection; and is inconvenient and expensive to the Merchant'; the second was that a lazaret should be erected; and the third that Chetney Hill was the proper location.[124] The House agreed with all three points, the first two unanimously, and resolved on 5 March 1752 to ask the King for plans of a lazaret, with estimates of cost and maintenance, to be laid before the House in the next parliamentary session.[125]

The plans were not delivered. The dichotomy between Parliament and Privy Council is plainly revealed by the registers of the latter, where there is no mention of contemporary parliamentary proceedings or of the plans for a lazaret. The fact was that the Privy Council, apart from their wider responsibilities, were extremely busy with urgent and practical issues of quarantine, among which the ponderous resolutions of Parliament were unwelcome. To some extent they would have seen them as an intrusion into the royal prerogative. If the King had been allowed to build lazarets before, why interfere with that now? And what did the term lazaret (to continue the Anglicism) mean? This was not a good time to quantify, within one year, the expense of a project of imponderable definition on land which the Crown did not own. The scope and purpose of a lazaretto in the Mediterranean sense needed discussion by all manner of interested parties before anyone could draw up a plan,

120 NA PC 2/102/300, 311.

121 For the warship being requested, see NA PC 2/102/451, 455.

122 *Journal of the House of Commons* [*JHC*], vol. 26, pp. 432, 447; British Library [BL] Add. MS 38351, fols 255–7.

123 NA ADM 106/2564, 8 & 13 Jan. 1752; *JHC*, vol. 26, p. 463; P. Froggatt, 'The Chetney Hill lazaret', *Archaeologia Cantiana*, 79 (1964), 5.

124 *JHC*, vol. 26, p. 478; BL Add. MS 38351, fols 255–7. Chetney was spelled 'Chedney'.

125 *JHC*, vol. 26, p. 478.

let alone a table of costs. A year earlier, when the Privy Council had only been vexed about goods from Barbary, the lazaret idea might have made some progress. But in 1752 it was a distraction.

It was the new regulations against Turkey that were making the Privy Council so much busier. It was one thing to face the Barbary merchants, who had no corporate unity, but quite another to take on the powerful Levant Company, nettled as its members were by growing attacks on their exclusivity. The recent episode of the foul-bill ships had led to all cargoes from the East being aired, with inordinate delays and some damage. The tactic was now to petition the Privy Council in the name of the Company, rather than any of its members, pointing out the need for more airing facilities.[126] Ideally, the Company wanted parity with the Dutch, having learnt that ships from Smyrna with clean bills of health could reach Amsterdam without opening and airing their cargoes.[127] The Privy Council were anxious to appease, even if it risked annoying the Admiralty. At the request of the Levant Company, they made a plea for more warships to assist with the airing.[128] There were then eight vessels under quarantine in Stangate Creek, but only two naval ships to receive their cargoes.[129] A strong hint was given to the Admiralty that if more ships were provided they would not be detained for long, as quarantine against Turkey was being reconsidered in the light of the attitude of the Dutch.[130]

The Levant Company felt the position in Holland was their trump card. In May 1752 they took occasion, when petitioning for the release of a ship called the *Thames*, to seek the removal of all quarantine against arrivals from Turkey with clean bills of health.[131] It was alleged that there had been no plague at Scanderoon and Cyprus, where the *Thames* had called, for more than eight years. Again they compared their own position with that of their near rivals, hoping trade could 'be upon as easy Terms as that of our Neighbours the Dutch'.[132] The Privy Council made enquiries in Holland and were told of a new placard, dated 1 May, under which ships from Smyrna with clean bills, and in obvious good health, were excused quarantine.[133] From elsewhere in the Levant, a quarantine of 20 days for ships with clean bills remained in force from an earlier placard.[134] On 28 May 1752 the Lords Justices agreed to virtually the same arrangement for Britain, in that quarantine against Smyrna (with clean bills) was abolished, although 20 days' detention and subsequent airing remained in force for arrivals from other Levantine ports.[135] This was an unfortunate decision. One plague hot spot was being treated differently from the others, on no sound basis, and the shipping route from Scanderoon and Cyprus, a favourite of the Levant Company, saw no advantage. The Privy Council paid the price of its illogical Order when

126 NA PC 2/103/73.

127 Ibid.

128 NA PC 2/103/73, 81, 82.

129 NA PC 2/103/73, 81, 82.

130 Ibid.

131 NA PC 2/103/72.

132 Ibid.

133 NA PC 2/103/98–101.

134 Ibid.

135 Ibid.

merchants importing currants from the Ionian Islands argued, in March 1753, for quarantine to be abolished for them, as it was for Smyrna.[136] If the Turkey merchants had this privilege, why should not they, who were 'less liable to suspicion'?[137]

Ironically, the main worry for the Privy Council towards the end of 1752 was again Barbary, or more specifically Algiers, which was in the grip of a ferocious epidemic. Some of the North African coast was already under 40-day quarantine in Britain, and in June this was extended eastwards to Cape Rusata.[138] That is to say, it stopped at the point where the Levant was conceived to begin. Having just made a new Order for the Levant, the Council were not inclined to alter it, but directed Customs officers that all ships from the Mediterranean were to be strictly examined.[139] Then came a report that the plague had spread to Rhodes, but the Council were still reluctant to upset the Levant Company by increasing the 20-day quarantine from places other than Smyrna. Instead, Customs were to make absolutely sure that no ship from the Mediterranean had touched at the island.[140] The Algiers plague, although not of the notoriety of the Messina outbreak, was to prove prolonged, troublesome and expensive.

Innovative legislation

Having established that a lazaret was desirable, Parliament, early in 1753, walked more deeply into the quagmire of quarantine. There was still the need to underpin the authority of the King in Council, as events in Bristol were bearing out. Six crewmen went ashore 'in a Mutinous manner' from a ship at the quarantine station.[141] If that had happened at one of the Mediterranean lazarettos the men, if caught, would have been killed or sentenced to a life in the galleys. As it was, the Law Officers of the Crown struggled to establish any basis for punishment, as all Acts of Parliament which gave extraordinary powers to the Crown and allowed summary jurisdiction were expired.[142] But this was only one aspect of a complicated subject which Parliament, for the first time, could ponder at its leisure. All previous quarantine Acts had been passed in a state of near terror. There was, of course, the plague in Algiers to cause background concern, but in 1753 the likes of Horace Walpole were not panicking at the prospect of a life-threatening epidemic in London.

---

136 NA PC 2/103/352.

137 Ibid.

138 NA PC 2/103/140.

139 NA PC 2/103/457.

140 NA PC 2/103/502.

141 NA PC 2/103/128. The ship was the *Constantine*. There was nothing new about seamen jumping ship under quarantine conditions. Customs officers in 1745 had reported 34 seamen on the run from one ship (*CTBP* (1742–5), p. 710). Many of these escapees were seeking to avoid the press gangs.

142 Ibid. The only route was by indictment or information. Magistrates, at the request of local Customs officers, could issue a warrant for arrest and the case would be heard at the next assizes. The real problems began then.

On 22 January 1753 the House allowed Viscount Barrington and five other members to bring in a quarantine Bill.[143] It is Barrington, therefore, who can be credited with at least some of the initiative for the parliamentary interest. Not yet a Privy Councillor (he was appointed in 1755), Barrington had been a Commissioner of the Admiralty since 1749.[144] His involvement suggests the navy were already worried that the Privy Council's policy for quarantine, and especially airing, would soon become troublesome. There was some irony in this, as the navy's press-gang tactics, when a ship was under quarantine, were a perpetual irritation for the Privy Council. The Bill reached its second reading on 20 February, when the sections of Act 7 Geo. I, c.3 which had enabled the King to force people into lazarettos and set up lines around infected places, and the whole of 8 Geo. I, c.10 which cancelled that power, were read.[145] The Bill was then committed by 92 votes to 49.[146] This division signalled that the parameters of royal power were at the heart of the new proceedings, and that a significant minority of Commoners did not want the balance of authority disturbed.

The Bill spent the next three weeks being discussed at various times by a committee of the whole House. On 12 March the several amendments were read, re-analysed and generally agreed.[147] But there were still concerns about the commencement of the Act and, more especially, how long it should stay in force. An amendment was proposed which would have limited the duration to five years.[148] This was defeated, and the Act was left indefinite – a significant milestone in quarantine history. After later minor amendments, some in the Lords, the Bill received the royal assent on 17 April 1753.[149] It became *An act to oblige ships more effectually to perform their quarentine; and for the better preventing the plague being brought from foreign parts into Great Britain or Ireland or the isles of Guernsey, Jersey, Alderney, Sark or Man.*[150]

The importance of this Act was that it radically altered the pattern and thrust of past legislation. There were new ideas and new procedures interspersed with the correction of old mistakes. The preamble dispelled any notion that Parliament wished to divest the King of his prerogative. The Act was necessary to enable offenders to be punished 'in a more expeditious manner than can be done by the ordinary methods of law'. It was also needed, as usual, to enforce compliance with such orders for quarantine as the Crown might think necessary. These orders were to be promulgated by Proclamation, as before, but also by publication in the *London Gazette*.

As if to emphasize the freshness of thinking, the Act began with a startling and unprecedented measure aimed at ships actually infected with plague. It was only recently that ships with foul bills of health had been the subject of anxious

143 *JHC*, vol. 26, p. 532.

144 *Oxford Dictionary of National Biography*; *Office-Holders in Modern Britain IV. Admiralty Officials, 1660–1870* (London, 1975), p. 23.

145 *JHC*, vol. 26, p. 607.

146 Ibid.

147 *JHC*, vol. 26, pp. 669–70.

148 Ibid.

149 *JHC*, vol. 26, pp. 671, 694, 742, 755, 773.

150 26 Geo. II, c.6. There is a useful commentary in Russell, pp. 446–53.

debate, *after* they had arrived. Now, the mood was proactive: Parliament had made a contingency plan. An infected ship, if north of Cape Finisterre, had to make for the harbour of New Grimsby in the Isles of Scilly, where the master would report to the officer of Customs. This was the first time the Isles of Scilly had featured in quarantine history. It would be the duty of the Customs officer to inform his colleagues on the mainland, who would notify a principal Secretary of State. Government would then take measures for the relief of the crew (who would not be allowed ashore) and to stop the spread of infection. The ship would remain at New Grimsby until the King decided otherwise. The penalty for disobedience would be death.

Next came rules for interrogating the master of a ship. This codified what had been, up to this point, a procedural matter within the Customs service. To establish whether quarantine was necessary, the delegated officer had to ask the name of the ship; the name of the master; the port(s) of lading; what other ports were visited; whether any of those ports had been infected with plague; the length of the voyage; how many people had been aboard when the ship sailed; whether any people had been or were then infected with plague; how many people had died on the voyage and from what cause; with what ships they had exchanged visits on the way; and what was the cargo. A deceitful master would normally be fined £200, but could suffer death if he lied about an aspect of infection. Forming a separate section, but very much a rider to the above requirements, was the need for a ship's master to produce a bill of health and manifest, as well as his logbook and journal. The fine for disobedience would be £500. This was the first time that bills of health, obtainable from British consuls, had been mentioned in a quarantine Act, some 23 years after their first appearance in a Privy Council Order.

Having established these radical points, the Act moved on to update, clarify or otherwise amend what were basically the provisions of past enactments. There were penalties (a long way short of death) for persons who left a quarantined ship without authority. Lazarets could be erected on common or private ground against proper rent or consideration; that was not a new measure, but this time the consent and advice of Parliament would be necessary. Russell noticed the significance of this provision, as also the requirement for any disputes to be settled ultimately by juries and not by magistrates.[151] The inhabitants of a lazaret were constrained to stay there under pain of death, and there was a section warning of 'disobedience or refractory behaviour' in quarantine stations. Customs officers and others were warned of the consequences to themselves for embezzlement or neglect of duty.

The next section was of interest as it extended quarantine to goods, deemed liable to retain infection, which had been transported from one country to another. Detention would apply even though the second country, and therefore the ships arriving from it, might not be liable to quarantine. Although that was unexceptionable at the time, a precedent had been created which would cause friction with commercial lobbies in due course. One departure which merchants and shipowners would have welcomed was the implication in section 15 of the Act that the opening and airing of goods could take place simultaneously with quarantine, rather than when it had finished. The importance of this concession has already been discussed. Discharge would

151 Russell, p. 449.

be by certificates from the Superintendent of Quarantine (an office not defined) and Customs officers. Now that the airing of goods was not post-quarantine, all involvement of the Privy Council in the routine discharge of ships and cargoes was theoretically at an end. Of course, that was far from how it would work, as most cargoes included enumerated goods and the complications which resulted produced a never ending series of petitions to the King in Council.[152] The Act included a rant, stronger than usual, against smuggling and showed the now customary suspicion of vessels less than 20 tons burthen, whose masters were required to give a bond in £300 against having contact with persons or goods in infected places. The commencement of the Act was to be 1 March 1754, that is nearly a year after the royal assent. The long delay was to allow the Act time to reach the Levant, so homeward-bound ships could acquire the necessary documentation.

The Act might have been more radical still had not one section of the Bill been rejected after much debate. The idea had been put forward that British consuls, especially those in the Ottoman Empire, should furnish a ship's master not only with a bill of health but also with a yellow, swallow-tailed jack. The master would hoist the jack on entering the English Channel, or any British port, as a warning for all other vessels, except the pilot boat, to keep away. There were, however, three arguments against the proposal. The first was that, in time of war, the jack would act as a signal to enemy privateers that the vessel was a rich Turkey ship; the second was that homeward-bound ships might hoist such a jack anyway to prevent press gangs from boarding; and the third reason was that smugglers would fly the jack permanently to stop Customs officers searching for contraband. Meeting such powerful objections, the idea was rejected.[153]

Before Parliament had given the Bill, resulting in the above Act, its second reading, another Bill had been introduced in the Commons which was significantly to affect quarantine. This other Bill received the royal assent on 15 May 1753, and became *An act for enlarging and regulating trade into the Levant seas*.[154] The main purpose of this measure was to relax conditions for entry to the Levant Company without throwing open the trade entirely. But the Act ended with two clauses that concerned quarantine, the first indirectly. This first clause stipulated 'That all rules, orders and regulations made for preventing infection, shall be, and remain in force and virtue as if this act had never passed'. The other clause was specific and much more important: it debarred goods 'liable to retain the infection of the plague', on ships from the Levant without clean bills of health, from being landed anywhere in Great Britain, Ireland or the off-islands, unless they had been sufficiently opened and aired in one of the following lazarettos: Malta, Ancona, Venice, Messina, Leghorn, Genoa and Marseilles. Russell was uncertain what the former clause meant, but assumed that the Levant Company had made their own rules for preventing infection, and these would stand.[155] The Company did indeed make rules, in that they prevented

152 The Act made no direct reference to enumerated goods.

153 The best summary of this episode is in *The London Magazine*, vol. 22, pp. 373–4. Mention is also made in Russell, p. 371.

154 26 Geo. II, c.18.

155 Russell, p. 447.

ships loading and leaving under certain conditions, but it would seem to have been Privy Council measures which legislators had in mind. It was almost an apology for the clause that followed it, which arrogated to Parliament a ruling that might otherwise have been made by Order and Proclamation.

Russell saw the foreign lazaretto clause as 'only a temporary expedient' until Britain had achieved its own land lazaret, then under discussion.[156] The difficulty with that view is that it assumes the British were minded in the first place to accept ships with foul bills. It would transpire later (after Russell was writing) that Britain had no such inclination. This was partly from fear of infection, but also from the inordinately long airing and quarantine periods which would ensue, and the knock-on inconvenience for the navy, who would need to send more old warships as airing hulks. The pressure on the navy would ease once the land facilities were eventually built, but those sheds or lazarets would be fully occupied with airing enumerated cargoes from ships with *clean* bills of health. Russell did not speculate on why the lazaretto clause was tacked on to the Levant Act, although the parliamentary progress of that measure was only one month behind the quarantine Bill. The clause did, of course, concern ships from the Levant, but the more logical place to include it was among other matters relating to quarantine. Perhaps it was just a massive afterthought, coinciding with the inability or refusal of the King to produce the plans for a lazaret which Parliament had requested in 1752. That conclusion would lend weight to Russell's view that the clause was a temporary expedient. But it was rather a recognition that any British lazaret could only be inferior and smaller to those of the Mediterranean, and that ships with the most suspect cargoes were best left to the experts. Whatever had been the thinking that induced the foreign lazaretto clause, its position in the Levant Act would, like so many other aspects of quarantine in the mid-eighteenth century, lead to complications in the years ahead.

On 1 March 1754, when the new quarantine Act came into force, the Privy Council issued an Order to supplement and clarify the rules.[157] They took the opportunity to confirm (but not rationalize) the existing quarantine restrictions against the Levant, excluding Smyrna, and against Barbary. The main point of the Order, however, was to make it clear that all goods liable to quarantine had to be aired for one week, except the usual list of enumerated goods which should be aired for two weeks. But at least this could be done during quarantine. It is interesting that even enumerated goods could then be released by a certificate from Customs officers, which indicated another and more determined effort by the Privy Council to free themselves from the minutiae of quarantine administration and the procession of Orders to the Treasury. Over the next few years there was, indeed, a marked diminution in this aspect of the Council's business, although they could never escape the ad hoc problems, or petitions via the King for relief from inflexibility. A sharp rise in the number of Orders to the Treasury (and from them to the Customs Commissioners) during 1759

156 Ibid. Russell assumed the whole Levant Act came into force on 24 June 1754, which was certainly the date from which certain sections were specifically mentioned to operate. But the Act curiously failed to pinpoint when the quarantine sections came into effect.

157 NA PC 2/104/69–76.

– an increase which continued over subsequent years – indicated that this policy of aloofness was unsustainable.[158]

Destruction of the Fowey

Early in 1754, a few months before the two Acts came into force, there happened one of the more bizarre and puzzling incidents in British quarantine history, when another ship was deliberately destroyed. This was the sloop *Fowey* (or *Fawey*) from Algiers. The events were publicized by a surgeon, Dale Ingram, as an appendix to his *Historical Account of the Plague*. This rare book, unjustly dismissed in his biographical memoir as 'a mere compilation', was a positive attack on contagionism.[159] Ingram did not believe that plague could be carried by goods: 'I am not afraid to say', he wrote, 'that the fear of the Plague being communicated by commerce and brought into England, has had almost as fatal effects as the Plague itself'.[160] He went on to worry that British commerce might be destroyed by quarantine and the recital of the *Fowey* incident, which he ascribed to 'superstitious absurdities', was his culminating indictment of national policy.[161] But even Ingram felt that unreasoned fear of the plague was not enough to explain the 'mysterious' decision to sink the ship and its cargo, and it is no easier today to ascribe the motive.[162]

Ingram went to great lengths to establish the sequence of events. Having tracked down Isaac Clemens, master of the sloop, and even interviewed his wife, Ingram published a paraphrase of the ship's log, followed by his own commentary which expanded on the basic facts.[163] The *Fowey* had left The Downs for Algiers in June 1753. She reached there on 9 August, and between then and 20 August the cargo was unloaded and the ship was kept in repair. On 21 August loading began (Ingram gives the various commodities in great detail), and some of the crew were occupied ashore at the merchant's house in packing bales of wool, which they compressed with their bare feet. Nine days later, on 30 August, the ship arrived at Gibraltar where she had other minor business. Despite a clean bill of health from Algiers, she underwent a precautionary quarantine of six days. On 3 November the *Fowey* reached Guernsey, her intended destination, but sailed on immediately to Weymouth which was

158 It is not clear which Order, out of so many, reinstated the Privy Council's commitment to discharge individual ships, but the index to NA PC 2/107 lists 223 ships which were the subject of Orders, a dramatic increase on the previous register. In PC 2/108 there are 208 indexed ships, in PC 2/109 there are 228, and so on.

159 See *Oxford Dictionary of National Biography*. Ingram was widely travelled. He had been to Smyrna, endured the lazaretto in Leghorn and worked in Barbados. Some of this experience is mentioned in annotations to the copy of his book in the Wellcome Library; there is no copy in the British Library.

160 D. Ingram, *An Historical Account of the Several Plagues that have appeared in the World, since the year 1346* ... (London, 1755), p. iii.

161 Ingram, pp. iv, 208.

162 Ibid. Ingram thought (p. 186) the *Fowey* incident 'will convince us that the dread of plague did strike us with such horrors, that we were ready to believe what we most feared'.

163 Ingram, pp. 187–208, from which all references in this paragraph and the next are taken.

probably where Clemens came from. There most of the crew went ashore, certain local dignitaries of the town, including the mayor's son and the postmaster, came on board, and a few gifts were distributed. The *Fowey* then went back to Guernsey, and on 6 November anchored in the road.

For two days all went well. Clemens reported to the Governor and received hospitality, and the ship was virtually in free pratique despite its port of origin. But the master was then accosted in the street by a gentleman who asked him for details of the voyage. Clemens replied, rather gruffly, that he had come from Algiers; the stranger then told Clemens he 'would make him to know who he was'. He turned out to be the local Attorney-General, and within a day an emergency meeting of the island's authorities had given the sloop 40 days' quarantine in the Great Road.[164] But on 8 November a boat came alongside, and the *Fowey* was ordered to get under sail immediately or the castle would open fire. Clemens protested to the Governor, and asked to wait for better weather. His request was refused, and in the teeth of a severe gale, the ship pitched and rolled out to sea. On 12 November, Clemens made it back to Portland Bay. Here the welcome had also disappeared, and the sloop was duly sent on to The Motherbank to perform her quarantine. She reached there the following day. For nearly four months which followed, during which all the crew were well and Mrs Clemens had joined her husband on board, the *Fowey* did not move. The master's log records the arrival, on 18 November, of the Collector from Portsmouth (to whom the story of the socializing at Weymouth was recounted), the abortive visit of a naval cutter seeking to impress crew, and the intake of victuals and coal. All this was pretty normal. And yet on 8 March 1754 the *Fowey* was taken out to sea, under the care of HMS *Arundel*, and sunk 13 leagues off Start Point.

The question which Ingram could not answer is why this ship was so harshly handled. Russell, who had only Ingram's account to go on, found the story 'very singular' and suspected 'reasons, which do not appear in the narrative, for such extraordinary treatment. If danger was apprehended, the destruction of the vessel was indiscreetly delayed: or was it necessary to wait the commencement of the Quarantine Act, which took place the 1st. of March?'[165] The obvious source for enlightenment is the Privy Council register, but there was no constructive reference until 10 January 1754, when the *Fowey* had already been at The Motherbank for nearly two months.[166] The Order, which recited from the ship's departure from Guernsey, was curiously normal. The cargo, however, was different from the usual Mediterranean shipments. It included 26 barrels of sugar, 50 bags of canary seed, 24 casks of wine, 1,000 buffalo and goat skins, 12 bales of flax, 1 pipe of beeswax, 10 bales of wool and 2 chests of linen. The master felt 'unsafe' doing quarantine at the location requested, and it was this that decided him to make for The Motherbank. The implication was a decision of seamanship. No mention was made of Gibraltar, Weymouth or Portland, or indeed of threatened gunfire. The purpose of the Order was to have the cargo aired on hoys for 14 days; casks were to be swabbed with salt water and vinegar; the ports and hatches of the sloop were to be left wide open for

164 Ingram, p. 203, admits this detail came from Clemens's wife.

165 Russell, pp. 430–31. He gives his source as 'Ingram's Historical Account, p. 197'.

166 NA PC 2/104/3, from which remaining references in this paragraph are taken.

airing; and the ship itself, after thorough washing, was to be 'fumed with Brimstone as hath been done on like Occasions'.

On 31 January the Privy Council considered a complaint from the Customs officers at Portsmouth about the difficulty of airing goods on hoys in an open roadstead, and another from the ship's agent that he could not find hoymen willing to face the risks.[167] The Council, therefore, ordered the enumerated goods to be sunk, as had been done with the silk and velvet in 1743, but they still wanted the non-enumerated cargo to be aired.[168] But there were more problems. The bales were nine feet long, difficult to manhandle from a wobbling ship, and the non-enumerated goods were mingled with animal skins still in the hair (and so deemed even more dangerous), which had been stowed loose.[169] Labourers could still not be found for the work, and nothing could be aired on the ship's deck in winter. The local Customs officers, therefore, made the bold suggestion that the ship with all its cargo should be sunk.[170] The Customs Commissioners agreed, which led the Privy Council to the same decision.[171] On 14 February 1754 the order was given for the ship to be escorted to sea by a warship, and drilled for scuttling; the hatches would first be secured by iron bars in case the ship 'blew up', and came to the surface.[172]

The Privy Council register does, at least, explain some of the delay which Russell found so strange. It was not a question of waiting for the commencement of the Act, which had no bearing on the destruction of ships; it was simply the time it took to respond to a developing situation, made worse when decisions proved impracticable. It is true that the Privy Council were slow to become involved, but perhaps no slower than they would have been for most ships. The conduct of quarantine for at least the 40 stipulated days was a routine matter for the Customs service until a report or petition sought the Council's involvement. The main point is why the *Fowey* needed to be destroyed at all. There must have been other ships arriving from Barbary with a similar combination of cargoes.

The answer was partly topographical. Had the ship reached Stangate Creek, its cargo would have been offloaded and aired in the normal way. For all its limitations, Stangate Creek was a sheltered anchorage. The Motherbank, however, was part of the Solent, and although screened by the Isle of Wight from the worst south-westerly gales, it was a roadstead and not a harbour. The ship itself might have been safer than off Guernsey, but there were real difficulties with offloading in a rough sea; also, the unwillingness of men to work with an enumerated cargo from a plague-ridden country was a significant factor. The *Fowey* was attracting bad rumours. In *The Gentleman's Magazine* a report was published, emanating from nearby Gosport, that the ship had the plague on board.[173] Stories like that were unwelcome in London

167 NA PC 2/104/33–4.

168 Ibid.

169 NA PC 2/104/43–5.

170 Ibid.

171 Ibid.

172 Ibid.

173 *The Gentleman's Magazine*, 4 March 1754: 'Gosport. The Arundel man of war, Capt. Lloyd, sailed from Spithead, to sink a ship and cargo which has been on quarantine sometimes [*sic*], at the mother bank, supposed to have had the plague on board'.

and limited the options for the Privy Council. The crux of the matter was the state of health at Algiers while the ship was there. Clemens had to swear before the Lord Mayor of London that he had not hesitated about entering Algiers, through fear of the plague, and that the town was healthy during his stay.[174] Ingram defended him on this point with some vigour, claiming that plague never struck Barbary in September.[175] True, the crew had trampled raw wool with their bare feet, but they were manifestly well. And had not the ship received a clean bill of health, and even done quarantine at Gibraltar?

It is difficult to avoid the conclusion that an example was made of the *Fowey* to encourage tighter procedures. The ship's master, and the Customs authorities at Weymouth and initially at Guernsey, had taken no account of quarantine requirements about which they could hardly have been ignorant. Whether the ship was really a health hazard had gradually become a secondary issue, as the practical difficulties mounted. This was a ship with enumerated goods from a hot spot of the plague; it had broken the rules twice, and the master, and indirectly the borough of Weymouth, would learn this would not be tolerated. In an era of quarantine when punishment by prosecution was so problematical, the destruction of property was a more efficient deterrent. But this line of action had expensive connotations, in that compensation was inevitable. The Privy Council might not have agreed to destruction with such alacrity had it involved another Turkey ship. As it was, this was a relatively small vessel with no costly fabrics from the Middle East. Even allowing for those differences, the low figures for compensation in this instance were strikingly at variance with the nearly £24,000 paid in 1721 for two ships and their cargoes, and even with the total of just under £2,000 for a part-cargo alone in 1743. The *Fowey* and her goods were owned by Joseph Littlefear & Co. of London, who petitioned for £1,247, 7s, but even this figure was disputed by Customs.[176] On 21 June 1754 the Privy Council ordered £1,031 12s, 6d to be paid for the cargo, and only £188, 4s, 6d for the sloop.[177] A further sum of nearly £159 was spent in sinking the ship, and the pilot was compensated by nearly £12 for the loss of his apparel.[178] In the end a total of just over £1,390 was paid out of the Old Subsidy, with no parliamentary involvement.[179]

The fate of the *Fowey* is one of the most unsatisfactory episodes in British quarantine history. It is doubtful whether, as a result, ships' masters and others paid any more attention to the rules. The episode did not mark the end of precautionary destruction in British waters, but for nearly half a century the Privy Council tried very hard to keep ships afloat. Perhaps the authorities on Guernsey were revealed in the worst light, and it would not be long before the responsibility of the Governor for quarantine would, at his request, become a matter for discussion with London.

---

174 Ingram, pp. 199–208.

175 Ibid.

176 NA PC 2/104/46, 112.

177 NA PC 2/104/163.

178 Ibid.

179 Ibid.

Messina: the mercantile perspective

A full list of ships affected by the regulations of the Messina crisis could be laboriously compiled from Privy Council registers, but the Quarantine Warrants, conveniently tabulated in Treasury papers, are a welcome, published alternative.[180] There is no reason to believe they are not comprehensive. They were essentially warrants to the Customs Commissioners to execute Orders from the Privy Council for the release of ships, or part of a ship's cargo, from quarantine. They exist over 30 months from mid-July 1743 (when quarantine started) to December 1745 (less than three months before quarantine ended). Some ships occur more than once, either because they were subject to more than one Order, or because they made more than one voyage.

To make a comparison with the statistics of the Marseilles crisis, the merchant ships mentioned in the Treasury warrants have been extracted using the same basis of ports of departure (arranged below, as previously, on a roughly geographical basis), number of ships from each port, and typical cargoes. When cargoes are not given they can often be guessed, and for only four ships is there no known port of departure. Scanderoon and Cyprus have been added to Smyrna, as Levant Company ships are known to have called there. The term Smyrna embraces ships from 'Turkey'. Warships are again excluded from the analysis, as are fleet auxiliaries such as tenders. Also ignored have been a few privateers and prizes, because the latter, although merchant ships, had not been intended for British ports. The table does, however, include two ships which ran aground off the Kent coast as they had apparently been making for the Thames estuary.

180 *CTBP* (1742–45), pp. 384–7, 593–9 [not indexed], 789–92. The tables for 1743 and 1745 are headed Treasury Warrants; that for 1744 is headed Treasury Orders.

Table 6.1 Voyage statistics of ships quarantined from the Mediterranean, 1743–1745

Port(s) of Departure	*Ships*	*Main Cargoes*
Smyrna, Scanderoon, Cyprus	19	Cotton, wool, silk, carpets, fruit
'Syria'	1	Cotton
Cephalonia	2	Currants
Zante	10	Currants
Zante, Cephalonia	1	Linseed
Trieste	1	Copper
Venice	6	Currants, manna
Venice, Trieste, Gibraltar	1	Drugs
Venice, Ancona	1	?
Venice, Zante	3	Currants
Venice, Zante, Cephalonia	1	Currants
Venice, Cephalonia	1	Currants, glass beads
Cesenatico	1	Sulphur
Ancona	1	Hemp
'Calabria'	1	Copper ore
Gallipoli [Apulia]	8	Oil
Gallipoli, Leghorn	1	Wine, silks
Gallipoli, Leghorn, Messina	1	Oil, silk
Belvedere	5	Raisins
Belvedere, Naples	2	Raisins, oil
Naples	5	Raisins, linseed
Naples, Leghorn	1	?
Genoa (1 ship via Dublin)	5	Oil, barilla, lemons, argol
Leghorn	59	Oil, wine, hats, stone, silk, fruit, argol
Leghorn, Belvedere	3	Marble, raisins
Lipari	1	Fruit

Milazzo	1	Silk
Messina, Leghorn	1	Silk
Port Mahon	5	Oil, naval stores (1 ship in ballast)
Port Mahon, Gibraltar	5	Prize goods, naval stores
Port Mahon, Oporto	1	Wine
Monaco	1	?
Gibraltar	9	Naval stores, prize wines, oil, figs
Algiers, Leghorn	1	?
Santa Cruz	2	Fruit, copper, leather, beeswax
Santa Cruz, Sallee	1	?
Villanova [Portugal]	1	Corks, brooms
'Altena' [? Altona, Germany]	1	Lemons

Source: Treasury Warrants in Calendar of Treasury Books and Papers (1742–45) pp. 384–7, 593–9, 789–92. The ship from Altona probably carried fruit trans-shipped from the Mediterranean. It is not clear why the ship from Portugal was quarantined, although cork was always a product deemed susceptible to carry infection.

In Table 6.1 there are 170 ships, to which the 4 must be added for which there is no known port of departure. Another small number of ships might also be added for the nearly three months of 1746 when quarantine subsisted, but the total of 174 ships over 30 months is convenient, as that was also, by happy coincidence, the length of time covered by the statistics of the Marseilles crisis. In comparing the statistics, however, the last five ships should be subtracted from the above table as their ports of departure were outside the Mediterranean. Thus a figure of 169 ships is set against the 335 from within the Straits which had been placed in quarantine in the earlier crisis. This marked decline in traffic over the 20-odd intervening years is consistent with the trend for imports into Great Britain over the same period, as revealed in the figures published by Whitworth. In the five years from 1720 to 1724 inclusive, the average value of imports from the Straits was roughly £70,000; for the same period the average value of imports from Turkey was roughly £298,000.[181] For the years 1740–44, the corresponding figures were about £36,000 and £125,000 respectively.[182] There are wide-ranging reasons for this decline, which impinge upon export markets, consumer trends and foreign competition, but the chief factor in the reduction of trade from the western Mediterranean was war with Spain.[183]

181 Sir C. Whitworth, *State of the Trade of Great Britain in its Imports and Exports ...* (London, 1776), part 2, pp. 33, 37.

182 Ibid.

183 Britain was at war with Spain in 1726–29 and 1739–48.

There is not necessarily a correlation between a lower value of imports and fewer ships, as cargoes could vary greatly in value and bulk; it has already been noticed that the cargo of a Levant ship would be hugely more profitable to a merchant than the cargo of a ship from elsewhere (unless that other ship carried silk). Also, one small part of a ship's cargo might be worth more than the sum of the other components. And, of course, ships came from places within the Mediterranean other than the Straits and Turkey, but these issues do not diminish the credibility of the Treasury statistics for ships in quarantine. Those figures suggest that quarantine in the 1740s had significantly less impact on the English mercantile scene, taken as a whole, than it had in the 1720s and markedly less than at the time of the scare from the Baltic. It might, however, be argued that quarantine itself played some small part in accentuating the decline of trade. The number of ships fell partly, one imagines, because fewer shipowners wished to venture into voyages where their assets might be inordinately delayed, and partly because that same delay meant ships which were regularly engaged on the same run had a longer interval between sailings.[184]

Some delays in the Messina crisis were very severe. The concession that airing could take place during quarantine did not always mean that a ship was released smartly once the 40 days had expired. Joseph Chitty was not the only merchant to fidget and fret while elements of a cargo went mouldy or rancid. At the least excuse, quarantine was delayed week after week. No one, for example, would take any risks with the *Italian Merchant* which had called at Messina, albeit before the plague had begun, and then completed her lading at Leghorn. In February 1744 she was again the subject of a petition for release, having already been detained for four months.[185] Any ship from the Levant could expect the same treatment. The worst delay was probably that suffered by the *Prince Rupert*. This ship had come from Santa Cruz (now Agadir) and Sallee, both in Morocco, and was therefore a victim of the plague scare in West Barbary rather than Messina.[186] The master had the misfortune to inform Customs officials at The Motherbank that around 50 persons were dying of plague daily at Santa Cruz when he took in his cargo.[187] The *Prince Rupert* appears to have been in quarantine for nearly a year, and the only surprise is that the ship, or at least its contents, were not sunk or burnt.[188]

When the ports of departure are compared between the crises of Marseilles and Messina, the main difference, of course, is the absence of shipping from Spain. Whereas Malaga was by far the main port of origin for ships quarantined in 1720–23, with Leghorn well down in second place, in the Messina crisis Malaga was irrelevant and Leghorn came to the fore. With 59 direct departures, and another 6 where it afforded a part cargo, this great entrepôt was involved in 37 per cent of all arrivals in England from the Mediterranean. No other port came anywhere near it.

184 If a ship generally carried fruit or oil, the delay was not too significant, given the dispensation for such cargoes in Privy Council orders.

185 *CTBP* (1742–45), p. 548.

186 *CTBP* (1742–45), pp. 679, 749.

187 *CTBP* (1742–45), p. 679.

188 *CTBP* (1742–45), p. 790, where the ship was subject to an Order in Council of 23 May, against which is the comment 'under quarantine since June 28 last'.

Leghorn was a collection point for goods from anywhere in the Mediterranean basin and made up for the unavailable ports of Spain. Venice and the Ionian Islands were still doing brisk business with English cooks. The cargo was invariably currants with the island of Zante involved in eight shipments, while Naples and Belvedere supplied raisins. These commodities were also, of course, available at Leghorn, as was olive oil, the staple of Gallipoli. While these and other cargoes were much the same as before, a feature of the above table is the first evidence of industrial cargoes: copper, copper ore and sulphur. Although the ratio of ships from the Levant proper had doubled from 6 per cent to 12 per cent since the Messina crisis – an interesting statistic given the decline in value of trade – it is ironic that the region where plague was endemic made such a relatively small contribution to the total of quarantined ships.

There is information in the Treasury records as to the port of quarantine for around half the ships detained.[189] The known figures indicate 59 ships at Stangate Creek (including 2 in 'the Thames') and 16 at Bristol. There were also 5 ships at Plymouth, 3 at Portsmouth (Motherbank), 2 each at Bideford (where they should not have been) and Hull, and 1 at Falmouth. Although it would be unsafe to speculate on this basis as to the whole picture, this is a more useful insight than the Marseilles crisis had afforded. The figures underpin the continuing maritime supremacy of London, but also the strength of Bristol. The character of quarantine in Devon and Cornwall is difficult to assess, not because the ports there lacked merchants who traded directly with the Mediterranean, but because they provided havens for ships which put in for repair or shelter. Quarantine at Plymouth was clearly a problem, as Customs there requested a dedicated man-of-war to oblige ships to follow the rules.[190] At the same port, prize-ships were another fortuitous and significant component among the quarantine detainees.[191] Some relief was afforded to the Customs service along the whole Channel coast by the decision of the Privy Council in September 1743 that ships from the Mediterranean, driven into port by stress of weather, could continue their voyage without quarantine.[192]

The welcome appearance of Hull among the quarantine harbours indicates that the north of Britain is poised, at last, to re-enter the narrative.

189 When these ports are not mentioned in the quarantine warrants from which the table is produced, they can sometimes be gleaned from elsewhere (e.g. *CTBP* (1742–45), pp. 302, 445 etc.).

190 *CTBP* (1742–45), p. 477.

191 These ships were not necessarily taken into the recognized quarantine harbours. Two, for instance, arrived in Dartmouth in May 1744 with a privateer from that port (*CTBP* (1742–45), p. 596).

192 NA PC 2/97/503; *CTBP* (1742–45), p. 370.

Chapter Seven

Indecision in Britain, 1756–1788

General discontent

For 40 years from the middle of the eighteenth century, bubonic plague was still the only disease against which Britain, and indeed other European countries, established preventive quarantine. It forebode badly for the 1790s, when a new disease was to be imported from a new direction, that those 40 years were characterized by inertia and indecision, punctuated by fits of panicky, heavy-handed authority. In that sense, little had changed from the first half of the century, but the difference now was the growing complexity of the management of quarantine, against which new and stronger mercantile interests were persistent and vociferous opponents. On the control side, policy (but not responsibility) eased away from the Privy Council towards Parliament and individual politicians; on the side of those affected, opposition, though still strong in London and Bristol, moved north where it would lay down roots. Manufacturers, especially in Manchester, saw no reason why a remote and theoretical risk should deprive them of their raw materials.

It was a mark of the instability of quarantine policy that the Act of 1753, the first considered and indefinite measure to underpin the King's authority, ran into immediate trouble over its choice of refuge for ships infected with plague. The Act had nominated the harbour of New Grimsby in the Isles of Scilly, a sheltered but narrow anchorage between Tresco and Bryher. In January 1756 the Commons considered a petition from the Scillies representing that the anchorage was a danger to the 500 inhabitants of the adjacent islands.[1] Local maritime experts claimed that New Grimsby harbour was no more than 400 yards wide and, being popular with homeward-bound ships, might contain more than 50 sail at any one time.[2] A less crowded proposition was St Helen's Pool, between the three uninhabited islands of St Helen's, Tean and Northwethel.[3] Being isolated and 'more open to the main Sea', the Pool was safer for both islanders and sailors, and it was claimed the island of St Helen's offered plenty of fresh water and a place to air goods.[4] In fact, the island was wholly unsuitable – a small, hilly wilderness of gorse, bracken and brambles. But knowing nothing of the local topography, and only too relieved that the principle of plague ships at the Scillies was not at issue, Parliament gave easy passage to a Bill

1 *Journal of the House of Commons* [*JHC*], vol. 27, pp. 372–3, 412.

2 *JHC*, vol. 27, p. 412.

3 The spelling was North Withell in the Act which ensued.

4 *JHC*, vol. 27, pp. 372–3, 412.

which substituted St Helen's Pool for New Grimsby. Royal assent was received on 9 March 1756.[5]

For the Privy Council, the preoccupation was not the contingency of plague but the reality of quarantine. As an urgent measure, better facilities were needed for airing at Stangate Creek. Early in 1754, HMS *Sandwich* was converted at Chatham dockyard into a quarantine hulk and became the first English floating lazaretto.[6] The difference between this warship and the two which had served earlier was that the *Sandwich* was stripped down and converted for airing, and so became unserviceable for the navy. The other two had been loaned simply for their deck space; they remained seaworthy and disposable, within the reserve fleet.[7] But the new arrangements at Stangate Creek were no consolation to the merchants of Bristol who, in March 1755, renewed their two-year agitation for the removal of quarantine, which still stood at 20 days, against arrivals from Venice and the Currant Islands.[8]

Anxious to appear even-handed, now that London merchants had airing facilities, the Privy Council pressurized the Customs Commissioners for a report which would enable the quarantine to be lifted and so appease the Bristolians.[9] More precisely, the Commissioners were asked by the Lords Justices to reconsider a previous report under which quarantine had been continued. But the Commissioners dug in their heels, pointing out they were not in a position to be helpful.[10] The receipt of accurate and up-to-date intelligence was not in their province; it was a matter for ministers who had access to consuls' reports and correspondence. If the Privy Council would arrange for the Commissioners to receive such documents, in this 'matter of infinite consequence', they could look at the problem again.[11] The Council inveigled Sir Thomas Robinson, Secretary of State for the Southern Department, into assisting, but by November 1755 the matter was still unresolved.[12] The merchants of London who traded to the Currant Islands now lent their weight to the faltering Bristol attack. They argued for parity with Holland and Hamburg, pointed out that Zante had its own quarantine against Turkey, and made the doubtful declaration that the islands had been free of any 'infectious distemper' for 40 years.[13] They ended with the cunning argument that the navy was being deprived of three to four hundred good seamen a year who could not be impressed from ships liable to quarantine.[14]

All this was to no avail, presumably because consular intelligence failed to give the necessary reassurance. A year later, in November 1756, the currant merchants petitioned again, and the Privy Council, recovering some of their recent confidence, dealt with it themselves by an internal committee.[15] The outcome, on 26 November,

5 *JHC*, vol. 27, p. 502. The resulting Act was 29 Geo. II, c.8.

6 National Archives [NA] PC 2/104/63, Feb. 1754.

7 HMS *Looe* was stationed in King Road near Bristol in 1760 (NA PC 2/107/313).

8 NA PC 2/104/359–60.

9 NA PC 2/104/411.

10 NA PC 2/104/462.

11 Ibid.

12 NA PC 2/104/462, 531.

13 NA PC 2/104/531.

14 Ibid.

15 NA PC 2/105/342.

was to put arrivals from Venice and the Currant Islands on the same basis as those from Smyrna – that is, quarantine was unnecessary if the ship had a clean bill of health.[16] Meanwhile, intelligence from North Africa suggested plague had returned there with renewed vigour. In April 1756 an Order and Proclamation enjoined strict enforcement of the subsisting 40-day quarantine against Algiers and Barbary.[17] Tired of these relentless precautions, two London merchants, Thomas Adams and John Hosier, petitioned in September 1757 for quarantine to be lifted from Morocco.[18] They made the extravagant claim that the kingdom had been free from infection since 1751.[19] But before the Privy Council could react, news reached London of plague in Lisbon, port of departure for packet boats to Falmouth, and a predictable frenzy ensued.

Lessons from Lisbon

The importance of the Lisbon scare (it was too brief to be called a crisis) is that it introduced William Pitt the elder, recently reappointed Secretary of State for the Southern Department, to practical issues of quarantine. This was to be the first sustained and significant involvement of a senior politician. On 25 October 1757 the Privy Council met in emergency conditions and summoned the Postmaster General and the Secretary of the Post Office to a meeting on the following day, when ideas would be expected for keeping plague out of the packet boats.[20] The evidence of plague at Lisbon was no better than hearsay, emanating from Corunna, but the Privy Council wanted their clerk to draft an Order for quarantine by the morning, while the Attorney General worked on a Proclamation.[21] On 28 October, Pitt, backed by a Privy Council Order, asked the Postmaster General to prevent the agent at Falmouth from bringing mail from Lisbon on shore.[22] The latest packet boat, however, had already landed its letters, and these were intercepted at Staines.[23] Ahead of the main post, one loose letter dated Lisbon, 13 October, had actually reached London and been opened.[24] Far from spreading alarm, this letter went a long way towards restoring normality, as it contained no mention of plague. The rest of the mail was fumigated at Staines, but the scare subsided as quickly as it had begun. On 31 October 1757, Pitt ordered all the mail at Staines to be delivered, and the Privy Council revoked their earlier Orders.[25]

16 NA PC 2/105/349, 355.
17 NA PC 2/105/150.
18 NA PC 2/105/587.
19 Ibid.
20 NA PC 2/105/609.
21 NA PC 2/105/610.
22 NA PC 2/105/612. Boats were to row continually around the packet to prevent landings.
23 Ibid.
24 Ibid.
25 NA PC 2/105/616.

While the Postmaster General had been stopping the mail at Falmouth, Pitt was in communication with Alexander Russell, then living in Lime Street, London.[26] This doctor was the half-brother of Patrick Russell and had served as physician to the English factory at Aleppo between 1740 and 1753.[27] Alexander Russell was asked to make practical suggestions for disinfecting money and mail from suspect ships.[28] He responded immediately and later went to Lisbon in a warship to investigate the rumours.[29] Russell, in his letter of 28 October 1757, advised that money needed no more than immersion in vinegar.[30] His precautions for mail were potentially far more troublesome. Letters which contained samples of cloth or thread should be returned to the ship and treated as part of the cargo. Other letters might be landed, but there was no escaping the vinegar: larger packets had to be opened and single letters slit on one side. It was then a job for the health officer, holding a pair of tongs, to dip the letters into a pail of vinegar and place them in a 'perfuming' case. Russell described this as a wooden box about 6 feet high and 4 feet wide. It consisted of shelves or partitions of wooden latticework, enclosed by a door. While the letters were placed on the shelves, a chafing dish should be lit at the bottom; this dish would contain charcoal and a handful or two of powder, consisting of one part of sulphur to five parts of deal sawdust. With the door shut, the letters would be smoked for one hour, with the operation repeated at will in cases of known infection.

Advice similar to Russell's was given by the Postmaster General, Sir Everard Fawkener, who was also a City merchant and one-time ambassador at Constantinople.[31] It is doubtful whether Russell and Fawkener had communicated with each other, as both men had been required to make a virtually instant response. In his submission to the Privy Council, Fawkener first sought to play down the danger, arguing that plague, to the best of his knowledge, had never been spread by infected mail or money.[32] He did, however, accept that immersion in vinegar and fumigation by sulphur were wise precautions. Indeed, he had 'known a very diligent and careful Person, who always mixed old leather in the fumigation ...' The importance of Fawkener's exposition is that he went slightly beyond his brief, by arguing for a quarantine station at St Just's Pool, upriver from Falmouth. This was the first time that this anchorage, destined to be well used, had been officially recommended. Fawkener suggested a pratique

26 The address comes from Russell's letter to Pitt, 28 Oct. 1757 (NA PRO30/8/54/277–80).

27 *Oxford Dictionary of National Biography*. He wrote a *Natural History of Aleppo* (1756), which dealt *inter alia* with the attitude of Europeans in Syria towards the plague.

28 NA PRO 30/8/54/277–80.

29 C. Maclean, *Remarks on the British Quarantine laws* ... (London, 1823), p. 13, states that Alexander Russell had been sent to Holland to investigate, but as his only source appears to have been Patrick Russell's book, this is presumably a mistake.

30 NA PRO 30/8/54/277–80, from which remaining references in this paragraph are taken.

31 *Oxford Dictionary of National Biography*; H. Robinson, *Britain's Post Office* (Oxford, 1953), p. 280.

32 NA PRO 30/8/83/1–6, from which remaining references in this paragraph are taken. Fawkener is not identified as 'The Post Master General' in the undated submission, but the attribution is clear.

house there, as well as lodgings for officials engaged in the 'purgation' of mail, all within a double barrier patrolled by soldiers from Pendennis Castle.

These two submissions spurred Pitt to a deeper enquiry into quarantine management. He asked Alexander Russell to prepare a model procedure but, in the opinion of Patrick Russell, these 'General Directions for Quarantine' were never finished.[33] But Patrick did come across, in his late brother's papers, a copy letter to Pitt, dated 28 March 1758, covering the despatch of a memoir which might have been sent. The memoir survived only as a 'corrected scrawl', but the copy letter was in better shape and Patrick published it in his *Treatise of the Plague*.[34] As none of this later material from Alexander Russell has survived in the Chatham Papers, it would appear Pitt had no time or inclination to follow up the advice, assuming that it ever reached him.

In the view of Alexander Russell, 'The present method of performing quarantine, in England ... is no security from infection; though perhaps it is attended with the same expence and inconveniency to the merchant, as if it were performed in the most effectual manner'.[35] Russell favoured a Mediterranean approach adapted for the British mentality:

> The whole of the health officers, throughout the kingdom, ought to be under the direction of a Board of Health in London, consisting chiefly of gentlemen who have seen something of quarantine abroad, and who would be induced by their public spirit to serve without salaries. To these should be added a secretary, and a physician, to assist in giving the proper directions, and to visit the Lazarettos, in cases of emergency.

Although he put lazaretto in the plural, Russell had positive ideas for only one, which would serve London, and accommodate the cargoes of ten or twelve ships at once. He gave a number of criteria for the site, which included security against smuggling, safety of anchorage, distance from passing traffic and healthiness of the air. His casual remark that perhaps some suitable location might be found on the River Medway was dismissive by implication of Stangate Creek.

Russell believed that the pratique house (to examine bills of health and examine ships' masters) should be separate from the lazaretto. He suggested Sheerness as a site for the Thames/Medway lazaretto, while another one at Deal would be 'absolutely necessary'. Other lazarettos or pratique houses might also be advisable around the country, particularly at St Helen's Pool. Russell went on to state, very broadly, the kind of jobs, such as guardian and gatekeeper, which these establishments might require. He made no estimate of costs in the letter, but reckoned outlay 'will not be considerable'. Perhaps it was this scarcely credible opinion which made Pitt lose interest, coupled with the unacceptable proposal for a Board of Health. The kingdom was not yet ready to emasculate its Privy Council.

---

33 P. Russell, *A Treatise of the Plague* ... (London, 1791), p. 438.

34 Russell, pp. 438–40.

35 Ibid., from which references in this paragraph and the next are taken.

Nervous years

The inaccuracy of rumours about plague in Lisbon made the Privy Council think twice when intelligence was received of disease even closer to home. In mid-March 1758 there was a rumour of plague at Brest, but no quarantine was imposed and ministers were unimpressed.[36] The only precaution taken was the suspension of the tobacco trade to Brittany, which involved cancelling the pass for a shipment from Whitehaven to Morlaix.[37] For the Levant, however, a tougher line was now felt appropriate. Later in March, the cosy arrangement with the Levant Company, which had seen no restrictions against Smyrna for nearly six years for ships with clean bills of health, was abandoned: reports of plague in the port led to the reimposition of a 40-day quarantine.[38] This was followed in June by an interesting quarantine, of like duration, against privateers returning to Britain from the Mediterranean.[39] The excuse was that privateers visited many neutral ships from Smyrna and the Levant, which might lead indirectly to the spread of infection. The same logic, of course, applied to ships of the royal navy, but they were not made the subject of a similar Order. The news went down badly with the privateers, who were doing lawful business under letters of marque; the *Royal George* refused initially to make Stangate Creek and sailed on for Deptford.[40] When she was eventually quarantined, more than 80 men from her complement, and a similar number from the *Volunteer*, absconded into the Kent marshes.[41] In a later incident, the master and 22 men from the *Leopard* privateer, which had taken a French ship from Smyrna, were recaptured after jumping ship.[42] A prosecution was successfully brought, with fines of £500 on the master and £200 on each crewman.[43] In any Mediterranean country, of course, they would have suffered death. It was a symptom of the volatility of public confidence that plague was rumoured to have broken out in the Borough, part of Southwark, caused by the escapees. This caused a large demand for rue and wormwood; the price rose 40 per cent overnight 'and the gardeners servants were employed all the day in taking those commodities to market'.[44]

With the focus on privateers causing such problems, the Privy Council extricated themselves by generalizing the application of the rule. They issued an Order, in June 1759, for all ships from the Mediterranean to do quarantine, as if from Smyrna, if they had had communication with any infected ship, or touched anywhere on the coast between Leghorn and Marseilles.[45] This measure was itself broadened in July, when all ships from the Mediterranean were ordered absolutely to perform 40 days'

36 NA PC 2/106/60–61.
37 Ibid.
38 NA PC 2/106/66.
39 NA PC 2/106/140.
40 NA PC 2/106/140.
41 NA PC 2/106/145–7, 170, 310, 321, 330, 337, 339, 358, 366.
42 *The Gentleman's Magazine*, 28 July 1760.
43 Ibid.
44 *The Gentleman's Magazine*, 29 July 1760.
45 NA PC 2/107/27, 39.

quarantine.[46] At the centre of policy, once again, was Pitt; he was receiving advice from Gibraltar, Venice and elsewhere that plague was causing other countries to extend their restrictions.[47] This was very much a long-term scare, with enough peaks of alarm, some scarcely credible, to cause petitions for relaxation to be ignored. In July 1760 Pitt was told by the British minister in Turin of a ship that had recently reached Marseilles from Syria: as soon as the hatches were opened, three people allegedly dropped dead.[48] The rumours and warnings continued well into 1761; the Venetian Resident in London told Pitt of even tougher quarantine in Venice against its own islands in the Levant.[49] It was not long before plague in Bosnia and Serbia added to the dangers of the Adriatic and caused quarantine to be reconfirmed by another Order.[50] Against this trend, the Privy Council did agree, in November 1763, to abolish quarantine for arrivals from Spanish ports within the Mediterranean, Gibraltar and Minorca.[51] One of the deciding factors, as usual, was parity with the practice of other countries, which in this case included Scandinavia. The several arguments adduced by the petitioners did not include the fact that two of the places were British.[52]

In England, Pitt was recognized as the prime mover of quarantine strategy, even beyond the limits of his ministry. He was solicited by the Corporation of Bristol to assist with their problems which, far from diminishing over the years, now threatened the credibility of national policy.[53] As the quays were some miles up the narrow Avon, quarantine was at moorings just within or outside the river mouth, and never far from shore. The escape of 98 men in July 1759, and similar episodes soon afterwards, prompted local Customs officers to seek military help.[54] The Privy Council, instead of sending soldiers, asked the Admiralty in April 1760 to supply a warship.[55] But the navy were part of the problem, as the men had been escaping to avoid impressment. A fight developed in the channel of the Avon, when one man was killed while resisting and another wounded.[56] The Corporation, to add to the confusion, wanted a warship, and it was the continuing absence of one which led

46 NA PC 2/107/78. Another Order that enforced subsisting quarantine was issued on 31 December 1760 (NA PC 2/108/130).

47 NA PC 2/107/23, 77.

48 NA PC 2/107/441.

49 NA PC 2/108/130.

50 NA PC 2/109/531.

51 NA PC 2/110/86, 133.

52 NA PC 2/110/133. The arguments were: restoration of peace makes British ships less liable to be stopped by cruisers (which had exposed them to infection); little trade subsists from the Levant and Barbary to Spain; regular quarantine is performed in Spain against arrivals from within the Straits; Dutch, Hamburgers, Danes, Swedes and others do not subject their trade from Spain to quarantine (and did not during the war); cargoes are often perishable; King is anxious to remove all obstructions to trade.

53 NA PC 2/107/336, 458.

54 NA PC 2/107/69,116. The 98 men escaped from the *Europa*. There were later escapees from the *Hopewell* and the *Penelope* (*The Gentleman's Magazine*, 8 Oct. 1759).

55 NA PC 2/107/336.

56 NA PC 2/107/358.

to their letter to Pitt. In July 1760 the Privy Council went along with their wish and the Admiralty were again asked to assist.[57] Ironically, the navy pleaded innocent of the problem; the captain of HMS *Looe*, now removed from Stangate Creek to King Road, claimed that seamen only absconded because there were too few Customs officers to enforce the rules.[58]

Later in 1760 the dread of plague reached almost a level of farce. On 27 September a large Algerine privateer went aground near Penzance, having lost all track of its position.[59] There were 170 survivors, who believed they had landed in Spain where they could expect slavery or cruel treatment. Their relief at finding the country was England was only matched by the terror of the Cornish who associated the vessel with plague. 'Nothing could equal the bustle and panic which this occasioned. Some ventured towards the beach, but quickly returned, affirming that they had smelt ... the plague smell', which was an excuse to drink brandy as an antidote.[60] When soldiers eventually arrived, the men were lodged at first on Penzance seafront, and later in a building more suited to quarantine, a little out of town.[61] In October the Privy Council asked the Admiralty for a transport to be made available, and the men were repatriated.[62] In May 1761, however, Algiers was the cause of another embarrassing incident. The Algerine ambassador, in quarantine at Stangate Creek, had contrived to send Pitt a letter. When this arrived in the common post with not the slightest evidence of fumigation, an angry Pitt sent it straight on to the Privy Council for an explanation.[63]

Over all these years, airing of goods during quarantine was straining the limited resources at Stangate Creek. There were, however, surprisingly few petitions for quarantine to be lifted, and none in relation to the Levant. It was only traders to the western Mediterranean who were at all persistent. Turkey merchants were beginning to accept that Britain was inevitably moving towards the position in the Mediterranean where quarantine, albeit for variable duration, was permanent against the East. Every piece of intelligence arriving at Pitt's desk from Italy and elsewhere accelerated the integration of Britain into the international exchange of warnings and advice, of which quarantine was the logical outcome. The problem was the inadequate range of facilities to meet the growing backlog of ships. By October 1762 the Customs Commissioners were warning that HMS *Sandwich*, which had been used as a lazaretto for airing since 1754, was in urgent need of expensive repair, and another ship was necessary.[64] But the Admiralty were far from happy, and felt the whole question of naval involvement in what was essentially a commercial issue, needed re-examination at the highest level. Thus, while Customs officers, merchants

57 NA PC 2/107/458.
58 NA PC 2/107/313.
59 *Naval Chronicle*, vol. 22 (1809, Part 2), pp. 295–6.
60 Ibid.
61 Ibid.
62 NA PC 2/107/501.
63 NA PC 2/108/329, 334.
64 NA PC 2/109/381.

and shipowners bemoaned the continuing deterioration of their airing hulk, the Admiralty prepared its case for an alternative solution on land.

Nearer a lazaret

There were two lines of attack, one through Parliament, the other at the Privy Council. The parliamentary tactic was to resurrect the resolution of the Commons, made on 5 March 1752, that a land lazaret should be built on Chetney Hill beside Stangate Creek.[65] On 20 March 1764 the House was moved that the old resolution be read, and a new request was made to the King for plans and estimates of the proposed construction.[66] The essential difference from before was that this request was made in the knowledge that the documentation now existed. The catalyst for action had been the deteriorating state of the airing hulk, as reported in 1762, and the paperwork had taken most of the following year to prepare. On 9 April 1764 Lord Charles Spencer presented to the House the desired plan, estimate and associated papers, which were ordered to lie on the table.[67] Four days later the House was given a report from the Navy Board, presented by Lord Howe of the Admiralty, on the expenses associated with the floating lazaretto in Stangate Creek.[68] Parliamentary records give no details of this report, but the register of the Privy Council makes up for the deficit.

The matter came before the Privy Council on 18 April, when a memorial from the Admiralty was referred to a committee.[69] The Admiralty paper included a report from the Navy Board – no doubt the same report as that presented to Parliament – which stated there was no three-deck warship at Chatham suitable for use as a replacement lazaretto.[70] The *Prince Frederick* was available, but that was a two-deck ship and Customs felt it would not provide enough room, 'they being often streightened for want of it in the Sandwich', which was of similar size. The Navy Board then outlined the real cost of keeping the *Sandwich* as a lazaretto. The initial expense of conversion and subsequent upkeep had amounted to more than £8,000; when the value of her hull, at least £6,000, was also taken into account, the ship's ten years of service as an airing hulk had cost nearly £15,000. The expense of converting and moving a three-deck warship would be greater, and this outlay would recur at roughly ten-year intervals. If facilities were built on shore, the Navy Board argued that they would be spared this expenditure, for which Parliament had made no provision, and work in dockyards would not be diverted from its proper role. The committee suggested that the Admiralty should insert in the ordinary estimate of the navy, for the next session of Parliament, the sum necessary for a shore lazaret, and

65 *JHC*, vol. 26, p. 478. See Chapter 6.

66 *JHC*, vol. 29, p. 967. See also Russell, pp. 435–6.

67 *JHC*, vol. 29, p. 1041.

68 *JHC*, vol. 29, p. 1050.

69 NA PC 2/110/412.

70 NA PC 2/110/423–5, from which remaining references in this paragraph are taken until otherwise stated.

that a floating lazaretto should continue until the facilities were built. On 9 May 1764 the Privy Council made an Order accordingly.[71]

There was some danger, now, that Parliament and the Privy Council were heading in different directions. It is probable that neither the Admiralty nor Parliament wished the building of a shore lazaret to be a matter for the navy. Over the next few months the momentum for action was checked, and the proposals might well have been dropped altogether had not an event in the Scillies drawn attention to the dire inadequacy of existing precautions. The incident, such as it was, occurred in November 1764. A ship from Naples had been forced out of Milford Haven and told to do quarantine in the Scillies.[72] This was arguably a wrong request, as there was no suggestion that the ship was actually infected, and St Helen's Pool was intended to be a harbour of last resort in an outbreak of plague, rather than an anchorage for normal quarantine. But the move served to test the system, and the system was found wanting. The commandant of the Scillies, who resided at Star Castle on St Mary's, complained to the Secretary at War that local officials had received no instructions as to how quarantine should be conducted.[73] Furthermore, St Helen's Pool was five or six miles from St Mary's, where the Customs officers lived, and might be unreachable in a gale.[74] A more pressing problem was that a number of coasting vessels bound for Ireland were using the Pool, as they often did, as a safe haven in bad weather. They would not willingly cede the anchorage to the uses of quarantine, and if the commandant were to force them out, they threatened to sue him for any damage they might incur in the open sea.[75]

From this episode it was clear that St Helen's Pool was no sanctuary, and that quarantine required expenditure as well as a sensible choice of location. If the arrival of a ship for routine quarantine caused such problems, it was as well that a plague-stricken ship, peopled by the dead and dying, had not already limped to anchor. St Helen's Pool was grotesquely inadequate. The tiny, barren islands surrounding the pool were suited only to seabirds. The pratique house or lazaretto which Alexander Russell had vaguely suggested in 1758 was out of the question. Communication with London could hardly be longer. It would be the best part of ten days before the authorities on St Mary's could even receive the Privy Council's instructions. And what sensible advice, what relief for the sick, what reassurance to the islanders could those instructions possibly contain?[76] St Helen's Pool was revealed for what it was – an 'out of sight, out of mind' solution to a national problem which the Establishment were reluctant to face. The Scillies were, *in extremis*, a sacrifice worth paying for the health of mainland Britain. The proof of that came four months later, when the Customs Commissioners were ordered to prevent all communication with

71 NA PC 2/110/430.

72 NA PC 2/111/39.

73 Ibid.; *Calendar of Home Office Papers of the Reign of George III* [*CHOP*] (1760–65), pp. 459–60.

74 Ibid.

75 Ibid.

76 The plight of infected crews was a worry to Russell (pp. 455–6).

the Scillies if a rumour from Barnstaple proved correct, that the islands were ravaged by some dreadful disease.[77]

The commandant's problem had reached the Privy Council via the Earl of Halifax.[78] Although it was relegated to the Treasury, the complaint brought home the weakness of Britain's resolve. If the Scillies had to muddle through, at least Stangate Creek, the main bastion of prevention and on the doorstep of London, could be made to give better protection. To this end, the question of a land lazaret should still be pursued, and the parliamentary process resumed its repetitious course. On 17 January 1765 the King was again humbly requested to have laid before the Commons the necessary plans and estimates.[79] These were evidently revised proposals, recently prepared. Four days later, during a wider presentation by the Admiralty on the naval estimates, the House received new plans, tables of reference, costings and a report on the best location adjacent to Stangate Creek.[80] These plans, which have not survived, were the work of a 'Mr. Stuart'. The knowledge of his identity was soon forgotten, and in 1805 his surname was written as 'Stewart' by the Clerk to the Privy Council, who described him as 'probably the Architect who had travelled much in the east, & was a Man of much Observation'.[81] It seems safe to conclude that this architect was James 'Athenian' Stuart, best known for his association with Nicholas Revett (which produced a seminal work on the antiquities of Athens), who had been appointed surveyor of Greenwich Hospital in 1758 and was associated with the Office of Works.[82] In 1755 Stuart had returned to England from a long visit to Greece and Constantinople, and had undoubtedly experienced life in a lazaretto at one stage or another in his journey. On 26 March 1765 a committee of supply recommended that a sum not exceeding £5,000 be granted to the King towards the building of a lazaret, and the House duly agreed.[83] There now seemed no obstacle to the removal of airing from sea to land.

Again the proposal was abortive. It seems quite bewildering that with money agreed and an impetus to proceed, no effort was made to bring the lazaret scheme to fruition. Patrick Russell was uncurious as to the reason, simply noting that the matter had 'rested'.[84] Froggatt ascribes the lack of progress to a variety of factors: a diminishing threat from plague in Europe; the increased cost of the Customs service; and the adequacy of the naval hulks.[85] But plague in Europe, so far from diminishing, was soon to threaten from areas which had been assumed for decades to be no longer a risk. In a few years, the airing hulks at Stangate Creek would be overwhelmed.

---

77 NA PC 2/111/127. Eleven days later, on 19 March 1765, the contagion was recognized as 'merely an inflammatory fever affecting the old', and the Order was revoked (PC 2/111/147).

78 *CHOP* (1760–65), p. 459.

79 *JHC*, vol. 30, p. 29.

80 *JHC*, vol. 30, p. 33.

81 NA PC 2/169/34–7.

82 Howard Colvin, *A Biographical Dictionary of British Architects, 1660–1840*, 3rd edn (London & New Haven, 1995); *Oxford Dictionary of National Biography*.

83 *JHC*, vol. 30, p. 309.

84 Russell, p. 436.

85 P. Froggatt, 'The Chetney Hill lazaret', *Archaeologia Cantiana*, 79 (1964), 6.

One specious reason for non-activity was that mentioned in the preamble to the Act of Parliament of 1772, which gave the Treasury power to treat for the purchase of a site. There it was claimed that doubts had arisen whether the King was 'sufficiently enabled ... to contract and agree for the absolute purchase of lands'.[86] But that problem could have been realized and dealt with rather sooner.

The main reason for inertia was more nebulous: it was a blend of anxiety for mercantile freedom and the uniquely British confusion between the boundaries of function. In most foreign countries, especially the smaller Italian states, an autocratic ruler or governing body, convinced of the need for a lazaretto, could simply get it built. In Britain there was still a niggling apprehension that quarantine went against the grain of legitimate trade. If the Levant merchants conceded it was unavoidable, merchants trading elsewhere saw it as a knock-on nuisance to comply with irrelevant Mediterranean principles. There had been no plague in England for one hundred years and, despite the occasional rumour in jittery London, no ship with a foul bill of health, or from anywhere in the Levant and Barbary, had landed a diseased seaman or an infected cargo. A land lazaret would have suggested the permanence of an institution in which the merchants had no belief and for which the Privy Council had no enthusiasm. As long as it remained more of a feasible option than a practical necessity, there was still a lurking desire to delay the construction from one year to the next.

The problem of demarcation compounded that of inertia. No agency of the Crown wished to take the lead in a pioneering venture which fell between every stool of responsibility. The enforcement of quarantine was an irksome task for Customs officers and lay only at the periphery of their mainstream duties. The Commissioners had already complained to the Treasury in 1761 that quarantine work was 'Burthensome'.[87] They did not influence policy, except when asked, and the building of a lazaret was not remotely within their brief. Once a lazaret on the best principles had been erected, the establishment would require permanent positions which Customs officers were unsuited to fill. If the Venetian precedent were followed – and details of the layout and functions of its two lazarettos had been published in London some years earlier – the posts of Prior and Sub-Prior would have to be created.[88] The Navy Board would be even less inclined to take on a responsibility that had nothing to do with the navy. The idea of a land lazaret was to free the navy's resources, not to embroil its management in extracurricular duties. As for the Office of Works, while they might be in a position to realize a building, they had to work with some other institution which would eventually run it, and in the mid-eighteenth century there were no volunteers. The crux of the problem was that Britain had no Board of Health, such as Alexander Russell had advised, and in its absence the administrative framework for a lazaret did not exist. It was Pitt who,

86 12 Geo. III, c.57.

87 E.E. Hoon, *The Organization of the English Customs System, 1696–1786* (Newton Abbot, 1968), p. 42.

88 The duties attaching to these posts were explained in *An Authentic Account of the Measures and Precautions used at Venice ...* (London, 1752), pp. 15ff.

as Secretary of State, had not acted on Russell's advice; it was now Pitt, among other Prime Ministers, who failed to press for the lazaret.

Enter the Board of Trade

The relentless quarantine against arrivals from the Mediterranean prompted a concerted revolt among merchants trading to Italy and Sardinia. The protest began modestly in February 1765, with a routine petition to the King in Council for taking quarantine off ships from the kingdom of Sardinia, which included part of what is now the south of France.[89] This prompted a lazy letter from the Privy Council to the Under-Secretary of State in Lord Halifax's Southern Department, asking for copies of such information as to health in the Mediterranean as shall be received 'from time to time'.[90] This indicated that the Privy Council were reluctant to reach a decision. In June various reports were read, but the Council's register noted nothing was ordered.[91] The matter might have ended there had not a scheme been hatched by merchants in England and on the Continent to involve the Board of Trade.

It was nearly 60 years since the Board of Trade (more correctly called the Council of Trade and Plantations) had played any part in quarantine, and as their role was still largely advisory, decisive action was not to be expected.[92] But an early function of the Board had been to receive consular reports on the state of trade with foreign nations.[93] The original idea had been that consuls or ministers would assemble the merchants in, say, Leghorn every six months and hear their ideas for improving or augmenting their business. These recommendations would then be passed on to the King, via the Secretary of State for the Southern Department, and to the Board of Trade.[94] From around 1718 this practice waned, but merchants now saw the resurrected procedure as an alternative line of attack. The British minister in Turin was persuaded to send Henry Seymour Conway (successor to Lord Halifax) some considerations for improving trade between Britain and the Continental possessions of the King of Sardinia.[95] In particular, he argued for a more direct communication with Nice and Villa Franca.

On 15 September 1765, at Conway's behest, William Burke forwarded the minister's paper to the Board of Trade.[96] The Board, as if sensing a trap, were slow to respond, but on 19 December they held a meeting with merchants trading from London to the relevant areas.[97] When the minister's points were explained,

89 NA PC 2/111/84.

90 NA PC 2/111/97.

91 NA PC 2/111/227.

92 *Office-Holders in Modern Britain III. Officials of the Boards of Trade, 1660–1870* (London, 1974), p. 4.

93 D.B. Horn (ed.), 'The Board of Trade and consular reports, 1696–1782', *English Historical Review*, 54 (1939), 476–80.

94 Ibid.

95 *Journal of the Commissioners for Trade and Plantations* [*JCTP*], vol. 12, p. 235.

96 Ibid.

97 Ibid.

the merchants replied that the direct communication already existed, and all that prevented the trade from growing was the quarantine imposed in Britain. They argued for this to be removed, as long as vessels carried no goods trans-shipped from the Levant, and pointed out 'that they had some time since presented a petition to his Majesty in Council ...'[98] In their toothless state, the Board of Trade replied to Burke with just a factual account of the meeting and no recommendations for the Secretary of State.[99]

Although the ploy had failed, the Board of Trade did not escape further involvement by having ducked the quarantine issue. Furthermore, the Sardinian question was now turning contentious: the British factory at Leghorn were also writing to Conway on matters of trade, and it was not in their interests to see Nice and Villa Franca developed. In April 1766 John Dick, the British consul at Leghorn, backed by 25 local merchants, sent Conway a memorial.[100] In one respect there was common ground with the Sardinian lobby, as the merchants argued strongly for the abolition of quarantine in Britain. They saw it as their greatest inconvenience. 'We are extremely unfortunate', they wrote, 'that we cannot make the Lords of the Privy Council sensible of the little Necessity of such a Precaution from a Port the best regulated in the Mediterranean, in Matters relating to the Preservation of the Health'. They went on to describe the complicated and lengthy quarantine process involving two lazarettos, between which goods for airing were distributed according to the bill of health from the place of origin. These precautions merited ships from Leghorn being admitted to free pratique anywhere in the Mediterranean, except in ports 'where ... an Emulation of Trade, and a political Reason joined to curb the Trade of Leghorn to their own Advantage'.

The merchants used time-honoured arguments to have quarantine lifted:

> The Prejudice ... arises from the Detention of their Goods, which often disappoint them in the Sale, or prevents their benefiting of the favourable Conjunctures that may happen, to dispose of them with advantage; besides submitting their Merchandise to an extraordinary Expence, it occasions a certain Restraint upon Trade, which stagnates the free Circulation of their Business, and hinders it from being so extensive as it might otherwise be.

The only reason they conceded for quarantine in Britain would be if a ship had communication with a Barbary cruiser during her voyage. Then followed the condemnation of the port of Villa Franca, from where the Leghorn factory assumed that quarantine had already been lifted. The merchants expressed their astonishment that such a favour could be granted to a port without proper quarantine facilities, where every ship was visited by a cruiser collecting dues for the King of Sardinia. Leghorn foresaw its own trade diminishing as Villa Franca, which had no English mercantile house, prospered in its stead. The factory warned of French machinations: cotton would pass from Marseilles to Villa Franca for trans-shipment to London; wine and oil from Toulon would do likewise, passed off as Italian produce. And there was worse yet. The 'Act' ships which brought cod from Newfoundland, pilchards

98 Ibid.

99 Ibid.; *CHOP* (1766–69), pp. 642–3.

100 NA PC 1/8/20, from which references in this paragraph and the next are taken.

from Cornwall, herrings from Yarmouth, and salmon from Scotland and Ireland to Leghorn, would no longer find silk from Turin there as return freight for London. While the silk moved to Villa Franca, the fish ships would load only 'Course & Rough Goods' at Leghorn, destined mainly for British manufactories; as the freight was less profitable, the shippers would increase the cost to industry, with a subsequent price rise for consumers.

As the Leghorn factory had been wrong in assuming ships from Villa Franca were excused quarantine in Britain, the Board of Trade were at least spared the prospect of a factional dispute. With the Sardinian question already dealt with as far as they were concerned, the Board, at Conway's request, focused on the question of quarantine against Leghorn.[101] They postponed the difficult question from week to week, but this gave the Italian merchants of London and Bristol time to perfect their case. On 12 June 1766 this was presented to the Board.[102] A week later the merchants submitted the cost to an act-ship of 21 days' quarantine, and a further letter was discussed from John Dick.[103] This letter enclosed memorials to Sir Horace Mann from the Court of Tuscany and from Marshal Botta, both seeking the abolition of quarantine for ships from Leghorn. In the face of such a powerful lobby, the Board of Trade could only show support. They deliberated about the text of a representation to the King, which reached the Privy Council on 11 July.[104] By coincidence, the Council were considering on that same day a petition from merchants at Liverpool for abolishing quarantine against arrivals from Italy, and another from merchants at London seeking the like against arrivals from the kingdom of Sardinia.[105] The factions had evidently made common cause. Both these petitions, and the representation from the Board of Trade, were delegated to the Committee for Plantation Affairs, where they were filed and forgotten.[106]

In late November 1766 the Privy Council were reminded of this outstanding issue by the arrival of two more petitions from the merchants who had business in Italy and Sardinia.[107] As if forewarned of their arrival, the Council had instructed the Customs Commissioners, a few days previously, to make an urgent enquiry into 'the nature and purport' of certificates carried by ships from Leghorn to prove they had undergone quarantine.[108] As for the petitions, they were also referred to the Committee, from which they instantly descended to the luckless Board of Trade. The reaction of the Board was to set up a meeting with representatives from both lobbies on 2 January 1767.[109] At this meeting Messrs Prescot and Godheard Hagen spoke for Liverpool, and Mr Matteux and others for London, and the Board asked them to expound on quarantine regulations in Italy and the trade it enjoyed with the Levant

101 *JCTP*, vol. 12, p. 285.
102 *JCTP*, vol. 12, p. 290.
103 *JCTP*, vol. 12, p. 293.
104 *JCTP*, vol. 12, pp. 294, 303–4; NA PC 2/111/714.
105 NA PC 2/111/715.
106 NA PC 2/111/714–15.
107 NA PC 2/112/103.
108 NA PC 2/112/95.
109 *JCTP*, vol. 12, pp. 349, 351–2.

and Barbary.[110] Four days later the Board sent a report, which can be assumed to have supported the abolition of quarantine, to the Committee for Plantation Affairs.[111] There is no evidence that it went any further. If it did, the Privy Council were far from minded to cooperate. For much of 1767 they received rumours of plague besieging the Italian peninsula: it was reportedly in Croatia, Montenegro, the Morea, Tunis and Malta.[112] During 1768 a French ship carrying the Tripoline ambassador to Holland was sent from Leghorn to the lazaretto at Marseilles under armed escort, as several deaths from plague had occurred on board.[113] With Sir Horace Mann now advising Britain to be constantly vigilant, the merchants of Leghorn could only bottle up their irritation.

There were two main outcomes to this abortive episode. The first was that the Board of Trade played no further role in quarantine until after its reconstruction as a committee of the Privy Council in 1786. The second was that it encouraged an anonymous writer, claiming a previous long residence it Italy, to publish the quarantine procedures at Leghorn in much greater detail. In 1767 *The Nature of a Quarantine as it is Performed in Italy* was published in London, seeking to correct and amplify the information given to the Board of Trade.[114] Compared with a previous anonymous pamphlet, which had described measures and precautions in Venice in painstaking detail, this was a slovenly and sensational work.[115] It was a pamphlet of confusing arrangement, designed to shock, drawing attention to the powers of death and destruction vested in the Health Office at Leghorn. It alleged that guardians placed to supervise ships showed more 'Fidelity' than Customs officers in Britain.[116] This was also a paper with contradictions, claiming that officials in the lazarettos were impartial, doing their job 'without any respect of Persons', yet the need to strip naked for medical examination was waived for 'People of fashion'.[117] *The Gentleman's Magazine* found other inconsistencies in a damning review.[118]

The same author must be credited with *The Immediate Necessity of Building a Lazzaretto,* published in 1768. This pamphlet, which reprinted extracts verbatim from the earlier one, was dedicated to Lord North, then Chancellor of the Exchequer, and claimed that the English defences were woeful. The writer was characteristically bloodthirsty, recommending that persons who salvaged goods from wrecked ships which were subject to quarantine, should be executed by the law or 'be shot, stabbed,

110 *JCTP*, vol. 12, p. 352.

111 *JCTP*, vol. 12, pp. 353–4.

112 NA PC 2/112/152, 473, 493, 530.

113 NA PC 2/113/195, 197. The first letter from Florence reached London in only four days. A fuller account of the episode is in *Annual Register*, 12 July 1768.

114 See Bibliography. The work begins: 'The Merchants trading to Italy, having lately been requested to attend at the Board of Trade, to give all the Lights they could in regard to the Nature of a Quarantine; and as there is Reason to imagine their Informations were neither so particular nor full as the Importance of the Object required …'

115 For the Venice precautions, see *An Authentic Account of the Measures and Precautions used at Venice* … (London, 1752).

116 *The Nature of a Quarantine as it is Performed in Italy* … (London, 1767), p. 25.

117 *The Nature of a Quarantine*, pp. 27–8.

118 *The Gentleman's Magazine*, vol. 37, p. 171.

[or] stoned' as they went about their work.[119] The rationale had echoes of his earlier pamphlet. There he had argued that 'Cruelty to the few, is yet an Act of Mercy to the many'; now he thought it 'better that some hundreds of villains be put to death on the spot … than that so many hundred thousands of innocent … people should be destroyed by the Plague', or even endangered by it.[120] Hidden in the rambling rhetoric was the suggestion that a main lazaretto should be built near Falmouth, with smaller ones elsewhere.[121] Neither pamphlet had any impact on national policy.

New Baltic alarm

With the next decade came a fresh and complex worry for the new administration of Lord North. The war between Russia and Turkey, which had repercussions over quarantine for Minorca, led indirectly to a menace from the Baltic which threatened the health of Britain in an insidious and rapid advance. Early in 1770 plague appeared in Moldavia and Wallachia and was conveyed inexorably westwards by returning troops and the movements of commerce.[122] It spread quickly into Poland and eventually reached Moscow in November. The weather was bitter and the infection appeared to lose its grip. But in February 1771 plague reappeared in a large factory making military uniforms. This was shut down and ringed by troops, but the disease burst through the cordon, and showed no sign of waning until October. By then, after riots and repression, the death toll in Moscow had reached 80,000, and mortality in outlying districts was proportionately as great.

The Privy Council took no action until 5 October 1770, when plague was within strike of the Baltic seaboard. On that day, a 40-day quarantine was imposed against Danzig and other ports in Prussia and Pomerania.[123] While no cargoes could escape airing for one week, enumerated goods were to be aired for two weeks on the floating lazarettos in Stangate Creek. As the situation in the Baltic deteriorated, the Council extended quarantine on 19 October to arrivals from Courland, Samogitia and Livonia.[124] Not wishing to be distracted by new rumours from the south, they also reconfirmed quarantine against the Mediterranean, extending it to Spanish ports within the Straits, Gibraltar and Minorca; these places had been in pratique with Britain for the last seven years.[125] Also on 19 October, worried about trans-shipments from infected countries, they imposed two weeks' airing on cotton wool and rags

119 *The Immediate Necessity of Building a Lazzaretto for a Regular Quarantine …* (London, 1768), p. 5.

120 *The Nature of a Quarantine*, p. 23; *The Immediate Necessity of Building a Lazzaretto*, pp. 6–7.

121 *The Immediate Necessity of Building a Lazzaretto*, pp. 8–9.

122 *Quarterly Review*, vol. 33, pp. 266–7; C.F. Mullett, *The Bubonic Plague and England: An Essay in the History of Preventive Medicine* (Lexington, 1956), p. 321, from which remaining references in this paragraph are taken.

123 NA PC 2/114/498–501.

124 NA PC 2/114/523.

125 NA PC 2/114/522.

arriving from anywhere.[126] These were the two products deemed most susceptible to harbouring disease. This was the first time that the power to air indirect imports, granted under the quarantine Act of 1753, had been exercised. Russell was critical of the logic, calling it an example of the Council's 'precipitation'.[127] The removal of cotton wool and rags for airing, from ships not liable to quarantine, struck him as 'a singular method of preventing infection'.[128]

Since the last crisis from the Baltic, 60 years earlier, imports from there and north Germany had somewhat altered. The Eastland Company was no more than a memory, and while naval stores were still vital to British shipping, a new commodity – rags for paper-making – was an increasing trade. One problem for the Privy Council was that rags were not, traditionally, an enumerated item, and the Order of 5 October had not added them to the list. Another problem was that administering to the needs of north Germany, the source of most rags, was diverting attention from the seat of the epidemic. On 27 October 1770 the merchants trading to Hamburg and Bremen petitioned for the Order of the 19th to be 'altered and explained', probably for the reason which troubled Russell.[129] After an informal session with the Clerk to the Privy Council, the merchants were invited to a committee meeting at the Cockpit on 30 October.[130] This had the disastrous effect of bringing about what the merchants feared most – the imposition of quarantine against Hamburg and Bremen for ships as well as their cargoes.[131] Rags and cotton wool were also imported in ships from America and the West Indies, but the Privy Council expressly excused them from quarantine.[132]

It was immediately understood that the *Prince Frederick*, the replacement hulk at Stangate Creek, would be swamped by the influx of rags from Europe.[133] Another ship, the three-deck *Newark*, had been made available by the Admiralty, but was still elsewhere, in the hands of the Customs service.[134] On 1 November the Treasury were asked to provide sheds or lazarets on shore, with proper houses and 'Centinel Boxes'.[135] This request was delegated to the Customs Commissioners who, within weeks, complained to the Privy Council of 'Obstructions' in their attempt to buy land.[136] They were told curtly to refer these to the Treasury.[137] There must have been a few small voices to query why the grander scheme for a land lazaret had not already been realized, as Parliament intended. There was certainly a voice wishing to contribute to the management of the crisis. Dr Mordach Mackenzie, a former physician to the British factory in Constantinople, had the ear of Lord

126 NA PC 2/114/524.

127 Russell, p. 460.

128 Ibid.

129 NA PC 2/114/535.

130 Ibid. The merchants were Messrs Blydesteyn, Vowell, Flower and Lessard.

131 NA PC 2/114/538–40. The Order was 1 November.

132 NA PC 2/114/573.

133 NA PC 2/114/541.

134 NA PC 2/114/562. It had been delivered to the Customs service in May.

135 NA PC 2/114/541.

136 NA PC 2/114/611.

137 Ibid.

Gower, President of the Council.[138] Gower persuaded his colleagues, at Mackenzie's suggestion, to ask the Admiralty for another ship to be available at Stangate Creek, this time with beds.[139] If a vessel were expected of harbouring plague, the crew would be stripped and taken naked to this extra lazaretto, where a change of clothes would be provided.[140] When the Admiralty baulked at the new demand, the Privy Council steered it towards the Customs service, but there is no evidence that Mackenzie's idea was put into practice.[141]

By late November 1770 the Council were in a muddle. The German merchants were still seeking clarity as to what products did, or did not, condemn a ship to quarantine.[142] The Council met a delegation and agreed that linens presented no danger – a view which their colleagues of 60 years earlier would have found most curious.[143] The result was an Order of 30 November which confined quarantine to ships from Hamburg and Bremen carrying only rags and cotton wool.[144] Russell was dismayed by 'such fluctuating orders' and went on to question the competence of the Council and the logic of their decision as to linen.[145] Early in December the Council had another change of heart; it now seemed to them inadequate that the country should be protected only against infection from rags and cotton wool. A new Order of 9 December extended a quarantine of 40 days to all ships from Hamburg and Bremen which carried also hemp, flax, human hair or feathers.[146] Restrictions were now encroaching on naval stores, giving the Admiralty a new cue for complaint. The small shipments from Germany were no great concern to them, but cargoes from the Baltic were crucial. The Admiralty sought exemption from quarantine for vessels carrying hemp from Riga, but the Privy Council could only promise to examine each ship on its merits.[147] Yet another concern for the Admiralty was agitation from Bristol for its own floating lazaretto. The Mayor had sought the assistance of Viscount Clare, to whom the Clerk to the Privy Council sent a letter, promising that 'a proper vessel' would be duly stationed.[148] This was a curious way to respond, especially as no Order was made. In a postscript to his letter, the Clerk mentioned that Lord North had been at the Council when the matter was discussed; some private understanding appears to have escaped the record.

The New Year saw no end to the Privy's Council's problems. It was still the importing of rags from the Continent which caused most dissatisfaction among merchants. Restrictions had crept south to Flanders, another main source of supply, and a committee 'appointed at a very numerous meeting of the paper manufacturers

138 NA PC 2/114/541.
139 Ibid.
140 Ibid.
141 NA PC 2/114/580, 585.
142 NA PC 2/114/597.
143 Ibid.
144 NA PC 2/114/603.
145 Russell, pp. 461–3.
146 NA PC 2/114/643.
147 NA PC 2/114/597, 601, 660.
148 NA PC 2/114/546.

of this Kingdom' was tasked to get quarantine lifted.[149] In late May 1771 the Privy Council agreed that ships with clean bills of health from Hamburg, Bremen and Flanders, as well as from the Baltic ports, would no longer be subject to quarantine unless they carried cotton wool.[150] Unpredictable to the last, the Council could now assume that the paper makers had been appeased.

News from Russia was still worryingly bleak and made the management of quarantine very difficult. Now that restrictions had been lifted against Danzig, except for ships with cotton wool, the British consul warned that linen brought there from Poland for export might not be safe from disease.[151] This upset a cautious confidence in Baltic precautions which had led the Privy Council, on 14 May, to allow two ships from Königsberg carrying hemp and flax to discharge without opening and airing their cargoes, as these had been previously aired at the port.[152] The Council were desperate for an accurate assessment of the general threat to commerce. This could only be reached from a better understanding of the steps taken locally to protect products and raw materials. They asked British diplomats at St Petersburg for an account of the plague in Moscow and the measures taken to contain it.[153] At the same time, they convened a meeting with Robert Nettleton, Governor of the Russia Company, and several of his colleagues, at which letters and reports from diplomats and others were read and discussed.[154] It transpired that the plague was largely confined to the lower classes, claiming around 500 lives a day. Merchants had left Moscow, but not in alarm; they were trying to avoid the inconvenience of the cordons sanitaires, imposed some two months earlier, which made normal trading impossible.[155]

The main exports from Russia deemed liable to infection were hemp, flax, linen, furs and bristles. There was, however, reason to trust the safety of the hemp, as it was the growth of 1769–70 and was subject to quarantine in St Petersburg before being shipped.[156] Furthermore, hemp was always repacked before export.[157] It was important to get agreement on quarantine now, as around a hundred ships were on their way from Russia, many having been forced into Norway by unfavourable winds.[158] But the Privy Council were still far from content. On 8 November 1771 a new quarantine of 40 days was ordered against arrivals from Russia and Riga.[159] A few days later the Russia Company were summoned back for a more detailed interrogation, when they assured the Council that no goods had left Moscow since

149 NA PC 2/115/222–3.

150 NA PC 2/115/220, 222; cf. *CHOP* (1770–72), p. 368, mentioning agitation from the Merchant Adventurers.

151 *CHOP* (1770–72), p. 369.

152 NA PC 2/115/184.

153 NA PC 2/115/421.

154 NA PC 2/115/419–21.

155 Ibid.

156 Ibid.

157 Ibid.

158 Ibid.

159 NA PC 2/115/424.

30 August.[160] They were asked many complicated questions about feathers and linen, and the marking, baling and packaging of goods.[161] But the Company had earlier written to Lord Suffolk confessing unease 'that those sorts of linens called manufactures' did not undergo the same precautions in St Petersburg as hemp and flax, and some had already arrived in London and been opened.[162] The Council must have felt vindicated, for once, in their cautious stance.

Choosing the quarantine ports

Russell believed that quarantine stations among the outports were appointed at the discretion of local officers of Customs.[163] He confessed not to know exactly when the Privy Council took over this responsibility, which, he knew, they had assumed by 1780. Enough has been written in this study to indicate that the Privy Council had long been involved in the approval of quarantine ports, if not in their selection. At Portsmouth, Plymouth, Falmouth, Bristol, Liverpool and Hull, not to mention a series of harbours strategically placed around Scotland, the Council had made quarantine lawful for ships with clean bills of health. That growth, however, had been somewhat haphazard, and only in 1772 did the Council make a systematic nomination of quarantine ports, defining the catchment area of each.

The prelude to this move was a sense that if Britain had escaped the plague in Russia, it was more from good fortune than preparedness. In his speech to Parliament on 21 January 1772, King George III hoped the danger from Europe had abated, but warned that vigilance and precautions were still most necessary.[164] The King later agreed with his Council that up-to-date reports from St Petersburg should be published in the *London Gazette*, along with a method of preventing infection.[165] The problem for Government was that precautions against plague were not well positioned. The dependence on Stangate Creek, with its overstretched resources, ignored the weak spots elsewhere which plague could exploit. From the Mediterranean as well as the Baltic, trade was increasing to the outports, and facilities for quarantine and airing needed to keep abreast of the trend. There was still a requirement, however, for the situation at Stangate Creek to be improved, and Government summoned up the energy to tackle at least one of the reasons why the land lazaret had been so long delayed. With a legal problem detected about the King's power to buy land, a Bill was brought before Parliament to 'explain and amend' the Act of 1753 and enable the Treasury to make the purchase and allow the site, limited to the purpose of a lazaret, to be vested inalienably in the Crown.[166] After a smooth Parliamentary

160 NA PC 2/115/429–31.

161 Ibid.

162 *CHOP* (1770–72), p. 370.

163 Russell, p. 454.

164 *JHC*, vol. 33, p. 409.

165 NA PC 2/116/234, 240.

166 *JHC*, vol. 33, p. 758. If the sum proved insufficient, the Treasury could make up the balance from duties on imports or exports.

passage of some three weeks, the Bill received the royal assent on 3 June 1772.[167] Perhaps the problem of powers was at the root of the 'Obstructions' of which the Customs Commissioners had complained, during their recent attempt to build airing sheds.[168] But the solution to a legal technicality was no remedy for the chronic lack of enthusiasm by which the scheme was blighted; for the underlying reasons already discussed, the lazaret remained an exercise on paper.

With the illusion of progress over Stangate Creek, the Privy Council now set about rationalizing the complicated arrangements for quarantine which had, wisely or otherwise, been ordered over the previous few years. On 8 July 1772 a new general Order made an historic advance in how quarantine was administered.[169] The Order began by reciting that quarantine was in force against arrivals from the Mediterranean, West Barbary, Russia and certain Baltic ports, and applied to ships from anywhere (except America and the West Indies) which carried cotton wool. Although the disease had abated in Russia, it might only be dormant until the summer, and the King thought it 'probable' that plague would then reach Britain. That was a more gloomy prognosis than he had made to Parliament. To maintain the defences, the new Order united the subsisting restrictions into one comprehensive measure. It then listed the quarantine stations for uninfected ships. In England, these were as follows:

1. Stangate Creek: for ships bound for London, the Thames and the Medway
2. Whitebooth Roads, Hull: for Ipswich, Yarmouth, Lynn, Boston, Hull, Newcastle and Berwick-on-Tweed
3. Hoylake, 'at the west End thereof': for Carlisle, Chester and the Isle of Man
4. King Road and 'Porshute' Pill: for Milford, Cardiff, Gloucester, Bristol, Bridgwater, Ilfracombe, Barnstaple, Padstow and St Ives
5. St Ives [*sic*] Pool: for Falmouth.
6. 'in some place between wood end and Saltash in the River Tamer': for Plymouth, Exeter and Poole
7. Motherbank: for [Portsmouth,] Southampton, Chichester and Sandwich.

Lynn had been overlooked in the original Order, but was added on 31 July.[170] Portsmouth appears to have been taken for granted. Certain large ports were omitted deliberately, many on the technicality that they were 'members' of a more senior port. This explains the absence of Liverpool, which was a member of Chester. When member ports were allocated a quarantine station other than that of their principal, this irregularity was pointed out. Ships bound to Padstow and St Ives, members of Plymouth port, and to Ilfracombe and Barnstaple, members of Exeter port, performed quarantine at King Road, an anchorage in the Bristol Channel near the mouth of the Avon. 'Porshute' Pill (usually written Portshute in later measures) can probably be identified with Portishead Pill, a creek (or pill) south of what is now Avonmouth.[171] A map of Somerset published in 1601 refers to the modern Portishead

167 *JHC*, vol. 33, pp. 767, 772, 777, 782, 785, 945–6. The Act was 12 Geo. III, c.57.

168 NA PC 2/114/611.

169 NA PC 2/116/358–66, from which all references are taken until otherwise stated.

170 NA PC 2/116/393, 400.

171 Portishead Pill is now lost in the complex of Portbury Docks.

Point as 'Portshut Poynt'.[172] In the far south-west, the provisions for Falmouth and Plymouth were to cause confusion and argument for years to come. The problem at Falmouth was not the location of the quarantine station, which was very suitable, as Sir Everard Fawkener had suggested, but its name. 'St Ives Pool' was a mistake for St Just's Pool and presumably came about from a mere slip of the pen; the scribe had recently written St Ives. It was to become an even worse aberration than 'Stowfort' Island, and for the rest of this study the misspelling will be ignored, but can be presumed to exist unless otherwise stated. As for Plymouth, the somewhat vague location in the estuary of the Tamar was probably introduced in a Proclamation some four years earlier.[173] Such imprecision would soon be irrelevant, as the navy wanted no truck with merchantmen which could spread disease.

For Scotland, the chance was taken to reduce to four the six quarantine stations chosen in 1743.[174] On the east coast, Inverkeithing Bay was now to serve ports between Leith and Aberdeen. For the north (as it was designated), Cromarty Bay was to serve everywhere from Inverness to Stornoway, including Orkney and Shetland. For the west coast, Lamlash in the Isle of Arran was to serve all ports between Wigtown and Oban; and Carsethorn was retained to serve Dumfries and Kirkcudbright in the extreme south-west. Following the quarantine against the Baltic and parts of north Europe, Scotland was now deeply affected by the disruption to trade. The ports in which ships were actually being quarantined, on the evidence of Privy Council registers, had little in common with the stations supposed to receive them. An analysis of Orders for discharge over two registers, covering 1 May 1769 to 31 December 1771, reveals 12 ships at Leith, 6 at Inverkeithing Bay, 4 at Dysart, 3 at Glasgow, 2 each at Ayr, Greenock, Firth of Forth, Dundee and Inverness, and 1 each at Dumfries, Clyde and 'Carolina Road'.[175] The main grouping, however, of 24 ships (63 per cent) was well poised to make use of Inverkeithing Bay.

In the Channel Islands, quarantine was to be done at Belle Croute (now Belcroute Bay) for Jersey, and in the Little Road for Guernsey, Sark and Alderney.[176] This decision followed correspondence between local commandants and the Earl of Rochford, Secretary of State for the Southern Department. Rochford had been informed in January that most ships bound for Guernsey had traditionally been sent to The Motherbank, 'which the merchants of the Island considered a distressing hardship'.[177] By Order in Council of 8 November 1771, a local place for quarantine could be designated by the Lieutenant-Governor, who had fixed upon the Little

---

172 Revd W. Phelps, *The History and Antiquities of Somersetshire …* (2 vols, London, 1835–39), vol. 1, frontispiece.

173 Bibliotheca Lindesiana, vol 8: *Handlist of Proclamations issued by Royal and other Constitutional Authorities, 1714–1910* (Wigan, 1913), has a Proclamation, 28 June 1768, making alterations to quarantine stations for ships bound for Plymouth, Exeter and Poole.

174 NA PC 2/116/358–66, from which all references are taken until otherwise stated.

175 NA PC 2/114 and 115, in which Orders for discharging ships under quarantine in Scotland are indexed collectively. As the Provost of Montrose was anxious for quarantine against Russia to be lifted (*CHOP* (1770–72), p. 413), other ports were no less involved in the Baltic trade.

176 NA PC 2/116/358–66.

177 *CHOP* (1770–72), p. 413.

Road.[178] From Jersey, Rochford was told that a mooring near St Aubin was the 'securest' spot, but the States preferred 'la Place sous Belle Croute', which was consequently adopted.[179] Rochford had also been in touch with the Governor of Alderney, who explained that neither his island nor Sark offered a suitable quarantine anchorage.[180] Ships bound for Alderney usually called first at Falmouth, Plymouth or Portsmouth to obtain pratique.[181]

Rochford had also written to the Isle of Man, which, it will be noticed, was included under Hoylake in the above list.[182] The Governor replied that 'orders and regulations for quarantine were as strictly observed in the Isle as possible, and Ramsey and Derby Haven Bays were assigned for that purpose; not that they were in any respect proper, but for want of any other commodious place'. From his ten years' experience of the island, the Governor knew nowhere he could recommend as a safe anchorage. This was a useful reason for moving quarantine to the mainland, and no doubt the island's reputation as an unofficial entrepôt for illicit goods added weight to the decision.

The Order of 8 July continued the necessity for cargoes to be aired for one week, and for enumerated goods to be aired for two weeks.[183] The list of these goods was now restated as hemp, flax, paper, books, silk (raw, thrown or wrought), linen, cotton wool, cotton yarn, manufactured wool, wool raw or anywise wrought, feathers, grogram or mohair yarn, human hair, goats' hair, Carmenia wool, carpets, cambletts, burdetts or other manufactures of silk and cotton, kid skins, skins in the wool or hair, sponges, wine and oil in chests, thread stockings, all goods packed with straw or cotton, straw hats, bristles, matting and artificial flowers. The inclusion of wine and oil in chests is difficult to understand. Customs officers at all the quarantine stations were expected to oversee airing. In the absence of naval hulks, and with no powers to build facilities on land, they could only order a master to go through the motions of airing cargo on the exposed deck of his ship.

Restrictions eased

With the Russian threat receding, the Privy Council found themselves dealing with petitions for easier trading from both the north and south. As matters stood, ships from anywhere in the Mediterranean and many parts of the Baltic were liable to quarantine, and at the first glimpse of a healthy horizon, merchants sought an end to restrictions. The move for relaxation from the south was headed by a lobby from Exeter. Merchants from there petitioned, early in 1773, that quarantine should be removed from ships which had left the Mediterranean with a cargo for some foreign port outside the Straits (from where quarantine in Britain was not required), and

178 Ibid.

179 *CHOP* (1770–72), p. 417.

180 *CHOP* (1770–72), p. 413.

181 Ibid.

182 *CHOP* (1770–72), p. 411, from which remaining references in this paragraph are taken.

183 NA PC 2/116/358–66, from which remaining references in this paragraph are taken.

where they had then loaded a cargo for England.[184] Their point was that Customs officers were imposing quarantine, even if the Mediterranean were one step removed in a ship's itinerary. This was not an easy issue, and the Privy Council referred it to a committee.[185] Within a month the committee reported that the Order of 19 October 1770 had not intended such ships to be included and, on 5 March 1773, quarantine for indirect arrivals was abolished.[186]

This success encouraged London merchants, led by George Wombwell, to petition for the removal of quarantine against ships arriving from Spanish ports within the Mediterranean.[187] On 7 April 1773 the Privy Council went along with that, and restrictions were also lifted against arrivals from Gibraltar and Minorca.[188] This only left Leghorn unappeased, and in July came another complaint from John Dick that the trade of the British factory was being prejudiced.[189] But by now the attention of Council was refocused on problems to the north. A difficulty had arisen at Hamburg, where the Admiralty no longer issued bills of health. John Hanbury, Deputy Governor of the Merchant Adventurers, had complained about this to the British Resident, who took it upon himself to issue them instead.[190] The Earl of Suffolk, Secretary of State for the Northern Department, took the matter to the Privy Council. On 9 June 1773 the Council ordered that ships from Hamburg, Bremen, Flanders, the Baltic and Russia should be able to land their cargoes without quarantine, notwithstanding the absence of a bill of health, as long as they carried no cotton wool, and their crews were in good health.[191]

This was helpful as far as it went, but there was soon a strong feeling among textile manufacturers that quarantine was unnecessary. In July 1774 the Committee of Trade and Manufactures at Manchester petitioned the Treasury for quarantine to be lifted against ships carrying raw cotton from Hamburg and Bremen, as it caused 'considerable delay and increases the price to the consumer'.[192] This was forwarded to the Privy Council, but appears not to have been read. Resistance was then orchestrated by Paul Amsinck of the Steelyard, agent for the Hanse towns. In December he petitioned on behalf of the merchants of Hamburg and Bremen, as well as Manchester.[193] Amsinck pointed out that the delay and expense were very detrimental, and that cotton was quarantined when it arrived in Germany, where it was landed and repacked for export.[194] As was usual at this period, the Privy Council referred this petition to an internal

184 NA PC 2/117/34.

185 Ibid.

186 NA PC 2/117/50, 76.

187 NA PC 2/117/105.

188 NA PC 2/117/142, 156.

189 *CHOP* (1773–75), p. 127. Dick had now been knighted.

190 NA PC 1/9/126.

191 NA PC 2/117/216.

192 NA PC 1/10/56.

193 NA PC 1/10/64; PC 2/118/317.

194 NA PC 1/10/64.

committee, which found in the petitioner's favour.[195] On 28 December 1774 the Council ordered all ships carrying cotton wool to be admitted to pratique, as long as they came from ports not subject to quarantine.[196] This formula, elusive as it was, satisfied the manufacturers of Manchester for the time being.

Over the next four years, bar routine trouble with the navy over press gangs, the Privy Council enjoyed a remarkable absence of issues of quarantine. The merchants at Leghorn, having skinned their knuckles by knocking fruitlessly at the Council's door, were apparently sulking quietly in the background. As long as British diplomats in the Italian states relayed stories of plague in and around the Levant – and those stories were frequent – there was no prospect of relief. On 11 December 1778, when Sir William Hamilton reported that plague had spread west from Salonica, quarantine was again extended to Spanish ports in the Mediterranean, Gibraltar and Minorca, but the Council declared they had no plans for any wider restrictions.[197] In 1779 the outbreak of war with the Bourbon kings of France and Spain heralded the end of the Privy Council's respite. The Customs Commissioners wanted quarantine hulks for Spanish prisoners of war, a request sure to upset the Admiralty.[198]

Of more pressing concern to the Council, during 1779, was a resurgence of pressure from Manchester. As very little merchandise was getting through the Mediterranean, the Committee of Trade and Manufactures now wanted cotton which had undergone quarantine in neutral ports, and then been re-exported, to be excused a further quarantine in Britain.[199] This seemed unexceptionable, given what the Council had allowed in 1774, when Paul Amsinck won the concession for merchants in Manchester and Germany. The problem now, however, was a growing belief in London that the quarantine precautions in some neutral countries might not be as good as they should be. For clarification, the Privy Council asked the British Resident in Hamburg for information on quarantine imposed in the Hanse towns against the Mediterranean.[200] The Resident asked the senates at Hamburg, Lübeck and Bremen to respond. Hamburg replied with an extract from their 'Register'. Rules were applied 'with the Utmost Rigour' when ships reached Cuxhaven from the Levant and Archipelago, but quarantine had been discontinued against the Straits, on reports of good health. The authorities promised to restore it if the Privy Council felt uncomfortable, and they ended with the hope that trade between Hamburg and England could be free from quarantine impediments. Lübeck confessed that no provisions existed, but they would now consider them; and Bremen omitted to reply.

195 NA PC 2/118/317.

196 NA PC 2/118/326.

197 NA PC 2/123/26, 85.

198 NA PC 2/124/219.

199 NA PC 2/124/380.

200 British Library [BL] Add. MS 38213, fols 22, 25, from which remaining references in this paragraph are taken.

From the Resident in Brussels, and the ambassador to the States General, similar information was gleaned about procedures in Flanders and Holland.[201] There was now the first hint to the Privy Council that quarantine in Holland, so often cited by the Levant Company as the model procedure for Britain to adopt, was not quite as good as it had been. By a placard of 1778, ships from Venice and Zante, and indeed any other 'unsuspicious' place of the Mediterranean, were allowed to enter port immediately, if they had no enumerated goods and a healthy crew.[202] Quarantine was performed only by ships from the Levant or Syria.[203] Holland had no direct commerce with Algiers, Tunis and Tripoli but, if that trade developed, those places would be subject to quarantine.[204] While the Privy Council were delegating these reports to the Treasury, the Levant Company weighed in, during January 1780, with a petition which was very much an echo of the one from Manchester.[205] But the Council were not to be rushed.

Errors and indecision

The decade of the 1780s was one of the worst in the history of quarantine management. Dissatisfaction was rife among merchants, both those who had a stake in a product and those interested in a particular port. The Privy Council, pushed one way and pulled in another, appeared unequal to the job. They made hasty and contradictory Orders, disorientated by the differing threats from north and south. International politics were in fast evolution, industry was developing with the help of steam, but the threat of a disease from the Middle Ages would not go away. And the principles of quarantine, like the plague itself, seemed out of place in a changing world.

Another scare from Turkey brought a mechanical reaction, and the first of a series of bad decisions from the Privy Council. On 20 September 1780 a brief Order imposed quarantine on all ships carrying any enumerated goods, without clarification of place of departure.[206] Within days, Customs officers at Portsmouth had put two ships from Guernsey into quarantine for carrying wine in chests.[207] The Council sent a hasty letter explaining the Order had been directed against goods originally brought from Turkey or the Levant.[208] With the Treasury advising caution, the Council had finally lost confidence in any of the quarantine measures in the ports of Europe from where cotton was re-exported to Britain. The ambassador in Constantinople, Sir Robert Ainslie, was bombarding Government with reports of plague, and the Privy Council

201 NA PC 2/124/447, 483. The Privy Council heard also from Hamburg (503).

202 BL Add. MS 38213, fol. 18.

203 Ibid.

204 Ibid.

205 BL Add. MS 38213, fol. 15, giving signatories; NA PC 2/124/481.

206 NA PC 2/125/381.

207 NA PC 2/125/392.

208 Ibid.

were taking notice.[209] Protests from merchants were virtually ignored; a report from the Customs service about the Manchester petition was marked 'nothing ordered'.[210] And worse was to come. Reports claimed now that plague was spreading rapidly from the Ukraine to Wallachia, which threatened a repeat of the horrors in Russia some ten years earlier.[211] On 15 December 1780 quarantine was imposed against Prussia, Pomerania, Courland, Samogitia and Livonia.[212] This Order was very much a replica of the one eight years before, which had settled the quarantine stations. These stations were now restated, with the usual instructions for airing.

The cotton merchants were saved from further petitioning when the Privy Council realized they had overreacted to the threat from the north. The medical assessment now was that 'the Distemper ... was no ways the plague ... but a Malignant Fever easily cured by proper Medicines'.[213] On 16 February 1781 the restrictions were therefore lifted, as long as ships brought no goods which were the produce of Turkey or the Levant, carried clean bills of health, and masters made oath that their crews were free from infection.[214] But from the Mediterranean, Ainslie, backed by Hamilton in Naples, confirmed that plague was rife.[215] An Order of 5 September 1781 reiterated quarantine on all ships from within the Straits.[216] It also reinforced the shaky measure of 20 September 1780, by reconfirming quarantine on enumerated goods from Turkey and the Levant.[217] Subsisting restrictions which, it might be argued, made the new ones unnecessary were recited to give extra weight.[218] But the contradictions continued. Ships from the Baltic countries named in the Order of 16 February were, in May 1783, excused the need to bring bills of health.[219] Yet on 25 July, following a rumour of plague in Crimea and the Polish border, quarantine against all arrivals from Danzig, Prussia and Pomerania was reimposed, along with stringent confirmation of the Mediterranean restrictions, following more bad news from Constantinople, via Ainslie.[220]

The Order of 25 July 1783 became notorious for its effect on the people of Edinburgh. It was cited by Russell in his criticism of the Privy Council, and later by Sir Gilbert Blane and then Gavin Milroy, although both were incorrect

209 Intelligence was regularly passed to the Customs Commissioners, for example NA PC 2/125/51, 257, 301, 334, 412, 521.

210 NA PC 2/125/450.

211 NA PC 2/125/470.

212 NA PC 2/125/470–76.

213 NA PC 2/126/120.

214 Ibid.

215 NA PC 2/126/509.

216 Ibid.

217 Ibid.

218 These were 8 July 1772, 11 November 1778 and 20 September 1780.

219 NA PC 2/128/254–5. This was as long as they carried no goods the produce of Turkey or the Levant.

220 NA PC 2/128/377, 385.

about the date.[221] The problem was that Edinburgh relied on Baltic corn and had less than three weeks' supply in the granaries.[222] If ships now on their way were quarantined, the city would run out. Encouraged by the view of two doctors that grain was very unlikely to carry infection, the Lord Provost wrote to London 'praying that such relaxation might be allowed in the discharge of all cargoes of foreign grain, as the distressed situation of the country so loudly called for'. It is interesting that the letter was sent to Lord North, then Secretary of State for the Home Department, who was expected to present it to the King and Privy Council. This was understandable, but it bypassed the proper route. Just as the merchants of Bristol, some years earlier, had targeted Pitt, now another letter to a politician was used as a substitute for petitioning the King in Council. Of course, it worked very well. On 8 August, the Privy Council abolished quarantine against grain ships from Danzig and Prussia, the register noting that corn, by the length of voyage and warm weather, 'is very much heated, and nearly in a state of Fermentation'.[223] This phrase, explaining that the reason for abolition was based on a process of nature, not on empty granaries, was curiously missing the point. A week later, when the Council discovered that plague had not reached Poland after all, restrictions against the Baltic were lifted altogether, subject to continuing good health.[224]

For the Mediterranean merchants, the swings and roundabouts of Privy Council policy continued to cause irritation. In April 1784 quarantine was taken off ships from Spanish ports within the Straits, Gibraltar and Minorca.[225] The reason had become almost a cliché: the King was 'desirous to remove all Obstructions upon Trade, so far as may be consistent with the Health and Safety of His Subjects'.[226] But in August quarantine was back, as loud rumours reached London of plague in Tunis and a suspect ship in Tangier.[227] At Marseilles, so it was claimed, six or seven people had already died of plague in the lazaretto.[228] Merchants put up with these restrictions for more than two years, before petitioning once again for quarantine to be removed from Spanish ports within the Mediterranean.[229] The Privy Council invited them to a committee meeting.[230] Evidently the merchants' case was strong, because, on 9 February 1787, an Order was made for restrictions to be lifted against all arrivals from the

221 Russell, pp. 456–8; Blane, *Second Report from the Select Committee Appointed to Consider of the Means of Improving and Maintaining the Foreign Trade of the Country. Quarantine* (1824), p. 53, and Milroy, 'Papers relating to quarantine', *British Parliamentary Papers*, vol. 58 (1861), p. 267, put the date at 1780.

222 The brief account which follows is taken from *Annual Register*, vol. 26, p. 212.

223 NA PC 2/128/419.

224 NA PC 2/128/440.

225 NA PC 2/129/77.

226 Ibid.

227 NA PC 2/129/388, 25 Aug. 1784.

228 Ibid.

229 NA PC 2/132/19.

230 NA PC 2/132/19–20. Two Commissioners of Customs were also asked to attend.

Mediterranean, including Gibraltar.[231] This was conditional on Spain keeping quarantine for ships from Turkey and Barbary. But the respite was brief. On 22 June 1787, reports of plague at Algiers resulted in quarantine being reimposed on all ships from the Mediterranean and the Straits.[232] This led, inevitably, to the merchants re-petitioning, but a committee of Council, in November 1789, could not agree to lift restrictions.[233] In February 1791 the merchants applied again and after much deliberation, to which the merchants contributed, quarantine was lifted from Spanish ports within the Straits, Gibraltar and Minorca on the same conditions as had applied in February 1787.[234]

In England, quarantine stations were causing some domestic disharmony. The main trouble centred on Plymouth, where the Admiralty were unhappy with merchant ships being anchored in the Tamar estuary, or Hamoaze, between Wood End and Saltash.[235] This was alleged to be too close to moorings for laid-up warships. The Privy Council asked the Customs Commissioners whether they could suggest some other location within the port.[236] A month later, when the Commissioners had not responded, the Council reminded them of the question and made their own suggestion of the Cattewater, which was the estuary of the Plym.[237] As this was a busy harbour for merchantmen, the Commissioners were, it would seem, unable to recommend it. On 28 June 1786 the Privy Council took radical action; they cancelled the status of Plymouth as a quarantine port and diverted all ships to St Just's Pool at Falmouth.[238] This infuriated Plymothians, who, in January 1787, alleged 'Detriment and Injury' from the June Order and suggested suitable sites within the port which would not prejudice the interests of the navy.[239] When this approach was ignored, the merchants narrowed their recommendation to Stonehouse Pool, an inlet of the Hamoaze just south of the naval dockyard.[240] With topography now all important, the Council, in February 1790, asked the Admiralty for local maps; these were sent on to the Customs Commissioners with the navy's view of the proposal.[241] It is probable that the navy were against it. A definite (and successful) objector was Sir William Young, the MP for St Mawes, who claimed Stonehouse Pool was inconvenient and dangerous.[242] This was early evidence of a protracted maritime jealousy between Falmouth and Plymouth, which was to leave the latter in a unique limbo in respect of its quarantine status.

---

231 NA PC 2/132/21, 30.

232 NA PC 2/132/374.

233 NA PC 2/134/271.

234 NA PC 2/135/454, 483–4, 486, 492. Meetings were attended by Customs Commissioners and Mark Gregory.

235 NA PC 2/131/18.

236 NA PC 2/131/32.

237 NA PC 2/131/134.

238 NA PC 2/131/325.

239 NA PC 2/132/22.

240 NA PC 2/134/479, 495.

241 NA PC 2/134/539, 546.

242 NA PC 2/134/539, 546.

The Plymouth merchants had claimed to represent their colleagues at Exeter and Poole, but it was already evident that for ships bound to Poole from the Mediterranean, carrying salt for merchants engaged in the Newfoundland fisheries, The Motherbank was proving more convenient.[243] It was not, however, ideal, and in December 1786 the merchants petitioned for a quarantine station at the South Deep in Poole harbour.[244] The Privy Council formed a committee to consider this, but as the merchants petitioned again in January 1787, they had not won the argument the first time and success was to elude them again.[245] The proliferation of quarantine harbours was not what the Council wanted. They were already having problems with Dover, where ships were guided into harbour by unlicensed pilots, known as hovellers. In May 1785 the Council had warned that Dover was 'not a legal place' for quarantine; they wanted the names of offending boatmen and warned that ships there would not be released in future.[246] But the practice continued. In October 1788 the Council had had enough and asked the Attorney General to prosecute the hovellers, if he thought the case were strong enough.[247]

Yellow flag adopted

At the end of the 1780s there were new parliamentary moves to tighten regulations and penalties beyond the scope of the powers of the Privy Council. The impetus for this appears to have come from self-proclaimed experts and those tasked with implementing the rules. The Customs Commissioners had been considering 'little defects' in the quarantine system, apparently on their own initiative.[248] Two of those defects – concerning letters out of ships and the airing of goods – had been raised by a Mr Thompson, who tried in vain for some salaried position.[249] Of more importance was John Pownall, a former secretary to the Board of Trade.[250] Pownall claimed he had been given permission by William Pitt, the younger, to write to him whenever he wished.[251] In September 1786, instigated by rumours of plague in Barbary, he exercised the privilege. Pownall dismissed the regulations that subsisted as 'perfectly nugatory', because 'the higher departments of Government' gave no orders or direction. Ships, he alleged, were not arriving as they should do at the quarantine stations, and passengers and goods for London were sometimes landed illicitly along the

243 NA PC 2/131/519.

244 Ibid.

245 NA PC 2/132/22.

246 NA PC 2/130/250.

247 NA PC 2/133/313.

248 NA PRO 30/8/181/11–12.

249 Ibid.

250 *Office-Holders in Modern Britain III. Officials of the Boards of Trade, 1660–1870* (London, 1974), p. 112.

251 NA PRO 30/8/168/246–9, from which remaining references in this paragraph are taken.

Channel coast. Pownall proposed that a ship, when approaching shore, should hoist some signal indicating its liability to quarantine, and that a warship or revenue cutter should then escort it to a quarantine station. If a ship's master faced death for disobedience, Pownall reckoned 'we might be tolerably safe'. Pitt, as Prime Minister, evidently felt there were elements in the letter to develop.

On 15 May 1788 George Rose and the Law Officers of the Crown were allowed to introduce a Bill in Parliament for the more effectual performance of quarantine.[252] Rose, as well as being member for Launceston, was Secretary to the Treasury, and had already corresponded with the shadowy Mr Thompson.[253] The Bill was not intended to be a major revision of policy, but an improvement to some aspects of practice. On 21 May the parameters of the Bill were widened to include issues affecting the dimensions of boats, a matter more connected with smuggling than quarantine.[254] After a short parliamentary passage, in which the scope was broadened further to include the abuse by ships' masters of certificates of registry, the Bill received the royal assent on 11 June 1788.[255] Entitled 'An act more effectually to secure the performance of quarantine, and for amending several laws relating to the revenue of customs', the new measure extended the questions which a master had to answer when his ship first arrived in a British port. Had he touched at Rhodes, the Morea, the African Mediterranean coast, the Levant, or the port of Mogador in Morocco?[256] Had there been any communication on the voyage with other vessels from those places? What pilots or other persons had entered the ship in British waters? Was there, or had there been, any sickness on board? The penalty for an untruthful answer was £200. It was no longer necessary to prove that an offender had been notified of any new regulation, as its publication in the *London Gazette* was considered adequate publicity, after a due lapse of time.

If Pownall had been dismayed by the continuing leniency of quarantine legislation, he would have been heartened that one of his own suggestions had to some extent been followed. From 1 January 1789 a vessel liable to quarantine, meeting another ship at sea or coming within four leagues of the British coast, was required to hoist a large yellow flag at the main topmast head.[257] At night, the flag would be replaced by a light. The penalty for non-compliance, once again, was £200, and there would have been many, besides Pownall, who found that quite inadequate. But at least the principle of a warning flag, first mooted and rejected for the Act of 1753, had been adopted. The rest of the Act, indeed the bulk of it, covered matters irrelevant to quarantine, but connected with the

252 *JHC*, vol. 43, p. 473.

253 NA PRO 30/8/181/11–12.

254 *JHC*, vol. 43, p. 492.

255 *JHC*, vol. 43, pp. 499, 515, 544; 28 Geo. III, c.34.

256 Mogador(e) was a new port laid out in 1760 by a French engineer. It rapidly became notorious as a plague hot spot, but why it was singled out for mention in this measure is not clear.

257 28 Geo. III, c.34, s.3.

responsibilities of the Customs service. This combination of subjects under the Commissioners' umbrella was symptomatic of the transition of quarantine from an occasional and peripheral chore to a permanent and mainstream activity, growing in scale and complexity.

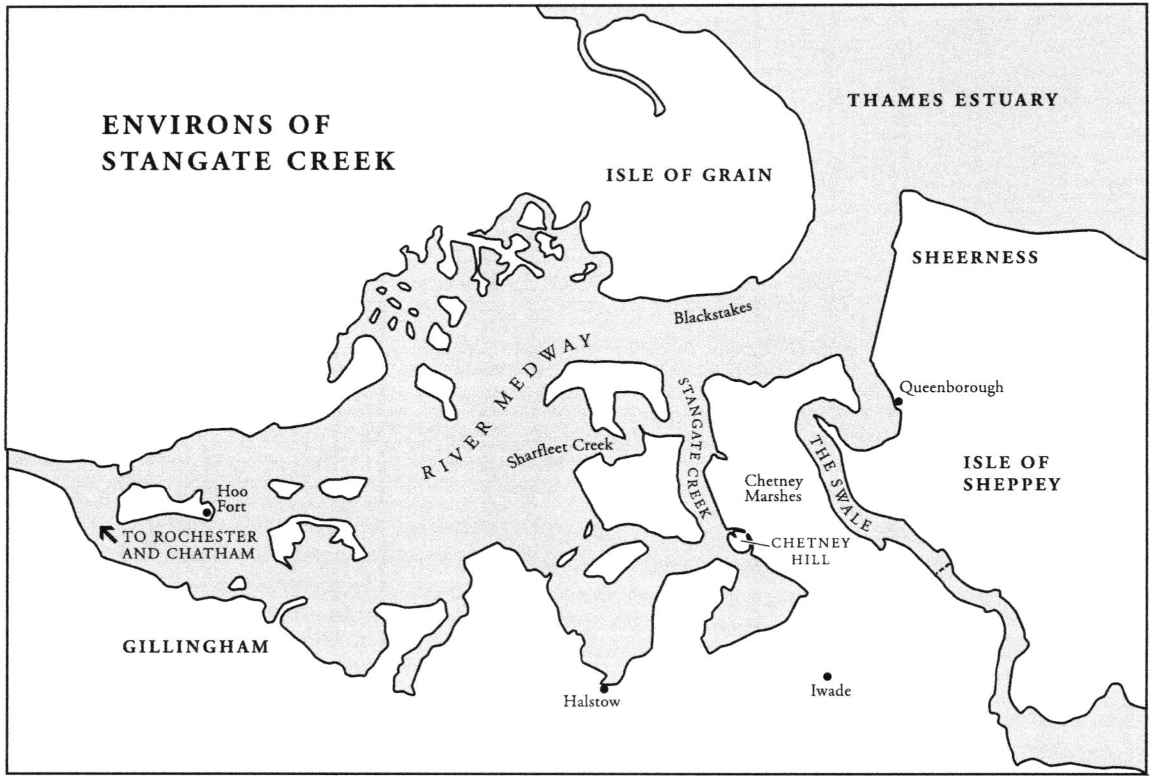

Map 7.1 The site of the abortive lazaretto on Chetney Hill, Kent

Chapter Eight

The Foul-Bill Dilemma, 1786–1800

Howard and Russell

The year 1791 is one of the milestones in the history of quarantine in Britain. It produced no radical changes in procedure (except within the Privy Council), but it saw the publication of what Mullett has called two 'encyclopedias of theory and practice'.[1] These books were John Howard's *Account of the Principal Lazarettos in Europe* and Patrick Russell's *Treatise of the Plague*, which together brought quarantine issues to a new level of public awareness. Mullett considered that Howard 'footnoted Russell's arguments', which in a way he did, as his work was a compendium of facts, but this tends to suggest that Howard's book was later, whereas the first edition of the *Account* had appeared in 1789.[2] Russell gave a handsome acknowledgement to Howard, who had died abroad in the previous year.[3] It is possible that the later edition of Howard's book, arranged by his executors, was inspired by the overlap with Russell's.

Howard was a philanthropist and reformer, who spent many years at home and abroad studying conditions in hospitals and prisons.[4] During his travels in Europe he encountered several lazarettos, which caused him to ponder the exposure of trading nations to plague and 'to reflect how very rude and imperfect' were our own defences.[5] Howard then set about a systematic visitation of Mediterranean lazarettos, beginning late in 1785, not because he was keenly interested in the principles of quarantine, but because 'establishments, effectual for the prevention of the most infectious of all diseases, must afford many useful hints for guarding against the propagation of contagious distempers in general'.[6] In looking for lessons to be learnt from the regime of a lazaretto, Howard allowed himself to be used by the Levant Company as an outlet for their pent-up frustration at the lack of any equivalent institution in

---

1 C.F. Mullett, *The Bubonic Plague and England: An Essay in the History of Preventive Medicine* (Lexington, 1956), p. 324.

2 Ibid.

3 P. Russell, *A Treatise of the Plague* ... (London, 1791), p. 404, noted 'It is with great pleasure I have it in my power to make this reference', i.e. to Howard's work.

4 *Oxford Dictionary of National Biography*. There have been memoirs or biographies by J. Brown (1818), E.C.S. Gibson (1901) and D.L. Howard (1958).

5 J. Howard, *An Account of the Principal Lazarettos in Europe* ... (London, 1789 & 1791), p. 1.

6 Ibid. In the third edition of his work *State of the Prisons*, published in 1784, Howard had made the observation in a footnote to p. 109: 'I wish some future traveller would give us plans of this Lazaretto [i.e. Leghorn], and that of Ancona and other places, as they might suggest some useful alterations in the construction of our hospitals and other public buildings'.

Britain. In so doing, he entered a commercial debate which was out of character with his disinterested reporting of the comments of foreign physicians on aspects of the plague, and on sanitary issues in general.

As Mullett's comment implied, Howard was a precise raconteur. His descriptions of the apparatus of quarantine extended to the exact measurement of buildings and the careful analysis of their purpose and usage. He was determined to inspect the Marseilles lazaretto but, being *persona non grata* in France, he faced the risk of arrest and passed himself off as a doctor.[7] It was remarkable that he gained access to the building at all, as Lord Carmarthen, the Foreign Secretary, had been unable to arrange it; not only were outside visitors strongly discouraged, but the French did not want the British to gain ideas for their competing Levant trade.[8] Howard succeeded in reporting arrangements at Marseilles, Genoa, Malta and Zante in some detail, although he dealt with Leghorn surprisingly briefly, despite accepting its status as the best in Europe. He did, however, publish plans of both the lazarettos there, as well as of others, namely Marseilles, Genoa, Spezia, Messina, Venice and Trieste, and for two of those (Genoa and Spezia) he included views.[9] He gave no plan or view of the lazaretto at Malta, and Ancona was entirely omitted, even from a description in the text. Howard's longest analysis by far was reserved for the system at Venice, partly from its seniority and status as a model for the others, and partly from his own detention there. He had deliberately left Smyrna in a ship with a foul bill of health, to undergo the full Venetian experience.[10] Howard was not impressed. He recognized the past excellence of the Health Office, 'but now, in almost every department into which I had opportunity to look, there is such remissness and corruption … as to render the quarantine almost useless …'[11] He felt, nevertheless, that their system had inherent merit. His full description of the practice and duties at Venice was provided by the British consul, and was evidently a copy of similar information sent to London in 1770, for the information of Government.[12] Howard was apparently unaware of the *Authentic Account* of Venetian quarantine, which had been published in London in 1752.

The deficiencies at Venice, and the knowledge gained from his many other visits, led Howard to suggest a model layout for a lazaretto. He had clearly found most of them dispiriting. 'Many lazarettos', he argued,

---

7 E.C.S. Gibson, *John Howard* (London, 1901), p. 135, explains that Howard had offended the French by a pamphlet on bad conditions in the Bastille, and by persuading English prisoners-of-war not to enter the French navy.

8 Revd J. Field, *Correspondence of John Howard, the Philanthropist* (London, 1855), pp. 96–9.

9 There is a photograph of the Spezia lazaretto in D. Panzac, *Quarantaines et lazarets. L'Europe et la peste d'orient (XVIIe–XXe siècles)* (Aix-en-Provence, 1986), p. 167.

10 Field, pp. 113–15.

11 Howard, p. 22.

12 Howard, p. 12.

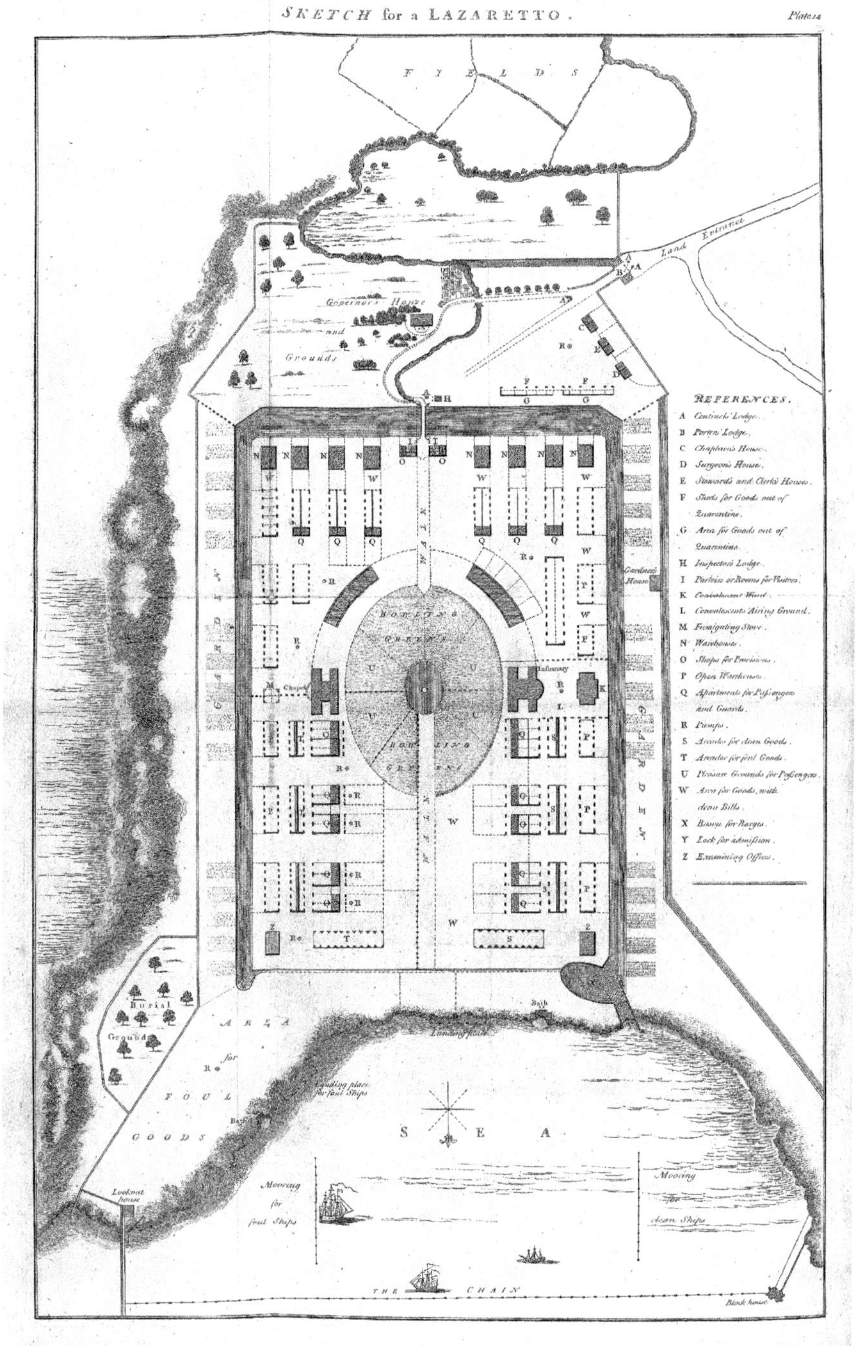

Illustration 8.1 Howard's sketch for a model lazaretto

> are close, and have too much the aspect of prisons; and I have often heard captains in the Levant trade say, that the spirits of their passengers sink at the prospect of being confined in them. In those of them which I have visited, I have observed several pale and *dejected* persons, and many fresh graves. To prevent as much as possible these disagreeable circumstances, a lazaretto should have the most cheerful aspect. A spacious and pleasant garden in particular, would be convenient as well as salutary.[13]

His utopian solution (Illustration 8.1), where water lay within the walls on three sides of a rectangle, relied on a happy coincidence of natural features and was presented without estimate of cost. In his accompanying observations, he made seven suggestions for procedure, which included a red flag to be shown by all ships liable to quarantine and a limit of 22 days' detention for passengers.[14] Howard emphasized the need for a strict segregation of detainees, arguing that infection was spread not so much by touch but by breathing 'the putrid effluvia' exhaled or given off by infected people and goods.[15] 'These effluvia are capable of being carried from one place to another, upon any substance where what is called scent can lodge, as upon wool, cotton, &c. and in the same manner that the smell of tobacco is carried from one place to another'.[16] Thus he revealed himself as a contagionist in the school of Mead.

Howard's trespass into the arena of trade was inspired, so he wrote, by the sight of three English ships undergoing a very long detention in Malta. It struck him 'that a lazaretto in England might save time and expense, and for this reason prove an advantage to our commerce'.[17] Such mercantile considerations, up to then, had been alien to his career and interests. From this position of commercial innocence, Howard asked British diplomats and expatriate merchants whether they agreed with him. For the factories in the Levant, this bolt from the blue was worth a dozen petitions to London. Here was an objective man of international reputation, respected by the House of Commons, willing to publicize the expense, delay and injustice to which, in their eyes, the Turkey trade had been subjected for far too long. Such a godsend would not be wasted. It was to transpire later that the Levant Company had already set up an enquiry into quarantine in Holland, but Howard would not have known that.[18] In a letter to him dated 3 July 1786, ten merchants of the Smyrna factory alleged devious motives and manoeuvres on the part of their competitors in trade.[19] They began, however, by suggesting 'that when the building of a lazaretto was agitated in England some time ago, the chief objection to it was the great expense it would be to the nation, which did not reap any adequate advantages by the Turkey trade.' The merchants looked at the problem the other way round, suggesting that if a lazaretto

13 Howard, p. 23.

14 Howard, pp. 23–4.

15 Howard, p. 24.

16 Ibid.

17 Howard, p. 26.

18 British Library [BL] Add. MS 38349, fol. 167: 'In the beginning of the Year 1786 the Company set on foot an Enquiry into the Mode of performing Quarantine in Holland ...'

19 Howard, pp. 26–9, from which remaining references in this and the next two paragraphs are taken.

were built, the Turkey trade would be a national asset. It must be queried, however, whether their analysis of the reason for inertia was correct, given that Parliament had made funding available.

The detail of the merchants' complaint centred on the hardship caused by the Act of 1753, which had forced ships with foul bills of health to perform quarantine in one of the named Mediterranean lazarettos before proceeding to Britain. The issuing of foul bills by the British consul at Smyrna was unavoidable, if even one case of plague in the city or its neighbourhood had been reported. As the native Turks took no cognizance of public health, the consul relied on the Greek community (the second largest) for information. But it was in the Greeks' interests, so the merchants claimed, to spread false reports; these would ensure that British ships were detained for inordinate periods in some Mediterranean lazaretto, and cotton would take seven months to reach England. During this time the Greeks, who managed three-quarters of the trade to Holland, could send Turkish cotton to England via Rotterdam which would arrive two or three months before the cargoes which had been sent direct. No ship could even load for Britain until 40 days had passed since the last case of plague.[20] The merchants stated that more than half the Levant cotton used in England arrived via the Dutch, 'to the great support of their Turkey trade, and the ruin of ours'. This was only possible because the quarantine arrangements in Holland were relatively lax. According to the British merchants, only cotton stored in the 'tween decks was offloaded to lighters for airing; the bulk of the cargo remained in the hold with the hatches open, but the air could only reach the upper bales. After 40 days all the cotton was unloaded into warehouses or trans–shipped for England. 'Thus you see, Sir,' the merchants told Howard, 'that one part of the goods perform a slovenly quarantine, and the rest may be said to perform none at all'. The danger to Britain which this represented was the merchants' trump card. Even greater alarm should be felt, as the ships themselves had been allowed to load when plague was rife, yet they had only to wait 40 days before sailing for Holland with clean bills of health.

The merchants acknowledged that Turkish cotton imported into Britain via Holland was now subject to quarantine, but claimed the Dutch had merely abridged their own rules, inadequate as they were, to compensate for the extra delay. When the idea of a lazaretto was mooted in Holland, the feeling prevailed that it would be time enough to consider one when the English had built theirs. Now, the merchants suggested, was exactly the time for London to steal a march. A foul-bill lazaretto would allow cotton shipped direct from Smyrna to beat the Dutch to the British market. Instead of sending only 5,000 bales a year, the factory could more than double that, which would result in more ships carrying a greater volume of British exports to finance the purchase of yet more cotton in Turkey. Even if the Levant trade were still considered of minor importance, the merchants felt confident that Government would accept the health case for a lazaretto, which even 'the most insignificant' Italian state had deemed necessary.

20 This was one of the self-policing regulations of the Levant Company. See Russell, pp. 344–5, for the six regulations of the Company which concerned quarantine.

Two merchants in Salonica wrote soon afterwards, endorsing the views of the Smyrna factory.[21] In his book, Howard summarized the arguments for a British lazaretto and added some minor comments of his own. He also listed the variety and value of goods exported from London to Turkey in 1786.[22] The striking point to emerge from the merchants' letters was the reversal of attitude towards the Dutch. The nation which had, a few decades earlier, been a role model for British practice, was now denounced as a danger to international health. The Levant Company, which had formerly wanted nothing more than parity of treatment with its greatest rival, now argued for its suppression with a vehemence reminiscent of Anglo-Dutch resentment in the seventeenth century. As for 'the benevolent Howard', as Maclean was to describe him (not without malice), he would have been less comfortable with the xenophobia of his correspondents than with the opportunity for preventing fatal disease which their intolerance might happily bring about.[23]

Russell's *Treatise* was distinctly more forceful than Howard's *Account*. It was designed to shed light on the medical history of the plague, suggest ways to prevent it spreading, and 'induce those who possess the power of correcting errors and supplying defects, to bestow some attention on the defensive measures which have been proposed, at different times, to the Legislature, and partly adopted'.[24] That smacked of Howard's reference to 'rude and imperfect' defences, but Russell was confrontational. The Government were on notice that the dismal record of British quarantine was about to be exposed. As a former physician to the English factory in Aleppo, Russell was well placed to draw on his experiences of plague in the Levant.[25] He divided his monumental work into six 'books', each divided into chapters: the first book was an historical journal of the plague in Aleppo from 1760 to 1762; the second dealt with plague in its clinical aspects, and with a method of cure; and the third argued the doctrine of contagion, drawing from many historical events, notably the plague at Marseilles. Book four was entitled 'Of Quarantines' and book five 'Of Lazarettos and Quarantines'. The last book dealt with 'the Police in Times of the Plague'.

Despite this elaborate structure, Russell's work was discursive with some overlap and repetition between sections. The title to book four was something of a misnomer, as the first two chapters continued the theme of contagion and susceptibility to infection, and the third focused on the regulations of the Levant Company. Only in book five did Russell produce a really useful discussion of how quarantine should be conducted and the anomalies of the British system. He began by refuting the arguments of those anti-contagionists who had opposed Richard Mead and seen no advantages from a lazaretto. Russell's technique was to quote extracts at length from their writings and then indicate in detail the fallacy of their views. But even in this

21 Howard, pp. 29–30.

22 Howard, p. 30.

23 The quotation is from C. Maclean, *Evils of Quarantine Laws, and Non-Existence of Pestilential Contagion* … (London, 1824), p. 28.

24 Russell, Preface [unpag.].

25 For Russell, see *Oxford Dictionary of National Biography* and Mullett, *The Bubonic Plague and England*, pp. 322–4.

opening chapter he stood corrected at one point by Howard: with reference to cotton being exported from the Levant, Russell reckoned that all European countries with which Britain traded had quarantine regulations, 'and this precludes the probability of the goods remaining all along unpacked'.[26] But Howard's correspondents had suggested otherwise, in the case of Holland. Russell acknowledged his mistake in a footnote, which might indicate that the *Treatise* was so far advanced in production when the *Account* became available, that Russell was unable to restructure his text. In the second chapter of book five, which centred on a 'General Sketch for a Lazaretto', Howard had pre-empted Russell almost completely, although the latter was magnanimous in deferring to Howard's precedence. As Russell had had experience of the Marseilles lazaretto, he used it as the exemplar for his own model institution, which he described in great detail while acknowledging that 'Mr. Howard has perhaps left little more to be desired on the subject'.[27]

Russell can be credited with bringing to general notice the idea of the 'touched' bill or patent. In Britain, bills of health were recognized as either clean or foul, whereas in Mediterranean countries there were intermediate stages. The touched or 'slightly tainted' bill should, in Russell's words, 'express the state of the circumjacent country and villages, which may have suffered, or be suffering, from the plague, though the place of the Consul's residence itself should remain sound'.[28] Russell argued that many clean bills should more properly be classified as touched, but there was no enthusiasm in the Levant Company for this more exact description. Similarly, there was no attraction for the Privy Council in making more obscure the definitions which were generally treated with suspicion in any case. But as the Act which forced ships to do quarantine in certain Mediterranean ports had based that necessity on bills of health which were other than clean (as distinct from foul), the notion of touched bills could have been introduced without affecting the legislation in force.

It was Russell's contention that a ship with a touched bill merited only a little more formality than one with a clean bill. But as his proposals for treating a clean-bill ship were severe, there was little comfort in the minor difference. Russell insisted that the crew of a clean-bill ship be quarantined along with the passengers and he referred vaguely, by footnote, to the 20 days required at Marseilles.[29] He made no recommendation for the length of quarantine for the cargo, but suggested that of the ship could be ten days less. In the case of a touched bill, he introduced another concept from Marseilles, that of the 'sereine'.[30] This was essentially a system of preliminary airing to test whether a cargo were infected. A few bales of cotton would be opened and thoroughly handled on the deck of the ship over three or four days. If none of the handlers were taken ill, that batch of cotton could be transferred to the lazaretto to continue airing, while its place on the deck would be taken by another

26 Russell, p. 399.

27 Russell, p. 404. He was also complimentary about Howard's own ideas: 'Mr. Howard has given a very full account of the regulations at Venice; and has also proposed some regulations of his own, which highly merit attention' (p. 408).

28 Russell, pp. 367, 372, 375.

29 Russell, p. 412.

30 Russell, p. 417. The origin of the word is obscure.

batch from the hold. This might continue, in France, until all the cargo had processed from hold to deck, but Russell suggested a ship might unload after the second sereine. Only when all the cargo was in the lazaretto would the quarantine for the ship begin. This might be 25 days, the same period as for the passengers and crew, implying that the cargo would be aired for at least 35 days.[31] Of course, if a ship carried non-enumerated goods, the precautions could bc cased, but not done away with.

In his discussion of procedure if plague were to break out on a voyage, Russell's theories collided with reality as Britain had, of course, designated St Helen's Pool for the reception of infected vessels and their occupants. Without criticizing the principle of this, Russell expected more from the nation by way of 'justice' and 'humanity'.[32] Unless St Helen's had a foul-bill lazaretto, it was useless. If a captain knew he was taking his afflicted crew to a safe harbour with facilities in place to receive them, the system might work. If not, Russell foresaw only a desperate attempt to escape a death more certain than the one ordained in law for breach of the rules. Lonely, terrified men, short of provisions and bereft of hope, would scramble ashore at the nearest mainland, leaving an infected ship to the mercy of pillaging locals, and threatening the spread of some frightful epidemic. Russell was adamant that change was needed at the top. After recounting, with his usual attention to detail, the history of quarantine measures in Britain, he rounded on the Privy Council,

> which, different from the practice in most other countries, constitutes the only Board of Health in Britain. But, considering the multiplicity of affairs claiming the time and attention of the Privy Council, and the important offices held by many of the Members, it can hardly be expected that the Board should find leisure sufficient for entering into a variety of minute enquiries, absolutely necessary to the establishment of permanent regulations, and for framing provisional directions for a number of emergencies, incident to the superintendence of quarantine. Hence it is not to be wondered if powers, which the Council ought alone to exercise, be too readily delegated to others; if orders be sometimes issued upon imperfect information, and unsteadily altered or revoked, without any fixed rule of decision; and lastly, if frequent delays happen unnecessarily, from an omission of making due provision for such exigencies as may be expected, in the ordinary course of things.[33]

Russell went on to justify his comments by a recital of events from 1770, and by a renewed swipe at the lack of forethought over St Helen's Pool. He concluded his arguments by suggesting 'that the management of quarantine should be entrusted to a Council of Health, distinct from the Privy Council'.[34] His late brother, who had argued for this more than 30 years earlier, would have been delighted. But for all his recommendations, Russell did not enjoy the full support of the mercantile lobby. Many of his ideas would have delayed ships for even longer. He was not so much pleading the case for a British lazaretto as pointing out how it should work if it were ever built. The problem for merchants was not the Privy Council but the

31 Ibid.

32 Russell, p. 431.

33 Russell, p. 453.

34 Russell, p. 466.

indirect system by which their orders were implemented by the Customs service – with the Treasury sitting awkwardly in the middle. A Board of Health might simply be a Privy Council by another name. In describing best practice once a ship was in quarantine, Russell had no suggestions for improving the line of command from the top. Furthermore, his comments about commerce were ambivalent. While he could describe quarantine at one point as 'a certain heavy tax upon commerce', he could accuse merchants at another of neglecting to mention plague in their correspondence in case 'an unguarded paragraph' might embarrass their ships.[35] In fact, Russell showed himself almost naive in understanding how both commerce and Government worked. He suggested that if a ship arrived from a place badly infected with plague, it might not be wise to unload it in July, August and September, the months of greatest risk. Recognizing the distress this would cause to commerce, Russell felt 'the equity of the legislature will not leave the merchant ... without some compensation for what he may suffer in consequence of the extraordinary length of quarantine, a measure equally intended for the public safety'.[36] The Privy Council might well have asked him how this generosity would be financed.

In the months ahead, it would be Howard who inspired the Levant Company to make their strongest representation for relief. Russell would be called upon by Government only for his medical advice, playing a disinterested role in relation to commerce.

The growth of trade

On two occasions in this study, tables have been presented to show the volume of shipping from the Mediterranean, the ports whence it came, and the main cargoes. The first table was in relation to the Marseilles crisis, beginning in 1720, and the second to the plague in Messina, beginning in 1743. Both tables covered two and a half years, and it was shown that in the earlier period 335 ships had been quarantined in Britain from within the Mediterranean, as against only 169 in the later period. The reasons for that decline were discussed. It will be appropriate now, before dealing with the years when the quarantine debate was at its most intense, to examine once again the volume of trade from the Mediterranean, and indeed from ports elsewhere against which (if only in relation to certain cargoes) quarantine restrictions applied. The most convenient source is Privy Council Register No. 29, covering the 13 months from 1 April 1791 to 30 April 1792. This reflects the period when the works of Howard and Russell became widely available, and when the Levant Company drafted their new petition. The statistics are shown in Table 8.1

35 Russell, pp. 373, 466.

36 Russell, p. 430.

Table 8.1 Statistics of ships quarantined, 1790–1791

Port(s) of Departure	*Ships*	*Main Cargoes*
Constantinople, Dardanelles, Smyrna	1	SC
Constantinople, Salonica, Smyrna	1	SC
Constantinople, Smyrna	1	SC
Smyrna (Gibraltar)	17	13 SC; 2 M'bank; 2 ?
Smyrna, Malaga	1	M'bank
Samos, Smyrna	1	M'bank
'Palmos' [?Patmos]	1	?
Scanderoon	1	?
Alexandria	3	1 SC; 1 Bristol; 1 ?
Alexandria, Cyprus, Acre	1	SC
Alexandria, Tunis, Gibraltar	1	SC
Zante	7	1 SC; 1 Hoylake; 5 ?
Zante, Cephalonia	2	1 Bristol; 1 ?
Zante, Cephalonia, Cadiz	1	Hoylake
Zante, Barcelona	1	Hoylake
Zante, Waterford	1	Hoylake
Cephalonia, Malaga, Gibraltar	1	Bristol
Trieste	3	1 SC; 1 ?
Trieste, Constantinople, Smyrna, Scanderoon, Acre, Cyprus	1	SC
Trieste, Zante, Cephalonia	1	SC
Venice	5	1 SC; 1 Hoylake; 3 ?
Venice, Trieste, Messina, Gibraltar	1	SC
Venice, Trieste, Zante, Gibraltar	1	Hoylake
Venice, Zante (Gibraltar)	10	5 SC; 2 M'bank; 2 Falmouth; 1 ?
Venice, Zante, Cephalonia	3	1 SC; 1 Bristol;1 Hoylake
Venice, Cephalonia (Gibraltar)	4	SC
Venice, Cephalonia, Zante	1	SC
Ancona	2	SC
Ancona, Smyrna, Samos	1	SC
Ancona, Trieste, Zante	1	Falmouth

Ancona, Trieste, Zante, Cephalonia	1	SC
Ancona, Leghorn	1	SC
Brindisi	1	?
Brindisi, Gallipoli	1	?
Gallipoli	9	2 SC; 2 Bristol; 1 Hull; 1 Falmouth; 1 M'Bank; 1 Hoylake; 1 ?
Gallipoli, 'Serejento', Gibraltar	1	Falmouth
Gallipoli, Gibraltar	1	Falmouth
Gallipoli, Messina	1	Bristol
Gallipoli, Malaga	1	Bristol
Salerno, Naples, Cirella	1	SC
Salerno, Naples, Gibraltar	1	SC
Naples	5	2 SC; 1 Falmouth (ballast); 2 ?
Naples, Gallipoli	5	2 SC; 2 Falmouth; 1 Hoylake
Naples, Gallipoli, Malaga	2	SC
Naples, Gallipoli, Gibraltar	1	SC
Naples, Cirella	1	?
Naples, Messina (Gibraltar)	3	SC
Naples, Cagliari	1	M'bank
Naples, Palma	1	SC
Naples, Gibraltar	1	SC
Civita Vecchia	1	IB
Leghorn	56	19 SC; 14 Hoylake; 4 Bristol; 5 IB; 2 M'bank; 1 Falmouth; 1 Hull; 10 ?
Leghorn, Elba, Smyrna	1	SC
Leghorn, Mytilene, Smyrna, Samos	1	SC
Leghorn, Zante	1	Bristol
Leghorn, Catania, Messina	1	Hoylake
Leghorn, Malaga (Gibraltar)	4	1 SC; 2 Hoylake; 1 Bristol
Leghorn, Genoa	1	SC
Leghorn, Trapani	1	M'bank
Leghorn, Gibraltar	7	3 SC; 2 Hull; 2 Hoylake
Genoa	5	2 SC; 2 Hoylake; 1 ?
Genoa, Smyrna	1	SC

Genoa, Leghorn, Nice	1	SC
Genoa, Alicante	1	SC
Messina	8	3 Bristol; 2 Hoylake; 2 SC; 1 ?
Messina, Lipari	1	SC
Messina, Lipari, Naples	1	SC
Messina, Terra Nova	2	1 Bristol; 1 Hoylake
Messina, Palma	1	Hoylake
Lipari, Messina	1	SC
Trapani	1	1 ?
Trapani, Malaga	1	Falmouth
Nice	2	1 SC; 1 ?
Nice, Leghorn	2	SC
Nice, Leghorn, Genoa, Gibraltar	1	SC
Nice, Genoa, Leghorn	3	2 SC; 1 ?
Nice, Carthagena	1	SC
Marseilles	10	7 SC; 2 Hoylake; 1 ?
Marseilles, Zante	1	Hoylake
Marseilles, Palamos	1	Bristol
Marseilles, Gibraltar	2	SC
Marseilles, Gibraltar, Guernsey	1	SC
Marseilles, Guernsey	1	SC
Sète	1	M'bank
Sète, Marseilles	1	M'bank
Barcelona, Genoa	1	SC
Barcelona, Leghorn, Palermo	1	Bristol
Barcelona, Marseilles	1	SC
Barcelona, Marseilles, Malaga	1	SC
Denia, Messina	1	SC
Alicante, Gibraltar	1	Bristol
Carthagena	1	?
Malaga	8	3 SC; 1 Bristol; 4 ?
Malaga, Ancona, Zante	1	SC
Palma, Messina	1	?
Ibiza	2	1 Port Glasgow; 1 Clyde
'Straits'	1	SC

Gibraltar	6	5 SC; 1 ?
Gibraltar, Malaga	1	SC
Gibraltar, Mogador	1	SC
Gibraltar, Cadiz, Guernsey	1	Leith Roads
Gibraltar, Lisbon	1	IB
Mogador	7	6 SC; 1 ?
Mogador, Sallee	1	SC
Nantes	2	SC
Rouen	1	SC
St-Valéry	1	SC
Dunkirk	1	SC
Ostend	5	SC
Amsterdam	17	13 SC; 4 Hull
Rotterdam	24	13 SC; 9 Hull; 2 ?
Bremen	1	SC
Hamburg	3	1 SC; 2 Hull

Notes:
SC = Stangate Creek; M'bank = Motherbank; IB = Inverkeithing Bay.
? means the quarantine station is not recorded.
When Gibraltar is in brackets, this indicates that one ship or more from the number given also called there.

Source: NA PC 2/136

There are 333 ships in Table 8.1, but the true total must be augmented to 336 to accommodate three vessels for which no part of departure was indicated, and which therefore could not be tabled. Of the 333, a total of 63 (19 per cent) were quarantined from ports outside the Mediterranean, leaving 270 from within the Straits. This figure, over 13 months, indicates a volume of trade far more brisk than during the longer periods of analysis mentioned above. When examining the ports, however, some allowance must be made in this table for a point which was relevant only slightly in the earlier analyses. In 1791 the Privy Council were more interested in the entire voyage of a ship through the Mediterranean than in its return passage. Thus some of the places in the table are those on the outward leg, especially when they are followed by ports in the Levant. But the onward voyage for cargo was not necessarily to the East, as is shown, for instance, by the ship which sailed from Leghorn to Trapani in Sicily and then to The Motherbank. The cargo was only salt, the staple export of Trapani, and so the ship must have arrived in Leghorn with a cargo and then sailed to Trapani for the return load.[37] Sometimes the start of the voyage is given as Newfoundland, which indicates an outward cargo of fish, but as transatlantic ports have no relevance to quarantine at this date they are not mentioned in the table.

It will be noted that the above analysis, unlike earlier ones, does not indicate main cargoes. It might be argued that the staples have been sufficiently indicated already, but the omission results also from the absence of information in the register. It was not, however, a complete absence, and when a ship carried a cargo of only one commodity (for example, oil from Gallipoli, fruit from Messina, or salt from Trapani or Ivica), the clerk sometimes made a note of it. This was especially the case with cotton wool which had originated from the Levant. Thus the quarantine for ships from French, Dutch and German ports was only if they carried that commodity. The inclusion of these western European ports makes a significant difference to the league table of places from where ships and cargoes were quarantined the most. While the hegemony of Leghorn was uncontested, with the port appearing in connection with 82 ships (although not necessarily, for the reason given above, with 82 cargoes), only Zante (33 ships) and Smyrna (27) were ahead of Rotterdam (24). Amsterdam (17) was beaten by Venice (25), Naples (23), Gallipoli and Messina (both 22), Malaga (21) and Marseilles (19), but when the two Dutch ports are combined (41), they are second only to Leghorn. Another interesting entry is the new port of Mogador in West Barbary, which had been mentioned in the Act of 1788 as a place from where caution should be exercised.[38]

The ratio of ships from the Levant (taking the definition to include the Archipelago, Egypt and Cyprus) as compared with elsewhere in the Mediterranean, was slightly higher at 16 per cent than it had been in the Messina crisis (12 per cent). In absolute terms, the number of ships had risen appreciably in the previous few years. The Levant Company produced statistics for 1740 to 1763, which showed that the average number of ships arriving from Turkey and Egypt in any one year was fewer than nine.[39] But in 1792 they reported that 37 ships had arrived and been entered with the company, a figure which is not inconsistent with the 43 ships over 13 months (including four months in 1792) revealed by the above table.[40] A few years later, the Customs Commissioners produced their own statistics, confirming the figure of 37 Levant ships in 1792, and indicating an annual average of 22 ships since 1785.[41]

The purpose of showing the quarantine stations is to give a rough idea of where ships were bound. Register 29 gave the information with some regularity, leaving only 14 per cent of stations unspecified. Of the 284 known arrivals, 60 per cent were at Stangate Creek, 13 per cent at Hoylake, 8 per cent at Bristol, 7 per cent at Hull,

37 But not necessarily in ballast. The movement of goods between Mediterranean ports was another reason for the Privy Council to worry that a ship might be infected.

38 28 Geo. III, c.34. Gibraltar has not been mentioned in the above commentary because the number of ships which called there en route for Britain is problematical, and some of them called only for water or intelligence.

39 National Archives [NA] BT 6/149, no. 7.

40 Ibid.

41 NA BT 6/149, no. 12.

and 4 per cent each at the Motherbank, Falmouth and Scotland. Hull is one of the very few ports where Customs records allow an alternative and precise look at the number of ships quarantined.[42] This material, which includes the name of each ship, the name of the master, the tonnage and the port of origin, is therefore a measure of how far Register 29 might be deficient. The Customs source indicates a total of 22 ships at Hull over the 13 months as against the 19 in the Register, which does not undermine confidence in the Privy Council source. Perhaps the most interesting revelation of the Register is the rise of Hoylake as a quarantine station, demonstrating the increasing trade of Liverpool with the Mediterranean. This trade was general in character, and the cotton imports from north Europe were confined to Stangate Creek and Hull, despite the proximity of Liverpool to the cotton mills of Manchester. In Scotland, Port Glasgow and 'the Clyde' each had a ship in quarantine, although the approved station had been removed to Lamlash. The growing importance of Inverkeithing Bay was demonstrated by its seven arrivals.

Register 29 is complemented by detailed statistics of the quarantine stations for England and Wales, produced by the Customs Commissioners for each of the three years from 1790 to 1792. The totals of ships which were quarantined is shown in Table 8.2.

Table 8.2 Ships at quarantine stations in England and Wales, 1790–1792

Quarantine station	1790	1791	1792	Total
Boston	-	-	1	1
Bristol	34	28	18	80
Dartmouth	2	2	-	4
Deal	-	1	-	1
Dover	5	3	1	9
Falmouth	17	11	6	34
Harwich	-	1	-	1
Hull	1	20	9	30
Liverpool	28	34	38	100
London	2	3	1	6
Milford	1	4	2	7
Padstow	-	1	-	1

42 NA CUST 92/24. This is a copy return, 10 May 1800, requested five days earlier by the Commissioners in London, of ships (excluding warships and transports) which had done quarantine in the port between 5 January 1790 and 5 January 1800. This information was, of course, requested from all outports, but no other copy return has survived in such detail.

Penzance	1	3	1	5
Plymouth	8	2	2	12
Portsmouth	28	25	8	61
Rochester	195	180	187	562
St Ives	-	1	-	1
Sandwich	2	7	2	11
Scilly	1			1
Swansea	-	1	-	1
Weymouth	-	-	1	1
Whitehaven	-	-	1	1
Totals	**325**	**327**	**278**	**930**

Source: NA BT 6/149, no. 12. Designated quarantine stations are shown in bold. The original table also included aggregate tonnages, albeit with a caveat as to the accuracy.

The first point of interest is the large number of minor ports where quarantine was evidently tolerated, despite the theoretical duty for a ship to proceed to the station for which that port was a feeder. Although the 63 ships at these 'illegal' ports made up less than 7 per cent of the total in quarantine, strategic harbours like Plymouth, Dover and Sandwich were always popular with masters who could argue that a ship was too leaky or damaged to sail on any further. As Plymouth merchants were so resentful at the loss of the town's quarantine status, and as the navy brought in prizes there, it is only surprising the total was not more. But when the figures are judged overall, the percentage of ships at the designated stations accords well with the analysis of Register 29, despite the absence of Scotland from the 1790–92 statistics. The ratio of ships at Stangate Creek over the three years was still 60 per cent of the total, while Liverpool (Hoylake) maintained second place at nearly 11 per cent, and Bristol was still third at almost 9 per cent. The Motherbank, however, at close to 7 per cent moved clear of Falmouth and Hull, which both dropped slightly below the 4 per cent revealed by the Register. The total of 20 ships for Hull in 1791 is shown to have been exceptional, and the local Customs records confirm that.[43]

Until November 1791 the Council were still in the habit of referring petitions for discharge to the Customs Commissioners, who then reported back with their recommendations. It might well be contended that, by law, the discharge of ships was within the competence of the Commissioners anyway, but the habit of petitioning the King in Council for the release of enumerated goods after airing, and of perishable

43 The figures in NA CUST 92/24, although produced several years later, confirm those in the table.

goods within as short a time as possible, had not died away. There was no such thing, whatever the law might ordain, as a standard release date, and the constant hope of merchants was that they could short-circuit the system. The Privy Council considered not so much the port of departure as the cargo. Eighteen days elapsed between the referral to Customs of the petition of the *Ann* from Messina (cargo unspecified) and the subsequent order for discharge; but only one day applied to the *Royal Tar* from the same port carrying fruit.[44] Even ships arriving from Leghorn, with its exemplary lazarettos, were uncertain how the Privy Council would react. The *Ulysses* from there, no doubt with Smyrna cotton (which would have been duly aired before trans-shipment), had to wait more than three months between the referral and discharge dates; but the *Diamond*, probably with currants, waited only four days, and the *Margaret* only two.[45] Even ships from Holland had contrasting experiences, despite their identical cargoes. The delay (that is, the interval between referral and discharge) could be as little as one day or as many as six.

As ships at Hull were discharged from quarantine as quickly as those at Stangate Creek, it is evident that the Hull merchants had agents in London who could handle the petitioning. That was not, however, the case for merchants in Scotland, who suffered a further disadvantage in that they were subject to the Scottish Board of Customs. The most prolific petitioner by far was Joseph Sherwin Gazeley, who imported rags and general cargo from Italy in ships which were quarantined in Inverkeithing Bay. The Privy Council treated these ships uniquely. Register 29 gives a precise description of their cargoes and how they were treated; the enumerated goods, which were rags in bags, were to be taken out and aired on lighters for two weeks; the non-enumerated goods, which could be anything from marble to sweetmeats, were exempt.[46] This formula was repeated, *mutatis mutandis*, every time that Gazeley petitioned, as though no standing instructions for routine cargoes could be entrusted to the authorities in Scotland. What the Council were doing was bypassing the stage of referring petitions to the Scottish Board of Customs (because of time and distance), and deciding for themselves how the ships should be handled.

It may have been from this precedent, or from Russell's criticism of constant delegation, that the Privy Council streamlined the system of referrals to the Customs service in England and Wales. The last referral in Register 29 was on 19 November 1791. The 142 ships which came later were apparently discharged by the Privy Council on their own initiative, but it is more probable that the petitions had been referred to Customs automatically, and that the Commissioners now reported back to the Council direct. This process effectively bypassed the Treasury. When the Privy Council were undecided, or wished for more information, they wrote to the Commissioners for further facts. They asked, for instance, when the cotton on board the *Jenny*, trans-shipped at Rouen, had been loaded in Smyrna, and from exactly which port in the Levant the *Jackall* had received her samples.[47] This was a big step forward for the Privy Council; in terms of quarantine, they had passed from

44 NA PC 2/136/10, 44, 46, 61.

45 NA PC 2/136/88, 184, 194, 282, 286.

46 NA PC 2/136/192–3, 250, 342, 356, 460, 585.

47 NA PC 2/136/595, 602.

adolescence to maturity, breaking with a century of tradition. It is indeed possible that the Customs Commissioners were now sidelined in the process of determining when a ship and its cargo should be released. There were advantages in this for the master and merchant, in that ships would be discharged all the sooner. The confidence which had arisen in the Council a few decades earlier, when they had felt able to refer difficult issues to an internal committee rather than to the Commissioners, was now confirmed. There was no question of the Council finding themselves too busy for quarantine, or of it becoming a humdrum matter beneath their corporate dignity. Not only did they make time for quarantine, but a casual inspection of their registers might lead to the conclusion that they spent little time on anything else. Indeed, in Register 29 there were 40 meetings of the Privy Council when quarantine was the only subject discussed. Faced with Russell's promotion of a Board of Health, the Establishment were standing their ground.

A meaningful Board of Trade

Fired by the publication of Howard's *Account*, and sensing an argument too strong for Government to resist, the Levant Company set about their case for the reception in England of ships with foul bills of health. The days of petitioning the King in Council were long past, and the Company directed a memorial to William Pitt, the Prime Minister, in his capacity as Chancellor of the Exchequer.[48] The exact date of the memorial is unclear. A copy in the Liverpool Papers was endorsed 5 June 1792, but two of the supporting papers were dated in the following November. This might indicate that the Company were advised to strengthen their submission before it passed to the Privy Council. The plea was for a lazaretto in which goods from Turkey might be accommodated 'under all Circumstances'. This would promote the Levant trade and, the Company claimed, lead to the employment of 6,000–8,000 tons of additional shipping. Because of the subsisting restrictions, more than 40 ships were detained in Mediterranean lazarettos, or unable to leave the Levant. These misfortunes were laid at the door of Parliament, which had enacted Section 12 of 26 George II, c.18, requiring all ships from the Levant without clean bills of health to perform quarantine in one of the Mediterranean lazarettos. The Company wanted Turkey ships, whatever their bill of health, to sail direct to Britain subject to such quarantine on arrival as Government might think necessary.

The argument for this change of policy was rooted in law much earlier than the infamous Section 12. By the Navigation Act of 1660, it was generally the rule that foreign commodities could only be imported, in ships English-built and mostly English-manned, from their country of growth; an exception, however, had been made for goods originating in the Levant, which might still be imported from those places in the Mediterranean whence they had traditionally been shipped.[49] In other words, ports such as Leghorn which had long been supplying England with, for example, Levantine cotton, could continue to do so. The Company claimed that this

48 BL Add. MS 38351, fols 243–57, from which remaining references in this and next three paragraphs are taken unless otherwise stated.

49 12 Chas. II, c.18, s.12.

was the law until another Act allowed cotton wool to be imported from anywhere, albeit in British ships, from July 1766.[50] In fact, an Act of 1719 had already removed the privilege in respect of raw silk and mohair yarn, but it was cotton wool which caused the Company their anxiety, because of the growing imports from Holland.[51] This was very much a reiteration of the points made public by Howard. Dutch ships could load during the plague and do 'a loose Quarantine of forty days, ... which is frequently mitigated'. The result was that goods via Holland were being sold in England while British ships were still performing quarantine in the Mediterranean, a procedure which could last at least 95 days, or more commonly from five to seven months.

In support of their claims, the Company had assembled a dossier of evidence and historical background. One ship's master swore that his vessel had been four months and four days in quarantine at Leghorn; another swore to four months and fifteen days.[52] While these facts were very recent, the testimony of Robert Wilkinson, a Smyrna merchant, about the quality of quarantine in Rotterdam, went back to 1788.[53] Wilkinson had taken passage in a Dutch ship, which left Smyrna during an outbreak of plague. When they arrived near Rotterdam, a physician boarded the ship, satisfied himself that the crew were healthy, and authorized the removal of the foul bill of health and some letters, after they had been lightly sprinkled with vinegar. The actual quarantine was only 30 days (although supposed to be 40), during which time four lighters came alongside. One took off fruit for immediate transfer to Rotterdam, while the other three loaded cotton and yarn. The remainder of the cargo, 791 bales of cotton wool, remained on board exactly as it had been stowed. After these 30 days, during which none of the goods had been aired in ship or in lighters, the whole cargo was landed in Rotterdam; had a British ship been nearby, wanting the cargo, it would have been trans-shipped for London there and then.

Next, the Levant Company supplied an extract of a letter from the consul and factory at Smyrna, which was virtually a copy of the letter which the merchants had sent to Howard in 1786, and was subsequently published.[54] Their dossier was made complete by a summary of measures taken in Parliament since 1752 to achieve the elusive goal of a lazaretto.[55] If Howard's *Account* had been the inspiration for their latest letter, Russell was also showing himself useful, as their summary was borrowed from his *Treatise*.

On 8 January 1793 Pitt forwarded the memorial to the Privy Council, who considered it the next day and referred the whole complex question to the Committee of Council for Trade and Plantations, the most recent manifestation of the Board of Trade.[56] This permanent body, although conceived as advisory, took over the

50 6 Geo. III, c.52, s.20 (quoted as s.25 in BL Add. MS 38351).

51 The 1719 Act was 6 Geo. I, c.14.

52 BL Add. MS 38351, fols 247–9; NA BT 6/149, no. 1.

53 BL Add. MS 38351, fols 250–51; NA BT 6/149, no. 1.

54 BL Add. MS 38351, fols 252–4; NA BT 6/149, no. 1.

55 BL Add. MS 38351, fols 255–7; NA BT 6/149, no. 1.

56 NA BT 6/149, no. 1; PC 2/137/306–7. The temporary Committee of the Privy Council for Trade and Plantations (superseding the earlier Council of Trade and Plantations) had been formed in 1784, to be replaced by a permanent Committee of the same name in 1786.

foul-bill question and managed it virtually without reference to the parent Privy Council. The President was Lord Hawkesbury, better known by his later title of 1st Earl of Liverpool.[57] On 12 January the Board met with Samuel Bosanquet, Deputy Governor of the Levant Company (or the Turkey Company, as they now preferred to be called), and two members, John Dunnage and Samuel Hicks Gribble.[58] There were also two representatives from the Commissioners of Customs. A paper was read to the visitors 'intended to serve as a Memorandum and a ground work for a plan of building a Lazarette, and for the better and more effectual performance of Quarantine'.[59] The author of this important paper was not revealed and cannot easily be guessed.[60] The style is too terse and pragmatic for Russell, and he can be ruled out for another reason in that he became, in a sense, a referee of the outcome. It seems reasonable to speculate that Pitt had asked for the paper to be prepared in the last months of 1792, before the petition of the Turkey Company had been seen by the Privy Council.

The author, whoever he was, began by suggesting that ships with foul bills should call first at some port at the entrance to the Channel, so that 'a medical Person' could examine the health of the crew. An infected ship should be sent immediately to St Helen's Pool in the Isles of Scilly, 'there to remain 'till such Ship shall be ordered to be sunk or otherwise destroyed, or shall be suffered to depart from thence by Order in Council'. A healthy ship should be given a certificate allowing it to proceed 'to the Lazaret of the Port to which … [it] is bound'. The surgeon there should have the power, even at that stage, to send the vessel to St Helen's Pool. The lazaret, set within high single or double walls, should consist 'of Apartments fit for Sailors within the Inclosure, and … the necessary Sheds for the purpose of airing Goods, and a building at the Gate fit for the dwelling of the Officers'. Regulations should take account of the length of the voyage, the change of climate, and the concept of enumerated goods. It was assumed that an Act of Parliament would follow, giving power to the Privy Council to make minor alterations in procedure. 'The charge of building this Lazaret and the annual Charge of maintaining it … [should] be borne in certain Proportions by the Publick, and by the Ships of the Port for the Convenience of which the Lazaret is built. All such ships paying a Tonnage Duty.' This should be levied on all ships trading to the Mediterranean and, by implication, to West Barbary, whatever their bill of health. Other ships should pay only if they carried enumerated goods which constrained them to quarantine. The author then recommended that penalties and punishment should stay roughly as they were; although these were less harsh than elsewhere, they were serving the purpose. Until a land lazaret was completed, he suggested hulks should be used according to the new regulations.

57 See *Oxford Dictionary of National Biography* under Jenkinson, Charles.

58 NA BT 5/8/349–51.

59 Ibid.

60 This memorandum appears to be the undated and unsigned paper forming BL Add. MS 38353, fols 176–8, from which remaining references in this paragraph and the next are taken. This paper is dated in pencil as '?1794', but must be two years earlier judging by the context.

Turkey ships bound to ports which were not given a lazaret should continue to perform quarantine in the Mediterranean.

The Turkey Company were asked to prepare a plan of action, based on the memorandum. They formed a committee of their members and set about the work with alacrity, while the Customs Commissioners researched certain statistics to assist them. By 18 January 1793 the Company had already 'framed a Sketch of a Plan'.[61] The idea had been that their report would be submitted first to the Commissioners for their comments, but Bosanquet lost patience waiting for confirmation that the site would be Chetney Hill. He therefore sent the interim sketch to Hawkesbury, 'that the Committee [of the Turkey Company] may be honoured with his Lordship's sentiments whether they have proceeded conformably to the ideas of the Committee of Privy Council'.[62] Hawkesbury merely forwarded it to the Commissioners, enjoining more haste in the acquisition of the site.[63]

On 27 February 1793 the Turkey Company produced their first report proper, correctly addressed to the Commissioners of Customs, although another copy was sent immediately to Hawkesbury.[64] The report began by suggesting that a ship without a clean bill of health should fly a yellow broad vane containing a circle of black not less than 18 inches in diameter. The Company were, of course, aware that ships with clean bills were required to hoist a yellow flag, and recommended that this should continue. They then followed the guideline from the Board of Trade, by suggesting that ships without clean bills should make first for St Just's Pool above Falmouth, where a doctor should make an initial assessment. If he suspected the ship carried plague, he should direct it, of course, to St Helen's Pool in the Scillies, but the Company declined to include the savage options recommended on arrival by the memorandum from the Board. If the ship were healthy, the doctor should, as the memorandum had suggested, provide the master with a certificate of the state of health on board and send him on his way to the lazaret in Stangate Creek, allowing no contact with the shore or any other ship on the way. No other lazarets were envisaged. The exact site at Stangate Creek was a matter for the Customs service, but the Company felt it should cover between six and ten acres of land with a double wall. Most of this area should contain wooden warehouses of three storeys, sufficient if possible to take 10,000 bales of cotton. The enclosure should also contain houses for the superintendent (who would be on 'a handsome salary'), for his deputy, and for the surgeon, with rooms for porters, and an infirmary. The Company conceded that the surgeon might not need to reside permanently in the lazaret, but it was essential that he met every incoming ship to examine the certificate from his colleague at Falmouth. There was no mention in the report of the surgeon having power, at that stage, to send the ship to the Scillies.

61 NA BT 6/149, no. 3.

62 Ibid.

63 NA BT 5/8/356.

64 BL Add. MS 38352, fols 179–87, from which references in this paragraph and next three are taken. Another copy is in NA BT 6/149, no. 5, which has covering letter from Bosanquet to Hawkesbury blaming delay in submission on the wait for information from the Customs Commissioners.

The long voyage time from the Levant 'to the Northward' meant that goods on ships with foul bills need not, in the Company's view, spend longer than 40 days in quarantine, despite the 52 days sometimes required at Marseilles. When hatches were opened, as many bales as possible should be taken on deck for 6 days, before spending 34 days in the lazaret. The porters should range the bales in the warehouses, in rows, each bale on its end with the seam ripped open; once every ten days, a bale should be repositioned, the seam should be sewn up, and another seam opened to allow maximum ingress of air. During this time, the ship and crew should be performing a quarantine of 14 days, reckoned from when the last bale left the deck for the lazaret. The seamen's clothes would need airing and fumigating. If the ship also carried non-enumerated goods, like fruit and drugs, these could be delivered into lighters only five days after the bales had gone ashore. The Company then introduced the principle of the touched bill, which Russell had recently publicized, recommending such mitigation of quarantine as the Privy Council might think appropriate, conforming broadly with the rules at Marseilles.

Boats with a distinguishing vane and tarred ropes should communicate between the ships and the lazaret, taking daily orders for the necessaries of life, which the Superintendent would supply, charging 5 per cent over his disbursements. Any person wishing to perform quarantine in the lazaret, rather than on shipboard, should be allowed to do so, although the Company had not mentioned passenger quarters in their brief description of the buildings. It should be possible to communicate with friends, under strict supervision, in a part of the lazaret called the parlour or 'parloir', a procedure understood in all the main Mediterranean ports. This was probably the first time the Board of Trade had been made aware of the term, although Russell had introduced the concept in his *Treatise*, and Howard had included one in his model lazaretto, as well as showing others on the plans of existing buildings.[65] All letters leaving ships or the lazaret 'should be struck thro' with a Kind of Chissel', immersed in vinegar, and then dried.

For ships with clean bills, the Company envisaged a procedure no different from that already in practice on the floating lazarettos. They were coy about punishment for neglect or breach of duty. Beyond suggesting a £200 fine for a ship's master who did not fly the quarantine vane, the Company could only hope 'a sufficient Penalty' would be introduced to deter masters from breaking bulk or communicating with other ships on the voyage up the English Channel. They mentioned the need for guards, perhaps soldiers, around the lazaret, although this issue and evidently the punishment for trying to escape were 'not for the Turkey Company to decide'.

65 Russell, p. 407: for Howard, see, for example, both plans of the lazarettos at Leghorn.

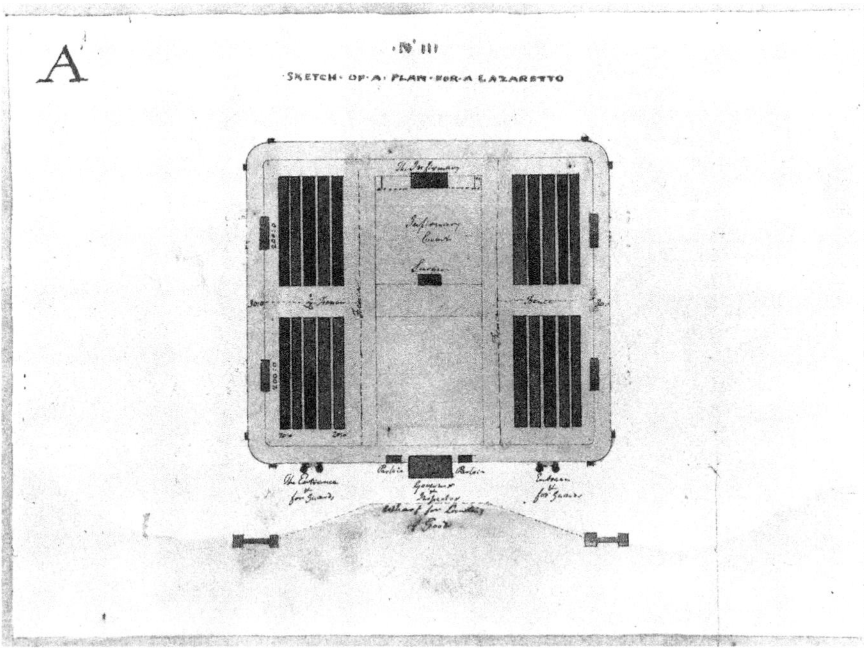

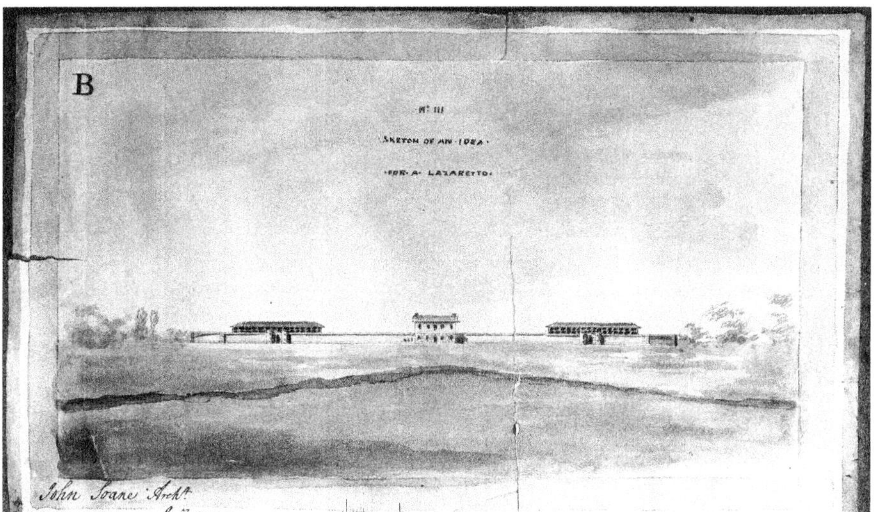

Illustrations 8.2 & 8.3 **John Soane's design for a square lazaretto, ground plan and elevation.**

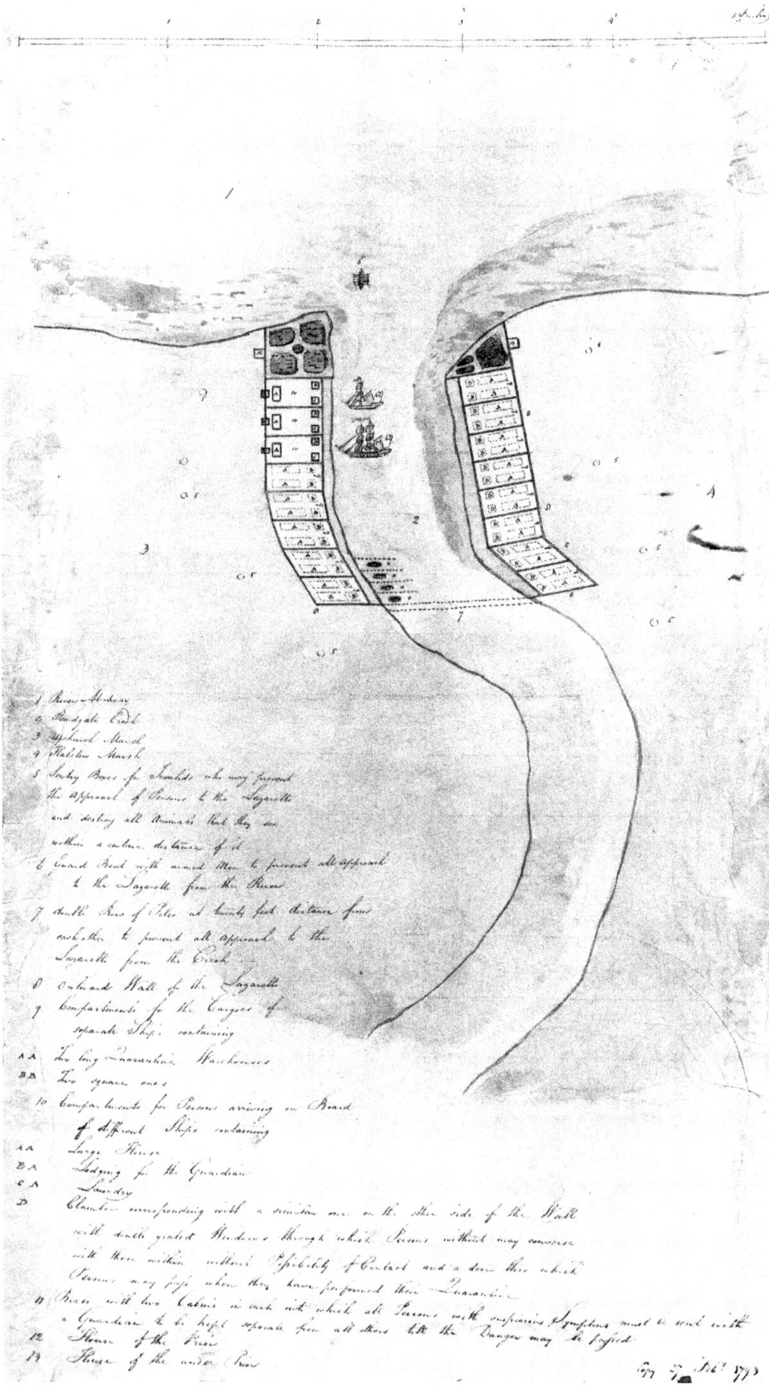

Illustration 8.4: John Soane's ground plan for a lazaretto off the River Medway

At this stage in their report, the Company introduced plans for a lazaret drawn by their surveyor, the now famous John Soane, later knighted.[66] Soane was also surveyor to the Bank of England and had received a Government position in 1791 as Clerk of the Works at Whitehall, Westminster and St James's.[67] Although he had visited Italy, there is no reason to suspect that Soane had any experience of lazarettos. He drew several plans and views of which the Company enclosed three sets, indicating a slight preference for the design which was square because it would hold the most goods. (See Illustrations 8.2 and 8.3).[68] This had faint echoes of Howard's model lazaretto in terms of the somewhat idealized access to a natural bay, but Soane included no accommodation for passengers or crew, despite two parloirs on either side of the building for the superintendent. If people other than guards were to enter the enclosure, only the infirmary awaited them. Soane did not explain how untreated goods were to be kept separate from the aired, but presumably one of the entrances might more properly have been termed an exit. The title of 'Governor & Inspector', repeated in another of the drawings, seems to have been his own creation.

Soane also made a ground plan for a spacious lazaret in Stangate Creek, at its junction with the River Medway (see Illustration 8.4).[69] This had a full table of reference, in which he used the terms Prior and Under Prior for the management, which must indicate the influence of Howard's description of the arrangements at Venice.[70] The word Prior had no religious significance in this context, as it denoted a magistrate in certain areas of Italy. The use of this term (in contrast to 'Governor & Inspector'), and the introduction of 'Compartments' with laundries for passengers, were two ways in which Soane displayed a knowledge and sophistication in this plan which contrasted with the austerity of the other designs. Only here did Soane attempt to make the lazaret fit a known topography, although he did not explain how goods were to be unloaded across the mudbanks. The other drawings assumed some site, as yet unconfirmed, to the east side of the creek near Chetney Hill. It was this uncertainty that made Soane cautious as to costs. 'He has therefore only stated to the Company that he apprehends, unless the Foundation should turn out uncommonly bad, that the Expence cannot exceed £50,000'.[71] That, of course, was ten times more than the sum which Parliament had allowed in 1772, but there had

66 H.M. Colvin, ed., *The History of the King's Works* (6 vols, London, 1963–82), vol. 6, p. 448. The plans have survived in the Sir John Soane's Museum, London.

67 H.M. Colvin, *A Biographical Dictionary of British Architects, 1660–1840*, 3rd edn (London & New Haven, 1995).

68 Sir John Soane's Museum [SM], vol. 60, p. 109.

69 SM, vol. 60, p. 105.

70 The key was as follows: 1, River Medway; 2, Stangate Creek; 3, Upchurch Marsh; 4, Halstow Marsh; 5, sentry boxes; 6, guard boat; 7, piles blocking entrance to the lazaret from the south; 8, outer wall; 9, storage for the cargoes of separate ships; 10, passenger (or crew) accommodation with house (A), guardhouse (B), laundry (C), and parloir with exit gate (D); 11, boats with two cabins to isolate those sick 'with suspicious Symptoms'; 12, house of the Prior; cabins to isolate those sick 'with suspicious Symptoms'; 13, house of the Under Prior. The letters A and B among the warehouses simply indicated whether the building was 'long' or 'square'.

71 BL Add. MS 38352, fol. 185.

been no suggestion then of a foul-bill lazaretto. As to the annual maintenance costs, the Company felt themselves 'not competent' to arrive at a figure, but suggested that it would not exceed (salaries included) the current expense of running and renewing the floating lazarettos.[72]

In the period, perhaps two years, while the lazaret was being built, the Company suggested that the old 90-gun warship then used as a lazaretto could be augmented by another of similar size, or two or three of smaller dimensions, or even ex-prison hulks from Woolwich.[73] They suggested that the regulations proposed for the permanent lazaret might apply to the hulks in the interim, promising, perhaps over-optimistically, that 'the Members of the Company will cheerfully submit to the Delays and Inconveniences … in Order to save the Government the Expence of providing a greater Number of Vessels'.[74]

As for the question of a tonnage duty, the Turkey Company, far from expressing dismay, suggested that a duty of one shilling per registered ton be levied on all ships entering quarantine.[75] This would be paid by the owners of the ships, who would then reimburse themselves from the owners of the cargoes 'at the same Rate for each Ton of Goods which shall be delivered from the Ship' – an ominous confusion between two types of tonnage.[76] The Customs Commissioners had informed the Company that 584 ships of 81,235 registered tons had performed quarantine in the previous three years, making a yearly average of over 27,000 tons. This figure, the Company reckoned, would rise to around 30,000 tons once the advantages of the lazaret were realized. With the triumphant forecast that this tonnage, at one shilling per ton, would produce an annual income of £1,500, the Company rested their case.[77]

Revision and discussion

Lord Hawkesbury's papers are frequently undated, so it is difficult to be sure which of his thoughts, or what comments of his advisers, applied at any one point.[78] But his basic reaction is clear enough: Hawkesbury was interested in detail. He reckoned a wooden building on brick foundations, with brick chimneys and hearths, would suffice, as 'most of the new Barracks … are built in this Manner, the Officers as well as Soldiers living in them with Comfort even in the Midst of Winter, and it is said they will last a Century at least if they are rough Cast'. He thought a wooden palisade around the lazaret might suffice, but did not rule out a brick wall. 'It is certainly not necessary that a Lazarett in this Country should be built as substantially, & upon

72 Ibid.

73 BL Add. MS 38352, fol. 186. This floating lazaretto was presumably the *Princess Amelia* mentioned in NA BT 6/149, no. 12, but that source suggests that the *Belle Isle* (or *Belleisle* / *Bellisle*) was also used, at least until 1791.

74 Ibid.

75 Ibid.

76 BL Add. MS 38352, fol. 187.

77 Ibid.

78 They may also be in draft form, which is the case with the comments which follow in this paragraph and the next, all taken from BL Add. MS 38354, fol. 104.

the same Plan, as those of Marseilles Leghorn & Malta, which are so much nearer the Place of Infection'. From his experience of barracks, Hawkesbury thought the lazaret 'may be finished by a Number of London Workmen in Six Weeks'.

As for the regulations, Hawkesbury suggested a meeting with members of the Turkey Company, certain of the Commissioners of Customs, and their surveyors, to put the proposals in a form suitable for submission to the College of Physicians. On the subject of costs, he considered the three issues were the expense of building, the salaries and maintenance thereafter, and the nature of the fund to be drawn upon. It was at the back of his mind 'that amongst the Papers at the Office There is some Information on all these Points', and he ordered a search of the files. Hawkesbury was convinced that the public, once they knew the financial arrangements, would only support one lazaret; thus he sided with the Turkey Company, rather than the author of the earlier memorandum.

Hawkesbury had another correspondent on quarantine, the same John Pownall, former secretary to the Board of Trade, who had bothered Pitt in 1786. From a letter that he sent Hawkesbury on 28 January 1793, it is clear the two had already met, but as Pownall had taken a hard line about punishment when writing to Pitt, he is unlikely to have been the author of the memorandum that acted as a brief for the Turkey Company.[79] In his January letter, Pownall expressed his background fears that the weakening of the exclusivity of the Levant Company had introduced a class of merchant who could not necessarily be trusted. Gone were the traders 'of a Rank and Character that induced Credit and respect in the Country where they resided', and in their place came 'Abuses & irregularity', with a consequent threat to the nation's health. The key to security from the plague should be a network of consuls who had no commercial interests, who held the keys of the warehouses, and who kept diaries about the incidence of plague, copied at intervals to the Privy Council for comparison with bills of health. In England, Pownall saw no merit in foul-bill lazarets at Stangate Creek, Hull or Liverpool. These would be 'not only useless but dangerous' because ships would be visited by smugglers before they got there. Pownall could only suggest a lazaret near Land's End, but not in the Isles of Scilly. Hawkesbury was not impressed by Pownall's intervention. The Board of Trade postponed consideration of the letter, and in fact ignored it.

Mindful that no site had been agreed for the lazaret, the Board were anxious for progress at Chetney Hill. The Commissioners of Customs put a brave face on their difficulties by admitting that the whole project was 'momentous'.[80] They hoped to gain more time for negotiation with the landowner by interesting the Board of Trade in another of their remits – the question of floating lazarettos as a temporary expedient for ships with foul bills. On 16 March 1793 the Commissioners reported that they had consulted two doctors, one being Patrick Russell and the other James Robertson, nominated by the College of Physicians. Both had been asked, separately, whether floating lazarettos in those circumstances would provide public protection. Russell

79 Pownall's letter is in NA BT 6/149, no. 4, from where remaining references in this paragraph are taken. There is no copy of the letter among the Liverpool Papers. The receipt of the letter was noted in BT 5/8/364.

80 NA BT 6/149, nos 6, 9, from which all references in this paragraph are taken.

had given a long-winded reply with a qualified yes; Robertson had been less prolix and more supportive. The Commissioners had then sent each of them a copy of the existing regulations at Stangate Creek (dated 1787) and of the Turkey Company's plan. Russell's reaction was that the regulations were fine for clean bills but not for foul; and that the Turkey Company's report was 'in general proper, though far from complete'. He worried that floating lazarettos would be too cramped for foul-bill cargoes, and only 'a distinct & separate Port' would do. As Robertson's reply was along the same lines, the Commissioners concluded that temporary lazarettos for ships with foul bills were not a good idea.

Hawkesbury took the report badly. On 26 March 1793 two of the Commissioners and their solicitor attended the Board of Trade and were told to discuss their doubts more fully and openly with the Turkey Company.[81] They were then asked to hold more talks with the physicians, 'to obviate or remove' the problems, 'in order to facilitate the dispatch of an Object of so much national importance'. To the same meeting, Bosanquet and other members of the Turkey Company had also been summoned.[82] From memory, they gave a list of their ships now in the Levant or Mediterranean, in quarantine at Leghorn or elsewhere, or likely to sail with clean or foul bills. They were asked to prepare more information. Now that war had broken out with France, what were the prospects for the Levant trade over the next two years, and what had been the effect on trade during the wars which had ended in 1748 and 1763?[83] On 3 April 1793 Bosanquet responded.[84] A list was submitted of ships from Turkey and Egypt which had undergone quarantine between 1740 and 1763. This was augmented by a reference to the most recent position, and a summary of how the wars had (or rather had not) affected their trade. In the current position, they referred to the need for convoys and listed ships in quarantine at Leghorn, others bottled up in Smyrna or Salonica, and a few nearer home. One ship had been lost to the French, carried as a prize to Marseilles.

With these time-consuming figures submitted, the Turkey Company set about preparing a second report on the concept of a foul-bill lazaret. This they dispatched to the Customs Commissioners on 8 May 1793, again with a copy to Hawkesbury.[85] The Commissioners had duly met with the Company's quarantine committee and come away with a vindication of their own stance against the concept of foul-bill floating lazarettos as a short-term expedient.[86] In the new report, the Company abandoned the idea and returned to the original proposition of a permanent land lazaret. Another reason for this change of heart had been a meeting with Russell and Robertson, who made it clear that the Company's first report contained significant omissions. The new report contained even more, but if the Company waited until the finer details had been settled, they claimed Government would miss the opportunity to bring

81 NA BT 5/8/410–11.

82 NA BT 5/8/409.

83 Ibid.

84 NA BT 6/149, no. 7, from which remaining references in this paragraph are taken.

85 NA BT 6/149, no. 8, from which all references in this paragraph and the next are taken unless otherwise stated.

86 NA BT 6/149, no. 9.

the new project before the current session of Parliament. The Turkey Company confined themselves, therefore, to mere 'Outlines of a Plan' annexed to their report; the report itself dealt with the vital question of a suitable location. The site had to be large enough to accommodate an enclosure for goods with clean bills; another for goods without clean bills; and a third for goods from infected ships, in the event of plague breaking out during the process of preliminary airing. That last misfortune would involve erecting 'some slight Building' for the crew. In the knowledge that negotiations for Chetney Hill were not going well, the Company suggested that 'land called Shaffleet or Sharpness, an island of very little value', be used instead. This land, now called Burntwick Island, had 'a Gut or Channel to the South', bordering on another island; this water was, in fact, Sharfleet Creek, which had been an alternative or overflow quarantine anchorage at the time of the Baltic crisis, although the Turkey Company seemed unaware of that. Their plan was to range the three enclosures along the north side of the channel, facing the ships themselves, which would be moored within booms at either end. They recommended that the site be surveyed, and urged the Commissioners to report with all speed to the Board of Trade, so as not miss the parliamentary session.

The 'Outlines of a Plan', annexed to the report and forming the bulk of the Company's submission, added little of substance to the recommendations in the first report.[87] The facilities at St Just's Pool (with the spelling at last rescued from the 'St Ives Pool' aberration), were to be enhanced by a proper pratique house. At the lazaret, there would be three types of enclosure, as mentioned above. The Company now envisaged a fourth grade of bill of health. To the clean, the touched and the foul bills, they introduced (without explanation) another intermediate stage: the 'suspected' bill. The significance of that variant would have been lost on the Customs Commissioners – as it soon would be on the Board of Trade – and in fact the difference between a touched bill and a suspected bill, such as it was, did not merit any differentiation in the handling of goods. In line, however, with the new terminology came a greater emphasis on the sereine, or preliminary airing on the deck of the ship, to see whether any of the crew succumbed to disease from handling the opened bales. These two Mediterranean touches, that is the new variant of bill and a rigid formula for the sereine, were probably the result of talking to the physicians, especially Russell.[88] The Company ended their report with an indictment of the absence of facilities at St Helen's Pool for ships which were actually infected. Here again was the voice of Russell. Not only were there no facilities at the Pool for the comfort and support of seamen, but no standing orders for what should be done. The Company could hardly have put it more strongly: they warned 'that if the Line Chalked out in the Act of Parliament of Communicating from one Custom House Officer to another and so to the Privy Council be adhered to the delay whould [*sic*]

---

87 There is another, undated 'Sketch of a Plan' as presented to the Customs Commissioners, in NA BT 6/149, no. 3. This would appear to have been a discussion document produced for the talks which the Commissioners had been told to have with the Turkey Company.

88 Although Russell did not discuss the suspected bill in his *Treatise*, he did refer (p. 367) to 'middle patents [in the plural], between the clean and the foul', while summarizing them as 'touched'.

be so great that many serious Evils might arise too obvious to render it necessary for the Turkey Company to point them out'.

Faced with such a decisive report, the Customs Commissioners had misgivings. It was not for them to endorse private criticism of Government policy about St Helen's Pool. But now that the Turkey Company had backed down on the question of temporary lazarettos for foul-bill ships, it was time to take the argument one stage further. In a letter to the Board of Trade dated 11 May 1793, the Commissioners reiterated their support for a land lazaret, but asked whether the admission of foul-bill ships was already Government policy, or were the Board of Trade discussing its expediency?[89] As for Shaffleet Island, one of their local officers found 'material objections' to the Turkey Company's idea, but they promised a proper survey.[90] The Commissioners agreed with the Turkey Company as to the urgency of a decision, so as to meet the parliamentary deadline.[91] In reply, the Board of Trade confessed that no national policy existed for foul-bill ships and requested the Commissioners to consider the question and make their own observations.[92] They also wanted the Shaffleet Island idea pursued at least to the next stage. As for the parliamentary deadline, Hawkesbury had already abandoned it.[93] The Board would only proceed on the basis of 'the fullest Information' from the Commissioners and the Turkey Company, and would then need to consult with the College of Physicians.[94] All that process was not to be rushed.

On 17 May 1793 the Commissioners were informed by the Turkey Company that John Soane, their surveyor, had another worry.[95] Soane noted that Chetney Hill was alongside the channel to the tiny port of Halstow, which would force ships under quarantine in the southern reach of Stangate Creek to anchor to one side, where the water was perhaps too shallow. Soane suggested that the survey of Shaffleet Island should also establish the depth of Stangate Creek. The matter was quickly resolved. A surveyor from Rochester, joined by the Master Attendant from Sheerness sent by the Navy Board, confirmed that Shaffleet Island was too low and marshy for quarantine purposes. After that report, there was no option but to make Chetney Hill, with all its disadvantages, into a working lazaret. On 19 June 1793 the General Court of the Turkey Company conceded that it was the best location.[96]

Tasked with reporting their views on whether the admission of foul-bill ships was necessary and advisable, the Customs Commissioners sought more information.[97] From the physicians they asked how the four kinds of bill of health varied in detail, and from the Turkey Company they wanted the number of ships which had arrived at foreign lazarettos over the previous five years with foul or touched bills.

89 NA BT 6/149, no. 9; BT 5/8/441–4.

90 Ibid.

91 Ibid.

92 NA BT 5/8/443–4.

93 The third session of the 17th Parliament ended 21 June 1793. The fourth session did not begin until 21 January 1794.

94 NA BT 5/8/443–4.

95 NA BT 6/149, no. 10.

96 Ibid.

97 Ibid., from which all references in this paragraph are taken.

Bosanquet replied immediately that the Turkey Company could not possibly supply such figures, and the Commissioners would need to ask Government. They wisely decided not to, but sought an equally impossible demand from the Foreign Secretary – copies of the quarantine regulations at Marseilles, Leghorn, Venice, Genoa and Malta. Other information could be gained more readily from sources broadly within the Commissioners' purview. From their Surveyor of Sloops, they asked for more facts about the geography of St Just's Pool, and whether it would be suitable for a pratique house. The Surveyor was encouraging, but recommended The Motherbank as an occasional alternative venue, as Falmouth harbour could not be entered in all weathers. From the Inspector General of Imports and Exports and the Registrar General of Shipping, the Commissioners sought a wide variety of other statistics requiring considerable research and collation.

On 30 July 1793 the Commissioners received answers from the physicians about the various bills of health.[98] According to Russell, a clean bill signified that a port of lading was free from plague and had been so for at least 40 preceding days. A touched bill meant a ship had arrived at that port from an infected place, but the crew were healthy. A suspected bill indicated either that the port was suffering from a less serious 'contagious distemper', or that it had frequent business with a definite plague spot. And a foul bill meant that plague was actually in the port, or its immediate vicinity. He admitted that the boundary between the two intermediate types was imprecise, and that they might at times be combined, as in the old regulations at Marseilles. But as the new printed regulations, dated 1788, differentiated between them, he reckoned England should follow suit.[99] Robertson's reply was consistent with that of Russell, lumping touched and suspected bills together. He based any distinction on the degree of probability of danger.

Now that the physicians had responded, the Customs Commissioners wondered whether they should now report back to the Board of Trade.[100] They decided, however, to wait until they had received the following main statistics: the number and tonnage of Turkey ships quarantined in Britain over ten years from 5 January 1783; the amount of goods imported from Turkey in the same period; and the amount of Turkey cotton wool imported during those years from countries other than Turkey. During the delay, the Commissioners were badgered by the Turkey Company to reveal what kind of recommendation they were prepared to make, but they would give nothing away.[101] Not until 16 November 1793 did the Commissioners convene to discuss their report, by which time they had still received virtually none of the information requested via the Foreign Secretary.[102] But the wait could not continue, and on 26 November the Commissioners sent the Board of Trade their considered report on the

98 Ibid.; NA BT 6/149, no. 12.

99 There is a paper, in French, distinguishing between the four types of bill of health, in BL Add. MS 38349, fol. 1. As this is dated 1788 it is evidently from the Marseilles regulations. The categories accord with Russell's views.

100 NA BT 6/149, no. 10.

101 Ibid.

102 Ibid.

expediency of admitting foul-bill ships.[103] Three days later they finally dispatched the full dossier of supporting statistics, in so far as they could be assembled from English sources.[104]

The Customs Commissioners had no doubt that foul-bill facilities were necessary.[105] They commented that Britain had made no provision for a diseased ship arriving from anywhere in the world. Technically that was wrong, in so far as St Helen's Pool was available, but the Commissioners were making the point that no shore establishment was in place. Such a ship might arrive at any time 'and ... a very recent Instance has not been wanting'. A foul-bill lazaret was essential for a country 'so eminently first in Commercial rank'. They were worried if Turkey cotton was receiving such a brief quarantine in Holland, but claimed not to have seen documentary proof that this was the case. They had discussed the Turkey Company's ideas for a land lazaret with the physicians, whose comments they attached. These ideas were now 'fit to be taken as the ground work of a Code of Regulations', but they noted that the Board of Trade were still intending to consult the College of Physicians for a wider medical opinion.

The statistical dossier forwarded on 29 November covered both quarantine and trade in England and Wales.[106] Many statistics were produced on the import of cotton wool from Turkey and elsewhere between 1783 and 1792. The amount of Turkey cotton wool received from Holland rose to more than 12 per cent of all cotton wool imports in 1785 and 1786, before dropping sharply to 0.5 per cent in 1788, presumably because quarantine restrictions in Britain were beginning to bite. The total rose to 8 per cent in 1791, when Hull was especially busy with ships from Holland, but by 1792 the amount had halved. The average annual cost of the quarantine service for the three years from 1789 to 1791 was calculated as some £6,582, but this figure did not tally with the breakdown of quarantine expenses by port over the same period (totalling £8,678). Also the costs were not proportionate to the number of ships using the quarantine stations. Thus, while the expenses at Stangate Creek were 52 per cent of the whole, at Liverpool (with its own floating lazaretto, but having only 10 per cent of all ships) they were nearly 25 per cent, leaving Bristol (9 per cent) as the only other port with significant costs; these were caused, at least in part, by the post of Superintendent of Quarantine (at £40 per annum) based at Portishead. Despite the popularity of The Motherbank, the only quarantine expenses at Portsmouth were for sloop hire, and it was this ingredient, along with the hire of extra men, which characterized the costs of the other ports, including Hull. The implication of these figures is that much of the routine work of quarantine was now considered as within the normal duties of a Customs officer, which undermined precision in allocating the proportion of costs directly attributable to quarantine.

It was 15 February 1794 before the Board of Trade were in a position to consider the report.[107] They accepted it immediately and instructed the Commissioners,

103 NA BT 6/149, no. 11.

104 NA BT 6/149, no. 12.

105 NA BT 6/149, no. 11, from which all references in this paragraph are taken.

106 NA BT 6/149, no. 12, from which all references in this paragraph are taken.

107 NA BT 5/9/172–4.

without delay, to join with the Turkey Company in producing a plan for a lazaret to accommodate ships with foul, touched, suspected and clean bills.[108] They had also to decide upon a port at the entrance to the Channel where these bills, and the health of crews, could receive a preliminary examination.[109] Finally they were to prepare estimates of building costs, and of the expense of running separate departments of the lazaret, and compare them with costs as at present.[110] On 22 March 1794 this report was ready.[111] It had been drafted by the Turkey Company, but was only presented to the Board of Trade, with a covering memorandum from the Customs Commissioners, on 2 May.[112] The delay came about because the Commissioners were a little worried by the Turkey Company's proposals and made marginal comments and annotations in red ink. They felt uncomfortable telling the Board that no fine distinction between bills had actually been made by the Turkey Company, despite the instruction; the Company had confined themselves only to foul bills, as precautions adopted for the greatest danger would naturally meet lesser ones, and if the principle of accepting foul bills were not accepted, they 'appeared to regard any alterations as a matter of indifference'. There was also no estimate of building costs because the land at Chetney Hill had still not been purchased.[113]

This third report of the Turkey Company began by assuming that land would be available near Stangate Creek.[114] The lazaret, to be enclosed by a high double wall and fosse, should have three enclosures or subdivisions: one for goods from ships with clean bills; another for goods from ships without clean bills; and a third for persons and goods from infected ships, or transferred because of illness from the other enclosures. In the first or second subdivision, there should be houses for the superintendent and his deputy and for the surgeon, with accommodation for the guardians and porters, along with a counting house and parlour for visitors. The Commissioners made an annotation here, suggesting that these buildings should be within the walls, but outside the enclosures. The Turkey Company wanted also a tavern and cellars for supplying provisions, an infirmary for the sick, and apartments for passengers who preferred to do quarantine on land. Sheds or open warehouses in the main two enclosures should be of three storeys, and a 'closet' adjoining the counting house should hold small parcels of monetary value. The third enclosure should contain only the infirmary and an open shed for delicate goods which would spoil if exposed to the weather. The lazaret should have its own wharf for landing goods and two entrances: one for goods into quarantine, the other for goods going out in free pratique.

108 Ibid.

109 Ibid.

110 Ibid.

111 BL Add. MS 38353, fols 58–72.

112 BL Add. MS 38353, fols 53–7.

113 The absence of this estimate made the Board's request for comparative figures irrelevant, but it is possible that the quarantine expenses discussed above were presented at this time, and not with the statistical dossier of 29 November 1793.

114 BL Add. MS 38353, fols 58–72, from which all references in this and the next three paragraphs are taken.

The senior staff should consist of a Superintendent (the word prior was never used by the Turkey Company), who would be responsible for losses between the times when goods entered and left the lazaret, although he could seek to be indemnified by the porters and guardians. It was envisaged that the Superintendent would be a single man, who would 'consider his Appointment a considerable Advantage'. At this point, the Customs Commissioners added an annotation that the salary should be adequate, and no person should be employed who had not had smallpox and measles. The Deputy Superintendent should be also the bookkeeper. There were then brief recommendations as to the post of surgeon (who need not be constantly resident), and the appointment of guards and porters.

Having sketched the administrative framework of the lazaret, the Turkey Company turned to procedure. Past recommendations were repeated, that ships without clean bills should hoist a warning signal before proceeding to St Just's Pool where a surgeon would examine the crew, and letters could be received, after fumigation or soaking in vinegar, in a small pratique house. As before, an infected ship should be sent to the Scillies, or if the weather was against that, it should continue to Portland Road or The Motherbank until able to return (unless allowed to stay where it was, by Order in Council). A healthy ship should continue to Stangate Creek, where the surgeon of the lazaret would confirm to the Superintendent that all the crew were well. The goods should then be sent to the enclosure appropriate for the bill of health. The Company had little time in their report for ships with clean bills, whose cargoes would be subject to such airing in the appropriate enclosure as the Privy Council should from time to time direct. It was deemed important that all goods from ships without clean bills, except non-enumerated goods in bulk or packed in wood, should undergo a preliminary airing (the word sereine was not used) of 14 days before quarantine proper. Then came the most elaborate instructions as to how this was to be achieved. When the physicians had considered the earlier reports deficient, it had evidently been preliminary airing which had caused concern. Bales were now to be opened, 'cutting up and turning down the Wrappers the length of one half ...', while chests with cotton should also be opened 'and these as well as the Bales should be left 24 Hours to evaporate without doing anything more to them'. There followed similar regulations for every variant of bale and for goods in double packaging. After the first 24 hours, it was important to rummage in the goods, leaving no part inaccessible to the length of a man's arm. After seven days of being 'agitated', the bales should be inverted and the process would then be repeated for a further seven days, on the other side of the packages. Only when this further week had elapsed should the quarantine period begin.

The period of quarantine should be 'decided by better Judges than the Turkey Company', but for bills other than clean they recommended 36 days from the end of the preliminary airings. The Superintendent should appoint two guardians for each ship and cargo, one guardian to stay on board, to ensure that clothes were aired or even lightly fumigated, the other to oversee the porters. At that point, the Customs Commissioners added an annotation, asking whether the guardians should be uniformed. Porters would unload lighters (which had taken goods from the ships) and take the merchandise to sheds. There, the bales should be stacked on end, while the ship and crew performed 14 days quarantine, reckoned from when the last bale or chest left the deck. The same period of detention should apply to passengers in the lazaret. After only five days of quarantine, any fruit on board ship could be offloaded on to lighters for market. Many of these points, and indeed the remaining regulations, had formed part of the earlier proposals. The Turkey Company ended their report by assuming any new Act would grant discretionary powers to the Privy Council to alter regulations to meet a change in circumstances. They also warned that rules would be needed for the conduct of officials, but not until the site and building plan were finally agreed.

On 15 July 1794 Samuel Bosanquet wrote to the Board of Trade asking whether they had yet considered what he called the joint report from the Commissioners and the Turkey Company; he wished Hawkesbury to be aware of his anxiety for progress.[115] In reply, he was sent copies of recent correspondence between the Commissioners and the agent for the landowner at Chetney Hill. It was quite obvious that the purchase was at an impasse, and Hawkesbury was adamant that no final plan or regulations could be put to the physicians until 'so many Obstructions and Delays' had been obviated.[116]

The defiant proprietor

The previous months had been characterized by a series of increasingly irritable letters from the Board of Trade to the Customs Commissioners, looking for progress in the purchase of the site for a lazaret, and the months ahead were to follow the same pattern.[117] The land was owned by a Mr Wildman (probably James Wildman of Chilham Castle), although negotiations were conducted by his brother Thomas, as agent. It was a bad omen that the Wildmans, in the mid-seventeenth century, had married into the family of the 4th Lord Teynham, whose descendant, at the time of the Baltic crisis, had obstructed plans to make airing grounds on the Isle of Grain.[118] When letters to Thomas Wildman were unanswered, the Commissioners' thoughts had turned, certainly by June 1793, to compulsory purchase.[119] But then a letter came from Wildman; the sale of the hill, he claimed, would be detrimental to Chetney Hill Marsh Farm and also to the Chilham Castle estate, as tenants would be inconvenienced and want lower rents. For the Customs Commissioners, any response was better than none. On 21 June they asked Wildman to give the acreage of Chetney Hill field and name his price. If he felt unable to part with only the hill, what was the price for Marsh Farm, and how big was it? Wildman's answer was evasive, stating only that he could not arrive at a figure, and an independent valuation would be needed. The Commissioners were happy with that: they told Wildman to get the land valued, and they would arrange for a surveyor to visit and review the price.

115 NA BT 6/149, no. 14; BT 5/9/254–5.

116 NA BT 5/9/254–5.

117 The first 'chasing' letter to the Commissioners had been 20 March 1793 (NA BT 5/8/400).

118 See Chapter 2.

119 NA BT 6/149, no. 10, from which remaining references in this paragraph are taken.

Wildman did nothing. Preoccupied with other aspects of the lazaret, the Commissioners did not harass him. A reminder from the Board of Trade that the next parliamentary session was approaching did not break the deadlock.[120] Even in February 1794, when the Board leant on the Commissioners by seeking the support of the Treasury, there was no breakthrough in negotiations.[121] It was not until mid-June that James Hume, clerk to the Customs Commissioners, revealed that he had written some time earlier to Wildman 'informing him that Mr. Hogben, a Surveyor at Rochester, will be directed to attend him, to see the Ground in question exactly marked out; but that no answer thereto had been received'.[122] On 18 July 1794 the Board of Trade showed signs of real impatience, embarrassed that the Turkey Company should see such ineffectual government.[123] Hume was to be reminded that the project was urgent; he responded with the news that Wildman was now asking, via Hogben, whether a smaller area (less than 25 acres) would not suffice.[124] Hume had already replied to Wildman that this 'was by no means more than will be necessary'.[125]

From that exchange it would have been painfully evident to Hawkesbury that the two sides, far from negotiating costs and dates, were still sidestepping like boxers, seeking the best position from which to land a punch. Summer turned to autumn; still the Board of Trade pressed for progress and still the Commissioners had nothing to report. When there *was* news, it fell, ironically, in a rare interval of more than two months in which the Board had no meeting. A letter from Hume dated 7 October 1794 was not read to the Board until 8 December.[126] Thomas Wildman was now objecting to the plan of 'insulating' that part of Chetney Hill wanted for a lazaret; unless the Customs Commissioners could 'furnish him with their whole plan in every respect', he could not proceed. The position was now reached where the plan for a lazaret could not be finalized until the site was known, but the site could not be bought until the vendor knew the plan for the lazaret.

Hume wrote another letter to the Board on 6 December.[127] He had recently had a further exchange with Wildman, who made new conditions on which he would be willing to treat for the sale. Hume complained of Wildman's 'guarded manner', and when he had increased the demand for compensation by another £23 per acre above the price fixed by his own surveyor, the Customs Commissioners had had enough. They acted only by delegation from the Treasury, and Hume informed the Board of Trade that without new powers the Commissioners could take the matter no further.[128] As the Board of Trade were equally vexed, the project might even then have been abandoned. But the Turkey Company would not let it drop. In late February 1795 Bosanquet and three of his colleagues attended a meeting of the Board and warned

120 NA BT 5/9/96, 7 Nov. 1793.

121 NA BT 5/9/173.

122 NA BT 5/9/238–9.

123 NA BT 5/9/255.

124 NA BT 5/9/256; BT 6/149, no. 15.

125 NA BT 6/149, no. 15.

126 NA BT 5/9/299.

127 NA BT 5/9/299–300.

128 Ibid.

that by the end of the year they would be in serious trouble: 'the Trade would be entirely at a stand or must be supported at the expence of Government'.[129] Pitt was in attendance and sympathetic to their cause; he told them the Treasury 'had given such Authority and Directions' to the Customs Commissioners as would obviate further delay.[130] It was now, at last, the time to consider stronger measures.

The powers vested in the Treasury by the Act of 1772, to treat for the site of a lazaret, allowed for a difference of opinion on the purchase cost to be settled by a jury at the general Quarter Sessions of the county affected.[131] This required a formal notice from the Crown to the landowner, at least 30 days before the Sessions began. In early March 1795 the Board of Trade urgently set about acquiring an instrument under the royal sign manual for giving Wildman the necessary notice.[132] The Customs Commissioners were asked to have it served without delay, or the 30-day deadline would be missed.[133] Presumably it was, as the subject was resurrected over a year later.[134] In June 1795 the Board of Trade came to the dismal conclusion that the last two years had been totally wasted and acknowledged the distress to the Turkey Company.[135]

The Board resolved to press on, but because many people whom they hoped to consult were 'out of town' for the summer, it was likely that yet another year would be lost.[136] This cryptic reference was perhaps to members of the College of Physicians, but also to certain experts in land law. It would appear that Wildman's title was yet another maturing obstacle to the purchase of land, and it brought about a further frustrating delay. On 30 March 1797 the solicitor to the Treasury informed the Board of Trade of the steps taken by Wildman to complete his title; he referred also to 'the refusal of the Judges to Report upon a Petition presented to Parliament for leave to bring in a Bill for that purpose'.[137] But what purpose? Perhaps there were complicated family trusts. The Board of Trade were clearly worried, conceiving that the opposition of the judges 'may be founded on Considerations merely of a private nature'.[138] The Board, apparently, thought the judges insufficiently briefed. They wanted the Treasury solicitor to wait upon them and try to have their objection to the Bill removed, as the land is 'for a great public use'.[139]

Thereafter, on the subject of the lazaret, the minutes of the Board of Trade are silent. Confusion deepens. Some land was bought from Wildman in 1797, for £5,250, but details of the eventual agreement appear to have been a matter only for the

129 NA BT 5/9/415.

130 Ibid. Pitt is not named, but the reassurance came from the Chancellor of the Exchequer.

131 12 Geo. III, c.57, s.3.

132 NA BT 5/9/420–1.

133 Ibid.

134 NA BT 5/10/67.

135 Ibid.

136 NA BT 5/10/55.

137 NA BT 5/10/358–9.

138 Ibid.

139 Ibid.

Treasury.[140] It is also unclear how far the third report of the Turkey Company was the plan finally adopted for the lazaret, and whether Russell and Robertson suggested further alterations. In 1795 the Turkey Company went back to Soane for further drawings, and although these too were probably not definitive, work at Chetney Hill did eventually go ahead.[141] This was not before 1800, when the final stage of parliamentary approval, so long accepted as necessary by the Turkey Company, the Commissioners of Customs and the Board of Trade, was finally obtained.

140 NA T 29/71, f.379, 21 Nov. 1797.

141 For the 1795 drawings by Soane, see Colvin, *History of the King's Works*, vol. 6, p. 448.

Chapter Nine

Land or Sea? The Lazaretto Debate, 1793–1800

Yellow fever

While the Board of Trade were engaged in policy, pondering the admissibility of foul bills of health, their parent body enjoyed no respite from the daily attention to detail which quarantine demanded. As well as orders for ships to be discharged, there were the usual instructions to Customs about vessels in distress while en route to elsewhere in Europe. As a rule the anxiety of the master to be on his way was matched only by the eagerness of the Privy Council to see him depart, especially if he had sick crewmen. But when a ship was stranded or wrecked, it might be necessary for salvaged goods, except wine and oil, to be aired at Stangate Creek. If the cargo were cotton wool, then the need for airing would be automatic unless the bales had been soaked in the incident. And the Council continually fussed and grumbled when ships had omitted, allegedly, to fly the yellow flag.[1]

With Britain now at war with France, the successive imposition and relaxation of quarantine, which had been a bewildering feature of policy some ten years earlier, did not continue to the same extent. The Privy Council still monitored reports of plague in the Levant, but a desire to get the cargoes safely to port overtook the tradition of tinkering with the delay once the ships had arrived. In March 1791 quarantine against Spain and Ivica was lifted under certain conditions, but in other respects the Privy Council were not minded to interfere with established restrictions.[2] In any case, the issues were now more sophisticated. In June 1793, when the Council considered a petition from the Turkey Company, the question was not the duration of quarantine but whether or not ships without clean bills, returning from the Levant in ballast or with part cargoes of non-susceptible goods, could arrive at British ports at all without calling first at one of the Mediterranean lazarettos.[3] But only in that one respect did the Privy Council allow themselves to be involved with a Company whose problems they had delegated to the Board of Trade. The Council had worries of their own, and

1 For sick crewmen, see National Archives [NA] PC 2/136/80 (ship from Spain to Honfleur at Bristol); for salvage and airing of cargoes, see PC 2/137/17, 149, 176; for yellow flag offences, see PC 2/136/596 and PC 2/138/272, 279, 283.

2 For the lifting of restrictions against Spain (which included arrivals from Minorca and Gibraltar), see NA PC 2/135/492. The context was helpfully explained in PC 2/146/523–6.

3 NA PC 2/138/297–300. Another question was how far the Privy Council were the proper judges of what goods were liable to retain infection.

they came not from the Turkey Company or even from the Mediterranean. A new disease was in the offing.

In the late summer of 1793 the Privy Council received intelligence that the ship *Hankey*, carrying cotton wool, had sailed from Grenada in the West Indies with several crewmen already ill.[4] Close behind her was the *Salus*, also with sick men.[5] When the ships reached Deal, the Privy Council learnt the disturbing news that both had been visited off the Lizard by the navy, who had impressed three crewmen from each.[6] While remonstrating with the Admiralty, the Council ordered that the baggage of customers who had died on the voyage and been buried at Bulam Island off the African coast, be sunk in deep water.[7] Five days later, on 22 October, both vessels were discharged from quarantine obligations without their cargoes being aired.[8] But on 11 November they were suddenly ordered to Stangate Creek where the cotton wool was to be aired for two weeks.[9] This change of heart had been caused by the arrival at Falmouth of two packet boats, the *Boyd* from Jamaica and the *Charlotte* from New York and Halifax.[10] The former had lost the master, ten seamen and a passenger on the voyage; the latter brought reports of 'a terrible disorder' at Philadelphia.[11] During November the *Boyd* was cleansed and fumigated in the course of a quarantine of 14 days, while remaining at Falmouth.[12] Meanwhile, the Privy Council issued an Order on 6 November, imposing a like quarantine of 14 days on all arrivals from Philadelphia, Delaware and New Jersey.[13] This was the first time quarantine had been imposed in Britain against the United States and the disease responsible for this precedent, and for the wider worries, was yellow fever.

This subtropical affliction had long decimated the crews of warships newly arrived in the West Indies.[14] It was probably the unspecified infection, emanating from Jamaica, which had worried the Privy Council in 1692. Unaware that the disease was caused by mosquito bites, naval surgeons struggled in vain to contain it and even to grasp its identity. In 1768 Lind reckoned that 'the black vomit, and the other symptoms which characterize the yellow fever, are often accidental though fatal appearances in [other] fevers of the West Indies'.[15] Nearly 20 years later Blane wrote that yellow fever differed in some respects from other fevers, but was not

4 NA PC 2/138/535, 552.

5 NA PC 2/139/20.

6 NA PC 2/139/21.

7 NA PC 2/139/23, 32.

8 NA PC 2/139/37.

9 NA PC 2/139/84. It was not until 4 February 1794 that Customs were told no further directions would be given about airing the cotton on the *Hankey*.

10 NA PC 2/139/61.

11 Ibid.

12 NA PC 2/139/93, 110.

13 NA PC 2/139/63, 65.

14 C. Creighton, *A History of Epidemics in Britain* (2 vols, Cambridge, 1891–94), vol. 2, pp. 102–3.

15 J. Lind, *An Essay on Diseases Incidental to Europeans in hot Climates* (London, 1768), pp. 112–13. In later editions (1771 and 1777) he made no significant changes.

so distinct as to form a separate species of disease like measles and smallpox.[16] He noted it broke out when men were 'exposed to unwholesome land air, or to the foul air of ships, whether from infectious effluvia, or proceeding merely from the putrefaction that takes place in neglected holds'.[17] On the other hand, it had been evident to Lind that patients with yellow fever in the Greenwich Hospital in Jamaica, built on a marshy site, tended to get worse rather than better, compared to the sick who stayed on the ship.[18] Both surgeons considered that the lifestyle of an individual newly arrived in the West Indies might render him particularly susceptible to catching the disease. Lind thought the symptoms arose 'sometimes from a gross habit of body, excessive drinking of spirituous liquors, and from being afterwards over heated in the sun'.[19] Blane simply warned the 'young, fat and plethoric' that they were at risk.[20]

For minds traditionally imbued with a dread of the plague, the prospect of yellow fever raised mixed emotions. A disease which required extreme heat to generate its deadliness would surely make no inroads in a British winter. But some uncertainty in the policy for defence was inevitable. Neither Lind nor Blane had discussed how far yellow fever was contagious in the way, or to the extent, that contagion was linked to the plague. In the absence of any lobby arguing that the disease could spread rapidly or even at all in the British climate, the Privy Council's response to the cluster of sickly ships had been far from timid. True, the *Hankey* and *Salus* had been dispatched to Stangate Creek to air their cargoes, but the Council had no intention of forcing packet boats to sail any further east than Falmouth for quarantine purposes, despite dreadful deaths in the course of their voyage. One reason was a disinclination to upset the Postmaster-General; another was the awareness that if disease did break out in Falmouth itself, it would be a very long way from London. The prospect of isolating the west of Cornwall appealed more than a cordon sanitaire around the Medway towns. But there was no serious belief in the Council that events would deteriorate to that extent.

It was alarming for the Privy Council, however, that although the disease had not come ashore in England, it was showing no signs of weakening its recent grip on transatlantic shipping. In December 1793 the *Tarleton* arrived at Liverpool from Grenada having lost many of its crew, to be followed in February by the *John* from the same island with a similar history.[21] Their cargoes of cotton wool, as well as the crews' wearing apparel, were landed at Hoylake for two weeks' airing, while the ships themselves were cleansed and fumigated.[22] But by now the automatic quarantine against North America had been found unnecessary and was revoked on 12 February 1794.[23] The Privy Council preferred to deal with arrivals on their

16 Gilbert Blane, *Observations on the Diseases Incident to Seamen* (London, 1785), p. 397.

17 Ibid.

18 Lind, pp. 173–4.

19 Lind, p. 123.

20 Blane, p. 398.

21 NA PC 2/139/168, 182, 332, 374.

22 Ibid.

23 NA PC 2/139/346–7.

merits, adopting the formula of airing and cleansing when it seemed appropriate, and ordering the baggage of deceased persons to be sunk in deep water. One outcome of this policy was the need to compensate widows and heirs for the compulsory loss of effects to which they were legally entitled.[24]

The latent menace of yellow fever would not go away. Off Newcastle, Liverpool and Lancaster, the chests and apparel of dead seamen were pitched into deep water.[25] At Falmouth, mail from the Jamaica packet was dipped in vinegar and smoked in sulphur before continuing its odoriferous journey to London.[26] In October 1794 the Privy Council at last had some reassurance, not that the scare was over but that their policy was on the right lines. They were attended by Beeston Long, chairman of the Society of West India Merchants, to whom they had already sent the opinions of the Garrison Surgeon of Fort Royal in Martinique and the Inspector of the Regimental Hospital in the West Indies, as to how the disease was spread.[27] Long produced his own evidence, which matched that of the army surgeons, showing 'That the Contagion was in the Air – and the Infection not otherwise communicable'.[28] Furthermore, on the voyages to England only those who had been ill at the time of sailing had died, and those deaths were relatively few. These comments were the more welcome because one Privy Councillor, the Earl of Charlemont, had received letters from Dr Alexander Haliday of Belfast very critical of the absence of quarantine against the West Indies.[29] He pointed out that cotton wool could easily convey 'infectious miasma' and called for stricter enforcement. 'Shameful negligence, with respect both to persons and goods', Haliday warned, 'has been on former occasions most notorious'.[30]

On 12 November 1794, when the yellow fever epidemic in North America had spread, the Privy Council introduced 14 days' quarantine against arrivals from Baltimore and Maryland.[31] The Order referred to a fever 'of the Nature of the Plague', similar to that which had raged in Philadelphia during the previous year. This form of words was necessary because quarantine had so far been envisaged only as a defence against plague, the one disease named in successive Acts of Parliament. It was unlawful, therefore, to institute quarantine against any other threat. This was not quite the problem it might have been because plague was still a generic name for any major disorder. Lind referred to scurvy as 'so consuming a plague', and it was not yet usual to qualify Levantine plague as bubonic.[32] In any event, the national mood was to put the health of the public before ambiguities

24 The first petition for compensation in the context of yellow fever occurred in November 1793, in connection with the *Hankey*; it was referred to the Treasury to act as they thought fit (NA PC 2/139/135).

25 NA PC 2/141/57–8, 111, 114.

26 NA PC 2/141/338–9.

27 NA PC 2/141/197.

28 Ibid.

29 Historical Manuscripts Commission [HMC], *Thirteenth Report*, pp. 220, 223.

30 Ibid.

31 NA PC 2/141/285.

32 C. Lloyd (ed.), *The Health of Seamen: Selections from the Works of Dr. James Lind, Sir Gilbert Blane and Dr. Thomas Trotter* (Navy Records Society, 1965), p. 83.

of language. The Foreign Office wanted clarification from the Privy Council about their quarantine policy towards the West Indies, an attitude which, as Haliday had noted, seemed none too severe.[33] Stephen Cottrell responded in confident tone that no general Orders had seemed necessary, but Customs officers had been told to pay special attention to ships from the Caribbean, and could insist on the airing of cargoes and the sinking of seamen's chests.[34] Yellow fever, by implication, was as much a matter for the Customs Commissioners as for the Privy Council, who defiantly reminded the Foreign Office that 'the Contagion is in the air and the infection not otherwise communicable'.[35] Only several years later did the Privy Council reveal that a general Order for quarantine against the West Indies had been proposed, but rejected immediately as too damaging for trade.[36]

During the first half of 1795, the yellow-fever scare appeared to subside. There were still worries about the safety of mail, and the West India merchants of London complained to the Duke of Portland that letters were being unduly delayed at Falmouth.[37] But North America seemed to be over the worst, and the Privy Council revoked quarantine against Baltimore and Maryland on 3 July.[38] Unfortunately, the respite did not last long. New reports of a 'Malignant and Epidemical Fever of the nature of the Plague' caused the Privy Council, on 14 October, to lay a quarantine of 14 days on all ships from New York and Norfolk, Virginia.[39] Before the end of the year, it was evident that these circumlocutions for yellow fever had to stop. At Hull, the master of an American ship had wrongly answered in the negative all the standing questions put to him about sickness of the crew, and whether or not his port of departure – Norfolk, Virginia – had been infected when he left.[40] The Law Officers of the Crown reported to Council that as the present quarantine regulations referred strictly to plague, the penalties against the master could not be enforced.[41] A paradoxical situation had therefore been reached in which quarantine regulations were justified by virtue of the vague meaning of 'plague', but that same imprecision provided a perfect defence against allegations that the rules had been breached. On 9 December 1795 the Privy Council wrote to George Rose, secretary to the Treasury, requesting that a Bill be put before Parliament to widen the definition of diseases against which quarantine might be enforced.[42]

While Rose dallied, the procession of Orders for enforcing and then relaxing quarantine against North America was becoming reminiscent of the stop-go

33 NA PC 2/141/319–21.

34 Ibid. Cottrell admitted that in August 1794 some tidewaiters had died in the Thames on ships from Jamaica but, as their deaths could not be linked to the ships themselves, quarantine had been removed.

35 Ibid.

36 NA PC 2/161/425, 11 Dec. 1802, in a letter to Sir George Shee for the information of the Lord Lieutenant of Ireland.

37 NA PC 2/142/391.

38 NA PC 2/143/363–4.

39 NA PC 2/144/321.

40 NA PC 2/144/474, 476, 489, 498. The master was Thomas Calvert of the *Friends*.

41 NA PC 2/144/498.

42 NA PC 2/144/506.

strategy which Britain had adopted against the Mediterranean. On 13 January 1796 quarantine was taken off ships from New York and Norfolk, Virginia, but reinstated on 18 October 1797 against arrivals from Philadelphia.[43] In the interval between those Orders, the confidence of the Privy Council had been tested and shaken by two unwelcome developments. The first concerned ships, and especially transports, from the West Indies. In May 1796 the Army Medical Board were worried that a too-hasty decision to remove quarantine from these vessels might endanger public health.[44] In response, the Privy Council ordered that, in future, quarantine should be removed from transports only when the Board considered it safe to do so. Unfortunately, the Board were not always informed of an arrival, or found it impossible to act before a ship had been discharged under local orders. The problem was brought to a head by the arrival at Spithead of HMS *Hebe*, which had lost seven seamen on the voyage from the West Indies; she had been preceded by two transports from Jamaica, with sick and injured, but quarantine for all three ships was only nominal.[45] The Privy Council might well have left the problem to Henry Dundas, Secretary at War, had it not been for the second unwelcome development.

This was the arrival at Falmouth of the *Sandwich* packet from Jamaica, with actual cases of yellow fever on board. In July 1796 two Commissioners of Customs were hastily summoned to the Council to consider whether the passengers who were well should be allowed to land.[46] In a confident decision, influenced by a brave opinion from a Falmouth surgeon named Trevossa, the Council decreed that they could.[47] But this episode only increased the Council's unease about transports. This time it was Sir Lucas Pepys, Physician-General of the Army, and two of his colleagues who were summoned to attend the Council. Under the influence of their cautionary words, and with the support of Secretary Dundas, it was agreed in late September 1796 that the Army Medical Board would appoint doctors at Plymouth, Portsmouth, Deal and Gravesend to go on board all transports from the West Indies and examine the health of the men before any decision would be taken as to quarantine.[48] It was inevitable that this measure would lead to confusion or even conflict with the Customs service, who would normally have made the judgement for themselves, at least in the first instance. The problem came to light at Plymouth where Dr Boone, local physician to the Forces, had been prevented by Customs officers from inspecting the sick men in the transport *Lady Jane*.[49] This was because the ship had arrived from Gibraltar and not from the West Indies, but the War Office now argued that the measure should extend to all transports from anywhere. It is not clear what the Privy Council decided.

On 3 January 1798 the quarantine against Philadelphia was lifted, but reintroduced on 28 September, and extended to New York and Boston on 24 October as yellow

43 NA PC 2/145/36; 2/149/278.

44 NA PC 2/145/525.

45 NA PC 2/146/405, 464.

46 NA PC 2/146/243.

47 NA PC 2/146/307.

48 NA PC 2/146/462–3, 473–4.

49 NA PC 2/149/322, 507.

fever continued to ravage.[50] In February the Privy Council had been astonished to receive a letter from George Rose, enquiring whether it was now proper to ask Parliament to make provision against the spread of ship-borne infectious diseases other than plague.[51] He was reminded that the Council's letter of 9 December 1795 had asked him to arrange just that.[52] This time Rose acted rapidly. On 12 February 1798 the Act of ten years earlier, in which changes to quarantine had been introduced as part of wider modifications to the Customs service, was read to the Commons.[53] On the next day a committee of the whole House discussed those parts of the Act which related to quarantine, but extraneous issues, such as the fraudulent import of glass, were added to their deliberations.[54] On 15 March the quarantine Act of 1753 was read to the Commons, and it was ordered that the committee of the whole House considering the 1788 Act should also make provision in the Bill for extending the application of quarantine to contagious diseases other than plague.[55] With no opposition, the composite Act received the royal assent on 5 April 1798.[56]

In terms of quarantine, the 1798 Act made three main amendments.[57] First, the rules for flying the yellow flag, introduced ten years earlier, were tightened and extended. It was now ordered that the flag was to be 'of six breadths of bunting', and the masthead light which replaced it at night was to be supplemented by a signal lantern, as used on warships. The flag was to fly constantly until the ship was discharged from quarantine. The penalty for a breach of the rules remained at £200. Secondly, pilots who took ships liable to quarantine into places other than designated quarantine stations were to be fined £100. Thirdly, quarantine provisions were extended 'to all such diseases or distempers, as his Majesty, by and with the advice of his privy council, shall judge to be probably infectious, and shall so declare by order in council notified by proclamation, or published in the *London Gazette*'. Despite this opportunity to be specific, the Privy Council continued to cite a disease 'of the nature of Plague' to justify quarantine against yellow fever in Philadelphia.[58]

The incidence of sickness in ships reaching Falmouth, far from diminishing, was soon calling for even braver decisions by the Council, who showed faith in the diagnoses of Cornish doctors. In October 1798 Dr Lowry of Falmouth suspected yellow fever in the *Triton*, arrived in ballast from St Bartholomew, four of the crew having died.[59] The local physician most trusted by the Council was Dr Luke, who

50 NA PC 2/150/5, 436, 509, 568, 573.

51 NA PC 2/150/173.

52 Ibid.

53 *Journal of the House of Commons* [*JHC*], vol. 53, p. 241.

54 *JHC*, vol. 53, p. 243.

55 *JHC*, vol. 53, p. 374.

56 *JHC*, vol. 53, p. 451.

57 38 Geo. III, c.33, from which all references in this paragraph are taken until the last. The point about 'main amendments' is that the Act also, in Section 3, decreed that offences against quarantine could be tried in any county within Great Britain or in the proper courts in the islands.

58 NA PC 2/151/436, 509.

59 NA PC 2/151/519.

came to prominence in July with the arrival of the *Princess Charlotte* from Jamaica.[60] This ship, on which eight had died, was released from quarantine well within the 14 days usually expected. It was Luke who supervised the removal ashore 'to proper lodging' of those who were well, and the transfer to a convalescent ship, presumably supplied at the expense of the Post Office, of the invalids.[61] But while the West Indies remained free of any general Order for quarantine, the North American states were still subject to a bewildering alternation between freedom and constraint. The quarantine against Philadelphia, imposed in September 1798, was lifted only three months later, to be reinstated on 16 October 1799 along with a new restriction against New York.[62] Reports of infectious fever in Virginia and Maryland led to an Order for quarantine on 12 November 1800, but this was rescinded five weeks later.[63]

In time of peace, the Privy Council would have been very troubled by reports that an epidemic of yellow fever had apparently crossed the Atlantic. In 1800 it was wreaking havoc in Cadiz, but as the port was blockaded their attitude was calm.[64] Had they known of contemporary correspondence between Sir Richard Bickerton, the blockading Rear-Admiral, and Lord Keith, they would have been even more relaxed. Bickerton thought that yellow fever 'is not so contagious as Gen. O'Hara [Governor of Gibraltar] imagines. I was in the W. Indies when it raged and always understood that a bottle of vinegar held to the nose was a sure preventive even in the room of an infected person'.[65] But Bickerton was safely at sea, while O'Hara saw the disease spread inexorably towards Gibraltar, where a visitor in 1800 noted a lazaretto on the Neutral Ground.[66] But the Privy Council made no quarantine Orders which expressly targeted arrivals from the colony. This was to prevent naval and military units from being taken out of commission in wartime, although a Proclamation was published on 29 July 1800 which reinforced quarantine for ships coming from or through the Mediterranean and from West Barbary.[67] But even that measure was aimed principally at plague, to which Gibraltar was so evidently at risk from the visible shore of North Africa. The traditional danger from that quarter was spelled out by Papon, also in 1800, when he advocated a permanent quarantine of 10–12 days against all ships from Gibraltar carrying susceptible goods.[68]

One of the most curious outbreaks of what was deemed yellow fever (the diagnosis must be in doubt), occurred in a ship travelling the Atlantic from east to west. In November 1802 the *Mary* put into Falmouth when a few days out of

60 NA PC 2/151/207, 245.

61 Ibid.

62 NA PC 2/152/82,419–20.

63 NA PC 2/156/121, 276.

64 NA PC 2/156/57.

65 C. Lloyd (ed.), *The Keith Papers* (3 vols, London, 1950), vol. 2, p. 139.

66 T. Walsh, *Journal of the late Campaign in Egypt ...* (London, 1803), p. 9.

67 Bibliotheca Lindesiana, vol. 5: *A Bibliography of Royal Proclamations of the Tudor and Stuart Sovereigns and of Others Published under Authority, 1485–1714 ... England and Wales* (Oxford, 1910).

68 J.P. Papon, *De la peste, ou Epoques mémorables de ce fléau, et les moyens de s'en préserver* (2 vols, Paris, 1800), vol. 1, pp. 218–19.

London on a voyage to Norfolk, Virginia.[69] She had many men ill of a 'malignant fever', and several of them had died.[70] Exactly when yellow fever was diagnosed is not clear, but Dr Luke let the sufferers come ashore 'to Sheds or Barns', a move of which the Privy Council later approved.[71] When the number of sick increased, they were transferred to a floating lazaretto.[72] This was presumably the same ship which had served in 1798 and was now a permanent feature in Falmouth harbour, or in St Just's Pool. There is no reason to believe that the navy were in any way involved with the choice of vessel or its conversion. There were diplomatic overtones to the incident, as the *Mary* was repatriating 73 Americans who had done service with the British military.[73] Rufus King, the American minister in London, was kept abreast of developments, and every effort was made to strike a balance between humanity and a natural desire to see the ship on its way.[74] The mayor of Falmouth was asked to provide relief.[75] Technically, the ship was not in quarantine, but the Privy Council were exercising a wider responsibility for public health, and only the master and one passenger were authorized to land.[76] On 8 February 1803 the *Mary* was allowed to set sail again, with permission to call at Ireland in the event of more sickness.[77] The shipowner looked for compensation over the delay, but the Treasury made an easy defence that Government had no case to answer.[78] Dr Luke was luckier and received an honorarium of £150.[79]

The chaos of war

While focused on the threat from across the Atlantic, the Privy Council could not neglect the difficulty of trade through the Mediterranean. War with France was interrupting the import of raw materials from Turkey, and quarantine delays were compounding the problem for manufacturers by preventing the release, in even and predictable quantities, of the cargoes which managed to arrive. In October 1795 the silk manufacturers of London complained that many workers were unemployed as a result, although some 12 ships were lying at Stangate Creek or Liverpool.[80] The Privy Council reacted by allowing Italian raw or thrown silk, if shipped from Leghorn or Genoa and not originating in the Levant, to be delivered without opening and airing.[81] Any benefit which this might have brought was quickly nullified by

69 NA PC 2/161/402.
70 Ibid.
71 Ibid.; PC 2/162/4, 17.
72 NA PC 2/161/438.
73 NA PC 2/162/18.
74 NA PC 2/162/17–8, 55, 122.
75 NA PC 2/161/403.
76 NA PC 2/162/17, 134.
77 NA PC 2/162/55, 82, 121.
78 NA PC 2/162/177.
79 This reference is indexed in PC 2/162 but not given a page number.
80 NA PC 2/144/368.
81 Ibid.

the decision of Spain, in 1796, to join France in the war against Britain. With the consequent withdrawal of the Royal Navy, the Mediterranean was effectively closed to British shipping in 1797. This led to a suspension of the Navigation Act, to allow goods from the Levant to be brought from any port in British or 'friendly' ships.[82] But when Napoleon acquired control of Italy, the catastrophe for the Turkey Company was virtually complete. The value of imports from the Levant fell from nearly £105,000 in 1797 to just over £42,000 in 1798.[83]

Very soon the desire to be helpful towards struggling mercantile interests put the Privy Council in collision with their duty to safeguard the health of the nation. When plague erupted in Corsica, early in 1798, the Council hoped an instruction to Customs officers to be extra vigilant might be enough of a safeguard.[84] But when the outbreak worsened, a full quarantine of 40 days was imposed on 24 January against arrivals from Minorca, Majorca, Corsica, Gibraltar and the ports of Spain within the Mediterranean.[85] A more intractable problem was soon to follow. The acceptance of cargoes from friendly ships annulled the long-standing precautions of the Turkey Company against departures for Britain in times of plague. Customs officers around the country were enjoined to put the Ottoman ship *St George* into strictest quarantine when and wherever she arrived.[86] The vessel had left Smyrna on 25 May with a foul bill of health and a cargo of cotton wool and yarn, ostensibly for Amsterdam.[87] She then called at Patras in the Morea to complete her loading and, so reports alleged, to acquire a clean bill of health for Britain.[88] Another ship with a foul bill from Smyrna was the *Princessa*, which arrived at Stangate Creek in August.[89] But as she carried non-enumerated goods – fruit, wood, nuts and drugs – the Privy Council felt able to agree with the importers, Messrs St Barbe, Green & Bignall, that they be delivered without airing.[90]

For the Turkey Company it was still evident that foul-bill facilities at Stangate Creek were a necessity, but they were now less convinced that a shore establishment was a better prospect than floating lazarettos. The extraordinary delays over acquiring the site and the uncertainties which remained about the costs and configuration had led them to consult Gilbert Blane of the Navy Medical Board as to which system would be more effective and about preventive measures in general. In December 1798 Blane corresponded with Sir John Coxe Hippisley, a member of the quarantine committee of the Turkey Company who had interests in Italy.[91] Although recognized as an expert on yellow fever, Blane was becoming increasingly drawn into questions

82 37 Geo. III, c.84 (royal assent 19 June 1797), to be in force until three months had elapsed since the end of the war.

83 A.C. Wood, *A History of the Levant Company* (Oxford, 1935), p. 179.

84 NA PC 2/150/68.

85 NA PC 2/150/86.

86 NA PC 2/150/571. The ship was also referred to as the *San Georgio*.

87 Ibid.

88 Ibid.; see also PC 2/151/139 for a report to Bosanquet (for the information of the Turkey Company) on how the ship had been dealt with.

89 NA PC 2/151/282.

90 Ibid.

91 *Letters, &c. on the Subject of Quarantine* (London, 1799), pp. 1–8.

of the plague. He was reaching the view that the two diseases had certain similarities, so 'the practical remarks are nearly the same …'[92] In separate correspondence with Rufus King, the American Resident in London, Blane was now unequivocal that yellow fever was infectious, and scornful of doctors 'paradoxical enough' to claim that the plague was otherwise.[93] The Turkey Company were little interested in yellow fever, but reckoned the twin interests of Blane gave him useful standing with the Privy Council who were vexed over both diseases.

The message to Hippisley from Blane was that ventilation and cleanliness were 'moral and religious duties'; which was why the 'cleanly' Dutch, despite 'the most slovenly and careless' quarantine procedures, had never suffered an epidemic of plague.[94] Similarly, argued Blane, London had escaped any visitation of the disease for well over a century because 'the advantages of spacious and airy habitations, of personal cleanliness, of dryness, and cleanliness from forming drains and common-sewers, are undeniable'.[95] The corollary was that quarantine had played little part in this protection, which led Blane to question whether the cost of a land establishment could be justified. He saw five advantages to the practice of using floating lazarettos.[96] First, they were more airy than buildings, which required high double walls, partly because the tide produced healthy draughts. Secondly, they were more easily guarded. Thirdly, they were less expensive. Fourthly, they could be moved. And finally, 'they admit better of being multiplied'. Their only drawback was that some passengers preferred to do quarantine on land, and Blane conceded the benefit of 'erecting some apartments on a small scale on the adjacent beach …'

The Turkey Company, before or after the letter to Hippisley, had consulted Blane and James Johnston jointly on wider aspects of plague prevention.[97] Johnston was another physician, and they replied as Commissioners for Sick and Wounded Seamen. It was their joint opinion that floating lazarettos were the better option, and they had had no hesitation in agreeing that the regulations at Leghorn could be appropriate for Stangate Creek.[98] Both men went there to see the floating lazarettos at work; the Privy Council appeared under the impression that their visit was at the request of the Admiralty.[99] The physicians suggested several ways to the Turkey Company for improving the lazarettos, by making the circulation of air more efficient. These measures, submitted in May 1799, included more gratings under foot, extra ports between the orlop and lower gun decks, and a cowl or 'turret, fitted with louvre boards' through the roofs.[100] At least one of the lazarettos was more like a floating building than a ship, and the physicians referred to the decks as 'forming the floors of the house'.[101] Among improvements to satisfy the needs of a foul-bill station, the

92 *Letters, &c.*, p. 1. Blane had been in touch with the Turkish ambassador.

93 *Letters, &c.*, pp. 10, 13.

94 *Letters, &c.*, pp. 3–4.

95 *Letters, &c.*, p. 17.

96 *Letters, &c.*, pp. 5–7, from which remaining references in this paragraph are taken.

97 *Letters, &c.*, pp. 21–9.

98 *Letters, &c.*, p. 25.

99 NA PC 2/152/146, 171.

100 *Letters, &c.*, p. 26.

101 Ibid.

physicians suggested a floating infirmary.[102] They were critical of existing legislation which obliged the Superintendent to refer to the Privy Council for directions if plague were ever to break out at the Creek.[103] In their view, he should have the authority to act quickly in a real emergency. That view, of course, followed the sentiments of Russell, whom Blane acknowledged as the expert.[104]

In their list of questions to Johnston and Blane, the Turkey Company had remarked that all the lazarettos of the Mediterranean in which their vessels without clean bills were legally obliged to perform quarantine were then closed to British shipping.[105] The Government, of course, were aware of this, and in the Commons a committee of the whole House was set up to consider and regulate the Levant trade.[106] On 12 July 1799 'An act to encourage the trade into the Levant Seas, by providing a more convenient mode of performing quarantine ...' received royal assent.[107] This Act (which also had a purpose unconnected with quarantine) did not repeal the problem section in 26 George II, c.18, but it empowered the King in Council 'to grant licence and permission' for goods without a clean bill of health to be landed in Britain direct from the Levant, subject to such regulations for quarantine as the Privy Council should decide upon. This formula was a temporary solution to a wartime problem, and implied that the obligation to air cargoes in the Mediterranean lazarettos would continue once peace returned. But as the end of the war was not in prospect, the Government had to face up to the immediate consequences of the Act. The Mediterranean had already reopened to British shipping, albeit under naval convoy, and so the provision of a foul-bill quarantine station at Stangate Creek was now inevitable and urgent. In line with the advice of Johnston and Blane, and with the confidence that airing in Mediterranean lazarettos would at some point resume, all parties moved away from the goal of a land lazaret and focused their attention on floating lazarettos.

On water or land?

Before July was out, the Turkey Company had delivered a memorial to the Privy Council urging that a framework for quarantine, under the new circumstances, be quickly established.[108] The reaction of the Council was to refer the matter to an internal committee, rather than delegate it to the Board of Trade.[109] Hawkesbury had been created Earl of Liverpool in 1796, but he was still the Board's President and had gained more expertise in quarantine matters than any other member of the

102 *Letters, &c.*, p. 27.

103 *Letters, &c.*, p. 28.

104 *Letters, &c.*, p. 8 (to Hippisley): 'For further information I beg to refer you to the work of Doctor Russell, who has deserved highly of the world for the intrepidity, ingenuity, and industry, he has displayed in his labors [*sic*] in this branch of his profession'.

105 *Letters, &c.*, p. 23.

106 *Journal of the House of Commons* [*JHC*], vol. 54, p. 656.

107 *JHC*, vol. 54, p. 738; 39 Geo. III, c.99.

108 NA PC 2/153/208.

109 Ibid.

Privy Council. More importantly, Liverpool had become acquainted with the leading figures in the Turkey Company, but that was perhaps part of the problem. Other members of the Council seem to have been irritated by the Company's memorial, and unwilling to continue the rather cosy but unproductive relationship which the merchants had enjoyed for so long with the Board of Trade.

The Privy Council committee returned the ball to the Company's court by asking what regulations they themselves had to propose, and whether these had already been mentioned to ministers or to the proposers of the recent Bill.[110] The Company might well have retorted that they had spent the last six years recommending regulations one after the other. It may be inferred that the Privy Council were unhappy to be landed by Parliament with this tricky and urgent responsibility, and had not been consulted as fully as they might have wished about the timing and text of the Act. Liverpool, in a letter dated 17 August 1799, confessed 'I knew nothing of this Act, 'till some time after it was passed ...'[111] This sentiment was echoed later in a letter from Stephen Cottrell, Privy Council clerk, to George Hammond, Under-Secretary of State in the Foreign Office. Cottrell mentioned that the earlier Levant Act 'had been rather improvidently repealed' before any lazaret could be established in Britain.[112] If 'repealed' was not technically correct, at least the adverb was appropriate. The new Act stipulated that the King in Council could allow a ship without a clean bill of health to head for Britain direct. But the King was usually in Dorset. Liverpool took the problem to Pitt 'and being sensible of the Impossibility of having a Council at Weymouth for every ship that may arrive, We agreed that it was better the Privy Council should take upon itself to exercise this Power at present ...'[113]

Any tension between the Turkey Company and the Privy Council evaporated when their respective committees met for talks.[114] There was no time for recrimination or another set of draft proposals. On 16 August 1799 a letter was sent to Pitt, via the Treasury, telling him that some Turkey ships were due immediately and that the floating lazarettos at Stangate Creek would be inadequate.[115] Did he approve of the navy making more hulks available?[116] And would he agree that the Commissioners for Sick and Wounded should be involved in the appointment of a surgeon to be stationed there?[117] Cottrell then sent a letter to the Treasury explaining that half a dozen Turkey ships with foul bills of health were expected over the next two months, with perhaps two in the ensuing week.[118] As the hulks at Stangate Creek (the *Princess Amelia* and the *Belleisle*) could scarcely air the cargoes of even four ships, they needed to be augmented by up to three old warships, with another to be fitted out as an infirmary, as Johnston and Blane had suggested. The Treasury were expected to discuss with the physicians the new post of surgeon and its salary and

110 NA PC 2/153/218.

111 NA PC 1/44/160.

112 NA PC 2/155/480–83.

113 NA PC 1/44/160, 29 Aug. 1799.

114 A minute of the meeting, on 14 August 1799, is in NA PC 1/44/160.

115 NA PC 2/153/259.

116 Ibid.

117 Ibid.

118 NA PC 2/153/276–80, from which remaining references in this paragraph are taken.

responsibilities; these included positioning and equipping the hulks, in consultation with the Superintendent of Quarantine. The Council were anxious to receive advice from any informed person at Stangate Creek about the drafting of new regulations.

Liverpool complained to a correspondent that Pitt was slow to respond.[119] In fact, Liverpool was far from happy with all aspects of quarantine at that juncture. His fellow Privy Councillors seemed to melt away in the summer months, leaving him to shoulder the burden of quarantine by himself, although 'this Business is of too much Delicacy and Responsibility to be transacted by one Person only'. Not only did the Lord President absent himself, but even Lord Grenville, who combined the posts of Foreign Secretary and Governor of the Levant Company, failed to attend the more important meetings.

On 24 August 1799 Liverpool learnt via Cottrell that Blane and Johnston had appointed Robert Newberry as the surgeon for the lazarettos.[120] Newberry, under their guidance, had rid the Russian fleet of infection while it was moored at the Nore during the previous winter.[121] He had a list of duties from his mentors, and others were to follow. Newberry, on Liverpool's advice, was not to have direct access to the Privy Council but could reach them if necessary via the Customs Commissioners, to whom he was to send regular reports.[122] At the end of the month, the Council were told that the Admiralty had ordered two old warships, the *Duke* at Portsmouth and the *Aboukir* at Plymouth, to be used as additional hulks, while the *Lizard* at Portsmouth could be fitted up as a hospital ship.[123] A little later the *Valiant* at Chatham was also made available as a lazaretto, probably instead of the *Aboukir*.[124]

The pace of activity was now taking its toll. If Liverpool were annoyed that his colleagues were unsupportive, he would hardly have been surprised. In the context of their wider responsibilities, quarantine was an immense and intractable difficulty. The issues were invidious, confusing and in rapid evolution, with an unspeakable disease as the cost of failure. In such a dense thicket of rules and decisions, mistakes could hardly be avoided. Cottrell, for instance, had ordered the *Sisters* from Smyrna to be detained on her arrival at Liverpool, before he realized that a foul-bill ship should only proceed to Stangate Creek.[125] For much of the time the Privy Council acted on rumour or doubtful intelligence; even the most reliable statement was delayed in the slow climb up the hierarchical ladder. News from Smyrna was painfully indirect, leaving the Council with little or no time to react. On 31 December 1798, when the *Withywood* sailed with a foul bill of health, the British consul warned the ambassador

119 NA PC 1/44/160, 17 Aug. 1799, from which all references in this paragraph are taken. The addressee is not revealed.

120 NA PC 2/153/299. The name was invariably spelt 'Newbery' at this period.

121 Ibid.

122 NA PC 2/153/299; PC 1/44/160.

123 NA PC 2/153/298.

124 NA PC 2/153/334. The register noted that the *Valiant* was in place of the *Conquerant* which was 'unfit to be removed', but that appears to have been an error. The *Conquerant* had not been mentioned, at least to the Privy Council, and the *Aboukir* at Plymouth, as well as being unfit, was probably regarded as too far away in wartime.

125 NA PC 2/153/301–3.

at Constantinople.[126] The ambassador wrote to Lord Grenville as Foreign Secretary, who referred the letter to George Canning, his Under-Secretary, who informed the Privy Council.[127] By then it was 3 March 1799. The message had taken 62 days, a normal voyage time for the *Withywood*. Luckily for the Council, she was delayed by a long call at Minorca, but other ships arrived direct.[128] This was, of course, a difficult period for mail, and war precluded the faster land route, but any Board of Health in the Mediterranean would have received intelligence from a consul direct.

In the face of such disadvantages, some new device was urgently needed to save the Privy Council suffocating under the pillow of quarantine management. Accordingly, the King was advised that a special Quarantine Committee should be established to consider the new regulations for foul-bill ships.[129] The Council had generated many quarantine committees in the past, but this one was to be exceptional in that the members would not be Privy Councillors. The instigator, of course, was Liverpool, who was also responsible for the membership.[130] He agonized into the small hours about the committee's size and balance. Hippisley gave him advice, but Liverpool found him 'rather a bustling intriguing Gentleman' and preferred the counsel of Sir Andrew Hamond, Comptroller of the Navy. At first he was wary of Hamond's preference for military doctors, as he (Liverpool) did not know them personally, 'and if they should not prove to be well disposed, they might create Obstruction and Delay'. But at least they would be preferable to delegates from the Royal College of Physicians, about whom Liverpool was scathing. He felt the College consisted 'of a number of Physicians of discordant Sentiments' and he had 'always been apprehensive that We should find great Difficulty in getting them to agree on any Opinion whatsoever'. Liverpool was minded, instead, to appoint one of the King's physicians. He also favoured the inclusion of Doctors Blane and Johnston, plus two members of the quarantine committee of the Levant Company, one Customs Commissioner who could appoint a colleague, and Stephen Cottrell, the Privy Council clerk.

In the event, Cottrell did not sit and the membership received other adjustments. The chairman was Sir George Baker, the elderly physician to royalty. The other ten members, according to Maclean, comprised eight physicians and two Levant merchants.[131] But if Maclean was accurate in identifying the merchants as E. Lee and J. Green, he was mistaken in assuming the other members were all physicians. A place had been found for Sir Andrew Hamond and there were two Commissioners of Customs, as Liverpool had intended.[132] Among the actual doctors were familiar

126 NA PC 2/152/343.

127 Ibid.

128 Because the *Withywood* had trans-shipped her cargo at Minorca, she was actually nine months on the voyage (NA PC 2/153/382).

129 NA PC 2/155/480–83.

130 NA PC 1/44/160, from which all references in this paragraph are taken.

131 C. Maclean, *Remarks on the British Quarantine laws …* (London, 1823), p. 16.

132 NA PC 2/155/480–83.

names: Sir Lucas Pepys, Patrick Russell and, of course, Johnston and Blane.[133] The earliest the committee could have met was late October 1799.[134]

In mid-November the Quarantine Committee reached an agreement with the Privy Council that huts or 'small cabins' should be erected at the northern corner of Chetney Hill in case anyone should fall sick in a vessel with a foul bill of health.[135] It is probable that these huts were intended to replace the hospital ship. Hamond now received a letter from the Privy Council in his official capacity, asking the Navy Board to carry out the work.[136] This implies that the Treasury had ducked involvement in the cost, although the Customs Commissioners and Superintendent of Quarantine had been consulted about the huts' location.[137] As the chosen site marked an agreement to keep clear of Sheerness, it would appear that the price to the navy for the inviolacy of the dockyard (and the cancellation of the hospital ship) was the work at Chetney Hill.[138] The committee were quick to make other points, including a recommendation that seamen should be exempt from impressment for ten days after quarantine had finished.[139] But their main work, and the *raison d'être* for their establishment, was the list of regulations to govern quarantine by foul-bill ships. On 20 November 1799 these urgent recommendations were accepted by the Privy Council, albeit on a provisional basis, and formed the substance of an important new Order.[140] The committee then reconvened to give the same topic their more mature consideration.

The first requirement of the Order was that ships should proceed straight to Stangate Creek. This did away with the long-standing suggestions that St Just's Pool at Falmouth should be provided with a pratique house for an initial assessment of health. No doubt the sickly state of Falmouth harbour, the only port in Britain where yellow fever cases were not uncommon, had a lot to do with that. Blane had favoured the Isle of Grain over Stangate Creek, but he would have been unaware of the problems which that idea had raised nearly a century earlier.[141] On arrival at the Creek, the master and mate were to go in the ship's boat, escorted by a guard boat, 'to certain Huts or Tents to be erected on the Beach' where they would answer the

133 The other members on 28 December 1800 were Thomas Gisborne, John Turton, J. Robertson Barclay and William Roe (*JHC*, vol. 55, p. 497). Baker's name did not appear in that list, but a letter from Fawkener to Baker (PC 2/153/ 458–9) confirms that he was convenor and president. Baker had wanted a Dr Robertson (presumably not Robertson Barclay) on the committee, but he was unavailable at Bath (ibid.). Maclean's list (*Remarks on the British Quarantine laws*) named Baker, Pepys, F. Gisborne [*sic*], Hamond, Russell, Johnston, Blane, Robertson Barclay, Thomas Boone, Lee and Green.

134 NA PC 2/153/458–9.

135 NA PC 2/153/532.

136 Ibid.

137 Ibid.; NA PC 2/153/592.

138 For the exclusion of Sheerness, see NA PC 2/153/592.

139 NA PC 2/153/568.

140 NA PC 2/153/453–51, from which references in the next five paragraphs are taken unless otherwise stated.

141 *Letters, &c.*, p. 6. To be more precise, Blane had favoured St Mary's, Isles of Scilly, or Falmouth for the Levant trade, and Hull, Yarmouth and the Isle of Grain for the Baltic trade.

standard printed questions and respond to certain others. The extra questions were: Was the cargo taken in at more than one port, and if so in what proportion? Were any letters or parcels exchanged with any other ship during the voyage? Were the crew and passengers the same as those who boarded at the port(s) of loading? Did anyone die, or fall sick, during the passage? The written answers, together with the foul bill of health, cargo manifests and any other letters, were then to be delivered to the Superintendent of Quarantine who would immerse them in vinegar, remove them with tongs, and then dry them 'in the Smoaking Case' for between 12 and 20 hours.

When the master and mate were back on board, the ship would be deemed under quarantine until further notice. The pilot, who had probably been picked up at The Downs, would then perform four days' quarantine either on the hospital ship (if such existed) or in 'a Hut or Tent constructed on the Beach', followed by a fumigation. The ship's boat or boats would then be delivered to the Superintendent of Quarantine who would guard them until the granting of pratique. There were then measures to ensure the ship was kept incommunicado under the watchful eye of guards, who would have powers to search lockers and chests for anything susceptible to infection and ensure that clothes and bedding were aired daily.

Passengers would be subject to the same quarantine as crewmen if they stayed on board, but the period would drop to 14 days if they hired another vessel for their comfort or convenience. That would not exempt them from being fumigated at release. Once the passengers had left the ship in which they arrived (assuming they took up the option), the hatches would be opened for a probationary airing of the enumerated goods. The word sereine was not used. As many bales as possible would be ranged on deck for three days, opened far enough for the crew to rummage within, and then re-sewn on the fourth day for delivery to the hulks by lighter, attended by a guard boat. Another batch of bales would then be hoisted from the hold to the ship's deck, but these would only be rummaged for two days before passing to the hulks. A third batch would have only one day's exposure. Of course, 'any suspicious Circumstances' would prolong the process.

Following this probationary airing, the ship itself would manoeuvre alongside the hulk, into which the rest of the enumerated goods, or non-enumerated goods in susceptible wrappings, would be transferred. The ship would then move away, with any other non-enumerated goods still on board, to perform a quarantine of 20 days elsewhere in the Creek. Then the ship, and presumably all those on board, would be fumigated before release. Enumerated goods, which would be aired on the hulks for 40 days, were defined as: hemp and flax; paper or books; silk raw, thrown or wrought; linen; cotton in wool, yarn or manufactured; wool raw or in any way wrought; feathers; grogram or mohair yarn; human hair; goats' hair; Carmenia wool; carpets; cambletts; burdetts or other manufactures of silk and cotton; kid skins and skins in the wool and hair; sponges; wine and oil in chests; thread stockings; straw hats; brushes; matting; and artificial flowers. This showed that no thought had been given to updating the list, where wine and oil in chests remained a curious anomaly. On board the hulks, the bales would be opened on one side so the porters could 'thrust in their naked Hands and Arms' over 20 days. The bales would then be re-sewn, turned over, and the process would begin again on the other side. Non-enumerated goods, except those packed in wood, glass or metal, were to be opened and aired on the hulks for 20 days. The excepted goods would still be opened and aired, but remain on the ship.

The Order also provided for 'a small Vessel, provided with one or more Assistants, and with proper Necessaries for the reception of sick persons'. That would seem to have been a substitute for the floating infirmary previously envisaged, and suggested something smaller and cheaper than the warship which Johnston and Blane had recommended. The relationship between this vessel and the primitive shore establishment was not explained, but it was still intended that 'a space of Ground of one hundred and fifty Feet' be enclosed and fenced at 'the Northernmost Corner of Chetney Hill'. This would contain three small wooden cabins, each about 12 or 15 feet square, and not less than 20 feet apart. Furnished to hold one sick person each, the huts would 'be erected on Shore near the Beach, with a Door on each of the Four sides, so that the sick Person may always be approached on the Windward side by those who administer nourishment and relief to them'. Also unexplained was the geographical relationship between these huts and the others, or tents, on the beach where a master would report the arrival of his ship. The word 'beach' was used – a misnomer in the context of the muddy creek – because the Crown owned the foreshore, and uncertainty perhaps existed about what land had been bought from Wildman. The Order ended with a stipulation that only the Superintendent of Quarantine could supply persons and ships with the necessaries of life, and that was to be in daylight. As these were strictly procedural regulations, there was no hint given as to how the foul-bill station would be paid for, whether by a tonnage tax or otherwise. Also, there were no concessions for ships with 'middle' bills between clean and foul.

These elaborate instructions were nullified from the start by the failure of the naval authorities to deliver the promised hulks.[142] Within a matter of days the situation at Stangate Creek descended into acrimonious chaos. Long before the Order of 20 November, foul-bill ships had been arriving; none posed an obvious risk in that the crews were healthy, but a queue was forming for the limited airing facilities on board the *Princess Amelia* and *Belleisle* lazarettos.[143] Early in November 1799 the situation quickly worsened. The convoy system through and from the Mediterranean meant that the Turkey ships *Ranger*, *Five Brothers*, *Catharina* and *Princessa* arrived virtually together.[144] The merchants immediately protested that the airing hulks could not cope with so many bales.[145] The passengers got together to hire quarantine vessels, but the problem concerned the crews. Their wages and maintenance exceeded £800 a month, and there were more men than were needed to air the cargoes on deck. Seamen could not be discharged until quarantine had

142 On 4 December 1799 the Superintendent of Quarantine reported that the new lazarettos would not be ready for a month (BL Add. MS 38355, fols 113–17).

143 The *Withywood* and *Minorca Packet*, both originally from Smyrna, had arrived 21 September (BL Add. MS 38355, fols 113–17).

144 Between 4 and 8 November (BL Add. MS 38355, fols 113–17).

145 BL Add. MS 38355, fols 113–17, from which remaining references in this paragraph are taken.

finished, but it could not even begin until all the cargo had been offloaded to the hulks. But the hulks were full.

Had the problem rested with Smyrna ships alone, the Privy Council might have shrugged their shoulders and told the merchants to be patient. Unfortunately, other ports of departure were also in the spotlight. Higher up the queue were three ships from Mogador, the notorious plague spot in West Barbary. The *Aurora* had arrived in Stangate Creek in late August 1799, by which time the British consul at Tangier had already warned of plague in Morocco.[146] In early October the ship's agents reminded the Privy Council that the *Aurora* had been in quarantine for more than a month.[147] A few days later two other ships, the *Mentor* and the *Lark*, sailed into Stangate Creek from Mogador, where the master of the latter had died during an outbreak of plague.[148] Their arrival roughly coincided with anonymous letters of warning, forwarded by Dundas to Lord Liverpool.[149]

All these events had been monitored by the Quarantine Committee, on whose advice the clothes of the late master of the *Lark* were sunk in deep water.[150] But the committee remained so deeply worried about the threat from Mogador that they recommended on 5 December 1799 that all three ships should be sunk with their cargoes.[151] The Privy Council were appalled. They asked the committee to reconsider and explain their reasons.[152] The physicians stood their ground. Much of the cargo consisted of bales of goats' skins, packed with the hair turned inwards and loaded in time of plague by natives, many of whom were thought to have died.[153] Skins were especially susceptible to harbouring infection, but it would be impracticable and highly dangerous to turn each item around to allow airing.[154] Even opening the hatchways would be dangerous, and the non-enumerated goods could never be separated with safety.[155] The committee also felt that if an outbreak of disease did occur, there would be a catastrophic loss of confidence in a quarantine system which the Government was trying to improve and enlarge.[156] And had not the Privy Council sanctioned the destruction of the *Fowey* in 1754?[157] But still the Council questioned their judgement. Could the destruction not at least wait until the next meeting of Parliament on 21 January, when the question of compensation could be raised?[158] No, replied the committee: the ships were overcrowded, there was a

146 Ibid.; NA PC 2/153/74.

147 BL Add. MS 38355, fols 113–17.

148 Ibid.; *JHC*, vol. 55, p. 244. The Privy Council had learnt of plague at Mogador in July (NA PC 2/153/393).

149 *JHC*, vol. 55, p. 244.

150 Ibid.

151 *JHC*, vol. 55, pp. 245, 497; BL Add. MS 38355, fols 113–17.

152 *JHC*, vol. 55, pp. 245, 497.

153 *JHC*, vol. 55. p. 497.

154 Ibid.

155 Ibid.

156 Ibid.

157 Ibid.

158 *JHC*, vol. 55, pp. 245, 498. Parliament adjourned between 12 October 1799 and 21 January 1800.

danger of embezzlement, and the skins were turning rotten.[159] All those on board who would not be needed in sailing the ships to their point of scuttling should be embarked on another vessel and then released after a further 21 days' quarantine if they remained in good health.[160] And so, on 7 January 1800, with no parliamentary sanction, an agonized Privy Council ordered the three laden ships to be scuttled by their own crews.[161]

More light was shed on the destruction of the ships when John Green, treasurer of the Levant Company, testified to a parliamentary committee in 1819.[162] Green made it clear that Pitt, either within or independent of the Privy Council, had taken a grip on events. The Quarantine Committee, on which Green had sat, had been summoned before him to explain their insistence that the ships with their cargoes should be sunk. Green remembered that Pitt 'seemed to be very reluctant' that the destruction should take place.[163] The extent of Pitt's concern can be judged by a memorandum in the Chatham Papers, ostensibly from Lord Liverpool.[164] This document explored the history of quarantine in so far as it affected countries rather than cargoes, and as it began by guessing what had been in the minds of the legislature when the Act was passed in 1799, it constitutes further proof that that statute had caught the Privy Council by surprise.

The thrust of the paper, however, was to point out the dangerous precedent which the Quarantine Committee had created by ordering the destruction of ships from Mogador. This was tantamount to an embargo of trade with a diseased port, although no quarantine Act had ever included such a prohibition, and the Privy Council had never recommended the King to institute such a ban, although he had been vested with the necessary powers in 1721 and 1733. The author felt the public should be made aware if ships were to be destroyed solely on the grounds that they came from an infected place. Merchants might 'become subject to great Losses; and they may think they have a right to claim Indemnification, and, if such Indemnification is allowed, it is possible that they may be induced to carry on the Trade even for the Indemnification; and, in such case, a very great and serious Charge will be brought on the Revenue of the Country'. The author recommended an urgent review by Parliament of the dangers which the precedent implied.

On 11 February 1800 Pitt read to the Commons a message he had received from the King, which recited the circumstances of the sinkings and recommended Parliament 'to consider whether any, and what, Allowance should be made to the Parties, for the Losses they may have sustained ...'[165] The message was referred to a committee chaired by Charles Bragge, the member for Bristol who had steered through the

159 *JHC*, vol. 55, p. 498.

160 Ibid.

161 Ibid.; NA PC 2/154/43.

162 *Report from the Select Committee Appointed to consider the validity of the doctrine of Contagion in the Plague* (1819), p. 41.

163 Ibid.; Green's evidence suggested that he himself played a leading part in the committee's decision making.

164 NA PRO 30/8/259, fols 338–42, from which remaining references in this and the next paragraph are taken.

165 *JHC*, vol. 55, p. 170.

Levant Seas Bill in the previous year. Other committee members included Pitt, Lord Hawkesbury (son of Lord Liverpool) and George Rose.[166] Bragge asked the Privy Council for sight of the relevant papers, and the Comptroller of the Household agreed on behalf of the Crown.[167] On 28 February 1800 William Fawkener attended the Commons and deposited 16 documents covering the whole episode from the institution of the Quarantine Committee to the Order for the ships' destruction.[168] It was a measure of the thoroughness of the committee's work that Bragge did not report to the House until 8 May. It was a measure of the constitutional importance of the findings that the report was published *in extenso* over 15 pages of the House of Commons *Journal*.[169]

Bragge reported every twist and complication of the outward and return voyages which led eventually to the ships' destruction. He then turned his attention to the course of the plague in Morocco, which was reckoned to have killed 7,500 people in Mogador, leaving only 1,500 alive. The committee had established not only that the skins had been loaded in the last three weeks before sailing, when the plague was especially virulent, but they had been stored in a warehouse uncomfortably close to a burial pit. Some skins as well as cow hides, another element of the cargoes, had been brought from places farther afield where plague had erupted weeks before it had arrived in Mogador. The sudden death of the master of the *Lark*, who had been employed with his crew in packing the skins, was the final incident to frighten the committee, although Bragge admitted that plague was not a confirmed diagnosis. Moreover, no other person in the *Lark* or in the other ships had been ill while at Mogador, or at any time since.

Arriving at the question of compensation, Bragge made a point which the Quarantine Committee had raised with the Privy Council: that contemporary moves to establish a lazaret – which he admitted had been sanctioned as far back as 1753 – promised to make similar destruction unnecessary for the future. In this instance, the committee had assessed compensation from the prime value of the goods, augmented by port and freight charges, plus extraordinary expenses, seamen's wages and the cost of provisions from the time quarantine expired until the destruction of ships and cargoes. Added to those totals came the value of the vessels, cabin furniture and personal effects. The precedent for this, explained Bragge, reverted to the burning of the Turkey ships in 1721; by implication, those out of pocket by the loss of the *Fowey* in 1754 had been less generously treated. Included in the legitimate charges, Bragge mentioned the cost of insurance premiums which were now considered 'an almost constant Mercantile Charge'.

Following a most thorough enquiry, the *Aurora* was valued by the committee at £2,300, the *Mentor* at £1,300 and the *Lark* at £1,200. When the other elements of compensation had been added, Bragge reported a recommended total of just over

166 Ibid. Robert Banks Jenkinson, eventually 2nd Earl of Liverpool, had become Lord Hawkesbury in 1796 when his father was honoured by the earldom.

167 NA PC 2/154/292, 411.

168 *JHC*, vol. 55, pp. 244–5.

169 *JHC*, vol. 55, pp. 496–510, from which references in the next two paragraphs are taken.

£41,007, which a Committee of Supply, on 26 May 1800, increased to £44,400.[170] Given this huge sum, the ease with which precedents had been recalled, and the fact of publication, it was remarkable that memory of the payout proved exceedingly brief. In 1819 neither John Green nor his parliamentary interrogators had any precise recollection of the figure. Green, when pressed, thought compensation might have exceeded £20,000, but he only spoke 'from conjecture'.[171] Even Maclean, a few years later, was curiously uninformed about the sinkings and could only latch on to Green's estimate as evidence of the squander of public money.[172]

The opening months of the new century brought only misery to anyone connected at any level with British quarantine. The floating lazarettos at Stangate Creek, despite the absence of the three ships from Mogador, were full. Part of the cargo of the *Boyne* from New York was aired on a hired lighter, at the merchants' request and expense, to save precious time.[173] On 30 January 1800 the Privy Council asked George Rose to organize crews for the *Duke* and *Valiant*, so the ships could assume their role of supplementary lazarettos.[174] Nearly a month later he was curtly reminded that nothing had been done.[175] On 10 February Dr Newberry was asked to report whether the huts had been built in the way that the Order of 20 November had requested.[176] From his reply, the Council were annoyed to learn that, while the huts had been built on a correctly sized plot of 150 feet by 75 feet, they were only 10 feet square and had an unauthorized window on each side as well as the requested door.[177] Sir Andrew Hamond was told to put things right.[178] On the water, fruit was rotting in the long wait, as the Quarantine Committee had taken no cognizance of perishable cargoes, and the Order, therefore, had made no concessions for early release. Messrs Smith, St Barbe & Marten petitioned for figs and other fruit on the *Magnet*, a foul-bill ship from Smyrna, to be offloaded to lighters for ten days' quarantine (as opposed to airing) at their own expense.[179] The Privy Council replied that they were 'not disposed to depart from the rules laid down by the Quarantine Committee', but within a month the latter had relented.[180]

On 2 April 1800 the Quarantine Committee presented a 58-page report to the Privy Council, giving their considered views on how foul-bill quarantine should be conducted, and making certain wider recommendations. The report seems not to have survived, but the text was known to Maclean when he published his *Remarks on the British Quarantine laws* in 1823.[181] It is evident from Maclean's comments that

170 *JHC*, vol. 55, p. 575.

171 *Report from the Select Committee* (1819), p. 41.

172 Maclean, *Remarks on the British Quarantine laws*, p. 8.

173 NA PC 2/154/83.

174 NA PC 2/154/173.

175 NA PC 2/154/293.

176 NA PC 2/154/219.

177 NA PC 2/154/244.

178 Ibid.

179 NA PC 2/154/572.

180 NA PC 2/154/572, 683, 693.

181 Maclean, *Remarks on the British Quarantine laws*, pp. 16–18, where he also mentioned the length of the report, and from which all references in this paragraph, concerning the report,

the committee had made much of the quarantine Act of 1753, the Levant Seas Act of 1799, and the description of quarantine practice at Venice in Howard's book on the lazarettos of Europe. Maclean's intention was to ridicule the committee for taking the doctrine of contagion for granted, but in so doing he gave invaluable insight into some of their recommendations. They suggested, for instance, that a frigate with 'medical men' be used at Stangate Creek as a hospital ship and that a smaller vessel should be stationed at St Helen's Pool for sufferers from the plague. The committee went on to recommend two levels of enumerated goods, based on their relative susceptibility to harbouring infection, and concluded with the advice that a lazaret at Chetney Hill, on land already bought by Government, would best meet the requirements for a foul-bill station. According to Maclean, the committee argued for a 'board of health, composed of competent persons, who should correspond with all British consuls in foreign parts, and to whom all quarantine questions should be referred in the first instance, for their report to the privy council'. Maclean was probably unaware that for Johnston and Blane, as well as for the representatives of the Turkey Company, the recommendation of a land lazaret was the antithesis of their earlier thinking.

As their report was urgently required, the Quarantine Committee had agreed that members with anything further to suggest should write a supplementary letter to the Privy Council.[182] Patrick Russell wrote two such letters to Fawkener, the first arguing that, as the foul-bill station would lack experienced personnel, 'two young Medical Gentlemen' should be sent to Constantinople, at Government expense, to learn more about the plague at first hand.[183] The second letter was more discursive, but in essence it argued that British bills of health, particularly for the 'middle' patents, should conform closely with the style and language accepted in the Mediterranean.[184] It is reasonable to infer from this energy and enthusiasm that Russell had played a leading role in deciding the committee's policy.[185]

The Privy Council accepted the main thrust of the report. Also on 2 April they thanked the committee for their 'diligence and ability' and asked them to prepare plans for a land lazaret, with those elements to be built first which would remedy the defects of the existing system.[186] The committee were to liaise with the Office of Works and consider the size of the establishment and the salaries and expenses which would follow.[187] But the Council then rejected the idea of a Board of Health. They argued, somewhat obscurely, that if the establishment at the lazaret were made 'more complete' it would answer the purposes of a Board of Health, and in any event 'Cases of considerable Difficulty and Emergency' would always require the attention of the Privy Council 'according to the Practice which has immemorially

---

are taken.

182 BL Add. MS 38234, fol. 29.

183 BL Add. MS 38234, fols 31–2.

184 BL Add. MS 38234, fols 33–5.

185 cf. Maclean, *Remarks on the British Quarantine laws*, p. 18: 'This report bears marks of having been principally the workmanship of Dr. Russell …'

186 NA PC 2/154/473–5.

187 Ibid.

prevailed'.[188] But then came a more meaty objection. The Council did not believe that Foreign Secretaries would countenance any correspondence between the Board and His Majesty's representatives abroad, unless the King approved in each instance.[189]

To assist the committee, the Privy Council launched letters in every direction. James Wyatt, Surveyor-General and Comptroller of the Office of Works, was asked to attend the Quarantine Committee and prepare estimates for each stage of the project.[190] George Rose was directed to get more statistics from the Customs Commissioners: these would include the annual cost of quarantine stations over the last ten years and the number of ships (with tonnages) which had been there over the same period.[191] Rose was also asked for a plan or survey of Chetney Hill, if such existed, as the Quarantine Committee were of the view that part had already been bought by Government.[192] This last, lame comment indicated how far the Privy Council had lost track of the negotiations with Wildman a few years earlier. Finally, the Council cast widely about for any plans of lazarettos which might already exist. Rose was to enquire in the Treasury, while Under-Secretaries of State were asked to research departmental archives.[193] The Privy Council recalled that Robert Wood, who had been Under-Secretary to Pitt, Egremont and Weymouth more than 30 years earlier, had been 'very active in proposing the building of a Land Lazaret', and his papers might be useful.[194] The most interesting request was sent to William Huskisson, asking for any plans which might be in the office of Henry Dundas, Secretary at War, as the Quarantine Committee believed those relating to the lazaretto at Mahon in Minorca had been lodged there.[195] That was a reference to the plan sent by James Johnston to London in 1767. Maclean noted scornfully that Sir Lucas Pepys of the Quarantine Committee had been an advocate of a lazaretto on the Mahon principle.[196]

On 24 April 1800 the Council wrote to Baker with the results of their many enquiries.[197] The Foreign Office had discovered nothing, and the Home Office could find only a paper from one Captain Blanket about quarantine in Mediterranean lazarettos, sent to the Home Secretary in 1788.[198] But Dundas did produce the Mahon plan, although it lacked a table of reference. It was felt that Colonel Lindenthal, then in London, might be able to assist in its interpretation.[199] Another important result of the trawl was a conveyance, with plan, of the land conveyed at Chetney Hill

188 Ibid.

189 Ibid.

190 NA PC 2/154/475.

191 NA PC 2/154/492.

192 NA PC 2/154/511.

193 NA PC 2/154/512–13.

194 NA PC 2/154/513.

195 Ibid.

196 Maclean, *Remarks on the British Quarantine laws*, p. 18. See further Chapter 5 above.

197 NA PC 2/154/559–61.

198 Ibid.

199 Ibid.

from Wildman to the Lords of the Treasury.[200] Unfortunately, no other details of this conveyance were given, so questions such as the amount of land bought, the cost, and even the date of the transaction, remain obscure. It is unfortunate for the historian that the ancient removal of this conveyance and of the Minorca plan from their proper custody has militated against their survival.

It then dawned on the Council that the Turkey Company had sent ideas for a land lazaret to the Customs Commissioners in 1793, annexed to a letter, and in early May the Commissioners complied with a request to make them available.[201] These were presumably the drawings prepared by John Soane, but the Privy Council were more impressed by the amateur efforts of soldier-governor Johnston. On 6 May 1800 the Minorca plan was forwarded to Wyatt with the instruction that he keep the Chetney Hill lazaret 'simple and economical'.[202] He was expected to begin by making his own survey of the site, a task in which the Customs Commissioners were asked to provide every assistance.[203] The Council then wrote to the Attorney-General returning a draft Bill for reducing the various quarantine laws into one new enactment.[204] They had missed out in the framing of the Levant Seas Act; they were not going to be bypassed in the discussions which lay ahead.

Focus on Chetney Hill

Fawkener made his next visit to the Commons on 24 June 1800, when he deposited four more solicited papers.[205] These were an estimate of continuing the present arrangement of floating lazarettos at Stangate Creek; statistics of quarantine around the country over the previous ten years; a table of tonnage duties proposed to be levied on ships under quarantine; and the plan and estimate of a land lazaret prepared by James Wyatt.[206] On the same day, the Commons were informed that the King recommended them to consider the building of the lazaret, and the House instantly formed a committee to discuss the basic points, especially the cost of building and the rate of the tonnage duties.[207] Charles Bragge was authorized to bring in the Bill and, despite amendments at every stage, its progress through both Houses was rapid. On 28 July 1800 royal assent was given to *An act for erecting a lazaret on Chetney Hill, in the county of Kent; and for reducing into one act the laws relating to quarantine, and for making further provision therein.*[208]

200 Ibid.

201 NA PC 2/154/586.

202 NA PC 2/154/598.

203 NA PC 2/154/614.

204 NA PC 2/154/716.

205 *JHC*, vol. 55, p. 695; NA PC 2/155/105.

206 Colvin, *Biographical Dictionary of British Architects*, lists the lazaretto at Chetney Hill under Wyatt's works. See also Colvin, *History of the King's Works*, vol. 6, p. 448.

207 *JHC*, vol. 55, pp. 695–6.

208 *JHC*, vol. 55, p. 784. The Act was 40 Geo. III, c.80, from which references in the next six paragraphs are taken unless otherwise stated.

The preamble acknowledged that three ships from Mogador had recently been destroyed at great public expense because no adequate facilities were in place for foul-bill ships and cargoes. Statutory permission existed, however, for the King to build a lazaret at Chetney Hill, where the Treasury had purchased land. Once the plan of the lazaret had been approved by the King in Council, the Act authorized £65,000 to be spent by the Treasury from the Consolidated Fund. The new building would be under the management of officers appointed by the Treasury, which placed it within the sphere of the Customs service. The salaries would be decided by the King in Council and paid for by a tonnage duty. Once the capital cost of the project had been recouped, the duty might be reduced. The rates would be 7s, 6d for every ton burthen of a ship from the Levant and Barbary with a clean bill of health, which would rise to 15s if the bill were foul. If the ship arrived from anywhere else, the rates would be 3s and 10s respectively. If any ship brought goods from Turkey or Barbary indirectly, especially from Holland, the rate would be 7s, 6d; but that would increase to 15s if the Privy Council took the view that the ship should perform the same quarantine as one from the Levant or Barbary without a clean bill of health. A further 1s per ton burthen would be paid by ships entering the port of London. By a brief Act later in the year, following constitutional doubts, it was confirmed that tonnage duty would be applicable also in the Channel Islands and Isle of Man.[209]

The duties were exactly those proposed in the preliminary parliamentary discussions, but the Act went on to make certain exemptions: these applied to clean-bill ships carrying salt or in ballast, unless they came from the Levant or Barbary, and to any ship which had performed quarantine in one of the main Mediterranean lazarettos. Tonnage duty was to be levied on shipowners, who could reimburse themselves from the importers or consignees of the goods for 'such sums of money as shall be equal to the just and reasonable contribution, which the proportion that such goods … bear to the tonnage burthen of the ship shall require, and no more, according to the usage of merchants in like cases'. But as some ships returned to Britain half full, or carried cargoes which were very light in relation to the vessel's deadweight, there was the potential in that clause for controversy.

The Act then repealed all the legislation relating to quarantine from 1753 up to and including the recent Levant Seas Act, before reinstating the significant milestones which those earlier Acts had represented. The first reinstatement was the power to the King in Council, by Proclamation, to declare any infectious disease 'to be of the nature of the plague'. This was followed by a statement of liability to quarantine for ships, goods and persons from infected places. Until the land lazaret should be built, a ship on which plague appeared was to make for some foreign lazaretto if she had not yet cleared the Straits of Gibraltar. If outside the Straits, the ship was to make for St Helen's Pool; but beyond a requirement for 'all possible speed' in the relaying of intelligence to London, the Act made no improvement to the creaking chain of communication, and made no provision for the sick until the royal pleasure would be known. The penalty for a disobedient master would be death as a felon. Once the lazaret was built, the need to use St Helen's Pool would cease.

209 41 Geo. III, c.30, which had received royal assent on 31 December 1800.

The obligation of a master to hoist a yellow flag within four leagues of the British coast was confirmed. If his ship did not have a clean bill of health, the flag would contain a circle of black; in both cases the flag would be supplemented at night by a light and a signal lantern. The flag would fly until the ship was released from quarantine. The penalty for non-compliance would be £200. A fine of half that sum would be payable by a pilot who took a ship to a port not designated as a quarantine station. The Act then authorized Customs officers to accost any ship entering a British port and demand answers, on oath if necessary, to the standard questions. A penalty of £200 would be incurred by a master who was less than truthful, but if he lied about coming from an infected place, or about disease on his ship, he would suffer death. Once in port, the master would surrender his bill of health, cargo manifest, logbook and journal, or face a penalty of £500. Then followed a new requirement: at the port of loading the master would have delivered a sworn and very detailed copy of the manifest to the British consul. This copy would have been sent to the Customs Commissioners in London, to act as a check against the one which the master delivered. For every missing item of cargo, the master would be fined between £100 and £500 unless he had a valid reason for the loss. This system, of course, was designed to prevent ships breaking bulk off the English coast, but as some ships with clean bills would be bound elsewhere than London, there was scope for much delay before a manifest arrived in, say, Liverpool.

A penalty of £500 would be incurred by a master who was slow to proceed to his quarantine station, when ordered, or who let some person leave his ship; anyone who did leave would not only be compelled to return, but suffer six months' imprisonment when the quarantine had ended and be fined £200. The same penalty would be meted out to a master who arrived from a foreign lazaretto with a clean bill of health, but neglected to give details of his manifest and quarantine to local Customs officers, for transmission to the Privy Council. In comparison with the fine and imprisonment for jumping ship, the penalty for someone refusing to go to the quarantine station, or escaping from it, would be death. The same severe fate would await a Customs officer who deserted his station, connived in an escape, or gave a false certificate that quarantine had been completed. For lesser misdemeanours, an officer would face dismissal and a fine of £100. There were three more occasions when death would be the penalty: first, when a person entered the lazaret unlawfully and then tried to escape; secondly, when any certificate was forged; and thirdly, when someone tried to conceal or smuggle out letters or goods from a ship or the lazaret.

Once a ship or a person had completed quarantine, the master and two other people, preferably out of the ship, would swear to this effect before a senior officer of Customs (or before a jurat or magistrate in the Channel Islands or Isle of Man), and the officer would give a certificate of discharge. In the case of goods, a certificate of completion of quarantine would be given by the temporary custodian, and this would be sworn as correct by two other persons, but the goods could not be discharged until this document had been produced to the Commissioners of Customs in England or Scotland, or to the Lieutenant-Governor or Commander-in-Chief in the islands. The Act did not neglect the customary discouragement to smuggling, and prohibited the sailing of boats under 20 tons burthen, during an epidemic, without a bond from the master in £300 against calling anywhere forbidden by Proclamation. If this prohibition were broken, the ship would be confiscated and every crewman fined £20. As had been established in 1753, the publication of any Order in Council or Proclamation in the *London Gazette* would be deemed sufficient public notice. The Act came into force on 1 October 1800.

Long before that, the Privy Council had set about drafting a new general Order to complement the statute. In this process they were assisted by the Board of Trade, who had also been consulted over the quarantine Bill.[210] Some of the 46 provisions in the Order covered much the same ground as the Act, but the Order went into details of procedure and borrowed heavily from the final report of the Quarantine Committee.[211] The quarantine stations around Britain were reconfirmed, but ships with foul bills were to go only to Stangate Creek. The questions to be asked of masters were laid out at length and, among other measures, a system was set up for collecting letters, subject to treatment by vinegar and fumigation, from people in quarantine. The Order also spelled out which goods would be classed as enumerated, this time at two levels of susceptibility as the Quarantine Committee had suggested. Goods in the first class, deemed the most dangerous, were substantially those which had always been enumerated, with the addition of more items of animal origin, such as hooves and furriers' waste, and the less understandable 'Liquor of any kind in bottles or flasks'. Items in the second class were mainly drugs, including some plants such as tobacco or their by-products, for instance coffee and cork. If the ship did not have a clean bill of health, goods in the first class would be aired for 40 days, as opposed to 30 for those in the second class. Although dated 29 July (the day after royal assent for the Act), the Order was not sent out to the Law Officers of the Crown for their final scrutiny until 13 August.[212] The backdating was caused by the departure for Weymouth of the King, who had approved an incomplete draft before he left. As this approval had been on 29 July, it was necessary for the Law Officers to pretend their reports had been made even earlier than that – which apparently caused them no difficulty.[213]

Even before the parliamentary proceedings, it had been evident to the merchants at Liverpool and the manufacturers of Manchester that foul-bill resources were being limited to Stangate Creek, and that they stood to lose business as a result. On 19 June 1800 the Privy Council responded to a petition for a land lazaret at or near Liverpool.[214] In an unusually thorough and reasoned response, the Council pointed out that as no foul-bill ships had been legally allowed to enter Britain before the Levant Seas Act of 1799, the outports were no more disadvantaged by the present proposals than they had been all along. As the building of a foul-bill station was very costly, they could not reasonably expect more than one. Even in France, with its extensive Levant trade, there was only one lazaretto. It was appropriate that the

210 NA BT 5/12/28, 50.

211 NA PC 2/155/333–68, from which references in this paragraph are taken until otherwise stated.

212 NA PC 2/155/450.

213 Ibid.

214 NA PC 2/155/73–4, from which remaining references in this paragraph are taken until otherwise stated. The petition was presented by Simon Cock.

English station should be near London as so many ships were bound there, and the proximity of Government meant that instructions could be frequently and easily sent out in an emergency. In gracious conclusion, the Council acknowledged Liverpool and Manchester as 'considerable and respectable' places. That would have been small consolation to the merchants there, when the *Christiana Elizabeth*, already at Liverpool, was ordered to sail round to Stangate Creek.[215]

The Office of Works made a promising start to the lazaret scheme. In July 1800 a plan, perhaps a revision of the earlier one, went before the Privy Council, who asked the Treasury to release money so the work could begin.[216] Meanwhile, there was interest in what use, if any, had been made of St Helen's Pool. Cottrell asked James Hume, clerk to the Customs Commissioners, for urgent statistics as Lord Liverpool was considering what establishment would be needed there in the light of the recent Act.[217] Cottrell himself was 'pretty certain' that no ship infected with plague had ever been sent to St Helen's Pool or 'great Grimsby', by which he meant New Grimsby.[218] When the records proved him correct, Lord Liverpool was inclined to have only one or two men stationed there, but the Treasury were asked for their view.[219]

Another task for Cottrell was to liaise with the Foreign Office. He felt it necessary to give George Hammond, Under-Secretary of State, a brief résumé of events from the time of the sinking of the ships from Mogador to the passing of the Act a month earlier.[220] Writing on 22 August 1800, Cottrell promised to send 50 copies of the Act, bound up with the recent Order into a quarto book. These were for the information of British diplomats and merchants abroad, which brought Cottrell to the invidious question raised by the Quarantine Committee of how intelligence from abroad should be received. The Privy Council, explained Cottrell, thought the committee's view that diplomats should correspond directly with the Customs service 'would not be proper'; yet the Council were concerned about the time and trouble to the Foreign Office in forwarding letters to the Customs or the Privy Council. He might also have mentioned the inevitable delay. Hammond was to seek Lord Grenville's view as a matter of urgency, before the new regulations came into force on 1 October. Grenville's response was not recorded, but there is no reason to believe he supported the view of the Quarantine Committee.

'Section 38'

There were two aspects of the Order in Council of 29 July 1800 which caused particular trouble, and they were often linked. The first concerned the wider definition

---

215 NA PC 2/155/595.

216 NA PC 2/155/300–301.

217 NA PC 2/155/466.

218 Ibid. It is only surprising there was not more confusion between Great and New Grimsby, and also between St Helen's in the Isles of Scilly and St Helen's in the Isle of Wight. The latter was a popular anchorage for the navy.

219 NA PC 2/155/509–11.

220 NA PC 2/155/480–83, from which all references in this paragraph are taken.

of enumerated goods; the second was the interpretation of Section 38.[221] The effect of this section was to send to a quarantine station any ship carrying enumerated goods of the first class which were the growth, produce or manufacture of Turkey or Barbary, and which were imported from any place, including Holland, where there was no 'regular Establishment for the Performance of Quarantine'. The master was expected to produce a declaration sworn before a magistrate at the port of departure, and attested by the British consul, certifying whether or not the goods were of Turkish or Barbary origin. If they were, the declaration would state whether the ship was or was not the one in which the goods had been originally loaded. If it were the same ship, the master was to produce the original bill of health; if it were not the same ship, the declaration would state whether or not the original vessel had sailed with a clean bill of health. If none of the goods emanated from Turkey or Barbary, the ship would be excused quarantine.

The immediate problem for the Customs service was knowing which ports had a 'regular' quarantine establishment, and the Levant Company were asked for a list.[222] But there were deeper concerns, coupled with the interpretation of enumerated goods and knowledge of their origins. The secretary to the Customs Commissioners asked for further explanation of the cargoes which would render a ship liable to quarantine; to which the Privy Council sent a testy reply that all in their view was 'clear and distinct'.[223] On 14 January 1801 the Privy Council were forced to add two extra questions to the standard interrogation of masters.[224] Have you any cotton wool, thread or yarn on board, or any of the other articles enumerated in the first class? If so, are they the growth, produce or manufacture of Turkey or Barbary? Further questions were added in March about any communication with other vessels on the voyage.[225] There was now a better basis for sending ships to Stangate Creek, or to one of the few other stations with airing facilities, where the proper declarations would be produced. But the onus of proof was gradually changing: masters were being challenged to prove that goods did not come from Turkey or the Levant, as well as being asked for the paperwork if they did.

Before running into trouble with the declarations, the Privy Council were forced into a concession about cork.[226] Being included as an enumerated product in the second class, cork was now subject to 30 days' airing; but the merchants and shipowners of London pointed out – as their forefathers had done in 1721 – that it was normally used only as dunnage, that is protective wrapping. Non-enumerated, perishable goods were being held up in quarantine as if the cargo consisted solely of cork. The Privy Council were thankful for Section 41 of their own Order, which allowed them to abridge quarantine as they thought fit. On 19 December 1801 ships carrying fewer than five tons of cork as dunnage were excused quarantine altogether, provided they brought a clean bill of health and the crew were evidently well.

---

221 NA PC 2/155/362–5, from which all references in this paragraph are taken.

222 NA PC 2/156/158, 201.

223 NA PC 2/156/294.

224 NA PC 2/157/87.

225 NA PC 2/157/398.

226 NA PC 2/159/579, from which all references in this paragraph are taken.

The cork episode was a warning to the Privy Council that the apparatus of quarantine was becoming too complicated. In February 1802 they were reminded of this by a letter from a committee of the silk merchants of London, who complained that their raw materials, imported from Leghorn as formerly, were now being subjected to quarantine at Stangate Creek despite arriving in ships with clean bills of health.[227] The bales had been opened in such a way that the silk was unmarketable and 'exposed to Plunderage', although the regulation for airing applied only to ships without clean bills.[228] The Customs Commissioners, who denied knowledge of the incident, were told to ensure their men kept to the rules but the mistake had been understandable. There was now a dichotomy in the treatment of goods, regardless of what they were, based on the status of the bill of health; that was difficult to grasp in the context of what was hailed as a foul-bill quarantine station.

From Hull, in January 1802, came evidence of mercantile sharp practice little short of fraud. Sworn declarations were being duly presented for attestation by a magistrate and British consul at the port of loading, but it dawned on the controller at Hull that certain goods enumerated in the first class were being added to the list at a later date.[229] This was particularly troublesome for the Privy Council as they relied on the Levant Company and the Foreign Office to relay instructions. They could only request that British consuls should not subscribe their name to any declaration 'unless the same shall recite in Words at length and in continuity, and not in the Form of a List or Account', and their signature should be as close as possible to the last word in the text.[230]

Another worry for the Privy Council was the continuing mercantile jealousy between the north-west and London. In April 1802 the mayor, merchants and shipowners of Liverpool complained of being disadvantaged.[231] They alleged that Section 38 was being ignored at Stangate Creek with respect to arrivals from Holland with Turkish goods. When Cottrell questioned their evidence, they cited a 'leaked' letter from Fawkener to the Customs Commissioners, but a flustered Cottrell could not find a copy. The merchants also petitioned that the oath of a ship's master when 'regular Documents may accidentally be wanting', should be sufficient evidence that cotton wool was not originally from Turkey or Barbary.[232] The Privy Council could only retreat. As much as they wanted the sworn declarations, it was hardly possible to prevent unloading when ships, for one reason or another, arrived without them. On 9 April the Council came to the view that the oath of a master would be acceptable, provided the Customs Commissioners 'shall be of Opinion that such a Discretionary Power may be safely lodged in the Hands of the … Principal Officers of the Customs at Liverpool'.[233]

227 NA PC 2/160/230.
228 Ibid.
229 NA PC 2/160/10.
230 Ibid.
231 NA PC 2/160/371.
232 NA PC 2/160/399.
233 Ibid.

Once this formula had been conceded, it was difficult to hold it in check. The Chamber of Commerce at Hull petitioned for ships to arrive from the Baltic without quarantine or declarations, as it was 'well known' that goods from that quarter, which comprised most of the port's trade, were produced locally.[234] The Privy Council agreed that Customs officers at Hull should receive the same flexibility as their colleagues at Liverpool, but only in respect of the Baltic. Ships arriving from Holland should still produce declarations. If they could not, then the oaths of the masters or other 'proof' of growth should be submitted by local Customs officers to the Commissioners in London for a second opinion. The Privy Council expressed their surprise that, so long after the Order in Council, ships were still arriving without declarations, an omission which the Hull Chamber of Commerce attributed to 'ignorance or inadvertancy'. The Customs Commissioners were asked to draw up a standard form of declaration, and a specimen certificate for the British consul, 'that may meet the Letter as well as the Spirit' of Section 38. It was not until August that they were ready for distribution to merchants and others at home and abroad.[235]

From Hull, the uncertainty among officials spread north. In May 1802 the collector and comptroller at Newcastle reported that ships were arriving there from the Baltic with corn in linen bags, and masters had no declarations to present about the provenance of the linen.[236] The Privy Council had no option but to allow Customs officers there the same privilege as their colleagues at Liverpool and Hull, and in September the concession was extended to arrivals from the Baltic at Boston.[237] But it soon became evident that masters were not always in a position to offer any proof at all of the provenance of their goods. In November 1802 merchants at Hull pointed out that goods shipped through Hamburg were baled in the interior of Germany without the shipper or merchant knowing exactly what was in them.[238] Lord Liverpool was asked for his view as to whether bales 'Contents Unknown' at Hamburg and Bremen might be excused altogether from the scope of Section 38.[239] Such concession could be justified by the belief that both ports had adequate quarantine facilities, but the relaxation merely prompted merchants trading to Hull out of Amsterdam and Rotterdam to argue for similar treatment.[240] This, in turn, resurrected the awkward question of the adequacy of Dutch quarantine, and led to yet another scrutiny of their regulations.[241] It was June 1803 before copies of these rules reached Fawkener, but he was at Bath at the time, being treated for gout, and the placards were still in Dutch.[242] It would be many months before the Privy Council

234 NA PC 2/160/424, from which remaining references in this paragraph are taken until otherwise stated.

235 NA PC 2/161/146.

236 NA PC 2/160/508.

237 NA PC 2/161/246.

238 NA PC 2/161/362.

239 NA PC 2/161/386.

240 NA PC 2/161/404. The Hull merchants were represented by Samuel Thornton.

241 NA PC 2/161/415.

242 NA PC 2/163/101.

could consider what to do, and in the interim they wallowed without direction or policy as the complexities of their own Order proved impossible to manage.

In December 1802 the Council received a memorial from merchants trading with Portugal, forwarded by a Mr Zornlin, arguing that cotton imported from there but emanating from Brazil should be exempt from Section 38.[243] The reason put forward was that a regular quarantine now existed at Lisbon, but the Privy Council were not at all sure that was right.[244] Then came pressure from Scotland, where the Board of Customs had been watching with bewilderment as various concessions nibbled into the integrity of the Order in Council. In June 1803 they asked for a summary of how the law then stood, supposing a ship arrived with cotton wool from a port with no regular quarantine facilities and the master had omitted or neglected to bring a declaration and certificate.[245] The Privy Council responded that the goods should be regarded as Turkish, unless it was apparent they had crossed the Atlantic.[246] That reply was tantamount to a confession that Section 38, as drafted, was now meaningless.

For much of 1803, the Privy Council strove to reach some formula which would satisfy the merchants of Glasgow, growing in voice and influence and seeking concessions which the Scottish Board of Customs were powerless to grant.[247] In May the Council had given in to a request from the merchants that cotton wool imported to the Clyde from the West Indies and North America should be exempt from the documentation demanded by Section 38, and therefore free of quarantine. Three months later the West India Board of Glasgow asked for the concession to be extended to hides and other enumerated goods, and the Privy Council made a weak attempt to stand their ground. It transpired that the Scottish Board of Customs, as early as 19 August 1802, had warned importers of enumerated goods that in exactly nine months' time they would need a declaration and certificate, but ships were still arriving without them. The Glaswegians were then joined in protest by the merchants and shipowners of Greenock and Port Glasgow, who reported that their agents in the West Indies never thought it necessary to send certificates of origin as it was clear from other documents that the produce was local. Despite stating they would never abandon the need for declarations and certificates for anything except cotton wool, the Privy Council agreed that if evidence were given on oath that such documents were unavailable at source, or that the need for them had not been known, and if the master swore that the goods were not the produce of Turkey, they would be admitted without quarantine. It might well have been queried under what circumstances Turkish goods could find their way to such remote parts with a view to being re-exported to Britain, but the Council claimed to know of rare instances.

243 NA PC 2/161/416.

244 Ibid.

245 NA PC 2/163/261.

246 Ibid.

247 NA PC 2/163/472–4, from which remaining references in this paragraph are taken. The memorial from Greenock and Port Glasgow was not formally considered by the Privy Council until 25 February 1804 (PC 2/164/539–42), when there is a useful summary of the history of Section 38 since September 1802.

The new system was tested and found workable when the *Benson* reached Glasgow from Trinidad in December 1803 with no declaration or certificate.[248] Although carrying cotton wool with the sugar and lime juice, she was allowed to unload without quarantine if the master swore that the goods were not of Turkish or indeed African origin.[249] But any satisfaction felt on the Clyde was short-lived, as new outbreaks of yellow fever in North America led in October 1803 to a general Order for quarantine against arrivals from New York, extended in November to ships from Philadelphia and Alexandria, Virginia.[250] This led to serious inconvenience at Greenock, in January 1804, when four ships arrived from New York.[251] Cotton had to be located and separated among the potash, turpentine, pork, apple and staves, and aired on lighters for a fortnight.[252] As the quarantine station was back at Lamlash, on the Isle of Arran, the merchants argued for the site to be moved to Holy Loch.[253] While this idea was referred for discussion by the Scottish Board of Customs, the scare from North America ended, and the Orders were revoked during February.[254] But the periodic reimposition of quarantine against North America would give the merchants of the Clyde no peace of mind.

For the sake of continuity, the story of Section 38 has been taken forward to a point where further parliamentary measures, backed up by a new Order in Council, were under consideration. It was no part of the Privy Council's intention, despite their humiliating experience of making the section work, to abandon either the paperwork or the control which it stood for. But decisions made in 1805 will only be meaningful when set against the backdrop of a resurgence of the threat from yellow fever, which must now be the focus of closer attention.

248 NA PC 2/164/340.

249 Ibid.

250 NA PC 2/164/271.

251 NA PC 2/164/373, 399.

252 Ibid.

253 NA PC 2/164/508.

254 Ibid.; PC 2/164/496.

Chapter Ten

British Board of Health and Kentish Fiasco, 1803–1820

'Gibraltar fever'

In the early winter of 1803 it came to the notice of the Privy Council that the Spanish port of Malaga was experiencing an epidemic of unusual ferocity. As the disease which had smitten Cadiz a few years earlier had not been too detrimental to British interests, the Council might have been excused for taking the news calmly. But there were several factors now which gave rise to disquiet. In the first place, information was arriving from two independent sources. British consuls were alerting Hawkesbury, as Foreign Secretary, and the navy were alarming the Admiralty, who rushed the news to Lord Hobart, Secretary of State for War and the Colonies.[1] As the navy had been a bulwark of reassurance about the yellow fever at Cadiz, their concern about sickness at Malaga could not be taken lightly. Secondly, the outbreak was spreading rapidly: Alicante and Carthagena were soon attacked, renewing fears for the health of Gibraltar. Thirdly, the identity of the new disease had not been established. And finally, Britain, even in wartime, had a considerable trade with Spanish ports of the Mediterranean. Merchants would be less tolerant of an impediment to business with accessible Malaga than they had been in 1800 in respect of blockaded Cadiz.

On 12 November 1803 the Privy Council took the unusual step of declining to discharge from quarantine several ships which had arrived at Plymouth under convoy from the Mediterranean, despite their clean bills of health.[2] The crews were to muster every day and be monitored 'for a certain time'.[3] Within two more weeks the situation had become far worse. The Customs Commissioners reported that thirteen ships which had loaded at Malaga during the epidemic were actually in British ports: five were at Stangate Creek, two at Bristol, one each at Ilfracombe and Liverpool, and four at Inverkeithing Bay.[4] In the last-named harbour, one of the ships, the *Dolphin*, had suffered five deaths. The master and two seamen had succumbed in Malaga, while two more men had died on the voyage, one as recently as 9 November.[5] Despite such worries, merchants were extremely anxious for the ships to be unloaded, as they carried perishable fruit.

1 National Archives [NA] PC 2/164/236.

2 Ibid.

3 Ibid.

4 NA PC 2/164/284–7. The Privy Council were not minded, in this crisis, to enquire why a ship liable to quarantine should have arrived at Ilfracombe.

5 NA PC 2/164/281, 284–7.

Uncertain how to act, the Council took the extreme step of summoning what was virtually a meeting of the Cabinet in the afternoon of 28 November 1803, in the Council Chamber.[6] Also in attendance were several physicians: the military were represented not only by Blane but by John Hunter, who had been a superintendent of military hospitals in Jamaica, and by a Dr Franks who had served with the army in Egypt.[7] Sir Francis Milman represented the Royal College of Physicians.[8] The doctors were asked whether oranges and lemons could safely be landed, but they would only recommend caution.[9] The legal position was shaky, as Malaga had issued clean bills of health to British ships after 26 September, when the sickness had erupted. Although a death during the voyage vitiated the clean-bill status, all the ships save one were in good health, and fruit was a non-enumerated cargo which would normally escape detention. The real problem was the lack of understanding about the disease itself, as consular reports failed to give the nature and symptoms. 'It might be the Plague – It might be the Yellow fever; or it might be neither'.[10] The meeting concluded that ships from Malaga should continue in the strictest quarantine and be treated as having arrived with foul bills of health.[11]

As usual with the Privy Council, their tough stance was modified within days, once commercial interests had geared themselves up for a protest. From 10 December 1803 the passage time could be deducted from the 40 days demanded by foul-bill quarantine, to protect fruit from rotting.[12] Furthermore, there was no obligation for a ship to proceed to Stangate Creek unless she carried enumerated goods of the first class or the crew had some contagious disease.[13] It was still necessary, however, for packages, baggage, bedding and clothes to be aired locally over 15 days. The exception to these rules was the *Dolphin*, for which quarantine had to continue.[14] There was an immediate problem at Inverkeithing Bay where Customs officers, confusing packages with packaging, were opening boxes of raisins and soft fruit to remove the paper wrappings.[15] The Privy Council made it clear that the Order applied only to baskets and other external protection.[16] Further problems, however, were obviated when Malaga returned to rapid normality over the winter. On 21 February 1804 the Council advised the Customs Commissioners that ships from Malaga need no longer be treated as foul-bill arrivals.[17]

---

6 NA PC 2/164/281.

7 NA PC 2/164/284–7.

8 Ibid.

9 Ibid. The doctors merely suggested that as little communication should be had with the ships as possible.

10 Ibid.

11 Ibid. The Privy Council were poised to place Cadiz and Alicante under the same restrictions.

12 NA PC 2/164/325.

13 Ibid. In the heat of the moment, on 29 November 1803, it had been ordered that even ships bound for Scotland should do quarantine at Stangate Creek (PC 2/164/290).

14 NA PC 2/164/325.

15 NA PC 2/164/354.

16 Ibid.

17 NA PC 2/164/529–30.

The respite was short. In the summer of 1804 another mysterious and deadly epidemic swept southern Spain and succeeded where the Spaniards had failed in breaching the defences of Gibraltar. The point of introduction, allegedly, was the arrival on the Rock of a shopkeeper who had been lodging at a house in Cadiz, to which city the disease had spread (or returned), causing a huge mortality.[18] Public health in Gibraltar was then in the hands of William Pym, the garrison surgeon, who was destined to become an increasingly central and controversial figure in quarantine policy as the nineteenth century progressed.[19] One of his later opponents, Gavin Milroy, argued that quarantine deficiencies in Gibraltar were the real reason for the epidemic's introduction, especially as Pym was on leave of absence at the time.[20] Wherever lay the blame, the disease revelled in the filthy, overcrowded streets of the Rock. Nelson was among those who wrongly placed confidence in the lazaretto on the Neutral Ground as a safeguard for the garrison.[21] Over three months, from late August 1804, there were around 6,000 deaths out of a total population, including the garrison, of fewer than 16,000.[22]

With a British colony now decimated, and newspapers reporting in consternation that the 'Gibraltar Fever' was ever more widespread and destructive, the Privy Council developed symptoms of the national panic.[23] There was a flurry of Orders and letters, mainly to the Customs Commissioners. One asked them to report what resources would be needed to make the outports as 'effectual and … secure' as Stangate Creek for ships with or without clean bills of health.[24] On 14 November 1804 the Council asked the Admiralty, beset as they were with the difficulties of war, to provide more ships equipped with beds and winter clothing.[25] These vessels would lie in Stangate Creek in readiness for crews and passengers arriving from Malaga and Gibraltar in ships with foul bills.[26] On the same day, the Council extended strict quarantine to arrivals from ports between Gibraltar and Cape St Vincent, or in other words against Cadiz.[27] Also on the same day (although the timing was fortuitous), a quarantine of 15 days was laid against ships from South Carolina, Georgia and

---

18 F. Brockington, 'Public health at the Privy Council 1831–4', *Journal of the History of Medicine*, 16 (1961), 14, quotes Milman's figure of 100,000 dead.

19 For Pym, see *Oxford Dictionary of National Biography* and W. Johnston, *Roll of Commissioned Officers in the Medical Service of the British Army … 1727 to … 1898* (Aberdeen, 1917), no. 1252.

20 G. Milroy, 'Operation and results of quarantine in British Ports since the beginning of the present century', *Association Medical Journal*, [1] (1853), 635.

21 Sir N.H. Nicolas (ed.), *The Dispatches and Letters of Vice Admiral Lord Viscount Nelson* (7 vols, London, 1845–46), p. 238: Nelson to Captain-General, Barcelona: ' … a Lazaretto camp was formed upon the Neutral Ground, and from the precautions taken it was hoped that the disease would not spread …'

22 Milroy, 'Operation and results of quarantine in British ports', 635.

23 D. Sultana, *Samuel Taylor Coleridge in Malta and Italy* (Oxford, 1969), p. 215, mentions that 'Gibraltar Fever' was even a name for yellow fever in New York.

24 NA PC 2/166/240.

25 NA PC 2/166/166, 184.

26 Ibid.

27 NA PC 2/166/167.

Louisiana.[28] But if yellow fever were the enemy there, there was still no certainty in London that the same disease was ravaging southern Iberia.

No sooner had the Admiralty supplied the *Guelderland* and *Haarlem* for Stangate Creek than the Privy Council wanted more ships, this time for St Helen's Pool.[29] They would lie there equipped for up to 200 infected people while another ship, holding military medical staff and guards, would be kept on standby at Falmouth, or some other close port on the mainland.[30] When the Duke of York, as Commander-in-Chief, cooperated in this new request, there were signs that the contingency plan for the Scillies, so long demanded by Russell and others, would at last be put in place. It was four months later, in April 1805, when the dockyard at Plymouth finished the conversion of the 44-gun HMS *Pandora* into the hospital ship for St Helen's Pool.[31] Also at Plymouth, the *Hornet* sloop was fitted out as accommodation for medical staff, but the personnel would not arrive until they were needed.[32] Once the *Pandora* was operational, it was envisaged that she would be manned like a floating lazaretto at Stangate Creek, under the control of the local Collector of Customs.[33] There was already a revenue cutter called the *Providence* stationed at St Helen's Pool, with a crew of 17.[34]

It was a source of frustration to the Privy Council throughout the Malaga–Gibraltar crisis that the land lazaret at Stangate Creek, which would have made the Scillies establishment unnecessary, was a long way from completion. It would appear from a contemporary map (see Illustration 10.1) that only four sheds were then built. After two years without news, the Council had written to the Treasury in August 1802 asking for a progress report and some knowledge of costs in relation to the budget.[35] They appear to have received no adequate response until March 1804, when the Treasury confessed that the full £65,000 had been spent and the building was incomplete.[36] Should Parliament, wrote the Treasury, be asked for more money? The Council wanted to know how much more.[37] On 26 April, Nicholas Vansittart presented to the Commons, on behalf of the Treasury, 'An Account of the Sum wanted to complete the Works at Chetney Hill', amounting to £30,000.[38] When this money, two days later, was granted to the King by a committee of supply, the Privy Council looked forward to a rapid completion of the troublesome project.[39]

---

28 NA PC 2/166/171.

29 NA PC 2/166/230, 330.

30 NA PC 2/166/330, 332.

31 NA PC 2/167/300. The Admiralty had initially chosen HMS *Experiment* but it was found she drew too much water for St Helen's Pool.

32 Ibid.

33 Ibid.

34 NA PC 2/168/256–9.

35 NA PC 2/161/145. Another question they asked was: when did Wyatt think the lazaret would open?

36 NA PC 2/165/2.

37 Ibid.

38 *Journal of the House of Commons* [*JHC*], vol. 59, p. 233.

39 *JHC*, vol. 59, p. 243.

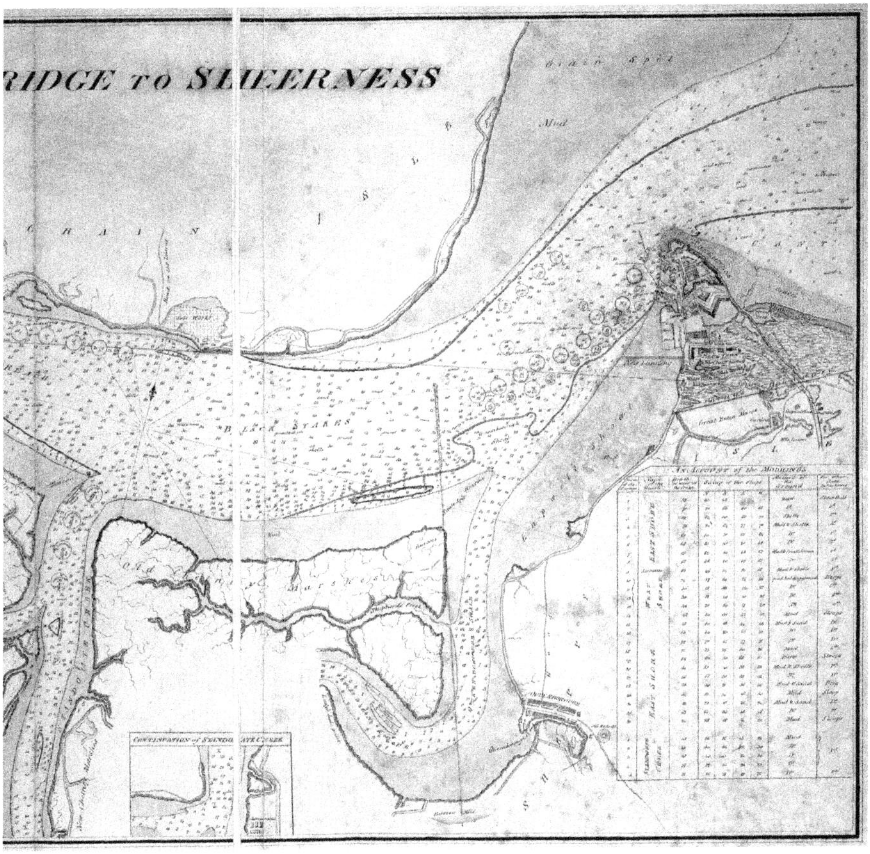

Illustration 10.1 Site of lazaretto (inset) and four airing hulks in Stangate Creek, Kent, 1803.

On 12 November 1804, with an influx of foul-bill ships expected daily and the new floating lazarettos not yet in position in Stangate Creek or St Helen's Pool, the Council asked Wyatt (via the Treasury) to report 'within the shortest possible time' when the land lazaret could accommodate people.[40] Were the beds installed, and how many would they hold? Would temporary huts help? If so, when could they be ready? Wyatt was to proceed 'with all possible Diligence and Dispatch'.[41] When no answer was received, the Privy Council asked the Customs Commissioners whether *they* had any idea of what was happening at Chetney Hill.[42] The Council summoned Wyatt, on 28 November, to a meeting in the Office of Trade.[43] In attendance also were Sir Lucas Pepys, President of the College of Physicians, and Milman, Blane,

40 NA PC 2/166/163.
41 Ibid.
42 NA PC 2/166/232.
43 NA PC 2/166/233.

Hunter and Franks.[44] It can be imagined that the physicians were ordered to instil in Wyatt a sense of the urgency of his task and the consequences of a failure of the quarantine defences. On 5 December 1804 the Council wrote directly to Wyatt, evidently not satisfied by his performance at the meeting.[45] They wanted an immediate report in writing as to how far the lazaret was complete. One-quarter of the existing warehouses should be converted temporarily for the reception of people, with some kind of palisade for security. How soon could that be done? On 10 January 1805 Wyatt was reminded of these requirements.[46] It was now explained that six huts were needed 'within the Stockade' for the isolation of the infected. Wyatt was unhappy with this, and in one of his rare constructive letters to the Privy Council, dated 28 February, he mentioned that a better configuration of huts had been arrived at in discussion with Dr Newberry.[47] On 6 March he was ordered to attend the Customs Commissioners on the following day to explain what he meant.[48] This was one of the few occasions when Wyatt appeared up to his job.

The Board of Health

Embroiled in the practical consequences of the Gibraltar trauma, the Privy Council felt a pressing need to clarify the character of the disease which they were facing. John Turnbull, a merchant trading to Spain, was summoned to the Council Chamber in October 1804 to see whether his knowledge could add anything to consular dispatches.[49] On 8 November, with the benefit of Turnbull's comments and before the meeting with Wyatt, the Council consulted Pepys and his fellow physicians about the widespread distress in Gibraltar and its neighbourhood.[50] In the following month the receipt of further advice from ministers and consuls, to the effect that the disease had spread to Leghorn and even Ragusa, induced the Council to take the unprecedented step of asking the College of Physicians for their help.[51] This was to be strictly a medical matter, with no merchants, military men or Commissioners of Customs playing a role. In a letter of 29 December 1804, Cottrell gave the College their brief.[52] How could the disease be prevented from spreading? To what extent was it proper to keep the public informed? And had they any general observations?[53]

On 10 January 1805 Pepys responded by letter.[54] The disease was 'Highly Malignant' and contagious, killing more quickly than the plague, and killing a greater

---

44 Ibid.

45 NA PC 2/166/257.

46 NA PC 2/166/389.

47 NA PC 2/167/140.

48 Ibid.

49 NA PC 2/166/84.

50 NA PC 2/166/153.

51 NA PC 2/166/350.

52 Ibid.

53 Ibid.

54 British Library [BL] Add. MS 38358, fols 232–7, from which all references in this paragraph and the next are taken unless otherwise stated. Brockington, 'Public health at the

proportion of those attacked. Having ruled out, by implication, Levantine plague, the College would not commit themselves to any alternative diagnosis. For doctors of a later generation, such as Gavin Milroy, there was no doubt that yellow fever was the culprit.[55] But by dismissing the suggestion that Britain might be protected from the disease by its colder climate, indeed by warning the Privy Council of the 'urgent necessity' of preventive action, the College appeared to exclude yellow fever, as well as plague. Pepys warned that war afforded little protection against seaborne infection, as neutral ships and prizes were still arriving. He recommended the strictest quarantine against all ships from anywhere between Cadiz and Leghorn and the coasts of Barbary. Magistrates, Customs officers, pilots and even coastal clergy should 'exert their influence to obtain the earliest Information of any Infringement of Quarantine'. While everything should be done to make detention 'as little distressing as possible to Individuals', with 'full and ample means of taking care of the Sick', quarantine stations should be provided with military guards.

With proper enforcement of quarantine, the College believed that the disease would not spread. In the event, however, of a physician meeting a suspicious fever, he should report it to a magistrate, who would arrange a second opinion from two 'of the most respectable practitioners of the ... Neighbourhood'. The magistrate, if alarm persisted, should inform the Privy Council. Should the disease break out, the College recommended the locality 'should be immediately placed under a Set of Regulations, approaching nearly to Martial Law', however 'repugnant' that would be to the population. In London and other centres, there should be detached houses to where 'any Accidental Case of the disease might be carried'. Then came the physicians' most important pronouncement: 'For watching over the regulations of Quarantine, correcting them where erroneous, perfecting them, where deficient, and, being ready to apply remedies to any unforeseen Evils which may arise; We do not know what better to recommend than a Board of Health ...' These bodies were proving very useful in North America. Pepys ended by recommending 'every exertion' to complete the land lazaret under construction, as the floating lazarettos were inadequate.

Such a report, a few years earlier, would have been politely dismissed by the Privy Council as unacceptably severe. Not since the Marseilles crisis, more than 80 years earlier, had ideas such as martial law, military cordons and compulsory isolation been mooted, and even in that desperate age they had been strongly opposed. But the real volte-face was over the prospect of a Board of Health. The Council were terrified by the thought of a disease more malignant than the plague, and informed the Attorney-General that they intended to recommend the establishment of such a Board to the King.[56] This would require a Proclamation. In a letter of 25 January 1805, the Privy Council asked the College of Physicians to submit a detailed plan for the establishment of a Board of Health, giving costs and terms of reference.[57]

Privy Council 1805–6', 25–7, publishes the full letter. His source is unreferenced.

55 Milroy, 'Operation and results of quarantine in British ports', 635

56 NA PC 2/166/578–80.

57 NA PC 2/166/557.

The College, however, were more concerned initially with the composition of the Board than what it should do. As the duties would depend on what was expected by Government, and as the question of remuneration for members depended on those duties, they did no more than recommend a membership of five physicians from their own number, plus one commissioner each from the Navy Board, Customs service and the Board of Sick and Hurt.[58] This meant a body dominated by doctors, in total contrast to the Mediterranean ports, where the Boards were controlled by merchants. Brockington refers to a dispute between Pepys and Milman as to who should preside.[59] In the event, the presidency was given to Sir Andrew Hamond, as Comptroller of the Navy.[60] Pepys and Milman were backed up by Hunter and two other colleagues, namely Henry Reynolds and William Heberden junior. Sir Alexander Munro represented the Commissioners of Customs, and Dr John Harness the Board of Sick and Hurt. The secretary to the Board was Dr James Hervey.[61]

The appointment of Hamond and Harness had been made by the Admiralty, at the request of the Privy Council; the Council also wanted the Treasury to choose the Commissioner of Customs.[62] While he was asking for this Commissioner, in February 1805, Cottrell could not overlook the opportunity to argue for the urgent completion of the land lazaret, as it had been mentioned in the same letter from the College of Physicians which had argued for the Board of Health. 'I am thereupon to desire', he wrote,

> that the strongest Injunction may be given to Mr. Wyatt by the ... Treasury (as has already been done by the ... Privy Council) to proceed with the least possible Delay in making Temporary Provision for the Reception of Persons liable to Quarantine in certain parts of the Building now erected at Chetney Hill, and to go on with all possible Expedition in compleating [*sic*] the whole according to the Plan which has been settled and approved.[63]

In fact, the Board of Health had nothing to do with Chetney Hill until the dying weeks of their existence. Formally established on 21 February 1805, their *raison d'être*, according to the announcement in the *London Gazette*, was 'to prepare and digest Rules and Regulations for the most speedy and Effectual Mode of guarding against the Introduction and Spreading of Infection, and for purifying any Ship or House, in case any Contagious Disorder should ... [occur].'[64] Maclean, on the other hand, believed that the Board had a more general remit 'to consider and report the measures which it would be appropriate to adopt, in case the plague or other infectious disease, attended with great mortality, shall pass the barrier of the quarantine, and actually

---

58 Brockington, 'Public health at the Privy Council 1805–6', 14; NA PC 2/167/54–6.

59 Brockington, 'Public health at the Privy Council 1805–6', 16.

60 Ibid.

61 For a discussion of those appointed, see Brockington, 'Public health at the Privy Council 1805–6', 15.

62 NA PC 2/167/53–6.

63 NA PC 2/167/54–6.

64 Brockington, 'Public health at the Privy Council 1805–6', 14–15. The full Proclamation establishing the Board of Health was published in the *Naval Chronicle*, vol. 13 (1805; Part One), pp. 144–5.

appear amongst us'.[65] He used this form of words, particularly the phrase 'barrier of the quarantine', as the basis for an attack on the Board's credibility. In one of their pronouncements, the Board warned 'that we must not risk the lives of our fellow-creatures, through a confidence in any speculative opinions, which want the sanction of experience'. This reference to 'speculative opinions', so Maclean assumed, was an attack on one of his own papers, and the Board's reliance on 'experience' was merely an implicit support for the system of quarantine, which Maclean thought unnecessary and detrimental.

It soon became clear that the terms of reference for the Board would be narrower than the members desired, as the Privy Council disagreed with them in one crucial aspect. There were three functions, or duties, which the Board put forward in a memorandum of 20 March 1805.[66] The first, and most important, was the superintendence of 'the whole Business of the Quarantine ...' That did not exclude reporting to the Privy Council any situations which might arise where the existing legislation was inadequate. Nor did it exclude the Commissioners of Customs from executing quarantine in a practical sense. The Board hoped, however, to be sent copies of all papers relating to specific ships at the same time as they were dispatched to the Commissioners. As that would put too much strain on the Privy Council office, the Board no doubt hoped that all the papers would be diverted to themselves. The intention, in so many words, was to usurp the whole management of quarantine, leaving the Privy Council as a channel to Parliament for new legislation, and the Customs service, in whole or in part, as a subordinate body to the Board of Health.

The second desideratum of the Board was the power to manage the public health of the country, especially the separation of the sick from the well, in the case of a major epidemic. In this respect, they confessed a liking for the drastic measures of 1603, which they believed might possibly remain in force to some extent and be capable of adaptation, as intervening measures had been of limited duration. The Board's third suggestion was for what Brockington has called a Centre of Epidemic Intelligence.[67] From diplomats, military doctors and other professionals working or living overseas, the Board would collect early news of significant diseases which might well pose a threat for Britain, giving time to increase vigilance and reinforce the defences. They argued that Gibraltar might have been spared the dreadful effects of the current epidemic if 'proper Information' had been received five years earlier, when the disease had first entered Cadiz. The Board concluded by quoting at some length from Russell's pioneering arguments as to why quarantine should be entrusted to a body independent of the Privy Council. As the Council had already conceded that such a Board was necessary, the reference can be taken as gratification to a frail

65 C. Maclean, *Remarks on the British Quarantine laws* ... (London, 1823), p. 19, from which remaining references in this paragraph are taken. It is evident that Maclean was quoting, but he does not identify his source.

66 NA PC 1/3646, published in Brockington, 'Public health at the Privy Council 1805–6', 27–9, from which all references in this and the next paragraph are taken.

67 It is not clear from Brockington's paper whether or not this term was contemporary.

and ailing Patrick Russell, who would not live to see the Board complete their short period of influence.[68]

On 5 June 1805, two and a half months after Hamond submitted proposals for the Board's terms of reference, a definitive reply was sent to Hervey by the Privy Council.[69] This was more than two weeks later than the date of their minuted decision.[70] The delay was an indication of prolonged discussion between the Privy Council and Government, and some disagreements. The main obstacle, undoubtedly, was the relationship between the Board and the Customs service. The Privy Council ruled out any extension of the Board's domain. It would be inconvenient to put the Customs service under any other body because of their excise duties.[71] Furthermore, the Customs Commissioners met daily and were best placed to supervise their own officials. Generally, it would be inexpedient that quarantine should be managed solely by a Board of Health, who should concern themselves with procedural issues. But 'suggestions and recommendations' would have to be made to the Privy Council – the Board were not to be vested with executive power. The Council, on the other hand, were by no means averse to the Board corresponding direct with consuls and military doctors abroad. This represented a distinctly more positive attitude than the Council had evinced in 1800, in the context of the Quarantine Committee. Now, they were prepared to recommend to Secretaries of State that consuls, as well as physicians and surgeons in the military, should be instructed to cooperate with the Board. The Council were also happy to let the Board have copies of all papers which they (the Council) received or generated relating to quarantine issues, and even to individual ships 'where any special circumstances shall arise'. But this was less than the Board had requested. Hervey was told that the Privy Council 'reserve to Themselves the authority which the Law has placed in their Hands of making such Orders and giving such Directions as may eventually be necessary in Cases not provided for ...'

Secretaries of State could not agree as to whether the Board of Health might correspond with individuals within their spheres of influence. The Earl of Camden, responsible for war and the colonies, had agreed in respect of governors in North America and the West Indies.[72] He was succeeded in July 1805 by Viscount Castlereagh, who was initially opposed to similar contact with consuls in Barbary, but later agreed.[73] The Foreign Secretary was Lord Mulgrave, who foresaw 'Inconveniences' if the Board of Health were allowed direct access to British consuls in general.[74] With only lukewarm support, the Board would have understood immediately that their aspiration to become a hub of intelligence, comparable with, say, their counterparts at Leghorn or Marseilles, would not be realized. Perhaps some small consolation

68 Russell died 2 July 1805.

69 NA PC 2/167/477–9.

70 Brockington, 'Public health at the Privy Council 1805–6', 17, 29, publishing PC 1/3654. He prefaces this minute as 20/3/1805, *recte* 20/5/1805.

71 NA PC 2/167/477–9 and Brockington, 'Public health at the Privy Council 1805–6', 29, from which remaining references in this paragraph are taken.

72 NA PC 2/168/53.

73 Ibid.

74 NA PC 2/168/53.

was a letter addressed directly to the Board, in autumn 1805, from the Council of Health at Naples, who reported an epidemic in the Ottoman fleet at Corfu.[75] This was perhaps the only occasion when the Board, via the Privy Council, alerted the Customs Commissioners to a menace of which they were otherwise unaware.

In 1805 the Board of Health produced five reports, of which the first two at least were printed.[76] The earliest report, dated 30 April, enlarged on the Board's interest in the precautions of 1603, and explained how an infected town might be run and controlled and what care and isolation might forcibly be visited on the sick.[77] The second, dated 15 May, dealt with infection itself and how to avoid it, for instance by fumigation and indirect contact with susceptible material.[78] The third report, dated 13 June, suggested ways to prevent fever in Gibraltar.[79] All three were approved 'with minor exceptions' by the Privy Council and were circulated to magistrates in Britain and to governors in the colonies.[80] The fourth report was discussed by the Privy Council on 1 August.[81] It suggested measures to mitigate the dreadful death toll in the West Indies from yellow fever.[82] In forwarding copies of the report to Government, the Council drew attention to two clauses: one argued for new troops to be sent to high and healthy ground; the other recommended that two companies of black soldiers should be attached to each infantry regiment, to do fatigues and guard duty on lower ground.[83] The rationale was that black people had shown themselves far less susceptible to the disease. The fifth report, submitted in September, was essentially a questionnaire, seeking the advice of local governors, doctors and military chiefs as to exact locations in the West Indies where yellow fever was least to be feared.[84] The Privy Council fully agreed that the questions should be put, but could only ask Castlereagh for his approval.[85]

As regards quarantine in Britain, the Board of Health were virtually excluded from decisions affecting particular ships. The exception was the incident of HMS *Africaine*, which had arrived at Cork from the West Indies, in November 1805, with many men sick.[86] Other ships in the convoy of 40 were also affected. There was nothing unusual in that, but alarm in the Irish station was such that the warship was ordered to St Helen's Pool.[87] Within days, when quarantine officers at Cork reported that the ship had actually lost no men in the voyage (although some had died before

75 NA PC 2/168/414.

76 Brockington, 'Public health at the Privy Council 1805–6', 20.

77 Brockington, 'Public health at the Privy Council 1805–6', 19.

78 Brockington, 'Public health at the Privy Council 1805–6', 19–20.

79 NA PC 2/168/59.

80 NA PC 2/168/23.

81 NA PC 2/168/132.

82 Brockington, 'Public health at the Privy Council 1805–6', 20, 30, publishing PC 1/3637.

83 NA PC 2/168/132.

84 Brockington, 'Public health at the Privy Council 1805–6', 20, citing PC 1/3666.

85 NA PC 2/168/328.

86 NA PC 2/168/506.

87 Ibid.

she sailed), it was realized that this might be an over-reaction.[88] The *Africaine*, therefore, was diverted to Falmouth where the situation could be reviewed. But no sooner had she arrived, than alarm was rekindled. On 17 November the captain reported 30 crewmen sick, including the surgeon, and one man had died that very morning.[89] The Privy Council, influenced by a diagnosis of yellow fever from Dr Luke, ordered the ship to proceed immediately to St Helen's Pool, which she reached on 23 November.[90] Somewhat later the hospital ship *Pandora* and sloop *Hornet* arrived from Plymouth via Penzance, where the medical staff and guards had finally been embarked.[91] The Privy Council sent a message to the personnel of the *Pandora*, expressing confidence that they would do their duty, and asking for daily reports on the number of sick and the progress of the disease.[92]

At this juncture of high anxiety, the Board of Health were informed of events and authorized to communicate direct with the medical staff in the Scillies, to whom they could offer ideas and advice.[93] The Board were also to receive duplicates of the reports from the *Pandora*.[94] But drama turned almost to farce, when Dr Baird, Inspector of Hospitals, arrived in the Scillies on 27 November to oversee the medical care. Baird found no fever on the *Africaine*: there were only eight men sick on board, of colds, rheumatism and ulcers.[95] Twelve others had been transferred to the *Pandora*, with complaints ranging from a diseased liver to 'Idiotism'.[96] None of this bothered Baird, who was even dismissive of chronic dysentery affecting another of the patients.[97] The *Africaine* was discharged from quarantine on 7 December 1805.[98] Ten days later the Privy Council agreed to the release of two local men from Tresco, whose unauthorized visit to the *Africaine* had resulted in a quarantine for themselves and their households.[99]

As a test of the contingency arrangements for St Helen's Pool, the episode highlighted failures. The warship had reached the Pool before the *Pandora*, and the Privy Council felt guilty for the 'extreme distress' this must have caused.[100] Even when the medical team did arrive, they were short of resources. On 6 December, when the crisis was over, the Comptroller of the Navy was still being pursued for

88 NA PC 2/168/520.

89 NA PC 2/168/545.

90 NA PC 2/169/5. Another ship, the merchantman *Queen Charlotte*, was also ordered briefly to St Helen's Pool, arriving 24 November. This vessel would seem to have been part of the convoy (NA PC 2/169/34).

91 NA PC 2/168/520, 547.

92 NA PC 2/168/564.

93 NA PC 2/168/567–9.

94 NA PC 2/168/564. These duplicates would be forwarded by the Privy Council.

95 NA PC 2/169/32.

96 Ibid.

97 Ibid.

98 NA PC 2/169/32.

99 NA PC 2/169/63. The men's names were given as James and John Odger.

100 NA PC 2/169/26.

beds and bedding.[101] The Duke of York was asked to consider having medical staff permanently on standby at Penzance or the Scillies.[102] There was also a question of demarcation of duties. A small, permanent garrison on St Mary's enjoyed the services of a doctor, who went to the aid of the *Africaine* before the hospital ship arrived.[103] For remuneration, he drew two bills on the Commissioners of Sick and Hurt, which they refused to pay.[104] This problem was deemed appropriate for the Board of Health who, in January 1806, recommended that a resident physician and assistant surgeon should be added to the quarantine establishment at St Helen's Pool, residing in the *Hornet* sloop.[105] The Privy Council went along with that, suggesting to the Treasury that quarantine on the Scillies should be 'nearly upon the same footing as it is now performed afloat at Standgate Creek'.[106] It was probably in 1810 that the *Hornet* was removed from permanent deployment in the islands.[107]

Shortly before pondering the problem in the Scillies, the Board of Health had become embroiled in the wretched mess at Chetney Hill. Having visited the building site on 21 September 1805, they wrote to the Privy Council in late October expressing their regret that such a location had ever been chosen.[108] For the Privy Council this was mortifying. Cottrell wrote to Hervey at great length on 7 December, reciting the history of decisions about Chetney Hill, since the site had been identified some 60 years earlier as the best with proximity to Stangate Creek.[109] As the story unfolded, it would have been evident to the Board that no medical opinion had ever been sought or offered about whether the site met sanitary requirements. Yet Cottrell was defending the hill for its 'Healthiness of Situation' as well as 'Safety of Anchorage, Space for the Ships … and Vicinity to the Metropolis'.[110] He stressed the last point, as most of the Turkey trade was to London. If the Board still felt the site objectionable, they were asked to consult with two Elder Brethren of Trinity House and two Commissioners of Customs, and report back as soon as possible.[111] The inclusion of Trinity House was novel, and resulted from their recent and successful cooperation with the Commissioners in the wider question of where quarantine harbours should be sited.[112]

101 NA PC 2/169/27, 77. It was noted on 29 November that beds and bedding had been ordered from the royal naval hospital at Plymouth (NA PC 2/168/597).

102 NA PC 2/169/26.

103 NA PC 2/169/117–18.

104 Ibid.

105 NA PC 2/169/309–11.

106 Ibid.

107 NA PC 2/187/318. The Admiralty announced that the sloop was unnecessary from their point of view and the Privy Council asked the Customs Commissioners whether they agreed. The response was not apparently minuted.

108 NA PC 2/169/34; PC 2/170/552.

109 NA PC 2/169/34–7.

110 Ibid.

111 Ibid.

112 This involvement dated from March 1805 (NA PC 2/167/129,139). See further below.

The Board of Health remained sceptical, and their resulting report so startled the Privy Council that it was April 1806 before a considered reply could be returned.[113] The main recommendation was that Chetney Hill should be surrounded by a canal, which would join Stangate Creek and allow an ebb and flow of water. Ideally, this canal would be able to take lighters, although it was conceived primarily as a large drain. Soil excavated from the canal bed would be used to heighten the hill, which would be under-drained and covered in gravel. The Privy Council were not averse to any of this, if it would at least bring the prospect of a completed and successful lazaret. They immediately asked the Customs Commissioners for estimates, telling them to 'employ some Surveyor of known Experience' in cutting canals. As he was to consult with Captains King and Woolmore of Trinity House as to the width and depth, it was clearly these Elder Brethren who been responsible for the radical proposals to the Board of Health. A separate estimate was requested for a canal capable of taking lighters, with a floodgate near the warehouses. This canal was 'to be subservient to the purposes of Drainage'. Among further estimates requested, was one for digging a well to the depth which had been found necessary at Sheerness.

After such useful work, much of it probably more impressive than the Privy Council had expected, the Board of Health came to a surprisingly rapid dissolution. Milman wrote a long, unsolicited letter on 5 July 1806 pleading for the Board to be made permanent, as the disease – he would still not refer to it as yellow fever – which had killed 100,000 in Cadiz alone could still devastate Britain.[114] Board members, he suggested, should receive four or five hundred pounds a year, less than was paid to similar appointees in North America.[115] Such remuneration was unlikely to have upset the Privy Council, and the reasons for the Board's dissolution must be found elsewhere. It must be remembered that the Council had been dealing with yellow fever for more than 12 years. Although they had not seen a case first hand, they had acquired a shrewd idea of how far north the disease could penetrate, and nothing in their experience justified the view that Britain was at risk. Certainly they had been alarmed when Malaga and then Gibraltar had been so dreadfully ravaged; indeed this alarm had created the Board of Health. But no report or advice from the Board had caused the Council to change their mind about the reality of infection. Now that Gibraltar was returning to good health, the Board had served their purpose.

Another factor influencing the Privy Council was the bickering relationship between members of the Board, which threatened to undermine their usefulness. Bad feeling between Milman and Pepys had led the King to appoint Hamond as President.[116] Although Milman had no quarrel with Hamond, and indeed thought he might make a good permanent appointment, he was dismissive of Hamond's successors as Comptrollers of the Navy, who acquired the presidency ex officio: 'Captain Nicholl hesitated to accept our Chair and Sir T. Thompson has actually

113 NA PC 2/169/485–6, from which all references in this paragraph are taken.

114 Published in Brockington, 'Public health at the Privy Council 1805–6', 22–3, citing PC 1/3736.

115 Ibid.

116 Brockington, 'Public health at the Privy Council 1805–6', 16.

declined it'.[117] Milman favoured a physician as President and suggested that the Comptroller of the Navy be removed from the Board altogether; he also reckoned the two Commissioners 'may be dispensed with'.[118] That would reduce the membership of the Board to five physicians, of whom, asserted Milman, only three were efficient.[119] Such infighting, to say nothing of arrogance, would have alarmed the Privy Council who had no wish to see a clique of society physicians, unchecked by lay appointees, acquiring the status of a department of state. And beneath the flurry of reports and letters of advice, lay the intractable issue of how far the Board could correspond with diplomats and others abroad. The more the Board became a cabal of physicians, the less chance they stood of winning direct and unmonitored access to persons responsible to the Secretaries of State.

One of the last decisions of the Board was to disagree with the Lieutenant-Governor of Jamaica about the wisdom of a floating hospital in Kingston harbour.[120] The Board, in a letter of 17 June 1806, preferred a healthier site on shore, but they had no time to continue the debate.[121] The Board of Health was formally disbanded on 14 August.[122] On 8 August the Privy Council had announced a parting gratuity of £500 to each member of the original Board, with the same sum to be divided between Nicholl and Thompson, the less-than-useful Comptrollers of the Navy.[123] The salary of James Hervey, as secretary to the Board, was continued for another year at £100.[124] On 4 September 1806 the members of the Board, no longer with any standing, wrote an unsolicited letter to the Privy Council urging the completion of the lazaret at Chetney Hill, hoping that healthier stations for the troops would be found in the West Indies, recommending further enquiry into the nature of contagious fevers, and pointing out that they had at least tried to establish a correspondence with consuls abroad.[125]

Brockington has defended the achievements of the Board of Health, but by European standards the body was a nonentity. Deprived of executive action, debarred from direct access with contacts abroad, forbidden to manage quarantine at home, the members were never more than a think tank to advise the Privy Council. Indeed, the Privy Council had never conceived that a Board of Health could be anything else. Its brief existence was an indictment of the British penchant for vested, autocratic interests and rigid hierarchical structure. There was a place for doctors in society and in the military, but not in Government. Ironically, the Mediterranean Boards of Health, steered by commercial and political lobbies, took a similar view. What set Britain apart from Europe was an attitude which deemed that both medical *and*

117 Brockington, 'Public health at the Privy Council 1805–6', 22.

118 Ibid.

119 Ibid.

120 NA PC 2/170/220.

121 NA PC 2/170/396.

122 Brockington, 'Public health at the Privy Council 1805–6', 30–31, publishes letter from Cottrell to Pepys.

123 NA PC 2/171/24.

124 NA PC 2/172/59.

125 Published in Brockington, 'Public health at the Privy Council 1805–6', 24, citing PC 1/3739. He refers to it as the Board's 6th Report.

mercantile interests, the two bodies which combined the necessary insight and experience, were unfit for the management of public health. And once the physicians became as autocratic and exclusive as their political masters – which is what Milman's unfortunate letter had revealed – it was time for the Establishment to halt them in their tracks.

Clarifying the rules

It was symptomatic of the irrelevance to Government of the Board of Health that Parliament passed a new quarantine Act without reference to the members. *An Act for making further Provision for the effectual Performance of Quarantine* received royal assent on 12 March 1805.[126] As Parliament had passed a comprehensive quarantine Act in 1800, repealing all previous legislation, the need for a large, new Act five years later appears far from obvious. Furthermore, the ostensible reasons are unconvincing. In moving the Bill, George Rose explained that the Act of 1800 had allowed the King to impose quarantine on ships arriving from countries afflicted with plague. 'The present bill', he continued, 'extended the like power with respect to ships coming from any countries infected with any other epidemical diseases which might be dangerous to the health of this country'.[127]

That wording seems bizarre when the whole point of the 1800 Act had been to declare any infectious disease 'to be of the nature of the plague', and therefore a reason why ships should be quarantined. The situation is only clarified when the exact words of the 1805 Act are examined: quarantine could now be demanded against 'the Plague, or any other infectious Disease or Distemper'. Thus a medical point was at stake. The disease which was ravaging southern Iberia was not, the physicians had decided, Levantine plague, and it was such a distinct illness that it was not even to be called 'of the nature of the plague'. Nor, apparently, was it to be called yellow fever, in case it might not be. A new disease for Europe needed a new form of words, simple and all-embracing, to ensure quarantine could be enforced.

Rose gave a second reason for the new Act and this resulted, very specifically, from the Iberian epidemic. The Privy Council had been induced to exceed their powers, with tragic results. A ship returning from Gibraltar had put in to Falmouth, but she was ordered out immediately to Stangate Creek.[128] On the voyage, the ship was wrecked off Chichester, but some of the crew scrambled ashore and were given assistance at an inn.[129] When these circumstances were discovered, the men were sent back to the wrecked vessel along with people from the inn, some of whom were drowned in the exercise. Rose justified this barbarism as 'a partial evil compared with the much more extensive and alarming one which the order was calculated

126 45 Geo. III, c.10; *JHC*, vol. 60, p. 132.

127 T.C. Hansard, *Parliamentary Debates*, vol. 3, p. 222.

128 Ibid.

129 *Naval Chronicle*, vol. 13 (1805, Part One), p. 153. This also states that the vessel had been ordered from Falmouth 'to Stokes Bay, the place appointed for the performance of Quarantine'. That was apparently a reference to The Motherbank, but as the ship had passed Portsmouth she was heading, it would seem, for Stangate Creek.

to prevent'.[130] The legal issue was that the men had not left their ship deliberately to avoid quarantine, but to save their own lives. As this broke no law, it raised a question as to whether they could forcibly be returned on board. The new Act was to make provision for that and, as regarded the Chichester case, the Privy Council and others acting under their orders were indemnified from any legal process which might otherwise have arisen from their treatment of those on shore.[131]

This indemnity clause gave no comfort to the Privy Council in a wider context. For whatever reason, the Act did not protect against an incident in December 1804 when the Council had illegally extended the quarantine of three ships from Leghorn (the latest place rumoured to have the Malaga–Gibraltar epidemic) by treating them as foul-bill arrivals when their bills of health were clean.[132] It can be deduced that this delay had ruined at least part of the cargoes, which contained a mix of enumerated and non-enumerated goods, and that legal action had already begun. On 2 July 1805 a Bill was presented to the Commons to indemnify the Privy Council and their agents, and stay the proceedings.[133] The Bill raced through Parliament and received royal assent on 10 July.[134]

After that brief deviation to July, it is now necessary to revert to the main quarantine Bill, introduced to the House by George Rose in February. The two reasons which he gave for the Bill have been explained. He might, indeed, have mentioned a third reason which, although it became of no importance, was initially the one that mattered. This was the repeal of the quarantine duties imposed by the Act of 1800. Despite little sign of mercantile dissatisfaction in the records of the Privy Council, there was evidently a lobby protesting either at the rate of the tonnage duties, or the fact that they were levied initially from shipowners rather than importers or consignees. The proof of this is a reference in the Board of Trade minutes, dated 5 February 1805, to a draft Bill for repealing the duties; the Commissioners of Customs were asked to comment on the Bill and arrive at an alternative system which might be incorporated into a Privy Council Order.[135] By then, the Commons in Committee had already considered the question of tonnage duties and had decided, on 1 February, that they should cease.[136] But then the House, for some reason, reversed their decision and the duty payments remained.[137] It was at this point that Rose introduced his Bill, giving the two reasons discussed above.

In most respects, the new quarantine Act differed only marginally from the legislation of 1800. Now, the Privy Council (not the King in Council) were empowered

---

130 Hansard, vol. 3, p. 222.

131 45 Geo. III, c.10, s.25, which contrived to refer to the incident without specifying when and where it had taken place.

132 These facts are known only from the preamble to 45 Geo. III, c.97.

133 *JHC*, vol. 60, p. 458.

134 *JHC*, vol. 60, p. 488; 45 Geo. III, c.97.

135 NA BT 5/15, p. 28.

136 *JHC*, vol. 60, p. 28.

137 This volte-face (if it was one) is evident from the fact that tonnage duties were then immediately resolved upon. But as there was at least one minor textual change (see next paragraph), it is possible that the duties had to be repealed in order to be reintroduced, albeit with the slightest of modifications.

to make Orders in 'any unforeseen Emergency', while pilots were to ask masters where they had loaded cargo or at which ports they had touched on the voyage. This would apply to ships arriving from anywhere in the world. The pilot would then notify the master, if necessary, of the obligation to quarantine. Tonnage duties were unchanged, although the references to Holland and to ports having no regular quarantine establishments were discontinued. The obligation remained for a master to deposit his bill of health, manifest, logbook and journal with the Superintendent of Quarantine, but the elaborate procedure under the 1800 Act, requiring a copy of the manifest to be deposited with the British consul at the port of loading, for independent transmission to England, was no longer required. No doubt this had proved unworkable in years of continuing warfare.

On 5 April 1805, the day when the new quarantine Act became operational, the Privy Council issued a revised General Order of great length.[138] There were few radical departures from the Order of five years earlier. During March they had met with Sir Lucas Pepys to tinker with the definition of enumerated goods of the first class, and they had asked representatives from Trinity House and the Customs Commissioners for advice on wider aspects, especially the enhanced role for pilots and the position of quarantine stations.[139] The latter showed some important changes. Holy Loch, instead of Lamlash, was now confirmed as the station for the Clyde estuary and for ports between Oban and Wigtown. Almost a year earlier, the Privy Council had intimated to the Customs Commissioners in Scotland that they intended to ask the King to agree to the change.[140] Ships bound for ports on the north coasts of Devon and Cornwall, and for places between Llanelly and Aberystwyth, were now to make for Milford Haven, which was also an option for ships bound anywhere further north, as far as the Isle of Man and even Carlisle.[141] The intention was to ease congestion at Hoylake, for Liverpool, where there were still no adequate facilities. Finally, the quarantine stations in the Channel Islands were abandoned, in favour of The Motherbank or Falmouth. This followed confusion at Guernsey as to the authority to release ships once quarantine there had ended.[142]

In designating a new quarantine station at the fine natural harbour of Milford Haven, the Privy Council envisaged an establishment second only to Stangate Creek. As the locality was relatively remote and unpopulated, it is likely that a foul-bill station was being pondered from the outset, although the Order in Council stipulated that all ships without clean bills had to make for Stangate Creek or The Motherbank, depending on their commercial or naval status.[143] But in May 1805 the Privy Council

138 NA PC 2/167/227–68. There is a printed copy in BL at 748.f.13(2).

139 NA PC 2/167/128–9, 139.

140 NA PC 2/165/231.

141 The Customs Commissioners were formally notified of Milford Haven's new status in a rider to a letter of 6 April (NA PC 2/167/292).

142 The confusion centred on whether or not the power to discharge ships under quarantine had been transferred to the Privy Council some ten years earlier at the request of the Lieutenant-Governor. Jersey had been unaffected by this quandary, but there were also fears about the safety of ships at quarantine anchorages in the islands (NA PC 2/164/432–4, 457–60).

143 Order in Council, 5 Apr. 1805, s.4.

convened a meeting with Wyatt, two Commissioners of Customs and two Elder Brethren of Trinity House, to consider a quarantine station near the entrance to the English Channel for ships with foul bills, in lieu of Stangate Creek.[144] The Council had St Just's Pool in mind, and Wyatt was asked whether any of the buildings erected at Chetney Hill could be removed there, and at what cost.[145] With the navy making increased use of Falmouth as a wartime station, this radical idea came to nothing, but it was evidence of the Privy Council's interest in the Western Approaches, and if Falmouth was not suitable for foul-bill quarantine, perhaps Milford Haven was.

During the spring of 1805 the Privy Council requested the Customs Commissioners to recommend what posts and salaries would be necessary for Milford Haven and St Helen's Pool.[146] It took the best part of three months for the Privy Council to reach a decision, based on the Commissioners' report. During that interval they waited for news of progress at Chetney Hill and wondered, it would seem, whether a foul-bill station could be maintained in the Scillies. But in August they reached a decision about the pay and duties of the crew of the revenue cutter *Providence* at St Helen's Pool, which indicated that the establishment at the Scillies would not be expanded.[147] As for Milford Haven, the Commissioners had proposed a Superintendent of Quarantine backed by an assistant, 12 mariners and a boy, based on board a sailing vessel in the harbour.[148] The Superintendent, in their view, should receive £200 per annum, the Assistant £150, and the mariners the usual salary of £18, 5s paid to men on the revenue cruisers, with an extra allowance of 1s, 6d per day when employed on quarantine duty. The boy would receive £10 per annum, plus 6d for every day on duty. Each floating lazaretto stationed there should have a master supported by a mate, two guardians, ten men and a boy. The master was recommended to have a salary of £150 per annum, as against £100 for the mate. The salaries paid to the mariners and boy would be the same as for those in the harbour vessel.

In the event, the Privy Council chose a more complicated scheme.[149] The Superintendent at Milford Haven was to get only £100, paid quarterly, but at the end of each year he would be given 20s for each ship which had performed quarantine. If the total remuneration were still less than £200, the difference would be made up against a certificate of good conduct from the Collector and Comptroller of Customs. The Assistant would receive only £80 paid quarterly, plus 15s per ship, with the same safeguard. As for the floating lazarettos, the Council could not agree that 'guardians' should be appointed anywhere except Stangate Creek, and their duties at Milford Haven and elsewhere could be performed by tidewaiters on a daily rate of pay. The master of each lazaretto would be paid £100, plus 10s for every ship which had passed quarantine; the mate would get £60, plus 7s, 6d per ship. The Commissioners recommended that these establishment and salary levels should

144 NA PC 2/167/464–5.

145 Ibid.

146 NA PC 2/168/193 makes it clear that the Customs Commissioners had responded to this request by early May.

147 NA PC 2/168/256–9.

148 NA PC 2/168/253–6, from which remaining references in this paragraph are taken.

149 Ibid. and PC 2/168/193, from which all references in this paragraph are taken.

apply at all major quarantine stations, and the Privy Council concurred. It was also stipulated that when no ships were performing quarantine, men would be occupied in cruising against smugglers.

The Order of 5 April 1805 produced the most elaborate questionnaires yet devised for ships' masters. The main one contained 26 numbered questions which grew progressively in length, so that towards the end there were several sub-questions to each number.[150] The information required went from the obvious ('Are you the Commander or Master?') to the problematical ('Do you know whether or not your Cargo, or any Part thereof, had been long in Warehouse before its being taken on board?'). As part of Question 8, the master was to be shown a list of enumerated goods of the first class and asked whether any were on board. If they were, he would be asked to specify whether they were 'of the Growth, Produce, or Manufacture' of Turkey, the African coast of the Mediterranean, or West Barbary. He would also be asked whether he had any declarations to prove or disprove his answer. This linked with Section 42 of the Order, which was very much a rehash of the troublesome Section 38 of the Order of 1800.

The main difference in Section 42 was the geographical application. Section 38 had applied to ships carrying enumerated goods of the first class from any place where there was no regular establishment for quarantine. The new wording applied only to ships from Europe outside the Straits, and from the continent of America, again if the port of loading had no recognized lazaretto. The declarations and certificates about whether or not the goods were from Turkey or Barbary in origin, and the information needed about bills of health, stayed the same. There was no mercantile outcry in the months that followed. Beyond a slight contretemps with the Russia Company, as to whether Archangel and the Baltic Russian ports might be exempt from the Section, the Privy Council had a smooth ride.[151] They did, however, extend the scope of the Order to Newfoundland, Cape Breton and other islands off North America.[152] In 1808 the Council met with representatives of the Customs Commissioners to consider abandoning the section in respect of enumerated goods of the first class from Europe outside the Straits.[153] On 8 August 1810 the section as a whole was suspended indefinitely, as long as the master made oath that the port of loading had been free of disease, and the importer or consignee made oath that the goods were not originally from Turkey or Barbary.[154] It was, admitted the Privy Council, just too difficult to insist on paperwork in times of war. No doubt many merchants felt that oaths might have been sufficient all along.

If the 1805 Act had resulted from confused origins, it had also borne the hallmarks of haste and inadequacy. Nothing condemned an Act more than the need for revision a year later. Lord Auckland, President of the Board of Trade, put a brave face on it. He informed Lord Grenville, Prime Minister, about 'final adjustment of a quarantine Bill, which we have prepared with great care and various advice, and which will not

150 Order in Council, 5 Apr. 1805, s.9.
151 NA PC 2/167/557.
152 NA PC 2/168/473.
153 NA PC 2/177/287.
154 NA PC 2/188/393.

have any opposition; Mr. Rose having contributed to it very materially'.[155] Auckland was correct about the non-opposition. On 16 July 1806, after the normal transition through Parliament at breakneck pace, royal assent was given to *An Act for making additional and further Provisions for ... Quarantine in Great Britain.*[156] This brief measure introduced a yellow and black flag, to be hoisted if a ship were actually smitten with plague or any other infectious and dangerous disease. The Act also made the recent legislation more meaningful, by requiring pilots to ask a master not only where he was from but also what cargo his ship was carrying. The pilot would then notify the master of an obligation to quarantine arising from the goods on board, irrespective of the port of loading.[157] It would appear, however, that there was not always the cooperation between pilot and Customs which the law had taken for granted. The amending Act revealed that some pilots and masters were not bringing to for the quarantine officer, so he could begin the formal interrogation. The penalty for this disobedience was a relatively modest fine of £100.

Another purpose of the amending Act was to waive tonnage duty for any ship, not otherwise liable to quarantine, which was detained purely because a person from some other vessel, which *was* liable, had come aboard. It also did away with the written proof of opening and airing of cargoes, and substituted a more simple system relying on oaths. It is not difficult to see, given this change, why the irksome paperwork required for Section 42 was eventually abandoned. But perhaps the most interesting section of the new Act was the power vested in the Privy Council to order ships from America or the West Indies, when yellow fever was prevalent, to 'come to an Anchor at certain Places to be appointed from Time to Time' by the Customs service, so the health of those on board could be checked. In effect, this meant ships could be directed to a quarantine station without necessarily a liability to quarantine. In one sense, this was no more than a regularization of existing practice as the Privy Council, on 18 October 1805, had ordered ships from parts of North America and the West Indies to undergo examination, to ascertain whether they had suffered any illness or death on board in the previous 40 days.[158]

The real breakthrough was that yellow fever was now, for the first time, honoured by a direct mention in quarantine legislation. The remaining sections of the amending Act dealt mainly with punishments for illegal intercourse between ships without clean bills at quarantine stations and the forging of certificates. The penalty for transgressors in the former case was a fine of £500; forgery, on the other hand, merited death as a felon. In a case of perjury, the Act relied on the punishments of subsisting law.

---

155 Historical Manuscripts Commission [HMC], *Fortescue*, vol. 8, p. 202.

156 *JHC*, vol. 61, p. 546; 46 Geo. III, c.98.

157 The Order in Council, 5 Apr. 1805, had made it clear (ss.12–13) that any goods whatsoever which were non-enumerated, and coming out of the Mediterranean or from West Barbary, even in ships with clean bills, would be aired on board for one week.

158 NA PC 2/168/418. The Order had also subjected ships from Pennsylvania and New York to 15 days' quarantine.

John Rennie and Chetney Hill

It will be recalled that in April 1806, on the recommendation of the Board of Health, the Privy Council had agreed to an estimate of costs for building a canal around Chetney Hill. The Commissioners of Customs, charged with finding a suitable 'Surveyor', targeted the engineer John Rennie. They looked forward to working with a more conscientious professional than Wyatt, whose half-hearted efforts at Chetney Hill left a legacy of chaotic accounting. In his official work elsewhere, Wyatt had also been found wanting. Colvin notes that 'as an administrator he was dilatory, negligent and irresponsible'.[159] Had he not enjoyed the support of the King, he might have been dismissed from his post of Surveyor-General and Comptroller of the Office of Works, as he was removed from his office of Deputy Surveyor of the Office of Woods and Forests.[160] As dissatisfaction with Wyatt peaked in 1805, the shambling project at Chetney Hill was evidently a principal factor.

Initially, the Customs Commissioners had some difficulty in getting Rennie to cooperate, as he was too busy to arrange an immediate visit to Chetney Hill.[161] The Privy Council appeared less aware than the Commissioners of Rennie's reputation, and took the delay of two or three weeks with irritation. They wanted to meet Rennie in early May but he was unavailable; by 21 May they were suggesting that Henry Eastburn, a surveyor working near York, should be approached instead.[162] But on 17 June 1806 Rennie sent a thorough letter to Cottrell commenting usefully on many aspects of the Chetney Hill project, and thereby disarmed the critics of his elusiveness.[163] He had contrived to inspect the site on 30 May in company with King and Woolmore, the two Elder Brethren of Trinity House who had suggested the perimeter canal. Rennie complained that no plans or sections for the project, or soundings of the creek, had been available to him, and that he had to send down a surveyor to make them.

Rennie reported that Chetney Hill had been levelled somewhat, and the summit was now about 14 feet above the level of an ordinary spring tide. The clay surface was soft after rain and the drains were incomplete. The marshland to the north and south was 'very low & full of small Creeks & Stagnant Pools of water' which 'in warm weather become very putrid & unhealthy'. The purpose of the canal, therefore, was twofold: it would cut off the connection with the marshes, as well as allowing barges to approach a wet dock at the foot of the hill. These vessels would carry goods from ships in Stangate Creek to the lazaret. The bottom of the canal would be two feet deeper than low water, while the sides would be six feet above high tide. The width of the canal was to be 24 feet. The wet dock would hold six barges, with

159 H.M. Colvin, *A Biographical Dictionary of British Architects, 1660–1840*, 3rd edn (London & New Haven, 1995), under Wyatt.

160 Ibid.

161 NA PC 2/170/42.

162 NA PC 2/170/242. The minute refers to Eastburn as 'a Mr. Eastborne at York'. For Eastburn, see S. Bendall, *Dictionary of Land Surveyors and Local Map-Makers of Great Britain and Ireland, 1530–1850* (2 vols, London, 1997), vol. 2, p. 162.

163 Institution of Civil Engineers [ICE], Rennie MSS, vol. 4, pp. 80–83, from which remaining references in this and the next paragraph are taken.

the water level held steady by lock gates. Granite quays would be 50 feet wide and furnished with iron railway lines rising by a gentle inclined plane to the 'Street', or north–south corridor between the ranges of buildings. This street would itself have railway lines, with branches into each of the warehouses, which would be equipped with cranes for offloading. The hill would need to be covered with a foot of gravel to ensure adequate drainage, a new well was essential, and there were concerns about the boundary wall. The rough estimate for that work was £40,670. Rennie could not be more precise as he lacked the original plans and, more importantly, because the route of the canal was imponderable. The land bought from Wildman amounted to 33 acres, but did not comprise the total extent of the hill. Unless the remaining 21 acres were purchased, the canal would have to be cut through the hill itself. Clearly, the longer route around the base was preferable, and probably no more expensive.

On receipt of this letter, the Privy Council were appalled at the expense, confused and rather angry; Rennie was summoned to an immediate meeting.[164] No strangers to humiliation and climb-down, the Council now faced up to the fact that Cottrell's confident defence of the location for the lazaret, made in his recent protest to the Board of Health and based on decades of complacent assumption, had been ill-judged. As usual in important matters, the Council took their time in making a formal response. Not until 5 July 1806 did they explain their thinking to the Treasury:[165]

> Their Lordships see great Cause to regret that the Situation chosen for the proposed Lazarette and Warehouses should appear by Experience to be liable to Objections so serious as are Stated by the Board of Health, and verified by the subsequent Examinations of the Elder Brethren of the Trinity House, and the Engineers …, and that these Objections should appear capable of no remedy, but at an Expence so serious as is stated in the Report of M^r^. Rennie.

But with so much investment already made at Chetney Hill, and no alternative site being put forward, 'it would not be now advisable to abandon the Works … as the Warehouses now erected are represented to be commodious for the Airing of Goods …'

There was, however, to be one concession to economy. Quarantine by people was to be performed afloat, either in the lazarettos used for airing or in some vessel fitted out for the purpose. Wyatt was to complete the buildings on Chetney Hill for the purpose originally intended, that is for airing goods, 'and to desist from carrying into Effect any further Part of the Plan or Building originally proposed for the reception of Persons'. As for the canal, the Commissioners of Customs were to ask Rennie to proceed, but on a limited scale. The canal would only be long enough to allow entry to the wet dock from the Creek, and the remainder of the site would be edged simply by a ditch to provide drainage and isolation. As there was no talk at this stage of asking Parliament for more money, it was hoped that the limitation to

164 NA PC 2/170/392. In fact, the meeting was asked for on 16 June, the day before Rennie wrote to Cottrell.

165 NA PC 2/170/552–5, from which remaining references in this and the next paragraph are taken unless otherwise stated.

Wyatt's work would roughly balance the extra costs envisaged by Rennie.[166] But the Commissioners were, at the same time, to treat for more land at the top of the hill and provide statistics of income and costs over the previous four years.[167]

Rennie was suspicious from the outset about the tenders for the new works. He wrote to the Commissioners of Customs on 2 September 1806, explaining that 'they appear so very various, that one would be apt to think many of the Offerers either mean to supply very bad Materials, or to do their work imperfectly, or that they have not viewed the Premises so as to enable them to judge what they are to do.'[168] Conscious of the sensitivity of the Privy Council to spiralling costs, he wrote a few days later to Cottrell, warning him that some thick layer of gravel or chalk was indispensable for the summit of the hill, and the cost would approach £5,000, a sum not to be deleted from his estimate.[169] Another worry for Rennie was the appointment of a superintendent of the works, as his own commitments countrywide left him no opportunity to monitor progress even from week to week. The obvious choice was William Pilkington, already Surveyor to the Commissioners of Customs, but he declined to take it on.[170] Rennie then recommended John Timperley, who had proved himself at London Docks, but he would not be responsible for Timperley's work: 'neither my Character nor Property', he told the Commissioners, 'shall depend on the actions of any other Person than myself'.[171]

On 29 September 1806 Rennie met Timperley at Chetney Hill and became anxious that he might be dragged into the architectural aspect of the project, as well as the engineering.[172] Wyatt's work, despite the wish of the Privy Council that he should complete the warehouses, was progressing slowly, if at all. Rennie noted that there was much still to do, including sewers, water tanks and surrounding walls. Only one painter was at work on the warehouses, yet another seven of them needed attention. Rennie wanted all these jobs finished as soon as possible as their non-completion would interfere with the engineering. He had already slightly exceeded his brief by ordering a temporary platform at the edge of the Creek to facilitate the unloading of even the most basic commodities. And underlying all these concerns was the greater worry that James Wildman was failing to cooperate. Indeed, he was being positively obstructive, by asking his steward to spy on the work. Rennie sensed that Wildman

166 In April 1806 the Privy Council had mentioned that the Treasury might be able to 'report' new costs to Parliament (NA PC 2/169/486).

167 In a letter, 7 August 1806 (ICE Rennie MSS, vol. 4, p. 97), to William Pilkington, Rennie stated that the acquisition of more land had been recommended by the Board of Trade. This is one of several references by him to the Board's involvement with Chetney Hill, but they are not borne out by their minute books.

168 ICE Rennie MSS, vol. 4, pp. 99–102.

169 ICE Rennie MSS, vol. 4, pp. 110–11. He estimated 14,000 tons of gravel would be needed.

170 ICE Rennie MSS, vol. 4, p. 121.

171 Ibid. For the identity of Timperley, sometimes confused with Temperley (who was another civil engineer), see A.W. Skempton, *A Biographical Dictionary of Civil Engineers in Great Britain and Ireland, vol 1: 1500–1830* (London, 2002), pp. 566, 708.

172 ICE Rennie MSS, vol. 4, pp. 167–8, from which all references in this paragraph are taken.

was trying to stop it altogether and reported to the Commissioners that he 'seems extremely unreasonable'. The contractors were ordered 'to proceed in defiance of him', but Rennie feared that yet another Act of Parliament might be needed to bring about a compulsory purchase.

The Privy Council appear to have revoked their earlier, irritable decision that the canal around most of the hill should be replaced by a ditch.[173] It was now to encircle it. The obstacle, however, was still Wildman, whose stubbornness meant the canal could not be realized in its logical position, as a simple cut around the perimeter. The sale of more acres was urgently needed to complete the project, but Wildman rebuffed every attempt to negotiate by imposing bizarre and impossible conditions. He now wanted a 30-foot wall between the lazaret and his own land, for sanitary reasons. Rennie explained to the Commissioners that this would not prevent infection (an indication, perhaps, that he was a non-contagionist), and the cost would be £13,800. It would be better, advised Rennie, to give him a sum approaching that figure in compensation and forget about the wall.

With negotiations by the Treasury and Board of Trade failing to achieve their object, the Privy Council resolved to tackle the problem themselves. On 30 June 1807 Fawkener wrote to James Wildman.[174] It is intriguing that the task was not visited upon Cottrell, whose style could be blunt. Fawkener's letter was little short of grovelling, pleading for Wildman to sell another eight or nine acres, as the project was in difficulty from causes unforeseen at the time of the original purchase. No reference was made to public health, national interest or patriotic duty. When Wildman ignored this letter, Fawkener wrote again on 10 July.[175] The Privy Council were prepared to offer him the same price per acre as before, with half that sum for every acre which would be covered by earth from the excavations. If the freshwater pond on Wildman's land dried up when the canal was cut, the Council undertook to create a new one. Then came the gentlest of threats. Would Wildman please reply by the 16th, the latest date on which the Council could arrange for a parliamentary Bill to vest the land in the Crown. In fact, Wildman replied by return, but only to ask for more money.[176] Fawkener responded by questioning the circumstances which had allegedly increased the value of the land, and asking for Wildman's final price.[177] Again, there appears to have been no reply. On 10 August 1807 Fawkener wrote a final polite letter, regretting Wildman's intransigence.[178] Parliament would be asked to consider a Bill for the compulsory purchase, at a fair price to be arrived at by valuation. That smacked of bluff, especially as the Act did not materialize. But Rennie, on 7 September, was still under the impression that a parliamentary Bill

173 ICE Rennie MSS, vol. 4, pp. 274–5,348, from which all references in this paragraph are taken.

174 NA PC 2/173/202.

175 NA PC 2/173/235.

176 Wildman's letter has not survived, but was evidently dated 12 July.

177 NA PC 2/173/281.

178 NA PC 2/173/464.

was in hand.[179] Backed by the Commissioners of Customs, he had argued for such a measure at a meeting of the Board of Trade.[180]

The absence of a Bill can be explained by the weariness of an impotent Privy Council and the distraction of natural disasters. On 1 October 1807 the exact anniversary of the beginning of engineering work, the incipient canal was overrun by a tide which Rennie called too high and too early.[181] Even this ill-omened setback he partly ascribed to Wildman's 'obstinacy', but the major contributing factor was sickness among the workforce.[182] A chronic and worrying disease had led to a shortage of manpower, resulting in the canal walls being too low. News of the illness had reached the Privy Council on 10 September, when they asked the Commissioners of Customs to send an eminent physician to investigate.[183] This was Dr Newberry, who had medical responsibility for the quarantine station in Stangate Creek. Before they received Newberry's diagnosis, the Council sent him a pamphlet on typhus fever.[184] Their unexpected familiarity with this condition was not explained, but there were mysterious and rather troubling diseases breaking out in such disparate places as Walcheren, Memel, Flushing and Folkestone, which brought home to the Council that they no longer had a Board of Health to fall back on.[185] On 14 September 1807 the Council were relieved to learn from Newberry's report that there was 'nothing peculiar' in the disease, which was also affecting nearby villages.[186] But six people had died, and Newberry was short of medicine.[187] The Privy Council ordered new supplies and port wine for the afflicted.[188]

The epidemic was distinctly more worrying to Rennie than it was to Newberry. Towards the end of the summer 'very few hands were able to work & scarcely any could be induced to go to a place where so Contagious a distemper raged with such violence'.[189] This meant that wages had to rise to 7s per day, with appropriate inducements for the gang masters who sought out the labour.[190] Timperley reported to Customs that out of more than 100 men on the site, only 30 to 40 were fit at any one time.[191] But Rennie battled on, turning his thoughts to other aspects of the project while the canal workings lay waterlogged. The flooding might have been pumped out by a steam engine, but he thought the slower alternative of an Archimedean screw

179 ICE Rennie MSS, vol. 4, pp. 390–91.

180 Ibid. The Board of Trade minute books are silent.

181 ICE Rennie MSS, vol. 5, pp. 24–7.

182 Ibid.

183 NA PC 2/174/56.

184 NA PC 2/174/119.

185 NA PC 2/174/124, 166, 318.

186 NA PC 2/174/69.

187 Ibid.; P. Froggatt, 'The Chetney Hill lazaret', *Archaeologia Cantiana*, 79 (1964), 13, refers to the burial of eight strangers in Iwade (the parish which included Chetney Hill) in 1806–7.

188 NA PC 2/174/171.

189 ICE Rennie MSS, vol. 5, pp. 24–7.

190 H.M. Colvin (ed.), *The History of the King's Works* (6 vols, London, 1963–82), vol. 6, p. 450.

191 ICE Rennie MSS, vol. 6, pp. 419–22.

would be adequate.[192] He understood that 20 beds had been ordered for the lazaret in addition to the 12 already there, plus 'an attentive Watchman' against fire. This man would be aided by 'an extinguishing Engine' and this time Rennie championed the cause of steam. If the appliance were a small four-horsepower engine, it would serve generally to pump water from the well, while it could also fight a fire in the lazaret if iron pipes were extended to each warehouse. But the cost, he warned, would be around £650.[193]

For much of the winter of 1807–8, the land around Chetney Hill remained under water and the half-finished works deteriorated. The excavation of the canal restarted tentatively on 11 January, but Rennie warned that more resources were needed to keep out the tide or the project would 'go to ruin'.[194] He still blamed Wildman for much of the problem and foresaw no real progress without an agreement. At the end of February Rennie's patience failed, and he wrote direct to Fawkener urging the Privy Council to intervene.[195] He explained that when he had set out his problems to the Commissioners of Customs he had been simply referred to the Board of Trade. Rennie needed more money for the project and some progress with Wildman. Failing both, he wanted to know what more he could do. 'I shall wait with impatience', he concluded, 'for their Lordships instructions'.[196]

But their lordships had no instructions. Rennie wrote again in late March 1808, warning that he would have no option but to lay off the workforce unless Wildman cooperated very quickly.[197] By chance, Wildman had written to the Treasury on the previous day, stating that if certain stipulations were met, he would sell the extra land for £3,750.[198] In guidance to the Treasury, the Privy Council suggested £4,000 should be offered for a sale with no strings attached, beyond an agreement for a supply of fresh water for cattle on the nearby marshes.[199] That sum, they pointed out, was much more than the land was worth. If Wildman were to reject this, the Treasury should consider a parliamentary Bill for compulsory purchase, or they could abandon the idea of acquiring more land, and cut the canal through the hill, according to an option originally proposed by Rennie.[200] There was no question of the project being abandoned.

Somehow the impasse was broken as, on 30 April 1808, a meeting on site took place between Rennie and Wildman.[201] Discussion centred on the canal and the disposal of excavated soil, which Wildman refused to have spread on his part of

---

192 ICE Rennie MSS, vol. 5, pp. 24–7.

193 Ibid.

194 ICE Rennie MSS, vol. 5, p. 120; vol. 6, pp. 419–22.

195 ICE Rennie MSS, vol. 5, p. 120.

196 Ibid.

197 NA PC 2/176/194. On 16 March, Rennie had also written to the Customs Commissioners, asking them to urge the Privy Council to come to terms with Wildman (ICE Rennie MSS, vol. 5, p. 118).

198 NA PC 2/176/227.

199 Ibid.

200 Ibid.

201 ICE Rennie MSS, vol. 5, p. 175.

the hill, except as an embankment against the tide.[202] In the end, however, Rennie negotiated an agreement more favourable than he had expected, which allowed the spoil to be spread over Wildman's land to the north and south, with stipulations as to the height and slope of the mounds.[203] But relief that engineering could soon restart was tempered by a bill for more than £1,500 from Hugh McIntosh, the main contractor, for losses allegedly sustained in the long delay.[204] Rennie saw merit in certain aspects of the claim and recommended an urgent payment of £1,005, as Wildman was expected to sign a new deed very shortly.[205] But with work poised to begin on 13 June 1808, Wildman made further demands.[206] The spoil was now to be deposited rather differently and covered in nine inches of topsoil or mould. There was also a request for a new wall.

Over the next four months Rennie and the Treasury persisted in exasperating and inconclusive negotiations with Wildman, while the canal made desultory progress. By the end of October 1808 Rennie was shown the draft of a new deed and expressed his concerns about the implicit costs, especially in supplying all the fresh water which Wildman demanded, and in erecting the eight-foot wall, coped in brick, which was now to encircle the hill.[207] As if his own worries were not enough, Rennie was soon being asked to certify bills submitted for work on the lazaret itself, although the buildings themselves were not within his brief. On 21 February 1809 he had this task transferred to John Sale, Wyatt's clerk of the works, recognizing that 'To Mr. Wyatt it is vain to make any application'.[208] Indeed it was, as Wyatt's financial disarray was now the subject of an inquiry, set up by the Treasury and led by the architect, George Saunders.[209]

In the spring of 1810 Parliament became involved for the last time in the Chetney Hill project, but not to the extent, or in the direction, which might have been expected. There was no involvement in the purchase of land from Wildman. Instead the House endured a reading of the 1805 quarantine Act, simply to agree that a Bill might be introduced so that the Treasury could appoint a Superintendent of Quarantine at places other than Chetney Hill.[210] The Act had not made provision for these appointments at any other quarantine station – a further indication of its hasty and careless composition. But on 30 April, some three weeks after royal assent for the brief new Act, the House was presented with an estimate of the money needed to satisfy outstanding claims for work on the lazaret.[211] Parliament did not demur and a grant of £21,000 to the Crown was made on 3 May 1810 from the

202 Ibid.

203 Ibid.

204 ICE Rennie MSS, vol. 5, pp. 210–11.

205 ICE Rennie MSS, vol. 5, pp. 212–13.

206 ICE Rennie MSS, vol. 5, pp. 219–21.

207 ICE Rennie MSS, vol. 5, pp. 294–5. The wall would cost £2,900 if continued around the land-edged perimeter.

208 ICE Rennie MSS, vol 5, p. 363.

209 Colvin, *Biographical Dictionary of British Architects*, under Saunders.

210 *JHC*, vol. 65, p. 178. The new Act was 50 Geo. III, c.20.

211 *JHC*, vol. 65, pp. 310, 581.

Consolidated Fund.[212] The project had now been voted a total of £116,000 of public money. Wyatt's total expenditure on the project was around £110,000 according to one parliamentary committee, but another found that he and later Saunders had been allocated the full sum.[213] This left nothing in the budget for Rennie whose initial estimate, it will be remembered, had been over £40,000. And since then, Wildman's demands had greatly increased Rennie's necessary spending. In 1811 quarantine was again before Parliament, but only to remedy yet another omission from the 1805 Act, which had not sanctioned Customs' officers to take the place of a Superintendent of Quarantine or his deputy who happened to be absent from his post.[214]

When Parliament had agreed the new funds, the Treasury asked Timperley for a progress report with detailed accounts. In October 1810 this document was passed to Rennie for his observations.[215] Timperley recounted in full the dismal sequence of events from 1 October 1806, when the work had begun. The uncertainties, chiefly occasioned by Wildman, had not only delayed the project but undermined morale. The fourth year of engineering 'was not begun upon with much more spirit than formerly …' There were never more than 50 men and 18 horses on site, and only half those numbers were present at the time when he was writing. Timperley shared Rennie's reluctance to become involved in the building of the warehouses, and the associated works, which he described as 'a separate Department'. He could only report generally that little extra had been done to the eight buildings erected, although some plumbing and joinery had been completed in the two originally intended to be fitted out for passengers. Another ten warehouses were destined to be built, as well as quarters for those in the quarantine service.

On 23 December 1811 Rennie submitted to the Commissioners of Customs a thorough and supportive appraisal of Timperley's report and accounts.[216] He explained also that Timperley had been ill for some time, and that he himself had met with a recent accident, both of which events had done nothing to advance the project. Rennie picked up on his own first estimate for engineering work, made with a lot of guesswork over five years earlier, and then repeated a series of further estimates by which a sum of under £41,000 had risen to over £55,000. Figures of actual expenditure, when set against the estimates, revealed an overspend of only £90, a near-balance of which Rennie was obviously proud.

212 *JHC*, vol. 65, p. 322.

213 Colvin (*History of the King's Works*, vol. 6, p. 449), citing a parliamentary public expenditure committee of 1810, quotes Wyatt's total expenditure at around £110,000. Froggatt, 'The Chetney Hill lazaret', 13–14, quoting NA AO 1/2499/434, puts the expenditure by Wyatt at £95,000 between 1801 and 1806; *Second Report … Quarantine* (1824), p. 110, lists the same figures as Froggatt, but adds £21,000 for 16 July 1810, being the sum required by Saunders 'to satisfy outstanding claims, on account of works executed at the lazaretto on Chetney Hill'. That makes the full £116,000.

214 The oversight was remedied by 51 Geo. III, c.46 (royal assent 31 May 1811).

215 ICE Rennie MSS, vol. 6, pp. 419–22, from which all references in this paragraph are taken.

216 ICE Rennie MSS, vol. 6, pp. 423–6, from which all references in this paragraph are taken.

For much of 1812, the work went along more steadily than at any time previously. On 6 August, Rennie announced to the Commissioners of Customs that the canal would be completed in two or three weeks, and the time was right for contractors to be chosen for the perimeter wall (to be ten feet high and coped with stone), the iron railways and stone blocks.[217] Now it was the turn of the Commissioners, doubtless worried about funding, to drag their feet. On 6 February 1813 a surprisingly patient Rennie reminded them that these tenders were outstanding, but if the contracts were placed in the spring, he foresaw no reason why all the works at Chetney Hill within his 'Department' should not be completed in the summer.[218] Rennie was on site on 9 and 10 September, and reported to the Commissioners on the 13th that the canal was virtually finished, all the gravel was spread, and most of the top of the hill (which was now evidently Government property) had been 'levelled and trimmed'.[219] But now there were other complications. Some of the dockside had slipped, leading to another month's work; also, a new 'expert' had arrived in the form of William Pym, who now, for the first time, began to influence Government in matters of public health.[220]

Pym was lately arrived from Malta, where he had served briefly as Superintendent of Quarantine, having been promoted out of Gibraltar.[221] Returning to England as a half-pay Deputy Inspector of Hospitals, he had no particular standing, but any doctor with experience of a Mediterranean lazaretto, especially one under British control, was valued by the Privy Council. Pym had also, of course, gained some useful knowledge of the infamous Gibraltar fever. It is not, however, clear by what authority he was in a position to recommend seven cranes for the dock basin at Chetney Hill.[222] The final stages of the project were now a matter for Rennie, Pym and David Laing, surveyor to the Commissioners of Customs. Laing wanted the railway system extended to the end of the warehouses, and Pym argued for the perimeter wall of the lazaret (as distinct from the wall dividing Government land from Wildman's) to be 18 or 20 feet high and within the canal.[223] Rennie did not dissent from most of this, but he did think the wall should be outside the canal, and he warned it would cost £11,500 if 20 feet high.[224] There were also formidable expenses to be incurred by the railway system and the seven cranes.[225]

On 7 December 1813 Rennie met Pym on site, but some disagreement lingered about the wall.[226] It seems likely that such a large, long structure was never even

217 ICE Rennie MSS, vol. 7, p. 126.

218 ICE Rennie MSS, vol. 7, p. 259.

219 ICE Rennie MSS, vol. 7. p. 314.

220 Ibid.; Rennie MSS, vol. 7, pp. 329–30.

221 W. Johnston, *Roll of Commissioned Officers in the Medical Service of the British Army* ... (Aberdeen, 1917), p. 78.

222 ICE Rennie MSS, vol. 7, pp. 329–30. Rennie had specified six cranes (cf. Colvin, *History of the King's Works*, vol. 6, p. 449).

223 Ibid.

224 Ibid.

225 Ibid. Rennie reckoned other remaining work, including the seven cranes, would cost £19,650.

226 ICE Rennie MSS, vol. 7, pp. 362–3.

started. It was certainly not regarded by Rennie as a matter for him, as he reported to the Commissioners of Customs that the only expense remaining within his purview concerned the seven cranes. The rest of the works, he wrote, lay 'within the department of the Architect'.[227] Who the architect was at that juncture is not clear. The railway lines, which Pym wanted reduced in number but increased in length, would cost another £5,850.[228] Although Rennie was distancing himself from the installation of the rails, he was happy both to estimate the expense and to remind the Commissioners, yet again, that they needed to enter into contracts for the supply.[229] It would seem they never did. During 1814 virtually nothing was done at Chetney Hill. On 31 May 1815 Rennie reported that: 'The original plan has never been completed & of course several parts are now in an unfinished state and therefore unless looked after will get much injury particularly the Entrances of the Canal into Standgate Creek'.[230] During 1816 work continued fitfully – Rennie insisted that Timperley should not be allowed to leave the site – but much of the correspondence was about past misfortunes, not least the chronic illness which still seemed to be a jinx on the site.[231] Workmen and their families who initially recovered 'were a long time in a very weak and feeble state', and many died prematurely.[232] In the spring of 1818 Chetney Hill was finally abandoned by its workforce, but for ten years previously the Privy Council had taken little or no cognizance of what was, or was not, being done there.[233] Pym claimed later that the Privy Council had sent him down to examine it, but if so they asked for no formal report.[234] As the expenses had mounted, it had become unthinkable to ask Parliament for yet more money. Only the Commissioners of Customs, the unwilling arm of a disenchanted Treasury, were exercising a half-hearted control. It was, therefore, from their own tight budget that a further and final sum of £55,000 was at some point made available to keep alive a project of which the Commissioners, as much as any other body, were utterly sick.[235]

In around 1820 the lazaret at Chetney Hill, such as it was, was demolished. Today very little remains of this once vast project, except the rough line of the perimeter canal and wet dock.[236] It is difficult to be definite about the date of demolition, and Froggatt and Colvin disagree. The main source for both is the *Second Report from the Select Committee Appointed to Consider ... Foreign Trade*, which took evidence concerning quarantine in the spring of 1824. The *Report*, in its preamble, referred to the lazaret as having been 'abandoned, and the materials disposed of by order of Government', but did not clarify when.[237] In an appendix, the *Report* indicated that

227 Ibid.

228 Ibid.

229 ICE Rennie MSS, vol. 7, pp. 401–2.

230 ICE Rennie MSS, vol. 8, p. 324.

231 ICE Rennie MSS, vol. 8, pp. 321, 383–4.

232 ICE Rennie MSS, vol. 8, pp. 383–4.

233 See Colvin, *History of the King's Works*, vol. 6, p. 450, for labourers leaving site.

234 *Second Report ... Quarantine* (1824), p. 68.

235 *Second Report ... Quarantine* (1824), p. 4.

236 Froggatt, 'The Chetney Hill lazaret', has two plates of Chetney Hill, one an aerial photograph showing foundations of buildings.

237 *Second Report ... Quarantine* (1824), p. 4.

this disposal took place by public sale and raised over £15,000.[238] One buyer was Henry Peto, who had contracted to build the Custom House in London and acquired materials valued at £1,592, 13s, 6d, a sum which was debited to his account with Government.[239] The rest of the proceeds (bar some £400 in auctioneer's commission) augmented quarantine duties.[240] The *Report* did not specify in what year the sale took place, but Maclean, who had a personal recollection of events, stated that advertisements for the public sale were placed in 1819.[241] Froggatt, based on his knowledge of how Peto's contract progressed, believed the sale had taken place in 1815.[242] He was not, however, aware of Rennie's involvement at Chetney Hill, where it has been shown that work continued into 1818. In any case, Froggatt did not make an association between the sale of materials and the dismantling of the lazaret, and he put the date for the final abandonment as between 1820 and 1824.[243]

Colvin stated categorically that the lazaret was demolished in 1820, and although this might be a little too exact, it seems reasonable to agree with his assumption that the sale of materials arose from actual demolition, rather than the disposal of an unused stock, which Froggatt's argument seems to predicate.[244] Unfortunately, one man who must have witnessed the demolition had a rather weak memory. On 6 April 1824 Charles Sanders, Superintendent of Quarantine at Stangate Creek, was specifically asked by the Select Committee: 'When were the works at Chetney Hill pulled down?' His reply, 'I think three or four years ago', was a curiously vague response from a man who had been working nearby for the previous 14 years.[245] It would appear impossible, at this remove, to be any more precise.

Sanders also confirmed, in his evidence, that the lazaret had never been completed.[246] It is unlikely that any more than eight or perhaps ten warehouses, essentially wooden structures perhaps with ancillary buildings, were erected on the hilltop, but Rennie appears to have finished the canal and the wet dock. It is a moot point whether the cranes and railway lines were ever installed; the stones lining the quayside were presumably among items taken by Peto for recycling in London. Leaving aside the medical issue of whether a lazaret was a sound idea, the impression from these few facts and assumptions, reinforced by the narrative of incompetence and procrastination, is that the whole Chetney Hill project was an expensive white elephant, and that its passing was a cause for celebration, and long overdue. There are, however, two considerations which argue otherwise. The first is an eyewitness account by Robert Semple, a seasoned traveller, of his experience when in quarantine at Stangate Creek, late in 1806, on arrival from the

238 *Second Report ... Quarantine* (1824), p. 4.

239 Ibid.

240 Ibid.

241 Maclean, *Remarks on the British Quarantine laws*, p. 18.

242 Froggatt, 'The Chetney Hill lazaret', 12.

243 Ibid.

244 Colvin, *History of the King's Works*, vol. 6, p. 450.

245 *Second Report ... Quarantine* (1824), pp. 41, 58.

246 *Second Report ... Quarantine* (1824), p. 58.

Mediterranean.[247] Semple reckoned the floating lazarettos were quite adequate for England, and he thought the idea to build on land was misguided. Nevertheless, he noted the plan to build 'a magnificent and extensive building now nearly completed, at the head of the Creek. It forms, indeed, a striking object in the middle of the flats and marshes with which it is surrounded …'[248] Semple was no stranger to lazarettos, especially at Leghorn, and his words cannot be disregarded.

It can be counter-argued, however, that the magnificence and extensiveness lay more in the proposal than in reality, and what Semple actually witnessed was 'striking' only from the contrast between flat, featureless marshland and a conical hill with buildings on top. But that viewpoint does not do justice to the concept. As soon as the project had entered its engineering stage, that is to say once Rennie had been appointed, the scheme was nothing less than spectacular. Chetney Hill came within an ace of being the most remarkable institution of its kind which Europe had produced. No other Mediterranean lazaretto, during the French Wars, had a basin controlled by lock gates, or cast-iron cranes, or an incline plane between levels, or a railway system to connect the dockside with the farthest warehouse. No other lazaretto in 1807 had a four-horsepower steam engine to pump water and fight fire. In other ways, of course, the project was lacking. The provision for passengers was aborted, and even if they could have been accommodated they would have had no exercise yard, chapel or onshore infirmary. It is also not at all clear what facilities, if any, would have existed on land for staff and guards. The lazaret might also have been inefficient, as there was little discussion about separating the aired goods from those newly arrived. But as a product of the Industrial Revolution, as a mechanized solution to a commercial problem involving ships, goods and changes of level, Chetney Hill would have had no equal. At Leghorn, Marseilles, Venice and the rest, no institution was so timeless, so immutable, so steeped in the customs and procedures of reactionary thought, than the lazaretto. If England did not quite produce her maritime wonder, she at least had shown the perspicacity to plan it by the latest technology.

What went wrong?

In 1824 the Select Committee of Parliament concluded that the situation for the land lazaret 'had been injudiciously selected'.[249] In fact, they had not gone into the question at all deeply. Sanders, for instance, had not been asked *why* the buildings had been abandoned, although the Committee did raise that point with Pym. He gave three reasons: the position was 'on the most unhealthy spot in England'; it would have taken great expense to complete it; and following peace with France, there were surplus warships to use as floating lazarettos.[250] The health issue had also been referred to by another witness, who called the location 'insalubrious', while a third

247 R. Semple, *Observations on a Journey through Spain and Italy to Naples* … (2 vols, London, 1808), vol. 2, p. 238.

248 Ibid.

249 *Second Report … Quarantine* (1824), p. 4.

250 *Second Report* … Quarantine (1824), p. 68.

(in answer to the question 'Do you know anything of the lazarette at Chetney Hill?') felt the ground had been 'so marshy, that they could not get a foundation, or attempt to erect a superstructure upon it ...'[251] The Committee did not attempt to establish how the huge funding for the project had been spent, or what occasioned such an inordinate delay once the money was in place. The name Wildman did not arise.

Colvin believed construction on the site stopped 'because all parties had lost faith in the value of the project'.[252] Froggatt went into the reasons more extensively.[253] In the first place, he argued that with a quarantine service becoming ever more costly to Government, they wished to avoid ongoing expenses, especially if the lazaret might not be needed in the future. 'There was growing popular distaste for international quarantine and a weakening in its enforcement on the Continent'. Froggatt also argued that anti-contagionism was growing, with its implicit scepticism that quarantine was effective. He then adduced Pym's argument, supported by one from Maclean, that the site was inherently unhealthy. But the main reason for the failure of the project, according to Froggatt, was the practical difficulty of laying foundations, to which one witness had alluded in his testimony to the Select Committee. Before these thoughts are analysed, notice must again be taken of Maclean, but from a work not quoted by Froggatt. He claimed credit himself for the abandonment of the project, having 'proved the absurdity of the doctrine of contagion before a committee of the House of Commons ...'[254] That, of course, fits neatly with Froggatt's third argument, about the strength of anti-contagionism.

The Select Committee to which Maclean referred sat in 1819 'to consider the validity of the doctrine of Contagion in the Plague'. It was typical of Maclean's bombastic prose that he should see success in failure. He had not 'proved' anti-contagionism to the satisfaction of the Committee, who heard many arguments for and against and reached a decision that the plague was contagious.[255] Maclean was, therefore, non-instrumental in the decision to demolish the lazaret. Whether or not the growing undercurrent of anti-contagionism was strong enough to persuade Government to abandon a project on the brink of completion is another matter. To a limited extent, it must have introduced doubts in some ministers' minds about the value of what they were doing. But whatever seeds of dissension were germinating in Britain, it must be remembered that Europe as a whole was still fiercely contagionist. It will be seen later how the plague in Malta, of 1813, had terrified the Boards of Health in France and Italy. Froggatt's suggestion that quarantine in Europe was weakening is questionable, and in England the Privy Council remained convinced of the need. Even without that conviction, it would have been commercial suicide to abandon the lazaret simply because quarantine against the plague was suddenly considered unnecessary. British shipping would have been punished by inordinate detention in the Mediterranean lazarettos where the principles of contagion and

251 *Second Report* ... Quarantine (1824), pp. 17, 39–40.

252 Colvin, *History of the King's Works*, vol. 6, p. 450.

253 Froggatt, 'The Chetney Hill lazaret', 11–12.

254 Maclean, *Remarks on the British Quarantine laws*, p. 18.

255 *Report from the Select Committee Appointed to consider the validity of the doctrine of Contagion in the Plague* (London, 1819), p. 3.

quarantine were staunchly defended. The Government were eventually to learn that a unilateralist approach in quarantine was a dangerous policy.

The argument that the site of the lazaret was too marshy for adequate foundations, was the one by which Froggatt set most store. The allegation had been made to the Select Committee of 1824 by a shipbroker, presumably a Londoner, but it must be questioned how much he knew about it.[256] It will be recalled that Pym did not include this problem among the three reasons he gave for the scheme being abandoned. The concept that marshland was unstable for building is readily grasped, but there appears to be little evidence of a significant problem in the context of Chetney Hill. For one thing, it was indeed a hill, and although of no great altitude the soil, according to Rennie, was clay. There was certainly a difficulty in making the hilltop drain, which is why Rennie advised a foot of gravel or chalk, but not because the ground was marshy. When the surrounding areas were so waterlogged that work could not continue, this was due to an influx of the tide, caused by a breached embankment, not by normal conditions. In his many letters and reports, Rennie does not complain that the land would not support buildings. True, the warehouses were not within his 'department', as he liked to call it, but the unsuitability of the ground would have been a wonderful excuse for Wyatt, had it been a factor.

That the marshland was unhealthy can be readily conceded, and this realization seriously undermined confidence in the suitability of the site. The hill was too low to escape the damp, stagnant air of the hinterland. This thought was not lost on Semple who, despite his admiration for the quality of the lazaret, noted that the surrounding marshes, 'if placed in the climate where plague originates, would soon convert it truly into a pest house'.[257] There was nothing new about such forecasts. In 1721 a pamphleteer had warned that Stangate Creek 'is the most improper of any [site] they could chuse, being in a low unhealthy Air, apt to breed Agues and Fevers, and therefore unfit for People that come from Sea to lie forty Days in'.[258] Yet the Privy Council, in 1806, had been almost offended and certainly surprised, when the Board of Health were so adamant that the site was unhealthy. Undoubtedly, the incidence of death and disease among construction workers and their families would have brought home the dangers to the Council and to Government. This was probably a factor, along with cost, which influenced the decision that the passenger quarters on Chetney Hill were to be discontinued. Quarantine was thought more healthy at sea than on marshes. But there was no school of thought to argue that Chetney Hill was unsuitable for airing goods suspected of harbouring Levantine plague. To suggest that the site was abandoned simply because it was unhealthy for people presupposes that Government were more concerned about the health risks to quarantine staff than the prevention of plague in London. There is nothing to support that. If the Chetney

256 Froggatt, 'The Chetney Hill lazaret', 12, believed the evidence was from Mr Levy, a merchant. The *Second Report … Quarantine* (1824), pp. 39–40, does not make it perfectly clear whether Levy or John Maude, a shipbroker, was speaking at the time, but there is a stronger case from the minutes for Maude.

257 Semple, vol. 2, p. 238.

258 *A Letter to a Friend from a Merchant who had Resided many Years at Leghorn …* (London, 1721), p. 19

Hill project were to be abandoned altogether because of the health risks, that would surely have occurred in 1807 when the deaths were at their height.

Mounting costs for the quarantine service were, as Froggatt suggests, a major reason why the project failed. Figures for income and expenditure will be examined later in this study, but it may be remarked at this stage that in any one year quarantine income was usually well below, and even less than half, the sum expended on the service in the country as a whole. The statistics produced by the Receiver General in 1824 showed that the Customs service were unable to answer in any meaningful way how far quarantine duties had been able to recoup the £116,000 granted to the Chetney Hill project from the Consolidated Fund.[259] When these ongoing costs are seen against the backdrop, described by Pym, of the sudden availability of redundant warships as airing hulks, then the abandonment of the lazaret begins to make sense. What Pym did not mention, however, was another advantage of the end of the French Wars, namely that the main Mediterranean lazarettos, so long out of bounds for British shipping, were now re-available for foul-bill quarantine. Indeed, the lazaretto on Malta was British-owned. Also, the destination of that shipping was another significant factor to doom the project at Chetney Hill. Much has been said in this study of the rivalry between the north-west and London, and the establishment of Milford Haven as a quarantine station signalled acceptance by the Privy Council that the cargoes deemed most susceptible to spreading infection – Levantine cotton – were now as likely to be bound for Liverpool as for London. That had not been the case in 1805, when Cottrell was responding to the Board of Health.

In around 1818, therefore, a picture emerges of a seemingly endless project, dogged by natural disasters, blighted initially by professional incompetence, drawn out beyond the patience of the Privy Council, pulling for ever on the purse strings of the Treasury, and stretching into an era when the danger it was designed to meet was heading in another direction. It made no logic to continue. Behind all these reasons was the procrastination of James Wildman who had been a self-centred nuisance over 25 years. Given a landowner with a better disposition, the land lazaret would have been completed many years earlier at a fraction of the cost, even allowing for Wyatt's mismanagement. If there were several factors which contributed to the abandonment of the lazaret, there was only one underlying reason why it had never been allowed to fulfil its role. That reason was James Wildman. Any foreign commentator, especially one conversant with quarantine in the Mediterranean, would have found his stranglehold bewildering and ridiculous. It was an indictment of the peculiarly English system of democracy which allowed the intransigence of an individual to delay indefinitely a scheme to protect the health of a nation. Wildman was a member of the county gentry – indeed he had been a High Sheriff of Kent – but he was not an aristocrat.[260] The senator in Venice, the merchant of Leghorn, the shipowner at Marseilles, the knight in Malta – none of them would have understood a culture which allowed Wildman to thwart the wishes of both Government and Parliament, and extort so much public money for land which was otherwise virtually useless.

259 *Second Report ... Quarantine* (1824), p. 17.

260 James Wildman, late High Sheriff of Kent, died 23 March 1816 in his sixty-eighth year (*The Gentleman's Magazine*, Apr. 1816).

None of them would have grasped the sensibilities which prevented Government from getting rough when it really mattered.

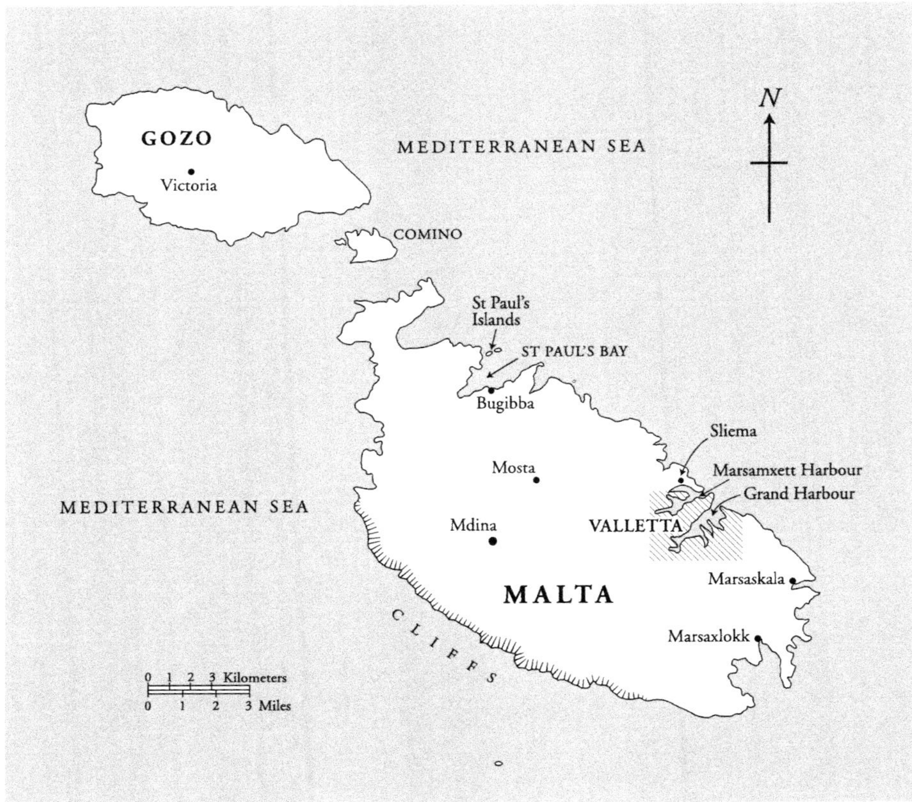

Map 10.1 **Malta and Gozo, showing the quarantine station of Marsamxett Harbour**

Chapter Eleven

Malta: War, Peace and Plague, 1640–1814

Quarantine before the British

The origins of the lazaretto on Malta are indistinct. Cassar refers to quarantine measures run by the Municipality of Mdina in the Middle Ages, but it was the Knights of the Order of St John of Jerusalem, who moved to Malta and the neighbouring island of Gozo in 1530, who established regular procedures based on their former arrangements on Rhodes.[1] Any discussion of quarantine in Malta from this point forward must be based on an understanding of the island's topography. The south side, and some of the west, are protected by cliffs; there are historic anchorages at Marsaxlokk Bay to the east, and St Paul's Bay to the north, but only the excellent natural harbours on either side of Valletta offer real security and shelter. It was in these harbours, therefore, approached from the north-east, that quarantine was enforced. The more southerly, known as Grand Harbour, is ribbed by peninsulas which jut out towards Valletta, creating a series of natural creeks which, when taken with Grand Harbour as a whole, form one of the deepest and most capacious natural havens in the world. Marsamxett Harbour, on the northern side of Valletta, is also a fine, deep-water anchorage, containing Manoel Island (now connected to the mainland), originally called Bishop Island.

In the early years of the Order of St John, both Grand and Marsamxett Harbours were used for quarantine. In 1640 an edict of Grand Master Lascaris directed all ships from the Levant and Barbary to either 'Marsa-Muscetto' or to a bay within Grand Harbour, where they should stay without communication with the shore until guardians of the health issued further instructions.[2] Any infringement would result in death by hanging and, if a ship's master were complicit in the offence, his ship would be forfeited; if a merchant were involved, his death would be supplemented by the confiscation of his cargo.[3] Before the end of the seventeenth century, quarantine in the Grand Harbour had moved to a wharf directly below the walls of Valletta and known as Il Barriera, or 'the barrier', from a row of bollards which separated the town's people from those in quarantine.[4]

---

1 P. Cassar, *Medical History of Malta* (London, 1965), pp. 285–6.

2 J.M. Pardessus, *Collection de lois maritimes antérieures au XVIII siècle* (6 vols, Paris, 1828–45), vol. 6, p. 355.

3 Ibid.

4 J. Galea, 'The quarantine service and the lazzaretto of Malta', *Melita Historica*, 4/3 (1966), 187; Cassar, pp. 298, 300 (eighteenth-century print of Valletta wharf showing Il

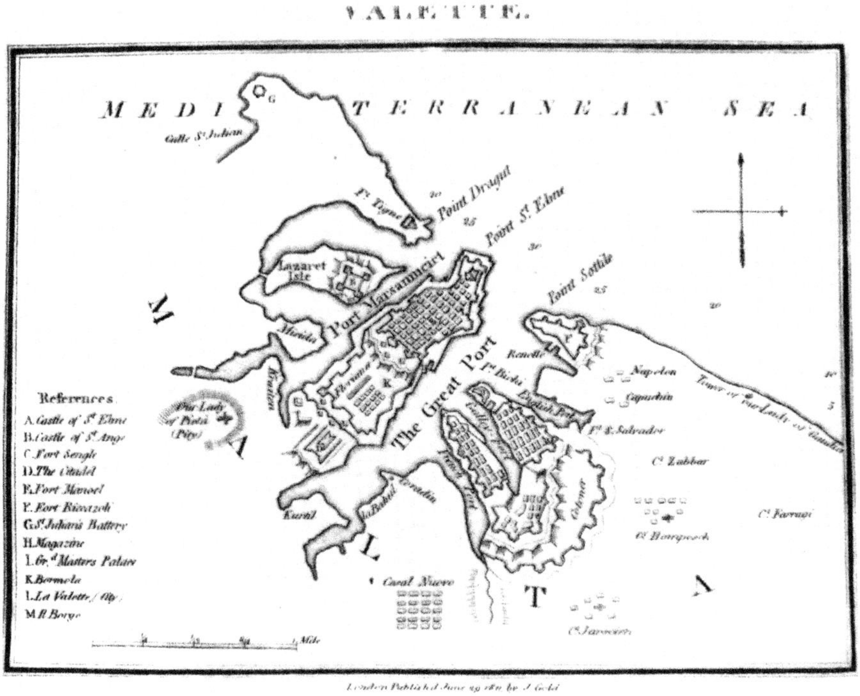

Illustration 11.1 The harbours of Valletta in 1811.

As Malta was periodically attacked by plague, despite such precautions, it made sense to move quarantine as far as practicable to Marsamxett Harbour, where isolation could be more effective. There is evidence of Bishop Island being used for the quarantine of infected persons from the sixteenth century, and it became the intention of Grand Master Lascaris to develop the island as a lazaretto.[5] In 1643 the land was bought by the Order of St John from the Roman Catholic Church.[6] According to Miège, the lazaretto was built in 1666, with Lascaris hoping to avoid further outbreaks of plague by endowing Malta with 'un établissement sanitaire semblable à celui de Marseille' [a sanitary authority similar to that at Marseilles].[7] New quarantine regulations were drawn up in 1724; dated two years later is the earliest surviving record at Marseilles of a letter from Malta giving the intelligence which was so much a feature of correspondence between sanitary authorities of the Mediterranean.[8]

Barriera).

5 Galea, p. 186; Cassar, p. 299.

6 Galea, p. 187; Cassar, p. 299.

7 M. Miège, *Histoire de Malte* (3 vols, Paris, 1840), vol. 2, pp. 416–17. Cassar, p. 299, believes the lazaretto was built on the island in 1643, but that would appear to be the date of the island's purchase.

8 Galea, p. 189, has summarized extracts from the rules which he cites from *Leggi e costituzioni prammaticali* (1724); Archives départementales des Bouches-du-Rhône,

In Britain, merchants and others who understood lazarettos held the Malta institution in high regard. Despite lacking the prestige of Leghorn, or the notoriety of Marseilles, the system maintained by the Order of St John was recognized as rigorous but not oppressive. The traveller Patrick Brydone, in 1770, was pleased with an official of the health office in Valletta who 'behaved in the civilest manner', while the fortifications and lazaretto in Marsamxett Harbour struck him as 'more like the works of a mighty and powerful people, than of so small a state'.[9] Howard explained that quarantine in Malta was of two kinds, petty and great: the former, for ships with clean bills, was undertaken by implication in Grand Harbour, while 'great' quarantine, for foul-bill ships, was performed at the lazaretto.[10] He described this building as having sixteen rooms over two floors; the eight on the upper floor opened on to a long balcony, but were 'very dirty'.[11] Indeed, he found all the old part of the lazaretto 'inconvenient' and 'less airy' than it should be, but the newer buildings, set within two courts, were much better, and could accommodate the cargoes of six or seven ships at one time.[12] Generally, Howard acknowledged that: 'The greatest care is taken to destroy infection should there be any'.[13] The captain of a Danish warship, who went so far as to commission a marble tablet in 1797 to commemorate his respect and gratitude to the health officials, would have gone along with that.[14] British merchants who used the lazaretto were a little less enthusiastic, but certainly not disgruntled; they experienced a wait of four months while cargoes were unloaded, aired and then reloaded, but that was no worse than the delay at Leghorn.[15] The only real concern for merchants using Malta was the way that cotton from widely differing parcels was indiscriminately rammed into bales after the long process of airing. Howard heard of this complaint first hand, and agreed that the cotton was 'rendered less marketable'.[16]

Statistics of the Maltese economy, published by French historians in the nineteenth century, show that in the ten years from 1779 to 1788 the *dritti di lazzaretto*, or lazaretto duties, produced a total income for the Order of 13,117 Maltese scudi (ten to the pound sterling), out of receipts of 13,611,422 scudi – a mere 0.09 per cent of the whole, and less than headings such as 'Presents' and 'Renounced Pensions'.[17]

Marseilles [ADBR], 200 E 463.

9 P. Brydone, *A Tour through Sicily and Malta in a Series of Letters to William Beckford, Esq. of Somerly in Suffolk* (2 vols, London, 1790), vol. 1, p. 333; vol. 2, p. 1.

10 J. Howard, *An Account of the Principal Lazarettos in Europe* … (London, 1789 and 1791), p. 8.

11 Ibid.

12 Ibid. Each court measured 101 feet x 63 feet and contained rooms and sheds. Work had just begun on two other buildings and a chapel. Howard also saw a burying ground, recently used, and a quarantine area for cattle.

13 Howard, p. 9.

14 Galea, p. 192.

15 British Library [BL] Add. MS 38349, fols 169–72.

16 Howard, p. 9.

17 L. de Boisgelin, *Ancient and Modern Malta* (3 vols, London, 1804), vol. 1, p. 305, giving annual breakdown. Miège, vol. 2, p. 440, arrives at the same total but states the years as 1778 to 1788, with no breakdown.

The duty was levied at the rate of 1 per cent of the value of goods which underwent quarantine.[18] On the other hand, the costs of the lazaretto (or more correctly in this case of the *Barriera e Lazzaretto*, thus including the arrangements in Grand Harbour as well) amounted in the same period to 28,083 scudi, which was 0.22 per cent of the total of 12,364,595.[19] The implementation of quarantine, therefore, cost more than twice what the system earned, but in either case the amounts were hardly significant. The accounts have a separate head for the *Sanità* or Health Office, which expended a further 12,532 scudi, but when this sum is added to the other, the true costs of quarantine were still only 0.32 per cent of total state expenditure and less than the Knights spent, for instance, on the purchase of slaves.[20] Yet even such modest outlay allowed for help to the neighbouring island of Lampedusa in the plague-ridden year of 1785.[21]

These accounts have been accepted by Galea, but the figures are very misleading.[22] The books of the Turkey ship *Smyrna*, which performed quarantine at Malta in 1786 on a journey to London, reveal that the lazaretto charges, exclusive of provisions, were 2,249 scudi or, at a rate of exchange (as it was then) of nine scudi to the pound sterling, just under £250.[23] Also in 1786 the *Diligent*, another Turkey ship bound for England, paid quarantine charges in Malta equating to £239.[24] From these two ships alone, therefore, the revenue was around 4,400 scudi, and yet the total income from the lazaretto duties during 1786, according to the published accounts, was only 1,812 scudi.[25] It would become apparent, early in the British administration, that much of the money levied by quarantine was being diverted from the Maltese Treasury into 'perquisites' taken in lieu of salary by the staff of the Health Office.[26]

It was consistent with the acquisition of Gibraltar and Minorca that the British found themselves masters of Malta, despite the absence of any strategic policy for the Mediterranean. The Knights of St John surrendered the island in June 1798 to Napoleon Bonaparte, who was on his way to Egypt. Napoleon lost no time in reorganizing the administration of Malta along the lines of revolutionary France. A Board of Health was one of the responsibilities visited on a new Commission of Government, and by an order of 16 June (only three days after the capture of the island), it was promulgated that 'Les lois de la santé à Malte ne seront ni plus ni moins rigoureuses que les lois de la santé de Marseille' [the health laws at Malta will

18 Miège, vol. 2, p. 432; W. Eton, *Authentic Materials for a History of the People of Malta* ... (London, 1802, 1805, 1807), p. 64.

19 Boisgelin, vol. 1, tables; Miège, vol. 2, p. 441.

20 Ibid. ; Eton, p. 64.

21 Boisgelin, vol. 1, p. 311.

22 Galea, p. 192, considers the lazaretto at this time to have been 'more or less self-supporting as regards current expenditure'.

23 BL Add. MS 38349, fol. 172.

24 Ibid.

25 Boisgelin, vol. 1, p. 305.

26 National Archives [NA] CO 158/2/263, Eton to Sullivan: 'The only change I have made [in the Health Office] is the abolishing of perquisites, and ordering all sums collected on account of quarantine under whatever denomination to be paid into the Lazaretto chest for account of Government'.

be neither more nor less rigorous that the health laws at Marseilles].[27] According to Miège, they had always followed Marseilles in any case.[28] At the same time, there was a feeling that the site in Marsamxett Harbour was inadequate, and a new lazaret for troops was requested.[29] Thus, also on 16 June, an order clarified that 'Le nouveau lazaret doit comprendre un espace de terrain de la valeur d'un quarré de 400 toises de long sur autant de large, et contenir différents bastides ou maisons de campagne' [the new lazaretto should comprise a land area representing 400 square *toises*, and contain separate fortified dwellings or country-style houses].[30] It would include barracks for 500 or 600 soldiers, and accommodation for a general and several other high-ranking officers.[31] A fine country house with a pretty garden was deemed essential. The new establishment was intended to provide quarantine, 'soit aux convalescents qui seraient obligés de retourner en France, soit aux différents détachements de l'Armée' [both for the convalescents who would be obliged to return to France and for the various divisions of the army].[32] The new buildings, therefore, would be something of a military hospital for troops wounded in the Egyptian campaign, as well as a lazaretto to supplement the facilities then existing at Toulon. But Napoleon's vision for quarantine was never realized.

The initial siege of Malta by the British had more to do with the claim to the island by the King of Naples, Nelson's friend, than with British hopes for a new base against France. As the siege progressed, Russia's interest in the island increased, with the election of Czar Paul as Grand Master of the Order of St John. In December 1798 it was agreed that the French garrison, once expelled, would be replaced by a joint force from Britain, Russia and Naples. Early in 1799 the Maltese Congress asked George III to assume sovereignty of the island, but the remainder of the year was occupied by the military and logistical problems of warfare by siege. Not until September 1800 did the French garrison in Valletta surrender to British forces. By then, London had wind of a worrying conspiracy over Malta between Napoleon and Czar Paul, which threatened to close the island to the Royal Navy.[33] The future of Malta was about to become central to British interests.

William Eton

The reduction of the French garrison had been achieved by Captain Alexander Ball, a friend of Nelson and a popular figure with the Maltese people. But as Ball's mandate was associated with the claim to the island by the King of Sicily, he was replaced by

27 H.P. Scicluna, *Documents Relating to the French Occupation of Malta in 1798–1800* (Malta, 1923), pp. 3, 89; W. Hardman, *A History of Malta* (London, 1909), p. 2.

28 Miège, vol. 2, pp. 416–17.

29 Hardman, p. 128.

30 Scicluna, p. 93. One *toise* was a little over six feet.

31 Ibid.

32 Ibid.

33 C. Lloyd (ed.), *The Keith Papers* (3 vols, London, 1950), vol. 2, pp. 156–7.

General Pigot, early in 1801.[34] Pigot combined the roles of Civil Commissioner and Military Governor, and made the British interest unambiguous. One month later Ball left the island and returned to his career, while urging London to separate the civil and military responsibilities, as only that would be satisfactory to the Maltese people. Ball also envisaged benefit to England from better trading links with Malta. On 6 March 1801 he wrote that 'When English Merchants and Warehouses with English Goods are Established in La Vallette, Vessels from all the surrounding Coasts of the Levant will come to Malta with their produce to barter them for these Goods, and return with the Woolens, Cotton and Hardware &c. of England'.[35]

This view of Malta as a potential entrepôt for Britain was novel. Even the military case for the island's usefulness was far from widely accepted and rested more on the negative instinct of denying the island to others. When Mark Wood, in 1796, tried to convince Pitt and Dundas of both the naval and commercial advantages of Malta, he was told by Dundas that the island was 'rather too high up in the Mediterranean'.[36] The most famous of the island's detractors was Nelson, who found it too remote from Toulon to be used as a base for blockading the French. In 1799 he wrote to Earl Spencer that 'the possession of Malta by England, would be an useless and enormous expense', although it was not to be held by the enemy.[37] He came to moderate his view, seeing Malta as, for instance, a staging post to India, but as late as 1804 Nelson wrote to a naval colleague that the island 'is a perfectly useless place for Great Britain; and as a Naval Port to refit in, I would much sooner undertake to answer for the Toulon Fleet from St. Helens [in the Isle of Wight], than from Malta'.[38]

On the commercial front, however, Ball's arguments were accepted. There was no attraction in the island's own trade, which consisted mainly in the export of cotton thread to Barcelona and a modest crop of oranges, but a British-owned lazaretto on the direct route from the Levant to London (and thus much better sited than Minorca) had obvious appeal.[39] As a first step towards raising the general commercial activity of Malta, Valletta was made a free port.[40] Lord Hobart, the new Secretary of State for War and the Colonies, appointed Charles Cameron as Civil Commissioner in May 1801, with instructions to make the lazaretto at Malta, already reputed 'the most compleat in the World', sufficient and effective for the Turkey trade.[41] The management of quarantine was to lie with one William Eton who, explained Hobart, was 'a Gentleman who by his personal observation in several of the Lazarettas [*sic*]

34 D. Gregory, *Malta, Britain and the European Powers, 1793–1815* (Madison & London, 1996), p. 141.

35 NA CO 158/1/19.

36 M. Wood, *The Importance of Malta considered in the Years 1796 and 1798 …* (London, 1803), pp. 11–15.

37 Sir N.H. Nicolas (ed.), *The Dispatches and Letters of Vice Admiral Lord Viscount Nelson* (7 vols, London, 1845–46), vol. 3, p. 315.

38 Nicolas, vol. 5, pp. 107, 341.

39 For Malta's native trade, see Hardman, p. 535.

40 The initial Proclamation was 30 July 1801. Others (for regulating trade) followed on 21 December 1803, 7 January and 25 November 1807, 15 March 1809 and 17 July 1812.

41 NA CO 158/1/44.

of Europe & by his Study of the Subject appears to have acquired a considerable degree of Knowledge respecting the Quarantine Laws …'[42]

Eton had solicited the post of superintendent with a letter to Dundas, Hobart's predecessor, in October 1800.[43] His earlier career was somewhat mysterious and very much involved with Russia. He claimed to have 'officiated' at St Petersburg while three treaties were negotiated, which were then drafted in his own handwriting.[44] Eton had also served Britain as a civil commissary in the Channel Islands, liaising between local people and Russian troops who were quartered there during winter months.[45] He claimed knowledge of Malta from a three-month residency, which had included a long stay in the lazaretto while on official business for the Russian Government.[46] Although there is doubt as to the exact nature of that business, it would appear that Eton was tasked with providing the Russians with information on the lazaretto, as well as on the island of Lampedusa which had potential as a quarantine station should Malta become unavailable.[47] London seems to have taken the view that, with Russia playing a devious role in relation to Malta, it was better to have Eton on the side of the British.

It also probable that Eton had sent Dundas or Hobart at least a draft of his *Survey of the Turkish Empire*, which was published during 1801. In this book, which advocated the abolition of the Levant Company, Eton added a fierce rider, 'Respecting the Inefficacy of the Quarantine Regulations in Great Britain', to a chapter on the British Turkey trade.[48] Having consulted, so he claimed, with health officials in Malta, Leghorn and Marseilles, Eton concluded (in block capitals) that quarantine in Britain was so ineffectual that it put the country in constant risk of Levantine plague.[49] He was a disciple of Russell and staunch contagionist, believing the disease might lie latent in cargo for longer than both the voyage time to England and the period of quarantine, and that airing, washing and fumigation were the only safeguards. The British approach, he claimed, was too timid and half-hearted. By contrast, the Mediterranean Boards of Health had summary powers independent of the local justiciary, and transgressors against quarantine were instantly, and quite properly in his view, shot dead.[50]

Eton's answer to this was not to improve the quarantine facilities in Britain, nor to educate the British into a better understanding of quarantine; it was sufficient to bar all vessels in the Turkey trade from entering Britain, whatever their bill of health, until they had performed quarantine in Malta, Leghorn, Marseilles, or

42 Ibid.

43 Hardman, p. 494.

44 NA CO 158/7 [unpag.], Eton to Penn, 7 July 1803.

45 Ibid.; Hardman, p. 494.

46 Hardman, p. 495.

47 W. Eton, *A Survey of the Turkish Empire* … , 3rd edn (London, 1801), pp. 490–91, includes a section 'Advantages to Russia in possessing this Island' [i.e. Lampedusa]. He states: 'A lazaretto must be built, and thereby the expences of quarantine will be saved to Russia'.

48 Eton, *Survey of the Turkish Empire*, pp. 472–7.

49 Eton, *Survey of the Turkish Empire*, pp. 473–4.

50 Eton, *Survey of the Turkish Empire*, p. 476.

elsewhere in the Mediterranean.[51] Of these ports, he claimed 'Malta is by far the best …; the regulations are even more to be relied on than at Leghorn, as they are in some respects more scrupulous'.[52] There, then, was the source of Hobart's belief in Maltese quarantine supremacy. As a philosophical contribution to the overall debate, Eton's comments offered nothing new. In fact, they were facile, reactionary and calculated to scare. But with Malta now in Britain's grasp, and the decision for a land lazaret at Chetney Hill making next to no progress, the pragmatic suggestion for all quarantine in the Turkey trade to be performed in the Mediterranean, was not unwelcome to ministerial minds.

Cameron was sent copies of specimen regulations prepared by Eton, as well as the report of the Quarantine Committee recently appointed by the Privy Council. He was told by Hobart to turn his attention 'so far … to the subject, as to be able to give every assistance in your power to Mr. Eton, and in some degree to judge of the Expediency & Propriety of the arrangements and regulations he may propose …'[53] Eton, for his part, was 'to enquire minutely into every circumstance and Regulation' affecting quarantine under the Order of St John, and how it had been conducted since the removal of the French.[54] His report and recommendations for the future, explaining why he deviated (if he were to) from past practice, was to be submitted to the military commander, but Cameron's sanction would also be necessary before Eton's plans were implemented.[55] In this role Eton was to be paid an annual salary of £800 a year (as against £2,000 for Cameron), with all proceeds of the lazaretto being credited to Government funds.[56] The two men were to travel to Malta together, although Eton had wanted to make another visit beforehand to the Black Sea and claimed that indecision by Government had cost him £600 already in his private affairs.[57]

The arrangements for Malta gave Eton a dangerous sense of self-importance which the Superintendent of Quarantine at Stangate Creek, on a quarter of the salary, would scarcely have believed. His incredulity might have been shared by the Privy Council, who had nothing to do with the appointment of Eton or, at that time, with any other aspect of quarantine in Malta. It was to be more a case of Cameron assisting Eton than the other way round. It would not have enamoured Eton to Cameron that, as early as 21 May 1801, he was ordered to pay the former £250 out of the island's revenues to meet his claims in relation to the aborted journey to the Black Sea, as well as to reward him for 'various Reports' requested in the past by Dundas.[58] Even when Eton was to make his recommendations on quarantine, Cameron was to be eclipsed by General Pigot, the military commander. In the event, Eton slighted both of them by sending letters directly to London.

51 Ibid.

52 Eton, *Survey of the Turkish Empire*, p. 477.

53 NA CO 158/1/45; Hardman, p. 495.

54 NA CO 158/1/45.

55 NA CO 158/1/45–6.

56 NA CO 158/1/46.

57 NA CO 158/1/45; CO 158/2/245–7.

58 NA CO 158/1/54.

Such action calls into question whether his job might not have been more than it seemed to be. According to Sultana, Eton 'was a confidential agent of the British Government for intrigue and espionage against the partisans of the Order'.[59] Gregory takes the same line.[60] Hardman, on the other hand, thought that Eton, 'if tradition does not belie him', was still a spy for the Russians.[61] He also referred to the 'reprehensible permission [given to Eton] to correspond direct with the Ministry in London'.[62] But was this permission ever given? Hobart's instructions to Cameron gave no hint of it. As regards Eton's orders to spy for Britain, he was certainly to monitor correspondence passing through the lazaretto – an exercise easily done in the process of fumigation – but not without the full knowledge of the Civil Commissioner. This is clear from a letter of September 1801 from London to Cameron, referring to correspondence happily intercepted in this way, but the credit for successful snooping was given to Cameron.[63] Hobart also told him: 'You will direct M^r^. Eton to continue the Examination of all suspicious Papers …'[64] That does not suggest a direct line between Eton and the ministry, and the absence of copied returns to his rambling dispatches would suggest they were largely unsolicited and increasingly unwelcome.

The official initially badgered by Eton was John Sullivan, Under-Secretary of State for War and the Colonies. On 5 July 1801 Eton reported that he and Cameron had just arrived on Malta, and that Cameron had been very well received.[65] The quarantine department exhibited 'the greatest confusion and disorder', and Eton announced his intention to revert to the regulations of Grand Master de Rohan.[66] Having thus established a postal link, Eton began to bombard Sullivan with letters, sometimes writing twice a day. On 10 July he informed Sullivan that it would be his (Eton's) 'duty' to lay before Hobart the requested report and recommendations on the quarantine service.[67] But the terms of reference from Hobart to Cameron had said nothing of the sort. Eton was alarmist, stating that the abuses of quarantine were such that islanders feared for their health, and merchants were worried that the ports of Italy would be closed to Maltese shipping.[68] He claimed to have already abolished the system of perquisites.[69]

Eton then mentioned to Sullivan that the 'beautiful' lazaretto in Marsamxett Harbour had 'not escaped the depredations of the French'.[70] The stages built for airing cotton and silk, as well as some doors, had been broken up for firewood

59 D. Sultana, *Samuel Taylor Coleridge in Malta and Italy* (Oxford, 1969), p. 4.

60 Gregory, p. 129: 'Eton was a partisan, employed by the government to spy on the Order …'

61 Hardman, p. 495.

62 Ibid.

63 NA CO 158/1/109.

64 Ibid.

65 NA CO 158/2/248–9. Some of this letter is transcribed in Hardman, p. 496.

66 Ibid.

67 NA CO 158/2/262.

68 Ibid.

69 NA CO 158/2/263.

70 Ibid.

during the siege. Repairs, and a new walled-in enclosure for cattle from Barbary, would cost up to £4,000.[71] Eton's intention was to send an estimate, survey and plan of the lazaretto direct to Hobart. But he would also 'furnish Mr. Cameron with the means of verifying the estimates, and judging of the indispensible necessity of this expence'.[72] Eton declared that it rested with Hobart to order the lazaretto to be restored to working condition, and to instruct Cameron to make the funds available. In the meanwhile, Eton proposed to spend an immediate £350, anticipating Cameron's approval, 'as there is no alternative'.[73] The specimen regulations which he had submitted to Hobart before departure coincided with those established by the Order of St John. Eton hoped to make use of part of Fort Manoel 'by the Quarantine corps', and claimed the approval of General Villettes.[74] But Villettes was at that time junior to Pigot, whom Eton was reluctant to approach on the grounds that his ideas 'cannot yet be prepared'.[75]

Eton's dilemma over Pigot was resolved when the latter, never a popular figure in Malta, was recalled to England in September 1801. The removal of Pigot had been one of the many matters, extraneous to quarantine, with which Eton bothered Sullivan. He ventured his views on most aspects of the civil administration and on the attitude of the islanders, and argued for British and Maltese ships to have the same navigational rights in the Black Sea as the Porte had granted to Russia and Austria.[76] Eton referred to his recent book, and the need to find new sources for corn and naval stores and open up a wider trade. He professed to be contemptuous of 'the narrow minded selfish sentiments, [of] some Jacobinial members of the Levant Company…'[77] Merchants trading within that same company might well have wondered, for their part, why they should put their ships through quarantine in a lazaretto run by such an ill-disposed superintendent. It was not only the Levant Company whom Eton upset. His appointment, as much as it was acceptable to the Maltese, was not entirely welcome with the British military. He complained direct to Hobart, in late July 1801, that Lieutenant Pemberton, the local agent for transports, had advised masters not to pay the new quarantine and port dues.[78] When the dispute between Eton and Pemberton looked set to worsen, Cameron stepped in to pay the charge of £1, 15s, 8d to the Health Office in respect of a transport due to receive pratique on the following day.[79]

71 Ibid.

72 Ibid.

73 NA CO 158/2/264.

74 Ibid.

75 Ibid. Gregory, p. 141, explains that Eton was not averse to Pigot, but the latter was 'not easy of access' and 'had neither taste nor capacity for civil administration …' Eton wrote to Sullivan in July 1801 suggesting that Pigot be recalled (NA CO 158/2/304–7).

76 NA CO 158/2/308–11, 29 July 1801. Eton had begun writing to Sullivan about political and civil issues on 10 July, and the letters became frequent. Only rarely did he touch upon quarantine, as CO 158/2/278–80 (also 10 July): 'I am the sole judge of the propriety or safety of giving pratique'.

77 Ibid.

78 NA CO 158/2/318–20.

79 NA CO 158/2/322.

When news reached Malta of the British success at Alexandria, Eton wrote a fawning letter to Sullivan, on 22 September 1801, offering his congratulations.[80] He was preparing to accommodate 20,000 men from Egypt in the lazaretto, an interesting echo of Bonaparte's intentions some three years earlier. One month later Eton wrote again to Sullivan displaying his most arrogant trait. He claimed that Cameron had wished him to become involved in Maltese politics. Now, with peace being discussed with France, Eton wanted a bigger role. He would take half-pay for the superintendence of quarantine (with £300 for repairs by Government to his rented house), and solicited in return a role of Commissioner, should a body be appointed to settle the affairs of the island before it was ceded.[81] 'I have stop'd all repairs of the beautiful Lazaretto', he continued, 'as we are ignorant of the conditions of the peace'.[82]

In fact, Hobart had already written to Cameron instructing that all expense on the lazaretto should cease. On 4 November 1801 Eton responded to a letter from Cameron giving him this news.[83] There is insight to be gained from this reply as to what Eton had been doing in his primary role. He referred, as he had done to Sullivan, of preparations having been made for receiving the army from Egypt, including French prisoners, some of them sick and wounded. Many men died in the lazaretto, which meant making a new burial ground. This entailed building a perimeter wall and bringing in earth, so that fresh graves could be a sufficient depth above the rock. In the lazaretto itself, new doors and windows had been vital. To facilitate the entry into Marsamxett Harbour, it had been necessary to invert old cannons along the water's edge. He had also acquired an old ship from the Admiralty to replace a guard boat ordered by General Pigot, which had proved unfit for service. In the Grand Harbour, Eton had enlarged the Health Office, which was now manned day and night. These were the expenses, defrayed by the island Treasury, which Eton claimed he 'could not avoid'. He did not quantify them for Cameron's benefit, but was at pains to point out that quarantine revenue had now increased by between £150 and £200 a month, all of which was now credited to public funds. Eton ended by noting that trade from the Levant was poor, because of rumours in Turkey that ships from the lazaretto in Malta would incur a second quarantine on arrival in Britain. That seems to have been his reward from the Levant Company for being rude about them.

The peace to which Eton had referred in October, transpired as the Treaty of Amiens, signed in March 1802. Within months of the surrender of the French in Malta, it was apparent that the Revolutionary Wars had reached an impasse, with the British supreme at sea, but the French all-conquering on mainland Europe. In the negotiations for the treaty, it was apparent by November 1801 'that the article relative to Malta was that which would present the greatest difficulties ...'[84] To obviate several problems, the French made a radical proposal which would have involved the Knights of St John reverting to an order of hospitality, so that the

80 NA CO 158/2/328.

81 NA CO 158/2/330–32.

82 Ibid.

83 NA CO 158/2/3–5, from which all references in this paragraph are taken.

84 *Cobbett's Political Register*, vol. 3 (1803), p. 1857.

military installations would be demolished: Malta 'should be converted into a great lazaretto, appropriated to the equal accommodation of all the different nations which trade in [the] Mediterranean and the Levant'.[85] This idea, however, was rejected by Britain, and negotiations continued into 1802. Among the provisions of the definitive treaty, Britain was to retain Ceylon and Trinidad, but the Cape of Good Hope was to be restored to the Dutch and Minorca ceded to Spain. The French agreed to withdraw from Naples and the Papal States, and Egypt was to be reunited with the Turkish Porte. As for Malta, the island was to be neutral and returned to the Order of St John of Jerusalem, with its independence guaranteed by France, Britain, Austria, Spain, Russia and Prussia. 'The ports of Malta', the Treaty continued, 'shall be opened to the commerce and the navigation of all nations, who shall there pay equal and moderate duties: these duties shall be applied to the cultivation of the Maltese Langue [or branch of the Order] ..., to that of the civil and military establishments of the island, as well as to that of a general lazaretto, open to all colours'.[86] British forces were to leave Malta within three months of the ratification of the Treaty, 'provided that the grand-master, or commissaries fully authorised according to the statutes of the order, shall be in the island to take possession ...'[87] This was the interim period to which Eton was alluding.

With the lazaretto marking time while the Treaty was finalized, Cameron sent Eton to Palermo to enquire about provisions for Malta and report on the commercial and political state of Italy.[88] Despite the ambiguities of their official relationship, they got on tolerably well, only falling out over an unauthorized correspondence between Eton and the Bishop of Malta.[89] Eton had told Cameron of his wish to stay on in Malta to further British interests when the island was restored to the Order of St John, and probably asked for his support. On 10 March 1802 Cameron informed Hobart that he could not offer a view on this, but he received daily assistance from Eton and could testify to his zeal and ability 'though mixed with much eccentricity'.[90] Hobart, before he could have read that, sent Cameron the conditions under which the Order was to be re-established in Malta, and it was evident that the lazaretto still featured in ministers' minds as a potential benefit to Britain, even when the island was given up.[91] Hobart continued to envisage Malta as 'the great Depôt of the Levant', which would 'draw from Leghorn and Genoa that Trade to which these Ports were indebted for the riches and active industry which so much distinguished them from the Towns of Italy'.[92]

With the treaty imminent, Eton became increasingly concerned for his own future. He solicited Hobart direct for a position as British 'minister or whatever title' in Malta, once the island was given up.[93] Two days earlier, on 6 March 1802, Eton

85 Ibid.; Hardman, p. 433.

86 Boisgelin, vol. 3, p. 251; Hardman, p. 434

87 Boisgelin, vol. 3, p. 250. The text in Hardman, p. 434, has slight differences.

88 NA CO 158/3/18–22. Cameron sent the report to Hobart.

89 NA CO 158/4/45ff.; cf. Gregory, pp. 248–9.

90 NA CO 158/3/26–9.

91 NA CO 158/3/34–8.

92 Ibid.

93 NA CO 158/3/262–3; cf. Gregory, p. 150.

had informed Sullivan that if he left the island then he would be relying on Hobart's patronage after a job in Malta well done.[94] As if to prove his success, he recounted that the British fleet and French prisoners had passed through Malta from Egypt without any health risk to the islanders, or any excuse for other countries to put ships from Malta into a precautionary quarantine.[95] At the same time, Eton confessed to have bent the rules 'for the good of the service' to shorten the detention of warships.[96] He even admitted that convalescents from the plague had been received in Marsamxett Harbour, and there had been a number of suspicious deaths.[97] Two of these had been diagnosed as from plague, but no one outside the quarantine department had been aware of this, except Cameron.

Hobart explained to Cameron that there was no intention of letting Eton act as minister to the Order of St John.[98] Gregory argues that Hobart had been warned against Eton by Ball, but it seems possible that he had had the measure of Eton all along.[99] In any event, it was Ball, recently honoured with a baronetcy, who was sent to Malta as the new British minister and plenipotentiary to the Order. When he arrived on 10 July 1802, he took over from Cameron.[100] The arrival of Ball was anathema to Eton, who had sought to poison Sullivan against Ball a year earlier.[101] As Eton also disliked Alexander Macaulay, the Public Secretary who was staying on the island, he engineered a return to England.[102] On 14 August 1802 Eton asked Ball whether he would intercede with Hobart on his behalf.[103] The ostensible reason was that Eton felt exhausted after overseeing the quarantine of some 9,000 vessels, many of them military, and giving assistance to Cameron from dawn to late at night.[104] Also, he had accounts to settle in London with the Boards of Transport and Sick and Hurt. His department, he claimed, would virtually run itself. Ball, only too pleased to see the back of such a devious man, went along with this, and Eton returned to London soon afterwards, having spent little more than a year in his post. He remained the nominal Superintendent of Quarantine on Malta and continued to draw the salary.[105]

Eton's figure of 9,000 ships under quarantine does not tally with his own statistics of vessels admitted to pratique from 1 July 1801 to 1 October 1802, which amounted to 3,748.[106] Most of these were evidently not detained in quarantine, and

94 NA CO 158/3/260.

95 Ibid.

96 Ibid.

97 Ibid.

98 Gregory, p. 150.

99 Ibid.

100 cf. Hardman, p. 497.

101 NA CO 158/2/248–9. Hardman, p. 496, reproduces part of the letter to Sullivan, in which Eton refers to Ball only as 'a certain person'.

102 For Macaulay, see Hardman, p. 496, quoting from same letter, Eton to Sullivan: Macaulay is 'abhorred for every species of vexation and insult'.

103 NA CO 158/3/140–41.

104 Ibid.

105 Ibid.

106 NA CO 158/5 has nine lists of total ships admitted to pratique in Malta during that period. The time interval between these lists is variable, but the grand total of 3,748 vessels

when they *were* detained the statistics do not indicate for how long. Eton claimed that revenue from the Health Office had recently risen to around £300 a month.[107] That was certainly more than in 1801, when Macaulay recorded an annual income of £1,613, 8s, 11d from the quarantine service, as against £3,007, 3s, 10d spent on the lazaretto.[108] But even those relatively poor figures meant that quarantine was now producing 10 per cent of the island's total receipts, while costing less than 6 per cent of the island's expenses. Macaulay was optimistic, now that Eton had made the necessary repairs and additions, that the lazaretto would more than pay its way in the years ahead.[109]

Eton's return to England did not mark, by any means, the end of his involvement with Malta, but he was not destined to return. This deceitful and manipulating man, castigated by posterity, can at least be credited with having applied himself conscientiously to the supervision of quarantine, although not to standards which would have satisfied the Boards of Health on the Continental mainland. How far Eton also worked to some clandestine agenda, and double-dealt the British, is not a matter for this study; but he may at least be forgiven for intercepting correspondence in the lazaretto, as this was nothing more than he was expected to do.

Ball wrote to Hobart in July 1803, asking for 'a confidential person' to be sent to the Levant to buy corn, of which Malta grew less than a quarter of its annual consumption.[110] It was probably not on Ball's mind that such a commission might be thought suitable for Eton, then back in England, although nearly two years previously the latter had advised Cameron, on Hobart's instructions, about the quality and availability of corn from the Black Sea.[111] But Eton was kept very well informed by his Maltese friends about all matters on the island. In England, he had found a new correspondent to harass: this was Granville Penn, Chief Clerk in the Office of War and the Colonies, and secretary to Hobart.[112] Although travelling periodically between London, Bath and Wales, where he owned a farm, Eton's immediate intention was to return to Malta, once his accounts for previous work had been passed by the Boards of Transport and Sick and Hurt.[113] Eton told Penn in June 1803 that he had now finished plans of the port and lazaretto for Hobart's information, and that sickness alone had prevented completion of the definitive compendium of quarantine procedures, presumably those which he had been asked to produce in Malta, originally for local approval.[114]

On his eventual return to Malta, Eton wanted a greater degree of independence than he feared Hobart would allow. Eton wanted 'an appointment from Government

---

was later confirmed by Eton in a letter to Penn (CO 158/7 [unpag.], 7 July 1803).

107 NA CO 158/5 [unpag.].

108 NA CO 158/3/229–31.

109 Ibid.

110 NA CO 158/7/359–63.

111 Eton, *Authentic Materials*, p. 239.

112 Penn was more receptive than Sullivan had been, and developed a particular interest in Malta. For his book of 1805, see below.

113 NA CO 158/7 [unpag.], Eton to Penn, 11 June 1803.

114 Ibid.

and only accountable to Government, as are the civil naval and military powers'.[115] He pointed out to Penn that, in the Health Office, he would be assisted by six experienced and prestigious men, which was more than could be said for Ball, Villettes, or even Nelson.[116] What he wanted was parity with Europe, where the Boards of Health were supreme and independent. This was a much tougher line than anyone had argued in the context of Minorca, and if any man could have persuaded the British Government to make a health authority so plenipotentiary, it was Eton. But Hobart was minded to make Eton even less independent than he had been under Cameron. On 7 July 1803 Eton protested to Penn that if he were not given sole responsibility for the quarantine service, the 'harmony' it had so far enjoyed could not continue.[117] It was his boast that: 'Neither the Admiral, General or Civil Commissioner ever interfered in my Department in anyway whatever', and he had received no complaints.[118]

For the future, Eton wanted the title Intendant or Intendant General, in order to match the French terminology, and suggested to Penn that this might be achieved simply by referring to him by such a name in official letters to Ball.[119] As the Quarantine Committee had recommended a title of Superintendent General within Britain, how much more necessary was it, argued Eton, for the title in Malta to reflect the dignity of the post.[120] But Hobart was evidently unimpressed by fancy Continental titles, as Eton was soon arguing for the title of Superintendent General; he was anxious to avoid the plain alternative of Superintendent, as he claimed to have 20 junior officers known by that title, for example a Superintendent of the Mole who stopped small boys looking for shellfish.[121] Eton also wanted 'a quarantine uniform' for the two commissaries ranked below him.[122] These men, from the Maltese aristocracy, traditionally served without salary, but after a few years' service they received payments from revenue known as 'commendaries'. As this system could not continue, Eton suggested they be salaried at £100 or £150 a year, a figure which he later dropped to £120.[123] It is to Eton's credit that, despite his isolation from Malta, he still felt keenly for the reputation of the quarantine service which, he would have argued, had been enhanced by his own reforms. Further evidence of this concern came in August 1803, when Eton sent Penn what was, in modern parlance, a press release to counter French claims that plague had spread from the lazaretto to the island and garrison.[124] His statement did not deny that plague had been diagnosed, but emphasized that the 'excellent' quarantine regulations had contained the outbreak and that the French had misrepresented the facts.[125]

---

115 NA CO 158/7 [unpag.], Eton to Penn, 17 June 1803.

116 Ibid.; he was referring, of course, to the Board of Health.

117 NA CO 158/7 [unpag.], Eton to Penn, 7 July 1803.

118 Ibid.

119 Ibid., postcript.

120 NA CO 158/7 [unpag.], Eton to Penn, 9 July 1803.

121 NA CO 158/7 [unpag.], Eton to Penn, 20 Sept. 1803.

122 NA CO 158/7 [unpag.], Eton to Penn, 7 July 1803.

123 Ibid.; Eton to Penn, 9 July 1803.

124 NA CO 158/7 [unpag.], Eton to Penn, 8 Aug. 1803.

125 Ibid.

While occupied with such administrative details, Eton was also planning the route of his return journey. His original intention had been to travel by Hamburg, the Tyrol and Trieste, as he could speak the languages along the route.[126] But in May 1803 he suggested to Hobart that his return should be via southern Russia, with a commission to buy naval stores and other provisions, and 40,000 quarters of wheat for Malta.[127] Hobart was reluctant to be drawn into this, and when Eton set off on 27 September, via St Petersburg, he was acting under the auspices of the Navy and Victualling Boards.[128] By then, Ball's request for corn from the East had been received and pondered in London, but given the mutual enmity between Ball and Eton, the latter was commissioned to buy only a token 2,500 quarters of wheat for the Maltese market.[129] Hobart informed Ball almost casually, in December 1803, that Eton was returning to Malta via the Black Sea, where he would be buying naval stores and making general enquiries about other produce for export.[130] There was no mention of corn for Malta, and in February 1804 Ball sent his secretary, Edmund Chapman, to order the quantity from Odessa which Eton had originally intended to send.[131] Eton knew nothing of this in advance and was outraged. The controversy which followed about quality and costs are not relevant to this study, but the episode explains why Eton never returned to Malta to continue his position as head of quarantine.[132] There was certainly no inclination in London to persuade Eton and Ball to come to terms. When Chapman reported from Kherson that Eton was dressing in the uniform of a general, Ball became adamant that he would not allow him back.[133] He wrote to Penn, in July 1804, that Eton's extraordinary conduct made 'him a very improper Person to be here'.[134] Ball went on to inform Lord Camden, Hobart's successor, that he had not heard from Eton since the latter had arrived in Russia; as far as Ball was concerned, Eton was on a commission from the Navy Board and had no business to transact for Malta.[135]

But Eton could not be dismissed from mind for two reasons. The first was that he was still nominally in post, and it was to be many more years before he was finally removed from office. The second was that, in 1807, he published the first four parts of what was claimed to be a history of the Maltese people.[136] On the title page, he styled himself 'Superintendent General of the Quarantine and Public Health Department in Malta', an inappropriate platform for what was seen as a political tract, masked by historical narrative, and a compendium of information on every aspect of Maltese life. Eton admitted to Secretary Windham in 1806 that Hobart had not wished the

126 NA CO 158/7 [unpag.], Eton to Penn, 11 June 1803.

127 Eton, *Authentic Materials*, p. 242.

128 Ibid.; NA CO 158/7 [unpag.], Eton to Penn, 28 Oct. 03.

129 Eton, *Authentic Materials*, p. 243.

130 NA CO 158/7/447.

131 NA CO 158/8/34. Gregory, p. 203; Hardman, p. 497.

132 See Gregory, pp. 203–5, for a summary of the events and accusations.

133 NA CO 158/9/17.

134 Ibid.

135 NA CO 158/10/56, dated 12 Apr. 1805.

136 W. Eton, *Authentic Materials for a History of the People of Malta …* (London, 1802, 1805, 1807).

first two parts of the history, drafted around five years earlier, to be published.[137] By the same letter, and by another one several months later, he alleged to Windham that Malta was being mismanaged and that Ball (by then a Rear-Admiral) should be recalled.[138] In February 1807 Ball had the opportunity to respond to Eton's remarks, which he repudiated at length, with wrath and vigour.[139] But it was April 1808 before Ball learnt that he had been entirely vindicated of Eton's accusations.[140] This good news was tempered by an admission from London that Eton could not be removed from his post, as this would inflame the Maltese people.[141] Ball retaliated against Eton by stopping his salary on the grounds that he was absent from his post without leave.[142] A protest from Eton to Secretary Castlereagh, Windham's successor (and predecessor), was to no avail.[143] But Ball died in October 1809, without having the satisfaction of seeing his adversary dismissed. This was to become a matter for the next Civil Commissioner, Sir Hildebrand Oakes, and will be discussed later in the context of his administration.

Mercantile pressures

In October 1802 Hobart informed Ball that the failure of Russia and Prussia to accede to the terms of the Treaty meant that the evacuation of Malta by the British had been suspended.[144] There were, of course, other reasons, among them the fear that a Malta restored to the Order of St John would become too affiliated to France, where Bonaparte was again giving cause for alarm. In May 1803 Ball became Civil Commissioner at the same salary, that is £2,000 a year, which had been paid to Cameron. One of Ball's early moves was to send Hobart a lengthy case for the military importance of Malta, as well as the commercial advantage it offered to Britain for extending her trade in the Levant, while restraining that of France.[145] This letter, dated 7 February 1803, anticipated by three weeks a report from Lord Elgin, British ambassador to Turkey, which concluded with the same view.[146] As Elgin was then in quarantine at Valletta, it must be suspected, despite the rules for non-contact, that Ball had discussed with him the wider opportunities for Malta. Ball elaborated on this argument a few months later, distancing himself in effect from Nelson by claiming that Malta was a better base than Minorca or even Gibraltar in bad winter

137 NA CO 158/12/245.

138 Ibid.; CO 158/12 [unpag.], 11 Oct. 1806.

139 NA CO 158/13/9–105.

140 NA CO 158/14/207–11.

141 Ibid.

142 NA CO 158/14/207–11.

143 Ibid.

144 NA CO 158/3/171.

145 NA CO 158/7/29–37.

146 J. Holland Rose, 'Lord Elgin's report on Levantine affairs and Malta, 28 February 1803', *English Historical Review*, 36 (1921), 236.

weather.[147] When ships were sent there for refit from the Toulon blockade, they could easily divert to the Adriatic should that become necessary.

Ball also re-stressed the commercial case for Malta, arguing it was well placed to take advantage of trade from the Black Sea, fed by the Russian rivers, which offered naval stores more quickly and cheaply than from the Baltic.[148] Ball himself was under some pressure from merchants, who at that time included 'Two or Three British', to increase the prospects for trade.[149] An undated 'Representation of the Merchants of Malta' has survived which, as it argues for the island to be a free port, appears to antedate Ball's appointment.[150] It is, nevertheless, an indication of the arguments to which Ball was receptive.

This 'Representation' was aimed at making Malta more useful for Britain, and it explained how this could be done. With the island a free port, ships from the East would unload 'in the Noble and Commodious' lazaretto, and immediately take on western goods for the return voyage. In the same way, ships from the West would arrive at the lazaretto to take on Levantine produce which had already been 'purified'. It would thus be cargoes but not ships subjected to quarantine. When this saving of time was allied to the shorter distances (as Malta was on the direct sailing route between east and west), no other port would be able to compete. The merchants felt that the 'celebrated' quarantine procedures in Malta would increase the sense of security in other countries so, by implication, ships bound for England should not undergo a further quarantine on arrival. As a free port, Malta could also expect extra trade with Italy, but the intention was very much to supersede Leghorn, Genoa and Messina as the routes into Britain for goods from Turkey. The merchants hoped trade with Turkey under the British flag would be possible, and that ships would be able to sail for England from Malta with the goods of other countries, if they could already do so from those countries direct. This would mean, they hoped, paying only one duty on arrival, which they asked should be no more than that paid by the Levant Company.

Malta would do even better, the merchants argued, if British-flagged ships were to be allowed to sail in the Black Sea. The export of naval stores to Britain would be invaluable, but so far only the French had profited. Malta could become a granary for the Mediterranean by stockpiling Russian corn. It annoyed the merchants that the Russians and Austrians already had this privilege of trade, and they foresaw fierce competition for Black Sea business once peace was restored. Nearer home, they wanted the navy to control the Barbary corsairs, who took prizes indiscriminately off the Maltese coast. To regulate the free port (which would embrace the whole island) the merchants drew up specimen articles, which included the imposition of a small tax on imported merchandise, but not on exports. The only commodity deserving central control would be corn, to be deposited in the *Università*, or state granary, and sold only by public order. Finally, the merchants wanted a Tribunal

---

147 NA CO 158/8/1–4.

148 Ibid.

149 The quotation is from 'General Observations on the Trade of Malta' by Francis Laing, Public Secretary, in NA CO 158/20 [unpag.].

150 NA CO 158/7/53–61, from which all references in next two paragraphs are taken.

of Commerce composed of the three main traders on the island, to resolve minor differences between themselves.

While backing the principle of greater trade for Malta, Ball was unhappy with the immediate loss of revenue which free-port status brought about. He complained to Penn, on 4 July 1804, that £40,000 had already been lost to Government by what he called 'the very injudicious Measure of taking off all the import Duties', and by trying to make Malta the equal of Gibraltar.[151] Ball wanted a system whereby civil expenditure would be met by revenue. Early in 1805 he returned to the same theme, admitting that he had revived some import duties, but only those acceptable to the Maltese.[152] He alleged Cameron had interpreted the term free port too generously by removing duties on goods both for consumption and in transit. Ball was confident that the geographical supremacy of Malta over Leghorn and Marseilles would 'soon reduce them to comparative Insignificance'.[153]

As the months passed, Ball became increasingly at odds with merchants both in England and Malta about exactly what duties were acceptable in a nominal free port. The London lobby, led by John Turnbull (Chairman of the Committee of Merchants trading with the Mediterranean) and supported by the Privy Council, fretted about inconvenience at Malta, and continuing discrepancies between duties in the island as opposed to those at Gibraltar.[154] Ball protested that he was still ignorant of what was happening at the Rock, and if there were any 'inconvenience' at Malta it was only on account of quarantine, which could not be avoided.[155] In any event, he argued that local circumstances might make it impossible to equate Malta and Gibraltar in every aspect of trade. Cameron, for instance, had made the tariffs at Malta conform largely with those at Leghorn, and local merchants had seemed happy enough at the time.[156] Indeed, the demand for mercantile property was high, and 'a few port-duties ... judiciously levied' were no impediment to trade.[157]

Within Malta, Ball's problems with the commercial lobby were not unsolicited. On 31 May 1806 he invited local merchants to tell him what restraints to trade existed in the island which were inconsistent with its status as a free port and entrepôt.[158] A week later 14 merchants signed a reply signifying they had problems with Custom House duties as well as the charges for the lazaretto and for taking on ballast.[159] Ball then convened a meeting attended by three delegates from the merchants. He declared his support for the desire shown by the Privy Council to increase Malta's trade and asked for a fuller memorial of the merchants' complaints.[160] This document, dated 28 June 1806, stressed the importance of making Malta an effective free port

---

151 NA CO 158/9/7–14.

152 NA CO 158/10/61–70. This report on the island's revenue and commerce had been requested by Camden in February.

153 Ibid.

154 NA CO 158/12/21–7.

155 Ibid.

156 Ibid.

157 Ibid.

158 NA CO 158/12/113.

159 NA CO 158/12/117.

160 Ibid.

at a time when its competitors suffered obstructed access because of the war.[161] The merchants then returned to the familiar theme of parity with Gibraltar, which had no Custom House and therefore no duties to impose. In terms of ballast, the request was for delivery at the rate of the lowest tender, and for payment to be made only for the precise amount taken on board. It was also felt that some of the Health Office charges 'bear heavy upon the Commerce'. The merchants wanted a reduction from 18 tari per day to 6 tari (there were 12 tari in 1 scudo) for the services of an official boat allocated to assist each vessel in quarantine, and that this charge should be removed altogether once the goods were in the lazaretto, as the only function of the boat in those circumstances would be to take provisions to the guards on the vessel. Finally, they wanted a reduction in warehouse costs once the goods were being aired. On 14 July, Ball conceded reform to the ballast charges, but little else.[162]

In August 1806 Ball was again defending himself to Windham against accusations by Turnbull and the Maltese merchants.[163] These covered the same ground as before, and there were signs of Ball's irritation. On the Gibraltar issue, he could only reiterate that he had never seen the regulations there, and so could not follow suit. He would certainly not concede that the lazaretto charges, in any respect, were too high. Ball would have none of the merchants' claims that goods held in the warehouses of the lazaretto were overcharged for their space, and felt that comparison with private storehouses was unfair. He countered that the merchants had not considered the high cost of overheads for the Health Office or the improbability of a dependable income. The wages of guardians needed to be high to compensate for the risks and privation. Ball dismissed the notion that the lazaretto was a source of revenue; in fact, it was 'rather a burden' on Government. He was, nevertheless, very proud of it, confident that Malta could 'boast of the most extensive and complete' establishment in Europe.

By now, the notion that the quarantine facilities in Malta were both excellent and vital had much support in Britain. Walsh, publishing in 1803, alluded to the 'remarkably fine lazaretto', and to the failure of Britain, before the chance acquisition of Malta, to appreciate the advantages well known to others.[164] This theme was developed a year later by Jackson, who followed Walsh in making a comparison with Minorca, and also reached the conclusion that Malta was better placed.[165] But while Walsh was arguing primarily from a military standpoint, Jackson stressed that Malta was well placed for the Levant trade, and 'affords excellent accommodation for shipping, both for those which have to perform quarantine, as well as those that have obtained prattick'.[166] In 1805 the influential *Edinburgh Review*, discussing the recent history of Malta by Louis de Boisgelin, felt that the importance of the island to Britain 'cannot be too highly appretiated [*sic*]', and joined those arguing for an

161 NA CO 158/12/125–9, from which remaining references in this paragraph are taken until otherwise stated.

162 NA CO 158/12/133–5.

163 NA CO 158/12/105–11, from which all references in this paragraph are taken.

164 T. Walsh, *Journal of the late Campaign in Egypt …*, 2nd edn (London, 1803), p. 19.

165 J. Jackson, *Reflections on the Commerce of the Mediterranean* (London, 1804), p. 8.

166 Jackson, p. 29.

entrepôt to assist the Levant trade, as Malta offered 'the most complete lazaretto in Europe'.[167] The most excited proponent, however, was Granville Penn, who felt that the authorship of a book promoting the island in all its aspects, also published in 1805, was not incompatible with his civil service position. He claimed that Malta,

> possessing a port in which the British navy might moor, and presenting a coast impregnable, if but moderately defended, by any assault; guarding the whole of the Levant, and effectually controlling the naval movements of France on the east, in that sea, is – whether we consider it with relation to the political interests of Europe, or with relation to our own naval and commercial interests, or with respect to its own local circumstances – absolutely singular and *one*, upon the surface of the globe.[168]

In the following year Napoleon Bonaparte issued the Berlin decree. By this measure, followed by the Milan decree of 1807, he sought to put Britain in a state of blockade and prevent the British trading with French allies and even neutrals. Britain retaliated by placing all countries allied to Bonaparte under counter blockade. From the ramifications of this mutual misery, Malta was uniquely positioned to benefit. War between Britain and Turkey led to Malta becoming a depot for neutral and British goods unable to reach the Levant and for Turkish goods destined for the Austrian states.[169] The American Embargo Act of 1808 led to Mediterranean goods being landed in Malta to make up for those debarred from America, while an increased demand in the Levant (deprived of goods from Saxony) for British cotton manufactures led to further stockpiles in the warehouses of Valletta. Gregory notes that in 1808 the value of British goods arrived in Malta exceeded by 30 times the value of such goods received in 1801, and merchants clamoured for more storage facilities.[170] As many as 40 British mercantile houses are said to have set up in Malta as a result of the Berlin and Milan decrees.[171]

Ball was anxious to get on well with the merchants. In the spring of 1807 he readopted the tactic of asking them to set out in a memorial what he already knew they wanted.[172] The merchants obliged with a paper dated 9 May, in which they asked for the wharves to be extended and for more warehouses to be built for British, colonial and foreign goods.[173] Those issues became somewhat sidelined later in the year, when Ball was empowered to license any ship from a friendly country to proceed to any non-blockaded port with the produce of Britain or her colonies, and to return to Malta with local goods.[174] This was far from straightforward for Ball, who was called upon by local merchants to recognize, without reference to London,

167 *Edinburgh Review*, vol. 6 (1805), p. 195.

168 [G. Penn], *The Policy and Interest of Great Britain, with Respect to Malta, Summarily Considered* (London, 1805), p. 16.

169 The position is well summarized in the 'Observations' of Laing in NA CO 158/20 [unpag.].

170 Gregory, p. 215.

171 Hardman, p. 537.

172 NA CO 158/13/331–5.

173 Ibid.

174 Following Order in Council, 25 Nov. 1807.

that the King in Council had not meant to exclude British-flagged ships from that privilege.[175] He was also under pressure from the consul and factory of Smyrna, who had decamped to Malta following the blockade of their base in the current hostilities. In March 1808 they reminded Ball of the advantages to the island from the Levant trade and suggested that the Jerusalem flag should be regarded as neutral; that move would enable them to withdraw property from Smyrna to Malta, in line with the declared wishes of ministers in England.[176]

Early in 1809 the Board of Trade instigated moves to allow Ball a discretionary power to release spare public warehouses for the use of merchants in Malta.[177] At that juncture, the awareness of certain British merchants trading to the Mediterranean about Malta's facilities appears curiously lacking. On 1 February 1809 the Privy Council considered a petition from Le Mesurier & Co., on behalf of themselves and other London traders, for a lazaretto to be established on Malta so that quarantine could be avoided in England.[178] The Council's response was no less bizarre, in that they asked the Customs Commissioners to report on the feasibility of such exemption, if a system for quarantine in the Mediterranean 'should be established'.[179] It was evident from this that the lazaretto on Malta was still regarded in certain quarters as an alien institution, nominally under British control but effectively self-regulating, and working hand-in-hand with the Continental Boards of Health. There was no attempt to integrate the Maltese lazaretto into British quarantine policy, not least because the arrangements there had nothing to do with the Privy Council. Yet British policy was not necessarily thought inapplicable to Malta. The island was, for a time, regarded as no different from Minorca which, as has been shown, received copies of Orders in Council affecting quarantine regulations in Britain, with the implicit understanding that these, however undesirable they might be in a regional context, should be incorporated into local rules. Ball religiously acknowledged receipt, from time to time, of Privy Council Orders affecting quarantine in Britain, including even the extension of Section 42 of the Order of 5 April 1805 (concerning certificates of the origin of goods) for arrivals in Britain from Newfoundland, Cape Breton and other islands off the coast of North America.[180] Some of these Orders were doubtless for information (as they affected goods from Malta arriving in Britain), but the revision of Section 42 was probably intended to influence quarantine policy in Malta.

On 26 October 1809, when Chapman wrote to England with news of Ball's death, he enclosed a resolution of a committee of British merchants on Malta bearing testimony to the esteem in which Ball had been held.[181] He had certainly been a champion of the Maltese lazaretto, and if the merchants still had grievances, Ball had at least been conscientious and heard their requests. There was always a grey area between commercial progress, military requirements and international relations, and

175 NA CO 158/14/163–5. For later developments, see Gregory, p. 215.

176 NA CO 158/14/229–33.

177 NA CO 158/14 [unpag.], Fawkener to Cooke.

178 NA PC 2/179/389.

179 Ibid.

180 NA CO 158/10/77, 135.

181 NA CO 158/14/541.

it was no fault of Ball, as Civil Commissioner, that he found the advancement of trade difficult to realize without upsetting other parties or stepping outside his brief. But the fact that a Committee of British Merchants, in other words an organized pressure group, was now established on Malta was an indication that Ball had failed to resolve basic issues. In the months of the interregnum, before Lieutenant-General Sir Hildebrand Oakes took up his post as the new Civil Commissioner, the committee maintained its momentum by lobbying London again through their colleague by proxy, John Turnbull.[182]

The substance of the merchants' latest complaints centred on the full warehouses in Malta and the problem of maintaining an effective and legitimate trade especially with Italy. This was, they complained, 'no ordinary war but a war that is carried on with implacable fury against every branch of Commerce of His Majesty's Subjects …'[183] As neither quarantine in general, nor the lazaretto in particular, were now a feature of mercantile dissatisfaction, the details of the letter to Turnbull need not be discussed. Suffice it to mention that a copy was also sent for information to Chapman, who forwarded it to Lord Liverpool, the new Secretary of State for War and the Colonies. As we shall see, when Oakes arrived on Malta in 1810, relations between the administration and the merchants became increasingly strained, with the lazaretto returning as a topic of contention.

Towards profit

The comment by Ball that quarantine was somewhat of a burden to Government sits awkwardly against the earlier claims by Eton, and indeed Macaulay, that the service was becoming a significant source of revenue. It has been shown above that in 1801 the lazaretto, while by no means in profit, was contributing more, proportionately, to the island's income than it was claiming as a share of the island's expenditure. Was that sustainable? The question needs examination against the background of how the lazaretto was run in the years between Eton's departure and his removal from office.

When Eton left for England in 1802, the management of quarantine devolved upon William Franklin, principal medical officer of the army in Malta.[184] Ball had set up a Board of Health in November 1804 and appointed Franklin as the representative of Government in what was otherwise a Maltese institution.[185] It was useful for Franklin to be a member, as many of the ships placed in quarantine were warships or transports. As he was the only person on the Council who spoke English, Franklin was frequently in demand and became considered as its president.[186] Ball

182 NA CO 158/14 [unpag.], Joseph Slythe, chairman of committee in Malta, to Turnbull, 21 Dec. 1809.

183 Ibid.

184 NA CO 158/17 [unpag.], Green to Oakes, 23 Nov. 1811. Franklin had a relatively distinguished career as a military doctor and was knighted in 1823.

185 Ibid.; Sultana, quoting Banda (official notice) 7 November 1804, calls it a Committee of Public Health.

186 Ibid.

was unhappy that Franklin should perform this role without remuneration, especially as quarantine benefited, at least equally, the commercial interests of the island who made no contribution to the pay of a military doctor. It was, therefore, in Ball's mind that Franklin should be paid a proportion of Eton's salary, but that did not come about.[187] Franklin himself declined remuneration on the grounds that from his military position 'it was his Positive duty to be Peculiarly watchful of every thing relating to the Quarantine', and because he did not wish to aggravate the rift which was publicly known to exist between Ball and Eton.[188] When Franklin left Malta in 1806, Ralph Green succeeded to his military duties and Ball duly made him de facto head of quarantine without the title of Superintendent. Green was offered the same prospect of remuneration as Franklin had been, but declined it for the same reasons.[189]

Under these military doctors, the rules of the lazaretto were vigorously enforced. Ball wrote to Cooke in January 1805, worried that rumours may have reached London that Malta was too accommodating to ships from Gibraltar. He admitted that one convoy had been granted pratique, but the bills of health had been clean, and despatches from the Rock had mentioned only 'a slight Fever prevailing'.[190] But once the position was known, all arrivals from Gibraltar, including warships and transports, were placed under a quarantine of several days, to the annoyance of the navy.[191] One Ragusan ship, with its crew dead or dying from yellow fever, was barred from entering the lazaretto at all and ordered back to sea.[192] Such cruel measures were justified by the knowledge that, without them, any ship from Malta would have been placed in punitive quarantine at such ports as were still accessible in the northern Mediterranean. Even as it was, ships from Malta arriving in Naples were quarantined for 40 days, and the detentions in Sicily, longer than those which applied to vessels from other neighbouring countries, annoyed successively Cameron, Ball and even Nelson.[193] In February 1805 Camden wrote to Ball congratulating him that Malta had been kept free of the contagion which had devastated Gibraltar and southern Spain, and reminding him that precautions could not be relaxed.[194]

As the lazaretto was handling such a high volume of traffic, an impressive income was to be expected. Receipts, however, fell short of the £300 a month which Eton had confidently predicted. His own published figure for 'Lazaretto Duties, and other sums collected by the Quarantine and Public Health Department' in 1802, was £2,000 out of a total revenue for the Maltese treasury of £287,765.[195] By that reckoning, quarantine in its widest sense contributed only 0.7 per cent to the island's income. But all the totals which Eton published for 1802 were inexact, because the island's accounts ran from 25 July in one year to 24 July in the next. On that basis,

187 Ibid.

188 Ibid.; the quotation, of course, is from Green, not from Franklin himself.

189 Ibid.

190 NA CO 158/10/3–4.

191 For complaints of naval officers, see Sultana, p. 256.

192 Sultana, p. 239.

193 NA CO 158/3/30; Sultana, pp. 17–18, 239.

194 NA CO 158/9/64.

195 Eton, *Authentic Materials*, p. 256.

the receipts from the lazaretto and Health Office for 1802–3 amounted to £1,321, which makes Eton's estimated figure look optimistic.[196] Furthermore, as expenditure on the lazaretto and Health Office for the same period was some £1,683, quarantine was actually in the red by around £362.[197] In 1803–4 (July to July) this shortfall was reduced to only £16: although expenditure on the service had risen by nearly £294 in comparison with the previous year (owing to quarantine for British and Maltese prisoners taken by the French and released in Barbary), profits exceeded the 1802–3 figure by more than £640.[198] For the year 1804–5, there was a confident prediction, made 12 months in advance, that receipts from the lazaretto and Health Office would reach £3,631, against expenditure of only £2,908, leading to the first-ever projected profit of around £723.[199] There are no actual figures for 1804–5, but Ball's disappointment that the lazaretto was something of a burden would suggest that this profit was never realized.

In the fiscal year 25 July 1805 to 24 July 1806, the lazaretto made less than £1,052, leaving a massive deficiency of £1,992 against expenditure.[200] Under the latter head, there were only three items: the salary to Eton, payments of more than £1,476 to other employees of the lazaretto and Health Office, and a bill of over £678 for repairs and maintenance.[201] This total of more than £3,043 was around 5 per cent of the island's total expenditure, whereas income from quarantine was only 2.7 per cent of total receipts. Thus the service was costing the island relatively the same amount as five years earlier, whereas the contribution of quarantine to the island's income had dropped by around three-quarters. In a sense, this was no more than a reflection of Malta's wider deficit in the balance of payments. When Ball reported the 1805–6 figures to Sir George Shee, Under-Secretary of State for War and the Colonies, he revealed that revenue was only a dismal 68 per cent of expenditure.[202] This was mainly because tenant farmers were defaulting on rents (as the war impeded their sale of cotton to Spain), but Ball also mentioned lower lazaretto receipts among other factors.[203] He did not comment on why these receipts should have dropped, but it may be surmised that Gibraltar was then in pratique with Malta as the epidemic in southern Iberia had petered out.

Following the Berlin and Milan decrees, the Health Office lurched quickly and dramatically into profit, in step with the rapid growth of Malta's trade. This was in contrast to the island's overall budget, which remained in deficit but by reduced amounts. In 1809, the last year of Ball's administration, the Health Office posted receipts of roughly £8,932 against an approximate expenditure of £5,643; these figures were 12.5 per cent and 6.5 per cent respectively of the national totals.[204]

---

196 NA CO 158/10/73.

197 NA CO 158/10/74.

198 NA CO 158/9/29.

199 NA CO 158/10/73–4.

200 NA CO 158/12/137.

201 Ibid. The salary to Eton was given as £888 17s. 9d. incorporating expenses of transmission.

202 NA CO 158/13/313–7, 319.

203 Ibid.

204 NA CO 158/19/155. These statistics were for the calendar year.

Ball did not live long enough to appreciate the extent of this reversal of fortune, but it would have been clear to him that quarantine was no longer the burden to Government which it used to be. One-quarter of the newly found profit margin could be attributed directly to Ball for his refusal to allow Eton, still in England, to continue drawing his annual salary. The problem which lay ahead was to maintain the income from the Health Office and lazaretto at such high levels once the artificial circumstances which had led to the increases were ended. In 1810 the level of trade declined with the repeal of the American Embargo Act, the restoration of peace with Turkey and the British occupation of the Ionian Islands.[205]

Quarantine under Oakes

When Oakes arrived in Malta as Civil Commissioner, the merchants were said to be 'living in a style of luxury suitable to princes'.[206] It was to become the misfortune of Oakes, a soldier with little experience in civil, commercial or economic matters, to preside over their slow decline.[207] One of the early moves by the Committee of British Merchants, in May 1810, was to test the attitude of Oakes to the lazaretto. For some years, under Ball, they had not felt the need or perhaps the inclination for change. Now, they complained of lack of covered space, which was causing ships to land their cargoes on open land, although quarantine was not deemed to commence until goods had been opened and aired in the sheds.[208] Also, it would appear that the wooden flooring within the warehouses, destroyed by the French (as Eton had reported many years earlier), had still not been replaced, whereby goods were being damaged by lying on the damp stones beneath.[209] Finally, the merchants queried the propriety of allowing persons from outside the lazaretto into rooms where passengers were under quarantine, with a risk of physical contact despite the theoretical vigilance of guardians.[210] This was a serious allegation which threatened to damage the merchants' own interests, if word of such careless practice reached Boards of Health elsewhere.

Oakes had no more experience of quarantine than of other aspects of civil administration. In June 1810 he confided in his friend Henry Bunbury, a more junior officer who had become Under-Secretary of State for War and the Colonies, that he would like to find new holders for the posts of Treasurer and Superintendent of the Health Office.[211] He recommended his friend, Samuel Tolfrey, lately a member of the Board of Revenue of Ceylon, as suitable for either position.[212] It was thereby evident that Oakes had more concern for personal favours than for the experience and savoir

205 'Observations' of Laing in NA CO 158/20 [unpag.].

206 [Charles L. Meryon], *Travels of Lady Hester Stanhope; forming the Completion of her Memoirs. Narrated by her Physician* (3 vols, London, 1846), vol. 1, p. 12.

207 For a discussion of the competence of Oakes, see Gregory, p. 174.

208 NA CO 158/18/127–9.

209 Ibid.

210 Ibid.

211 NA CO 158/16/89–91.

212 Ibid.

faire which the control of quarantine demanded. He was not, however, unaware that the job was a specialty, and he acknowledged the 'talents and experience' which Eton had displayed, while campaigning at the same time to have him replaced.[213]

In seeking the early removal of Eton, Oakes ran into the same diffidence in London which had thwarted the wishes of Ball. Oakes tried a two-pronged attack: he wrote directly to Lord Liverpool for a new Superintendent of Quarantine on the grounds that Eton, after eight years absence, would surely never return.[214] At the same time he asked Bunbury to have a quiet word with Liverpool to promote the interest of Tolfrey, but the matter was not concluded.[215] It was another seven months, in May 1811, before the question re-emerged, this time with some urgency: Oakes learnt that Eton's imminent return to Malta was being rumoured on the streets of Valletta.[216] On 30 July 1811 he stressed to Bunbury the absolute necessity of having Eton superseded, and the importance of barring such a dangerous man from returning to Malta.[217] Oakes had not lost hope that the appointment would pass to Tolfrey. In August, after Eton had had the temerity to write to Oakes, the latter sent a tirade to Liverpool in which the intrigues of Eton were roundly denounced.[218] This, at last, gave Liverpool cause to dismiss Eton from office. It was 22 November 1811 when Oakes thanked Bunbury for this welcome news.[219]

By the same post from Bunbury, Oakes had learnt with regret that Tolfrey was not to be Eton's replacement. Instead, the position had been given to William Pym, Deputy Inspector of Hospitals at Gibraltar, an indication that London wished quarantine in Malta to be under the control of a man with medical experience. Pym had done 13 of his 20 years' service in the quarantine department at Gibraltar, but had only received payment since 1804.[220] The news of Pym's appointment prompted Ralph Green, still nominally in charge of quarantine and the lazaretto, to solicit the assistance of Liverpool, via Oakes, for promotion to the permanent rank of Inspector of Hospitals.[221] Green claimed that he would not have sought Eton's job, even if he had known it would be vacant, and that he merely wanted to advance his career, which had already spanned 24 years.[222] Oakes was happy to go along with that, although Green was not promoted immediately. Liverpool would have been relieved that Green was not another applicant for Eton's job. On 15 August 1811 William Keith Ball, son of the late Civil Commissioner, had written to Liverpool soliciting the post of Superintendent of Quarantine at Malta, in lieu of a pension of £600 per annum to which he was nominally entitled by virtue of his father's services.[223]

213 NA CO 158/16/365–9.

214 Ibid.

215 NA CO 158/16/373–5.

216 NA CO 158/17 [unpag.], Oakes to Bunbury, 6 May 1811.

217 NA CO 158/17 [unpag.]; some of this letter is quoted in Gregory, p. 176.

218 NA CO 158/17 [unpag.], 1 Aug. 1811.

219 NA CO 158/17 [unpag.].

220 NA CO 158/23 [unpag.], Pym to Bunbury, 15 Apr. 1813. Pym claimed that from 1804 quarantine fees produced an income of roughly £800 a year for the Gibraltar Government.

221 NA CO 158/17 [unpag.], Green to Oakes, 23 Nov. 1811.

222 Ibid.

223 NA CO 158/17 [unpag.].

There must be a suspicion from this letter that Ball junior conceived the post as a sinecure. If Oakes did not quite share that view, he was far from convinced that it merited the high salary which Eton had commanded. In December 1811 Oakes wrote to both Liverpool and Bunbury to express his dismay that the salary available for Francis Laing, the new Public Secretary, was only £700.[224] This was £100 less than the salary of the Superintendent of Quarantine 'whose duties', he told Bunbury, 'however important, are but little laborious, and ... fall very short indeed of those of the Public Secretary, and it certainly never could be intended that this Officer [the Superintendent] who is called upon for no other expense in living than what he chooses to be at himself, should possess a larger Income than that Gentleman who is second in rank ... to His Majesty's Commissioner ...'[225] It rankled Oakes that Liverpool would only agree to a combined salary of £1,400 for the two posts of Public Secretary and Treasurer, to be divided as Oakes thought fit.[226] The outcome was £800 for the former post and £600 for the latter, but Oakes remained dissatisfied that the Public Secretary was not elevated in salary as well as rank above the Superintendent of Quarantine.[227]

On 3 March 1812 Oakes informed Liverpool that Pym had arrived in Malta a few days earlier.[228] On 1 May he told Liverpool that Pym wanted two months' leave of absence for personal reasons.[229] It might be conjectured that, after such a brief sojourn in Malta, Pym was risking Oakes's displeasure. In fact, that was not the case, and he recommended Liverpool to agree. Pym, who was suffering from a chronic liver complaint, had made a rapid reorganization of the Health Office. He stated later that he had 'found it a Mass of Confusion and Plunder', which paid no compliments to his fellow officers in the medical division of the army.[230] Pym's reforms promised to produce more revenue, and Oakes had formed a good opinion of his capabilities. But in a letter to Bunbury, Oakes suggested that Pym was anxious to find a better situation for himself as he was finding the Malta job 'inferior' to his previous post in Gibraltar.[231] The worry for Oakes was that Pym might be allowed to retain the post as a sinecure, following the precedent of Eton, with the day-to-day running entrusted to a deputy. In the meanwhile, the superintendence of quarantine in Malta devolved upon Joseph Thomas, garrison surgeon.[232] Oakes was still comfortable with army doctors, and Thomas gave him no cause for complaint.

One of Pym's improvements had been to extend the covered area of the lazaretto in line with the merchants' requests nearly two years earlier. In order to pay for this, he imposed a levy of 0.5 per cent on the value of goods which underwent quarantine

224 NA CO 158/17 [unpag.], Oakes to Liverpool, 23 Nov. 1811, and Oakes to Bunbury, 29 Dec. 1811.

225 NA CO 158/17 [unpag.], Oakes to Bunbury, 29 Dec. 1811.

226 NA CO 158/18/85–7.

227 Ibid.

228 NA CO 158/18/41.

229 NA CO 158/18/61.

230 NA CO 158/23 [unpag.], 15 Apr. 1813, Pym to Bunbury.

231 NA CO 158/18/75.

232 NA CO 158/22/223–4.

on board ship, rather than in the lazaretto.[233] These cargoes had traditionally escaped any kind of levy, and the British merchants were upset by the change. They were now a force to be reckoned with – an organized society up to 60 strong who met in general assembly and voiced forceful opinions through their standing committee of 16 members.[234] In June 1811 they had not thought it beyond their brief to petition for the Revd Francis Laing to be made Public Secretary in place of Chapman, who had returned to England on health grounds.[235] On their home turf, they bothered Oakes with technical problems around commercial law, bills of exchange and the inadequacy of measures for insurance.[236] With regard to the new quarantine levy, they would not back down – but neither would Oakes.[237] The merchants protested in vain that this was an arbitrary tax incompatible with free-port status.[238] The general rule among lazarettos, they argued, was that income should simply be enough to meet expenditure. They viewed the new levy not as a Health Office fee but a tax to augment the island's revenue.[239] Oakes did no more than send their views to Lord Liverpool for information.[240]

These comparatively minor events took place against a background of extreme disquiet among sectors of the Maltese people, orchestrated at a distance by the malevolent Eton. Beneath lies and false accusations, many denigrating the memory of Ball, lay basic concerns for political representation, freedom of the press, and an independent and effective judicial system. Late in 1811 a Maltese nobleman, the marquis Nicoló Testaferrata, arrived in London having made no headway with his approaches to Oakes.[241] Following a meeting with Liverpool where the alleged grievances were aired, the minister agreed to send a Commission of Enquiry to Malta to examine legal, civil and military responsibilities and the wishes of the populace. Such political issues are largely irrelevant to this study, but the Commissioners' report, dated 30 August 1812, embraced questions of trade and quarantine and produced useful comments and statistics from knowledgeable informants.[242] One of the three Commissioners was Oakes.[243]

The main informant on commerce was Laing, who pointed out that the island's trade had somewhat improved during 1811.[244] Speculative exports to Britain had now ceased, so that ships arriving with cargoes sometimes returned in ballast, but the import of colonial produce, especially coffee, was 'immense' and found a strong

233 NA CO 158/18/101–5.

234 The figure of 'not fewer than Sixty' is in 'Observations' of Laing in NA CO 158/20 [unpag.].

235 NA CO 158/17 [unpag.], 17 June 1811.

236 NA CO 158/19/244–50.

237 NA CO 158/18/119–23.

238 NA CO 158/18/107–17.

239 Ibid.

240 NA CO 158/18/101–5.

241 See Gregory, pp. 176–7.

242 The report constitutes PRO CO 158/19.

243 The others were William à Court and John Burrows.

244 'General Observations on the Trade of Malta', in NA CO 158/20 [unpag.], from which all references in this paragraph are taken until otherwise stated.

market. An entrepôt trade in English woollens, sold mainly in Malta and Sicily, had the potential for growth if manufacturers would do what their colleagues in the cotton business had already done, which was adapt their goods 'to the taste of the Levant market'. Laing described the trade of Malta with Marseilles, the Italian ports and Trieste as 'forced' and 'more or less active in proportion to the rigour or flexibility of the French Government'. By contrast, commerce with Barbary was unfettered, but not large in volume. The main trade to the east was with the Levant, but business with the Ionian Islands and the Morea was on the increase, and much British and colonial produce found its way into Europe through the ports of Albania and, more recently, through Salonica. While most of this business was conducted by the British merchants, Laing reported the existence of 20 or 30 Maltese houses 'of large capital and of considerable enterprise'. There were also German, Italian and Greek concerns, and itinerant merchants from Sicily, Albania and farther afield. In an earlier memorandum, Laing's predecessor, Edmund Chapman, had remarked that the commercial lobby 'now form the Bulk of the better order of Society in Malta. Nearly all the Wealth, Energy, & Information ... belong to this Class'.[245]

The Commissioners reproduced much of Laing's official paper verbatim, but added pertinent comments on the problems of free-port status. They were critical of duties payable to the Custom House on each bale, package, barrel or bundle of merchandise. These duties, they reckoned, should be *ad valorem*, in line with practice at Leghorn and Messina.[246] They expected the merchants to remonstrate in principle about any change whatever to the system, while privately conceding that the new basis was better.[247] As regards the Health Office, the Commissioners confirmed the new fees and regulations imposed by Pym.[248] These had been found acceptable to the merchants, with the exception of the 0.5-per-cent levy paid on goods held in quarantine on board ship, which they acknowledged had been the subject of an acrimonious exchange with Oakes. It will come as little surprise that the Commissioners upheld the levy and found the merchants' concerns 'greatly over-rated'. The justification for the levy, however, was set more against the need to increase salaries among the 21 employees of the Health Office for their 'interesting and important duties' (now that private fees and perquisites had been abolished), and the importance of maintaining the general expenses of the office when income from quarantine fluctuated, than against the cost of extending the quarantine sheds. The Commissioners summarized the amount of the levy – £25 on a cargo valued at £5,000 – as 'too trifling to merit consideration'.

The regulations and fees which the Commissioners endorsed were badly printed in English on the island.[249] They exhibited the normal obsession with enumerated goods of the first and second class. In fact, the wording of these lists, and the three opening questions to be put to a ship's master, were lifted without change from the Order in Council of 5 April 1805. Similarly, the yellow-flag rules smacked of British

245 NA CO 158/18/23 [unpag.], 13 Feb. 1812.

246 NA CO 158/19/85–7.

247 Ibid.

248 NA CO 158/19/142–3, from which remaining references in this paragraph are taken.

249 Copy in NA CO 158/19/218–26.

practice, and many extracts from the Order had been, so to speak, cut and pasted into the Maltese rules. For example, clause 32 of the Order, so far as it related to the probationary airing of goods, was identical with clause 17 of the rules.[250] Likewise, clause 39 of the former, dealing with the date quarantine should commence, had been virtually reproduced in clause 23 of the latter. There were, nevertheless, significant changes. The main distinction was that authority and discretion lay with the Maltese Board of Health, rather than with the Privy Council in London.

The Maltese rules had to cover both Grand and Marsamxett Harbours, as well as a hierarchy of officials. For instance, there was a Captain of the Port responsible, if necessary, for sending ships from Grand Harbour into Marsamxett for the attention of the Captain of the Lazaret, and a Chancellor of the Health Office who dealt with paperwork and payments. Also, quarantine times in Malta were significantly longer than in Britain. To give two instances: the duration for a ship with a clean bill of health (and, of course, for all those on board) was 25 days, as against 15 in Britain; and the main airing of enumerated goods of the first class lasted 60 days, as against 40 in Britain. Finally, the Maltese rules included punishment for misdemeanours, whereas in Britain that was always a matter for Parliament, and never a feature of Orders in Council. It is interesting that, while transgressions against the discipline of quarantine were punishable by death, officials of the Health Office, even those who embezzled items in quarantine, stood only to lose their job and pay a fine of £100.[251] As Eton had left Malta before the Order of 1805 existed, and as the military superintendents who succeeded him were no more than deputies, it must indeed have been Pym who introduced these semi-Anglicized rules during the brief period of two months when he was on the island. It is very doubtful whether the primitive lazaretto in Gibraltar was operating at that time by such rigid principles, but Pym would have had access on the Rock to relevant Orders in Council from London.

The Commissioners were heartened to learn that in 1811 the island's balance of payments had moved for the first time from deficit to a modest surplus of nearly £4,000.[252] Oakes would have been especially happy that the Health Office was maintaining its profitability. Receipts in 1810 were roughly £9,200 against costs of only £4,463.[253] These figures represented 12.8 per cent and 5.2 per cent respectively of the island's income and expenditure, percentages comparable with 1809, when quarantine had first shown a profit. In 1811 receipts reached £11,555, against costs of £5,058, representing 11.3 per cent and 5.1 per cent of the respective island totals.[254] For 1812, the Commissioners could only make use of the figures for the first six months, which showed the Health Office income making up 8.4 per cent and expenditure 5.3 per cent.[255] It is difficult to concur with the Commissioners' opinion that the new tariffs were responsible for 'highly productive' interim figures for 1812,

250 With the trifling exception that the enumerated lists in the rules were before-stated (rather than hereinafter-stated as in the Order).

251 That leniency did not apply, however, to guardians placed on ships.

252 NA CO 158/19/75.

253 NA CO 158/19/155–7.

254 Ibid.

255 Ibid.

but clearly the Health Office was in much better shape than it had been under Ball.[256] It was still impossible, however, to lower the percentage claimed by the maintenance of quarantine from the overall annual budget.

Rejection of their request for cancelling the new Health Office levy did nothing to make the merchants more comfortable with Oakes. The fateful year of 1813 began with more complaints, this time centred on measures to prevent the free export of specie.[257] In February, Oakes complained to Bunbury that the merchants were addressing him with 'impropriety' of style and 'disrespectful' language.[258] There was little, however, in the opening months to draw quarantine to the attention of either side. Perhaps the only question to trouble Oakes was how far quarantine should be extended to the neighbouring island of Lampedusa. It had been suggested by Lord Liverpool, in 1811, that its fertile fields might become a growing-ground to help feed the population of Malta.[259] Although the Commissioners had found obstacles and disadvantages to acquiring a lease of the island, Oakes took it upon himself to send a detachment of soldiers there early in 1813, with a view to building a fort and clearing the ground for cultivation. On 15 January, Oakes sent the commanding officer a set of instructions, which concluded with the order that if a branch of the Health Office were to be established on Lampedusa for quarantine purposes, he should consider himself bound by the directions of the official in charge.[260] All this came to nothing, as British involvement with the island ceased in 1814. But the issue of quarantine harked back to the earlier interest in Lampedusa expressed by Russia. There was clearly an advantage in possessing a remote yet habitable island during an outbreak of Levantine plague. In the case of Oakes, it was as if he had had a subconscious premonition of the ghastly months ahead. But, in fact, they took him and everyone else by total surprise.

Plague

On 8 April 1813 Oakes wrote two letters to London. One was to Earl Bathurst, the new Secretary of State for War and the Colonies, informing him that he had appointed Bunbury as the Public Agent for Malta in England, at £600 a year from the island's revenue.[261] The other was to Bunbury himself, a serious and confidential letter which revealed just a hint of alarm.[262] Bunbury was warned that reports of plague in Malta would soon reach London, and they would be correct. A ship had recently arrived in the island from Alexandria with two people dead, and two more of the crew had died in the lazaretto. The rest had not yet shown symptoms. Utmost precautions had been taken, wrote Oakes, 'and you are aware how completely our

256 NA CO 158/19/158.
257 NA CO 158/22/24–8.
258 NA CO 158/22/67–8.
259 For the history of British interest in Lampedusa, see Gregory, pp. 283–6.
260 NA CO 158/22/79–84.
261 NA CO 158/22/88–9.
262 NA CO 158/22/92–3.

Lazaretto is insulated, so that I trust there is nothing to apprehend'.[263] The Board of Health had suggested that the ship and cargo be destroyed, but by the quarantine laws of Malta the owners had the option of removing it, and the ship was returning to Alexandria that day.

One month later Oakes wrote to Bunbury again.[264] He did not go into details, but any trace of complacency had passed. The plague was now a 'dreadful calamity' and he confessed himself unequal to the job of containing it. He had been periodically ill for months, and his own sickness was now acute, but had no connection with the plague. He was giddy and vomiting and needed to be replaced with urgency. But despite his own weakness of body, he would stay on in Malta if he could offer 'either consolation or confidence' in the crisis.[265] A few days later, on 12 May 1813, Oakes wrote to Bathurst recounting the circumstances of the epidemic, the measures being taken, and the competence of the Board of Health.[266] But before the end of the month he was forced to acknowledge that the disease was still spreading. On 22 May he confided in Bunbury that he was again very ill.[267] The plague, it was hoped, would cease in the summer, and he intended to leave Malta by the convoy arranged for 1 July. That journey was not to be. In June, Oakes was still complaining to Bunbury of his weakness in body and mind, but he would 'not scruple' to remain on Malta if the 'public Voice' thought his presence would do some good.[268] A week later he sent Bathurst an update of the horror which the island was experiencing, and copies of the many edicts he had issued to impose control.[269] It had been necessary, since 5 May, to embargo all shipping in Valletta's two harbours. [270]

It will be helpful at this point to explain the outbreak in more detail. There have been few epidemics since the Great Plague which have been so exhaustively analysed, but the way the epidemic got ashore remained a contentious issue. A vessel called the *San Nicola* arrived at Valletta on 29 March 1813 from Alexandria, where (not unusually) plague was rampant. Two crewmen had died on the voyage, one with a bubo. On the day following the removal of the survivors to the lazaretto, the master was taken ill with plague-like symptoms and died quickly. His servant died a few days later, but the rest of the men remained in good health. A new crew took the ship out of harbour and back towards Alexandria, and it was widely believed at that point, as Oakes's letter had shown, that the danger was past. But on 19 April a local doctor was concerned for a sick child in Valletta, the daughter of a shoemaker named Salvatore Borg. Following the child's sudden death, with a bubo on her chest, her pregnant mother fell ill and also died, having been delivered of a premature stillborn baby. Then another child in the family became sick, but recovered. When Borg himself was attacked by fever, with swellings in his armpit and groin, he and

263 Ibid.

264 NA CO 158/22/106–7.

265 Ibid.

266 NA CO 158/22/110–12.

267 NA CO 158/22/138–9.

268 NA CO 158/22/140.

269 NA CO 158/22/142–8.

270 NA CO 158/22/116.

his remaining family, as well as their close associates, were removed by the Board of Health to the lazaretto.

Again there was hope that the outbreak was contained, but the disease found a route to the people via the midwife who had delivered Mrs Borg. Within a few more days she was dead, along with the man who had found her body and a girl who was accustomed to stay at the midwife's house. Even at that stage, the diagnosis was by no means agreed upon and 'dread of the quarantine police' induced people to mask their symptoms.[271] It was widely held that Borg was more of a smuggler than a shoemaker and had received goods from the *San Nicola* removed from quarantine by corrupt guardians. Dr Burrell, whose official report on the Malta plague, commissioned by the General Board of Health in London as late as 1852, found no evidence to support this, and concluded that the story rested on such hearsay statements as Borg's alleged lament on his deathbed: 'Oh! the linen, the linen'.[272] Even if contraband from Alexandria had caused the outbreak, it was by no means impossible that cargo from some other vessel was responsible.

Cassar points to 16 May 1813 as the date when the epidemic 'began to assume alarming proportions', so that Oakes was forced to order every head of family to make an immediate report of sickness in his household, under pain of death.[273] Rewards were offered for information about undisclosed illnesses, and for reliable evidence of how the disease was spreading. Many people still refused to believe that the epidemic was plague. Valletta was divided into districts, supervised by local guards who struggled to ensure that the disease did not pass by direct contact between inhabitants, and between people and susceptible items. First churches were closed, then shops during hours of darkness, and a night-time curfew was imposed on individuals. But at the end of May, with the death toll already exceeding 100, the disease broke through to the satellite towns around Valletta, and then on to Mdina. The Board of Health recommended tough measures, including the virtual isolation of communities except for the delivery of supplies, but Oakes was hesitant. He did, however, agree that the districts within Valletta should be cordoned off more tightly, and teams were organized to cleanse properties in which occupants had died.

When the lazaretto was full, the sick were taken to the adjacent Fort Manoel. The whole population of two of the poorest districts of Valletta were shepherded there en masse for their own safety. When the fort was full, the sick were conveyed to makeshift huts around the outskirts of Valletta. In Mdina, part of a convent was used as a hospital. Convicts were used to escort the living, clear out the dead, bury corpses and strip out infected houses. As they died, prisoners were imported from Sicily to take their place. The number of dead overall reached around 1,600 in early August.

At that nadir of despair, it had been understood for some months in London that Pym was not prepared to return to Malta. As his letter of resignation to Bunbury was dated 15 April 1813, he could have had no knowledge at that time of the outbreak

271 W.H. Burrell, 'Report on the plague in Malta in 1813', in General Board of Health, Appendix V to Second Report on Quarantine, in *British Parliamentary Papers*, vol. 45 (1854–55), p. 15.

272 Burrell, p. 13.

273 Cassar, p. 178.

of plague.[274] Again, Pym cited a chronic liver complaint picked up in warm climates abroad as the reason to stay in England. He had hopes of holding the Malta job through the services of a deputy (as Oakes had feared), but realized this might not be acceptable.[275] It would have enhanced Pym's reputation if he had withdrawn his notice once he knew, as he must have done within days of writing, that plague had struck the island. Oakes, it would appear, was kept in the dark for some time about the Superintendent's intentions. Only on 1 September 1813 did he tell Bathurst that news had reached him of Pym's decision.[276] Oakes made no comment beyond pointing out that Joseph Thomas had devoted himself unstintingly to the lazaretto during the 18 months when the Superintendent had been away.[277] He went so far as to recommend Thomas for Pym's job, and Thomas himself sent a memorial to Bathurst on 10 September, soliciting the appointment.[278] Also still on Malta, despite his earlier appeal for promotion, was Ralph Green; he had sent the Chief Inspector of Hospitals a clinical assessment of the epidemic.[279]

On 3 October 1813 Lieutenant-General Sir Thomas Maitland arrived at Malta in the role of Governor. The title Civil Commissioner was no longer relevant, as the island had just been annexed to Britain. This, of course, cleared the way for the departure of the ailing Oakes who, despite his infirmities, lived until 1822.[280] Maitland, nicknamed 'King Tom', was of a much different stamp than Oakes.[281] He was recently arrived from Ceylon, where he had been Commander-in-Chief, bringing back a reputation as a tough and able administrator. Maitland knew his own mind and spoke it. One biographer has described him as 'a benevolent despot', but when he arrived on plague-ridden Malta, breathing the infected air 'through a medium of arsenic and brimstone', his benevolence was not manifest to the Health Office.[282] Whereas Oakes had been comfortable with military doctors, admiring their conscientiousness and insouciance for reward, Maitland blamed them for the island's misfortunes. His startling antipathy stemmed from an early meeting at which he claimed they knew no more about the plague than he did.[283] On 16 November he told Bunbury that he had had 'more trouble with the Medical People than with any other Sett – but we have got them now into pretty good Order – but the thing will not go on well till we expurgate them out of the Island, Green &c. &c. of the nature

274 NA CO 158/23 [unpag.].

275 Ibid.

276 NA CO 158/22/223–4.

277 Ibid.

278 NA CO 158/22/270.

279 NA CO 158/22/112.

280 See *Oxford Dictionary of National Biography*.

281 For Maitland, see especially C.W. Dixon, *The Colonial Administration of Sir Thomas Maitland* (London, 1939) and W.F. Lord, *Sir Thomas Maitland: The Mastery of the Mediterranean* (London, 1897). Gregory, *passim*, is also useful.

282 Dixon, pp. 131, 139; Lord, p. 142, Hardman, p. 18. The full quotation is: 'We breathe very much through a medium of arsenic and brimstone at present, but I am told when I get accustomed to it, it will be quite delicious'.

283 Cassar, p. 184.

of whose Conduct to Oakes you can have no idea'.[284] Oakes would not have agreed with him.

A few days later worse was to follow. Maitland expressed his annoyance to Bunbury that the Army Medical Board had sanctioned 'the absurd and useless idea' that Green should remain in Malta.[285] He wanted him and 'Mr. Staff Surgeon Thomas' removed, for as long as medical men were 'interfering with Government and dabbling with our Merchants', the health of the island would always be at risk.[286] Maitland intended to reform the lazaretto, which he acknowledged as 'the most important Department in this Island', as it had 'been uniformly neglected in a most shameful manner, & been considered as a Sinecure Place ... and generally jobbed away by the Holder who was not present, to some Deputy – selected not from his fitness, but for the cheapness for which He would undertake to do the duties of His Principal'.[287] This was an attack on Eton and his deputies, but also to some extent on Pym, as Maitland wanted the regulations which he had introduced to be changed as well. He was also annoyed that the merchants of Malta had 'presumed' to write to Bathurst in support of Thomas's bid for the superintendence of quarantine.[288] Maitland's own view was that both Thomas and Green had 'done much to confuse and embarass [*sic*] – and little indeed to Systemize or Regulate'.[289] He told Bathurst that the lazaretto, had 'been governed with a degree of laxness that by no means makes it astonishing the very first time the Plague prevailed to the Eastward, that it should get into this Island'.[290] It was not, of course, the first time that plague had appeared to the east, but Maitland was dismissive of detail.

By that time, Maitland would have known that Pym's successor was to be Robert Grieves, another Deputy Inspector of Hospitals, who had been appointed in July 1813.[291] Grieves arrived on the island during November, but Maitland did not 'register' him in office until 1 October 1814, when all trace of plague had been removed.[292] He kept the military doctors as far removed from public health as was practicable. On 23 October 1813 Maitland confirmed Green as responsible for the health of the garrison, but nothing more.[293] The health of the islands in general was a matter for the 'Proto-Medico', or head of the College of Physicians.[294] The lazaretto and all matters of quarantine continued under the Acting Superintendent of

284 NA CO 158/24 [unpag.]; cf. Gregory, p. 242.

285 NA CO 158/25/444–5.

286 Ibid.

287 NA CO 158/24 [unpag.], Maitland to Bathurst, 16 Nov. 1813

288 Ibid.

289 Ibid.

290 NA CO 158/24 [unpag.], 13 Apr. 1814.

291 This was to be a permanent job during good behaviour, a normal formula (NA CO 158/29 [unpag.], Grieves to Goulburn, 5 Aug. 1817).

292 NA CO 158/29 [unpag.], list of office-holders.

293 *Proclamations, Minutes and other Official Notices, published by the Government of the Island of Malta, and its Dependencies, From ... 1813, to ... 1820* (Malta, 1821), pp. 3–4. As Green was still referred to as Deputy Inspector of Hospitals, Maitland was evidently unaware or dismissive of his promotion.

294 Ibid.

Quarantine; Thomas was not mentioned by name.[295] (It can be assumed that Grieves superseded Thomas in this role, but played little or no other part in controlling the plague). These three men were to attend the Governor's palace daily to make their report. In an emergency, or if the Proto-Medico discovered any new case of plague, they were to place themselves under the orders of Lieutenant-Colonel Rivarola, the Inspector General of Police.[296] This was a humiliation, especially for Green and Thomas, but in Maitland's view they had been responsible for the outbreak.

To the people of Malta, the Governor came across as blunt and decisive, but his self-confidence was reassuring. Master of his island, Maitland took all matters by the scruff of the neck. He set himself the task of balancing the island's books as well as defeating the plague. The matters were connected, as the Treasury had spent £60,000 in fighting the outbreak, while its revenues were severely depleted by the constant disruption.[297] On 16 October 1813 the Governor announced that a temporary loan account had been opened at the Treasury, to which the Maltese were invited to contribute in multiples of 1,000 scudi against debentures.[298] Some confidence returned slowly to public life. Encouraged that their isolation might soon be ended, now that no case of plague had been reported for 15 days, the people of Valletta and Floriana were told how every house, store and magazine would be systematically cleansed.[299] Free pardons were offered for a limited period to those who had hoarded possessions after knowing their house had been infected. On 17 November 1813 the process of cleansing was extended to other towns, with the exception of three communities where the disease was still in evidence.[300] Within another ten days, only the village of Curmi, cordoned off from the rest of the island behind two new walls patrolled by soldiers, was not promised an imminent return to cautious normality.[301]

On 29 November 1813 Maitland disbanded the island's Council of Health.[302] This was a recently established body set up by Oakes to replace the Board of Health, who had resigned in June in protest at the Civil Commissioner's lack of enthusiasm for their radical suggestions.[303] Rivarola was again a beneficiary, dealing now with passes and applications for changes of residence. As the gratitude for the Council's work, which Maitland thought fit to proclaim, exceeded polite convention, it can be concluded that the doctors had proved more useful to the Governor than he had expected. The dissolution of the Council was a sign that Maitland felt the plague was defeated. It is not clear what relationship had existed between this now defunct body and the triumvirate who had been ordered, a month earlier, to report to Maitland daily; but the removal of the Council left Maitland to his own devices. He fell out immediately with Rear-Admiral Langhorne – 'so very odd a Man' – about assistance

295 Ibid.

296 Ibid.

297 NA CO 158/24 [unpag.], Maitland to Bathurst, 6 Oct. 1813.

298 *Proclamations, Minutes and other Official Notices* (1821), p. 2.

299 *Proclamations, Minutes and other Official Notices* (1821), pp. 5–7.

300 *Proclamations, Minutes and other Official Notices* (1821), pp. 7–8.

301 cf. Gregory, p. 243.

302 *Proclamations, Minutes and other Official Notices* (1821), pp. 9–10.

303 Cassar, p. 182; Gregory, p. 240.

for HMS *Partridge*, a sloop from Gibraltar with 17 crewmen ill with yellow fever.[304] With the plague raging, it was impossible to land the men at the lazaretto so the ship was sent to St Paul's Bay. Maitland thought of setting them down on an island there, but the locals were reputedly more afraid of yellow fever than the plague, and if foreign nations learnt of this arrangement they would keep Malta in quarantine, reckoned Maitland, for 'God knows how long'.[305] The disagreement arose over whether the ship should, instead, cruise indefinitely offshore accompanied by a transport. The Admiral was unhappy with that, and the compromise was for the *Partridge* to sail for Lampedusa to land her sick.[306] This was the first and only time that the quarantine potential of that small island was actually realized by the British, although no facilities were built there.

The road to good health proved faster and smoother as the months passed, but there were still diversions. At Curmi, Maitland resorted to martial law, convinced that the continuing plague arose from the pilfering or secretion of infected clothing, and the village was converted to a lazaretto.[307] There was still an occasional scare in Valletta, and it was 3 January 1814 before normal intercourse was allowed between the towns around the harbours and the ships.[308] On 27 January, Maitland felt 'happily enabled' to declare that, after 54 days without infection (except in the lazarettos), the quarantine throughout the island would be replaced by general pratique in two days time.[309] As a gesture of the humanity of British rule, one Felix Camilleri, a lazaretto guard sentenced to death for breach of quarantine, was ostentatiously pardoned.[310]

In February 1814 the post-plague celebrations were dampened by an epidemic in neighbouring Gozo which had, until then, escaped attack. The cause was attributed to infected clothing allegedly from Curmi, but again the disease was no match for Maitland and his policy of segregation. The deaths on Gozo exceeded 100, but these were few in relation to Malta, where the final death toll was 4,572.[311] It was to be another seven months before Maitland could at last tell the world that the plague in his domain was 'completely extinguished', and that no further Proclamations would be issued.[312] This last message was terse, with none of the thanksgiving and euphoria which had accompanied the announcement in January. The commercial life of Malta had been virtually ruined. Maitland had beaten the plague but not the economic consequences, especially the excuse which certain countries used and prolonged to keep ships from Malta in a defensive and quasi-political quarantine. As early as May 1813 Oakes had warned Bunbury that enemies of Malta were characterizing the

304 NA CO 158/24 [unpag.], Maitland to Bunbury, 28 Dec. 1813.

305 Ibid.

306 Ibid.

307 cf. Gregory, p. 243.

308 *Proclamations, Minutes and other Official Notices* (1821), pp. 14–15.

309 *Proclamations, Minutes and other Official Notices* (1821), pp. 19–20.

310 A tablet recording this pardon, on the grounds that Camilleri was the first person condemned to death after the British assumed sovereignty of Malta, was erected beside the gibbet on Fort Manoel. The full Italian text is quoted in H. Luke, *Malta: An Account and an Appreciation* (London, 1949), p 100.

311 Cassar, p. 186; Gregory, p. 244.

312 *Proclamations, Minutes and other Official Notices* (1821), pp. 63–4, 8 Sept. 1814.

plague as Britain's fault.[313] In November that year Maitland took up the complaint, informing Bathurst that the commerce of the island was suffering 'from certain Measures that have been adopted down the Mediterranean upon what grounds and principles I am not aware …'[314] Such naivety, if that is what it was, would not last.

313 NA CO 158/22/106–7

314 NA CO 158/24 [unpag.], Maitland to Bathurst, 16 Nov. 1813.

Chapter Twelve

Anti-Contagionism in Britain, 1805–1825

Defying the sceptics

If the epidemic in Malta in 1813 encouraged debate as to whether or not the plague was contagious, the British Government had long been aware that traditional reliance in the efficacy of quarantine, based on the acceptance of contagion, was not universally accepted. It will have been apparent from references in this study to contemporary criticism of Richard Mead that a certain body of opinion had been denying for nearly a century that any connection existed between touching infected goods and the spreading of plague. Even in the middle of the eighteenth century, with the publication of Manningham's *The Plague no contagious Disease* ..., the analysis of the Marseilles crisis continued to inspire doubters and undermine the principles on which quarantine depended.[1] But these anti-contagionists were not sufficiently organized and vociferous to influence either public opinion or the minds of ministers, and when Howard, and more especially Russell, adopted a contagionist stance in the 1790s, the British entered the nineteenth century with the attitude that national policy for quarantine was correct, even if plans for a lazaret were proving difficult to achieve.

The Privy Council had not regarded yellow fever in the same light as plague, first because the disease was thought unable to propagate itself in a relatively cold climate, and secondly because the contagious aspect, in the literal sense of being spread by touch, was widely doubted. These views, however, had not prevented quarantine being used as a system of defence, because no other safeguard was available. It became increasingly irksome to merchants, importers and to the American authorities that quarantine was routinely imposed on transatlantic shipping when each report of yellow fever reached London ears. In America itself, there was a growing lobby which argued that neither plague nor yellow fever was contagious and, although quarantine was still practised in North American ports, there was a greater inclination than in Britain to question its relevance.[2]

In July 1805 the Privy Council had the awkward task of replying on behalf of Lord Mulgrave, Foreign Secretary, to a letter from the American chargé d'affaires, who had complained about the restraints to commerce which quarantine in Britain

1 cf. C.F. Mullett, *The Bubonic Plague and England: An Essay in the History of Preventive Medicine* (Lexington, 1956), p. 310.

2 Mullett, *The Bubonic Plague and England*, p. 330.

had brought about.[3] The Council stood their ground, arguing that British policy rested on 'unquestionable authority' and that yellow fever had caused Philadelphia to institute quarantine against Charleston. The Americans were concerned about the length of time ships were detained, in what seemed an overzealous application of the rules. But whereas quarantine in Britain for arrivals from North America was set at 15 days, with the same period to follow for the cargo, it had become customary to release ships and people as soon as goods were offloaded for airing into lighters. The Council admitted, however, that in the previous winter they had insisted on the letter of the law. It was unreasonable, in the Americans' view, to detain a ship and crew in quarantine for that length of time once the cargo had been removed. The Council, on the other hand, reserved the right to impose whatever period of quarantine they thought appropriate. Although they noted 'with great satisfaction' that Customs officers in American ports had, since 1801, granted bills of health, the Council felt the bills were not to be trusted. Intelligence suggested that passengers arriving at Philadelphia from the West Indies were allowed to land too quickly from the lazaretto station, and that new passengers were allowed to embark on what was probably a diseased vessel. As it was, Britain had always been more lenient with ships arriving from North America than from the Mediterranean because of the longer voyage time. The grumpy stalemate with the Americans was set to continue.

It was in Philadelphia where Charles Maclean, the great British champion of anti-contagionism, discovered the first receptive market for his radical views.[4] Maclean had experienced his first contact with yellow fever in Jamaica in 1790. His observations there, coupled with a study of the outbreak in Philadelphia in 1793, led him to the conclusion that 'no general disease, which is capable of affecting the same person repeatedly, is ever propagated by contagion'.[5] Maclean found employment as a surgeon on East India Company ships and, having arrived in Calcutta, published a dissertation on epidemic and pestilential diseases in 1796. Two years later, still in Calcutta, he was surprised and gratified when an American sea captain showed him a copy of his own book and other tracts which had been reprinted in Philadelphia in 1797. From this event, Maclean claimed credit for steering some American physicians on the path of anti-contagionism, although when these same publications reached London, 'they underwent', in his own words, 'a sort of regular medical excommunication'.[6]

The excommunicators were the College of Physicians, who had the ear of the Privy Council. It is improbable that the Council were even aware of Maclean's existence when, following the physicians' advice, they had agreed to set up a British

---

3 National Archives [NA] PC 2/168/90–92, from which all references in this paragraph are taken.

4 Maclean has been the subject of an essay by C.F. Mullett ('Politics, economics, and medicine: Charles Maclean and anticontagion in England', *Osiris*, 10 [1952], 224–51) and also has an *Oxford Dictionary of National Biography* entry. Much of the material comes from autobiographical anecdotes in his writings, which are also the source for most references in this paragraph.

5 C. Maclean, *Evils of Quarantine Laws, and Non-Existence of Pestilential Contagion* … (London, 1824), p. 41.

6 Maclean, *Evils of Quarantine Laws*, p. 43.

Board of Health. The Board, of course, acted wholly in accordance with contagionist principles and if the members had deviated for one moment from that stance, then its brief existence would have been shorter still. The Privy Council remained convinced that quarantine was the only effective way of preventing the importation of plague, and if its efficacy against yellow fever was more problematical, its use was at least evidence that the threat was taken seriously. Far from winding down other quarantine stations, in reaction to the hugely expensive debacle at Chetney Hill, the Council were receptive to ideas for strengthening the establishments elsewhere. The area to benefit most from this positive frame of mind was Scotland.

Apparently on their own initiative, the Customs Commissioners in Scotland drew up plans for land lazarettos both at Holy Loch, which had succeeded Lamlash as the quarantine station for the Clyde, and at Inverkeithing Ness.[7] These plans were sent to the Treasury who, in July 1805, forwarded them to the Privy Council.[8] The Council were happy to agree with 'Plan B' for Holy Loch, at an estimated cost of £9,110.[9] They were less convinced, however, of the need for a lazaretto at Inverkeithing and questioned the extent of trade to eastern Scotland from Turkey and the Mediterranean. If a lazaretto were needed, they wondered if one of the islands in the Forth estuary, for instance Inchkeith, might not be preferable.[10] The matter might have rested there had not the Danish minister in London, early in 1806, complained about quarantine delays in British ports, especially at Leith, which relied to a large extent on the facilities at Inverkeithing.[11] In their reply, dated 3 April, the Privy Council confirmed that land lazarettos had been authorized at both Holy Loch and Inverkeithing Ness, but the case for this expenditure, when no similar building had been deemed necessary at, say, Milford Haven, remains far from clear.[12] To offset the costs, the Council gave orders in July for the closure of quarantine stations at Cromarty Bay and Carsethorn.[13] Having given their decision for land establishments in Scotland, the Council, mindful of ongoing problems at Chetney Hill, had no wish to become further involved and were intolerant of complications. When a question was raised concerning the contractors at Inverkeithing, the Treasury were told emphatically that the Council had no view.[14] When the company who owned the airing hulk already stationed at Inverkeithing objected to a land establishment, the Council dismissed their petition.[15]

---

7 The idea for Holy Loch came first. When the Scottish Customs Commissioners were arguing for Lamlash to be superseded, they submitted a proposition for a land lazaret 'at a place pointed out by one of the Officers employed in the Quarantine Service …, in preference to a floating Lazaret' (NA PC 2/165/38, Mar. 1804)

8 NA PC 2/168/21.

9 Ibid.

10 Ibid.

11 NA PC 2/169/492–4.

12 Ibid. It would appear from PC 2/170/293 that the order to build the land establishment at Inverkeithing was dated 6 February 1806.

13 NA PC 2/170/428, 628.

14 NA PC 2/172/423.

15 NA PC 2/173/167, 408.

The lazaretto at Inverkeithing Ness, of which no trace remains, is well documented, owing to the work of a minor American writer named James Simson.[16] In 1882 Simson published his reminiscences of a childhood spent at the lazaretto, where he had been born in 1826, son of the Superintendent.[17] By then the institution was winding down, but Simson recollected that rags were occasionally still aired there, and indeed rags (for the paper industry) were why Inverkeithing Bay had long been the station for a Dutch-built airing hulk, some of whose ballast contributed to dry dykes around the new building.[18] Simson published a fine illustration of both the lazaretto and the dwelling house alongside.

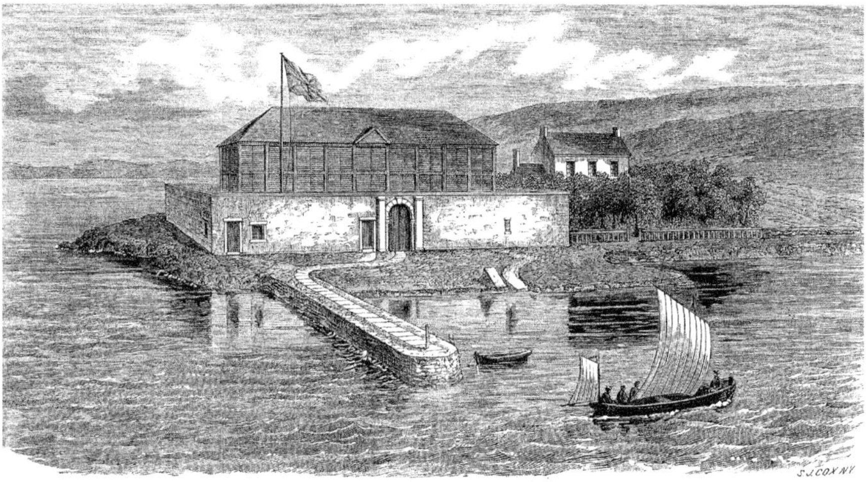

LAZARETTO, INVERKEITHING BAY, FIFESHIRE (1829.)

Illustration 12.1 Print of lazaretto

The engraving, made in New York, was taken from a photograph of a pencil drawing, made by the wife of an Ayrshire man to whom Simson's father had rented his house in around 1829.[19] It is difficult to exaggerate the importance of this authentic and unique view, which shows a kind of miniature fort far removed from the impressive and multifunctional Mediterranean precedents which Russell and Howard had recommended.

Simson recollected that the lazaretto was three storeys high and built of Memel timber. 'It was placed upon a number of square stone supports, some of which

16 See Bibliography. The title-page of his *Reminiscences* explains that he was also the editor of *Simson's History of the Gipsies* and author of four other works.

17 He was Walter Simson, mentioned in a parliamentary return of 1823 (*Journal of the House of Commons* [*JHC*], vol. 78, p. 999).

18 James Simson, *Reminiscences of Childhood at Inverkeithing, or Life at a Lazaretto* (New York, 1882), p. 5.

19 Simson, p. 6. The engraving was reproduced in smaller format in William Stephen, *History of Inverkeithing and Rosyth* (Aberdeen, 1921), p. 350.

were continued inside of the building to the beginning of the roof, to steady the structure'.[20] The supports were therefore like staddle-stones holding up a barn, and the infant Simson could move around beneath the lazaretto, while barely stooping. The three floors were slatted to allow a circulation of air. 'The sides and ends of the building were composed of a frame, and slats that opened and shut laterally; so that the structure could be thoroughly ventilated from below and all around, and have its contents exposed to the air outside'.[21] The illustration does not make it clear, but Simson refers to a stone building 'apparently intended for passengers' behind the wooden one.[22] In fact, it housed the labourers who aired the rags, and their regime was strictly controlled. Simson remembered that their food 'was passed in through an aperture in the wall, on what looked like the half of a barrel cut lengthwise, with shelves, on which the food was placed; and this on being turned on a pivot reached the inside, when the outside door was locked'.[23]

It would appear that goods were offloaded from ships in the bay into lighters, which moored alongside a pier protruding inland from the end of the ness, or headland. Simson refers to merchandise being moved 'on hand trucks, along a flagged way from the pier till it reached hoisting apparatus connected with the building'.[24] The smaller entrances in the perimeter wall were technically for passengers, but Simson was probably correct in assuming that the lazaretto was used only for airing goods. There was no road to it from Inverkeithing, which was about a mile away, and even the footpath petered out. When Simson's father had business in the town, he crossed the shallow entrance to the bay at low tide, walking on stilts.[25] This manoeuvre took him from the west ness to the east, from where he could walk to the town along the foreshore. He was paid £130 a year, but £90 of that was for the simultaneous post of Deputy Comptroller at Inverkeithing.[26]

In contrast to this east-coast institution, the lazaretto erected at Holy Loch is scantily documented. The site is not in doubt, marked by the modern 'Lazaretto Point', a small promontory to the north-west of Hunter's Quay, on the western side of the loch.[27] It seems that the establishment was rather larger than at Inverkeithing, and the superintendent received £130 a year for that post alone.[28] A description of 1845 referred to 'an extensive and complete range of stores, suited to receive infected goods of every description. The buildings are surrounded by a high wall; and close to them is erected a range of houses for the use of the Superintendent of

20 Simson, p. 5.

21 Ibid.

22 Ibid.

23 Simson, p. 6.

24 Ibid.

25 Simson, p. 8.

26 *JHC*, vol. 78, p. 999.

27 The monument shown at this location on Ordnance Survey maps is a war memorial and has no association with the lazaretto.

28 *JHC*, vol. 78, p. 999, which reveals that in 1823 the Superintendent was Andrew Pitcairn.

the quarantine, and the men employed in its service'.[29] There was no mention there of passenger accommodation, but by 1845 that would have been discontinued in any case. In later years there was an understanding within the Privy Council that the Holy Loch lazaretto had been envisaged expressly with yellow fever in mind; while such precision is not borne out by the Council's minutes of 1805, it is certainly true that the Clyde estuary at that time was receiving more ships from North America than from the Mediterranean.[30]

It was perhaps knowledge of the developments in Scotland that prompted shipowners and pilots at Liverpool, in December 1806, to agitate for better quarantine facilities in the Mersey.[31] They suggested that Bromborough Pool would be safer and less expensive than Hoylake, but there was no call for a shore establishment. The Privy Council were wary of initiatives from Liverpool, having been embroiled in the past in commercial jealousies between north-west England and London, and the Customs Commissioners were equally reluctant to express a view. Nearly two years passed before the latter were prompted to comment on the proposal, and only on 18 October 1809 did the Council appoint Bromborough Pool as the new quarantine station for Liverpool.[32] The only other change to quarantine arrangements in England at this period concerned a reduction in the size of The Motherbank station, authorized in 1811, as it was proving difficult for ships not to stray within the limits under certain weather conditions.[33] No changes were made at Milford Haven, but in July 1813 it was made an alternative foul-bill quarantine station to Stangate Creek for ships from the Mediterranean and West Barbary.[34]

Ireland

Little has been said so far in this study about quarantine in Ireland. As the systems in Ireland and Britain were not unified until 1825, it will be useful to look now at the Irish practice before that date. Stated briefly, the thinking in England was to leave Ireland to its own devices. There was a general understanding that those in authority in Ireland, subordinate to and dependent on policy in London, would follow the national lead over quarantine as they did in other matters relating to Customs. Ironically, during the seventeenth century, Ireland produced quarantine arrangements which were distinctly tighter and more precise than those in England. In 1625, to counter the arrival of plague from London, a Proclamation of the Lord Deputy and Council required goods to be aired for 30 days and passengers to be

29 *New Statistical Account of Scotland* (15 vols, Edinburgh & London, 1845), vol. 7, pp. 611–12.

30 NA PC 7/4/49–50 (1832).

31 NA PC 2/171/560.

32 NA PC 2/178/469; 2/183/407.

33 NA PC 2/190/375; 2/191/155; 2/192/298, 314, 321–4.

34 NA PC 2/194/509. But it was not to be used by ships which had the plague on board.

detained for 20.[35] The farmers of the Customs were to build wooden houses near Dublin, one for goods and the other for people, who were to be provided with the necessaries of life.[36] In the Irish outports, similar arrangements were to be made at the farmers' expense.[37] Forty years later, the same periods for airing and detention were re-enacted, and the Proclamation referred to two houses for this purpose having been erected on the island of Clontarf, at a cost of £300 borne by the city of Dublin.[38] It was also possible for Ireland to act independently of provisions in England. In 1681 Sir John Temple, Solicitor-General for Ireland, suggested to the Marquis of Ormonde that he might wish to follow the lead of France in making quarantine compulsory for arrivals from plague-stricken Cadiz.[39]

When England, under Anne, introduced quarantine measures against the Baltic, Ireland followed suit, with the Proclamations of the Lord Lieutenant (or Lords Justices) and Council in Dublin lagging a few weeks behind those of the Queen in Council in London. Again, the Irish were better organized. They appointed 'pratique masters' at Cork and elsewhere to certify when quarantine had been done.[40] While the English were frantic for the protection of London, leaving the outports to manage for themselves in deliberation with the Customs authorities, the Irish introduced seven quarantine stations around their coastline in 1711, with a roughly regular spacing and no particular emphasis on the port of Dublin.[41] In a clockwise rotation, beginning with the northern coast of Ireland, the station for ports between Tory and Rathlin Islands was Ballymastoker Bay off Londonderry; for ports between Rathlin Island and Carlingford Lough, it was off Kilroot in Belfast Lough; between Carlingford Lough and the Tuskar Rock, it was Poolbeg off Dublin until 10 April 1712, and thereafter Dublin Bay; between the Tuskar Rock and Mizen Head, it was near Spike Island in Cork harbour; between Mizen Head and Loop Head, it was Scattery Road in the estuary of the Shannon; between Loop Head and Blacksod Bay, it was off Hare Island in Galway Bay; and between Blacksod Bay and Tory Island, it was Killybegs harbour.[42] Unfortunately, such exemplary precision would not last.

Some bad incidents in the quarantine service, including the death of several men in 1720, brought home to the Irish authorities the fragility of an operation which functioned only on the basis of legislation passed in London.[43] While the preamble to every general quarantine Act passed at Westminster up to 1753, lumped Great

35 Bibliotheca Lindesiana, vol. 6: *A Bibliography of Royal Proclamations of the Tudor and Stuart Sovereigns and of Others Published under Authority 1485–1714 … Ireland and Scotland* (Oxford, 1910), p. 28.

36 Ibid.

37 Ibid.

38 Bibliotheca Lindesiana, vol. 6, p. 92 (28 July 1665).

39 Historical Manuscripts Commission [HMC], *Ormonde*, vol. 6, p. 134.

40 Bibliotheca Lindesiana, vol. 6, p. 202.

41 Bibliotheca Lindesiana, vol. 6, p. 198.

42 For some stations, this is a slightly abbreviated description.

43 Archbishop Marsh's Library, Dublin, MS.Z2.1.7 and MS.Z3.1.1 record payments amounting to £156 to six widows of men lost in a wherry employed in the quarantine service. In 1720 the Lord Lieutenant of Ireland had asked the Treasury for 'several armed wherries and sloops' (*Calendar of Treasury Papers* [*CTP*] (1720–28), p. 26).

Britain and Ireland loosely together, it was difficult to establish any relevancy for the Irish who, for instance, had a limited trade with the Baltic. Because their interests were so little affected, an Order of 1712 lifting quarantine from places outside The Sound was made applicable in Ireland, but such a ruling was most unusual.[44] Indeed in 1721, following the scare at Marseilles, and in the knowledge that Irish ports traded strongly with Spain and the Mediterranean, it was deemed appropriate for the Irish Parliament to pass their own quarantine Act.[45] This was to be in force, however, for only one year. Its main purpose was to empower the Lord Lieutenant, with the consent of the Irish Privy Council, to proclaim the prohibition of trade with an infected place. This statute was, in effect, delegating powers given to the King by a contemporary Act of the Westminster Parliament; but the Irish Act also raised for the first time questions suited to the local dimension, such as punishments (death for those who smuggled goods ashore out of quarantine, and a fine of £500 for those whose carelessness allowed it) and the erection of watch houses.

The next Irish quarantine Act was not until 1743, following the plague at Messina.[46] Most of the provisions were to have a currency of only two years, from 1 May 1744, but measures intended to restrain commerce in times of infection were indefinite. This Act fell in the middle of a 20-year period in which no quarantine Act was passed at Westminster, even in the face of the crisis at Messina. That omission, caused to a large extent by dithering in the Regency, has already been discussed. In Ireland, the constitutional issues were less daunting and the crisis was clearly in focus. It brought about the first Act systematically to cover the duties and responsibilities of ships' masters and Customs officers, and the procedures for quarantine and airing. Penalties for neglect or disobedience were detailed at every stage, and the English anti-smuggling tactic was adopted of banning ships under 20 tons burthen from sailing without lodging security in times of infection. Most clauses smacked of the Westminster precedents – there were powers to erect lazarettos on waste ground for airing goods and 'the receiving and entertaining of persons obliged to perform quarantine' – and if the Act gave the Irish power to act without reference to London, there was no appetite in Dublin for a divergent policy.

The Privy Council in London routinely sent copies of quarantine Orders to lieutenant-governors or military commanders in the Channel Islands, the Isle of Man and Ireland. In the off-islands the Orders were to be obeyed, while in Ireland they were for guidance, with the idea 'that the necessary Directions may be given for laying a like Quarantine in that Kingdom'.[47] There is ample evidence from the sequence of Proclamations that Ireland was happy to comply, but this did not give the Privy Council in London any inclination to intervene in the management of Irish quarantine. The point is illustrated by a petition in 1759 from Irish merchants to the

44 NA PC 2/83/443.

45 *Statutes at Large. Ireland*, vol. 5: 8 Geo. I, c.3, from which remaining references in this paragraph are taken.

46 *Statutes at Large. Ireland*, vol. 6: 17 Geo. II, c.12, from which remaining references in this paragraph are taken.

47 For example NA PC 2/100/313 (1747) & 2/101/303–4 (1749).

King in Council.[48] They wanted three ships at Dublin from Leghorn to be released from quarantine in the same way as were ships recently arrived at The Downs and bound for London.[49] The Privy Council returned the petition to Ireland, and re-explained their thinking for the benefit of the Lord Lieutenant.[50] In 1770 the Irish Privy Council were briefly troubled by the legality of their own Orders, as the Irish quarantine Acts had long expired, and Proclamations in Ireland did not reflect the authority of the royal prerogative.[51] But this was a constitutional nicety that no one felt inclined to explore.

As the eighteenth century progressed, the system for informing Ireland of quarantine initiatives in Great Britain tended to break down. This was due partly to the increasing tempo and complexity of decision-making (for instance, as bills of health acquired extra categories), and partly from the changing protocol attached to referral. Whereas the Clerk to the Privy Council had traditionally sent copies of Orders direct to the secretary to the Lord Lieutenant, they became channelled through the new post of Home Secretary from 1782, when the geographical departments of the Secretaries of State were abandoned. The bureaucratic inefficiency of this system can be illustrated in 1796, when papers recounting at great length (but with some urgency) the attitude of the Privy Council since 1772 to arrivals from Spain and the Mediterranean were sent from London to Dublin in four stages, one of which involved the Duke of Portland.[52]

For the Customs service in Great Britain, the extent to which Irish quarantine met British requirements was sometimes in doubt. The queries which arose, although few in number, give reason to believe that the uncertainty would have been far greater had Irish ports been a regular stopover on the trade run from the Mediterranean to England or Scotland. The position was not made easier by the attitude of the British Privy Council. When the English Customs Commissioners wished guidance, in 1771, on the treatment of the *Hero* from Malaga which had left quarantine in Baltimore Bay (south-west of Skibbereen), they were told by the Privy Council that she could not dock in the port of Chester before a thorough examination.[53] It might be argued that Baltimore Bay was not a proper quarantine station, but only late in the eighteenth century did the Privy Council come round to the view that 40 days' quarantine in an Irish haven were worth 40 days' quarantine in England.[54] In fact, there had never been solid reasons for suspecting that the quarantine service in Ireland was any less efficient or conscientious than its British counterpart. In the Marseilles crisis, the Irish played their part in burning suspect ships, and five of their Customs officers were taken against their will to Amsterdam in a French vessel, having been barred

48 NA PC 2/107/161.

49 Ibid.

50 Ibid.

51 *Calendar of Home Office Papers* [*CHOP*] (1770–72), p. 8.

52 NA PC 2/146/523–6. The sequence was PC to John King to Duke of Portland (Home Secretary) to Thomas Pelham to Lord Lieutenant of Ireland.

53 NA PC 2/115/99.

54 For example NA PC 2/135/76 (1790): letter from PC to Customs officers in Falmouth confirming that a brig with oil from Gallipoli need not be quarantined, having performed 40 days at Castle Haven in Ireland.

from returning to shore when the master refused to stop for quarantine.[55] It could be objected that the Irish were not too insistent that ships underwent quarantine at an approved station, but the same charge could often be levelled at the British. Another mark in Ireland's favour was that the Lord Lieutenant, whenever in doubt or confusion, asked the Privy Council in London for guidance. An instance of that came in 1781, when the Irish were perplexed by an Order in Council which allowed hemp ships from the Baltic to enter British ports without airing.[56]

If the flow of information from London to Dublin meant that the Irish were, sooner or later, apprised of British policy, the absence of any information in a reverse direction meant that the Privy Council had little knowledge of how quarantine was conducted in Ireland. By 1800, although not dissatisfied with the competence of the Irish, the Council were in the mood for assuming greater control. The question arose, in a roundabout way, from Scotland, where the Customs Commissioners, for reasons not apparent, had queried *inter alia* whether foul-bill ships were accepted in Ireland.[57] The Council replied defensively:

> With respect to Ireland, no answer is returned, because it is presumed that no Ships will come from Turkey to the Ports of Ireland, with Goods liable to Infection, or without clean Bills of Health. It will be time enough to give an Opinion on this Subject, whenever the Case arises; it is presumed there is some Establishment in Ireland, probably the same as here, for the performance of Quarantine by Ships coming with clean Bills of Health; this Subject, however, will necessarily come under the consideration of Parliament in the next Session, and it is probable the Quarantine Laws will then be made the same in Ireland as in England.[58]

But the 1801 Act of Union, which abolished the Irish Parliament, made no such provision. Ironically, a quarantine Act had recently been passed in Dublin which annulled two earlier Irish Acts (of 1771 and 1799) and formed the basis for subsequent Proclamations.[59] The new Act echoed the provisions of 50 years earlier and made no reference to foul bills of health or the course of action if a ship were actually infected.

There was now a danger that Ireland was operating under a quarantine system which failed to meet the complexities of the age. The Privy Council continued to dither as to how far Ireland should or should not be incorporated under the rules for British quarantine. When the Bill of 1805 was before Parliament, the intention was to extend the measures to Ireland, 'but on further consideration it was felt that some Provisions might not be suitable to its local circumstances'.[60] The practice, therefore, continued of updating the Lord Lieutenant at intervals of new British initiatives, and of the Lord Lieutenant, or Lords Justices, and Council of Ireland

---

55 J.W. Joyce, *Daniel Defoe and the Plague in Marseilles (1720–1722)* (Leeds, 1957), p. 5; HMC, *Eleventh Report*, p. 107.

56 NA PC 2/126/103–5.

57 NA PC 2/156/22.

58 Ibid.

59 Irish Act, 40 Geo. III, c.79.

60 NA PC 2/167/117.

issuing Proclamations in the wake of those from the King in Council. This archaic system did not strengthen confidence among British Customs officials in the efficacy of Irish quarantine. They were once more reluctant to allow pratique to ships which had allegedly performed quarantine at an Irish station.[61] It was not until June 1824 that the Privy Council drafted an Order directing that any ship which had been quarantined in Ireland would be exempt from further detention in Britain.[62] Given the knowledge of Irish quarantine which had just been imparted to a Select Committee of the Commons (as will be explained below), it is possible that the Order was never in fact issued.

Militant Maclean

From around 1809 the declining incidence of quarantine in the Privy Council's registers suggests that their lordships were set in their ways. The years of agonizing over yellow fever were deemed to be over and the management of the Chetney Hill project was delegated to the Treasury, acting through the Commissioners of Customs, and to Rennie. Some questions of quarantine were handled by the Board of Trade, to whom petitioners increasingly looked for support. By the end of 1812 the traditional lists of ships seeking release from quarantine, and the subsequent orders to that effect, disappeared from the Council's registers. As the Council were still responsible for releasing ships, the conclusion must be that clerks were considered competent to reach a decision when no complications were apparent. There were, of course, times when the Council could not delegate. A good example was the scare which caused a brief imposition of quarantine on ships from Sweden in April 1809, and there were occasional problems with arrivals from North America, and more especially from Spain and Gibraltar, when yellow fever erupted once more in 1810.[63] But the guidelines for prevention had been established and there were few issues of quarantine to cause the Council to break their stride. Even the plague in Malta raised no new emergency measures. In Britain, these were times to be lenient with minor transgressions. The Council took pity on five poor fishermen, rescinding hefty fines imposed for straying within the perimeter of The Motherbank station and rescuing them from prison when they were unable to pay.[64] Many transgressors petitioned for prosecutions to be dropped if they agreed to pay costs incurred by the Crown; others volunteered to join the navy.[65]

In these years of complacency, a heretic like Maclean was most unwelcome. He had gone to Germany in 1800, waiting for an opportunity to visit Paris where

61 For example NA PC 2/191/578 (1811), concerning a ship which had done 16 days' quarantine at Kinsale.

62 NA PC 2/205/489. This was the summary of the substance of the Order in the margin of the register. But as the text alongside was blank, either the Order was not actually made, or it was simply not fair copied.

63 For Sweden, see NA PC 2/180/427, 444; 2/181/330; for Gibraltar, see NA PC 2/189/305 asking Customs officers to be vigilant.

64 NA PC 2/190/254.

65 NA PC 2/182/567; see also 2/181 index for quarantine punishment.

he expected his 'long-meditated plan for the investigation of the plague' would be best received.[66] The preliminary peace treaty with France allowed him to propose to the Minister of the Interior that an institution for research and treatment should be established in Constantinople, funded by voluntary contributions from governments and individuals, and supervised by foreign ambassadors as well as a member of the Porte. Unfortunately for Maclean, the minister referred his idea to the French School of Medicine, who at that date were no more enamoured of anti-contagionist thinking than were their colleagues in England. Maclean attacked all such institutions as reactionary and self-protective, 'always the first to denounce, and the last to adopt, any useful innovation'.[67]

Thwarted in France (and briefly interned), Maclean returned to England in 1804 and resigned himself to a career as a military doctor.[68] This failed to give him the opportunities he had expected to progress his cause, and he technically deserted the army, although the authorities were not minded to prosecute. But neither were they prepared to accept his offer to volunteer for a medical role in the expedition to Walcheren in 1809, and he regained a role with the East India Company, for whom he lectured on diseases in hot countries. From this background, Maclean found favour with the Levant Company, under whose auspices he travelled widely in Turkish territory from 1815 and studied plague at the Greek hospital in Constantinople. In January 1816, returned to Greenwich, Maclean sent the Foreign Secretary, Lord Castlereagh, an unsolicited commentary on the Ottoman attitude to plague and British absurdities in seeking its prevention.[69] He argued it made no sense to keep a ship unproductive, a crew idle and a cargo wasting during 40-odd days of quarantine, 'on account of a chimera'. Maclean was not dismissive of all attempts at prevention; he praised the lazaretto lately introduced at Odessa by the Duke de Richelieu, and thought Maitland's tough approach in Malta 'cannot perhaps be surpassed in excellence of organisation' – a unique tribute to a confirmed contagionist. His main purpose, however, was to place in Castlereagh's mind a version of the idea he had floated unsuccessfully in Paris some 14 years earlier, for an institution to examine the plague. He claimed support from abroad, but now he was looking for Britain rather than France to take the lead.

At this point in his letter, Maclean turned to self-interest. He wanted to be the principal of the new institution at an annual salary of £2,000, with liberty to retire on full pay after an agreed period. When he died, he wanted half his salary to pass to his widow. The establishment would require three 'ambitious, intrepid, & well educated Young Men' as assistants, one a physician, another a surgeon and the third an apothecary. They would be paid £300 a year, and the total annual establishment expenses, by Maclean's reckoning, would approach £5,000. The site of the institution

66 Maclean, *Evils of Quarantine Laws*, pp. 47–8.

67 Ibid.

68 References are taken from *Oxford Dictionary of National Biography* and Mullett, 'Politics, economics, and medicine: Charles Maclean and anticontagion in England' until otherwise indicated.

69 NA BT 6/247 (which is an unpaginated compendium of Maclean's papers), from which all references are taken until otherwise indicated.

need not be in Turkey. He now favoured a more central Mediterranean position to benefit the Ionian Islands, Malta and Gibraltar, and it would be helpful if the staff could be peripatetic, ready to move in wherever plague were to strike. In this event, he envisaged that unusual expenses could be met by a tax on local inhabitants, which he expected 'they wld. cheerfully pay'.

It is doubtful whether Castlereagh even bothered to reply, as one month later, on 10 February 1816, Maclean sent a revised proposal. Although the estimated costs of the institution were now between £5,000 and £6,000, Maclean offered his services without remuneration. Castlereagh decided, after another month's delay, to refer the idea to the Privy Council, who delegated it without discussion to the Board of Trade. A less persistent campaigner than Maclean would have heard nothing more about it, as the Board were indifferent to medical proposals. But there was something reminiscent of William Eton in Maclean's arrogance and manipulative skills. In March 1817, exactly a year after his proposal had been delegated by Castlereagh, Maclean wrote directly to the Board of Trade. He asked for facilities to demonstrate that the plague was not contagious and might be cured, and that quarantine and lazarettos were 'worse than useless'. But earlier plans for an institution had been watered down, and Maclean's latest request was for the experimentation to take place on shipboard 'at an expense to government not exceeding the maintenance of an ordinary sloop of war'. The success of his demonstration (which he took for granted) would save Britain around £100,000 a year – a sum which he doubled in later correspondence.

The Board of Trade were no more persuaded by this scheme than they had been by the one earlier, but Maclean would not go away. On 20 August 1817 he wrote to them again, pointing out that it was 19 months since he had first approached Government and 5 months since he had written to the Board, and yet he had had no constructive response. He suggested he was misunderstood and thought to be pushing for private gain. In fact, he was simply disadvantaged, he claimed, by 'want of influence and connection in the State'. He hoped each member of the Board would examine his conscience if it were to transpire that, by 'slighting' his proposals, some four or five thousand lives were lost in Gibraltar alone. If Britain did not like his ideas, other countries would. The first volume of his researches was now printed, and would soon be published. This time Maclean received his reply, but not the one he wanted. The Board's letter has not survived but they had evidently taken Maclean's request as a piece of impertinence. In October 1817, nothing daunted, Maclean expressed brief regret that his tone had caused offence and resubmitted his case.

On still being ignored after that, Maclean showed signs of a crusading paranoia which the democratic principles of Government found it increasingly difficult to defeat or contain. Exasperated by the lack of comment, he pursued the Board of Trade for some reasoned response. But at the same time, he lost the coherence of his own argument and rambled about the millions of lives annually sacrificed for nearly 300 years following a papal 'delusion' about the nature of epidemics. An acrimonious stalemate was avoided by the diplomacy of Frederick Robinson, who became President of the Board of Trade early in 1818 at a formative stage in what was to be a long and renowned career. Robinson met Maclean in the Board's offices and explained why the proposals were difficult, and that they needed a more rational presentation. He was undoubtedly responsible for the gradual introduction to the impasse of the Privy Council, who could no longer remain aloof while their subordinate body was besieged by an obsessive physician.

Maclean's medical credentials suggested a way for the siege to be temporarily lifted, but it was a measure of last resort. In February 1818 the Privy Council asked the College of Physicians to comment on Maclean's ideas.[70] He was informed of this by Viscount Chetwynd and told that in the meanwhile the Council did not feel justified in recommending to the King that quarantine should be abolished.[71] Chetwynd, of course, would have known that the College were fiercely opposed to anti-contagionism. Maclean was predictably incensed. His two-volume book summarizing his researches, and arguing that the plague was not contagious, had recently been published and run into immediate trouble with the medical elite. Maclean felt it time to turn spiteful. In a letter of 16 May, he wished to place on record his 'distinct and exclusive claim to national remuneration, for having been the first and only person to refute one of the most stupendous errors ... to aggravate the lot of man'. He had applied to the Chancellor of the Exchequer for a reward recommended by the British ambassador to the Porte, and would take further action in ten days' time if there should be no response in the meanwhile. This completely altered the character of the debate, and reintroduced a massive dose of self-interest. Chetwynd would have been taken aback, and the Privy Council retreated to a traditional response in the face of insolence, which was to ignore it.

Again, Maclean might have been left at that point with no further opportunity to argue his case. But his work for the Levant Company gave him a route to Lord Grenville, the Governor. Grenville was a Privy Councillor, and his array of past employments, which included Home Secretary, Foreign Secretary and Vice-President of the Board of Trade, enabled him to supply the high-level support which Maclean had lacked and coveted. On 30 June 1818 Grenville saw to it that a supportive letter from Bosanquet, the Deputy Governor (with a letter of 30 May from Maclean to Grenville attached), reached the Privy Council. The Levant Company, as Maclean's writings had made evident, had funded his researches in Turkey. Maclean was now arguing that this support had been recommended by the Duke of Kent and Lord Grenville. If that were literally true, it is not easy to understand why such useful patrons had not been paraded earlier. Correspondence between Bosanquet and Grenville, which was openly copied to the Council, made it clear that the former was prompting the latter into supporting Maclean's demand for new research funds and 'some present reward'. It was probably Bosanquet who had supported Maclean in the first place, and the peers had put their signatures, as required, to necessary documents. Bosanquet's interest can easily be explained: as quarantine caused so

70 This is referred to only incidentally in BT 6/247. Mullett, *The Bubonic Plague and England*, p. 43, believed that the Privy Council were 'hailing the importance' of Maclean's theory, but that is unlikely. In 'Politics, economics, and medicine', 248, Mullett mentions that the Privy Council found in Maclean's work 'so much importance to the welfare of mankind in general', but their loyalties were still with the College of Physicians.

71 NA BT 6/247, from which remaining references in this and the next paragraph are taken.

much difficulty for the Levant Company, it was logical that they should sponsor work on a policy which would make it unnecessary.[72]

Maclean's letter to Grenville of 30 May had not so much solicited his backing, as complained that the Privy Council were withholding the grounds on which the College of Physicians had rejected the anti-contagionist viewpoint. There were, therefore, three issues now to be tackled: the conservative attitude of medical opinion; Maclean's wish to study the plague at public expense; and his claim for reward on account of past research and its outcome so beneficial to mankind. The Council, for their part, had no inclination to get involved, and on 3 August 1818 Grenville notwithstanding, Maclean was once more referred to the Board of Trade.[73] But this was no solution. Maclean's recent book had started controversy, and although the contagionists far outnumbered the disbelievers, there were grounds for an objective enquiry. Indeed, the closing months of 1818 gave no scope for any other outcome, as the parties entered deadlock: the College of Physicians found nothing in the second volume of Maclean's book which led them to change traditional views; the Board of Trade had made no meaningful reply to Grenville; and Maclean had browbeaten Under-Secretaries of State, but to no avail.[74]

Early in 1819, Parliament appointed a Select Committee to consider the validity of the doctrine of contagion with reference to the plague. The driving force here was Robinson, who saw no alternative way to relieve his Board of Trade of their tiresome correspondent. When he was pressed to explain why this subject was more suitable for the House than for the College of Physicians, Robinson conceded ground to Maclean by admitting that the quarantine laws were rigid, inconvenient and expensive, and that 'recent inquiries' had undermined the doctrine by which they were justified.[75] He acknowledged that the College of Physicians were unmoved, but it so happened that a recent committee considering prevalent epidemics in London had raised doubts as to contagion in cases of fever.[76] This was enough to persuade the House, and a Select Committee was established of 21 members, one of whom was Robinson.[77]

Soon afterwards Robinson received a published open letter from Augustus Bozzi Granville, a society doctor who had once served as a naval surgeon and had more recently travelled in the Levant.[78] Granville was a witness before the Committee and timed his 'letter' so that it followed his evidence. From his own observations in Turkey, heightened by an examination of Mediterranean lazarettos (in three of which he had undergone quarantine), Granville felt able to savage Maclean's recent book

72 cf. *Quarterly Review*, vol. 33 (1825–26), 239: 'The Levant Company, finding the quarantine laws inconvenient, resolved, a few years ago, to take a medical opinion upon the necessity of the restrictions which they imposed'.

73 NA PC 2/200/469.

74 NA BT 6/247.

75 T.C. Hansard, *Parliamentary Debates*, vol. 39, pp. 424–5.

76 Ibid.

77 See *Report from the Select Committee Appointed to consider the validity of the doctrine of Contagion in the Plague* (London, 1819).

78 For Granville, see *Oxford Dictionary of National Biography* and all works by Mullett.

and champion the case for contagion.[79] The Committee took oral evidence between 15 March and 18 May 1819. The chairman was Sir John Jackson, who had supported Robinson in the Commons debate. There were more than twenty witnesses, of whom three were heard twice. Maclean was both the first witness and the last, but only Dr John Mitchell and Sir Robert Wilson gave him unqualified support.[80] Of the rest, most were doctors whose uninformative evidence, admitting inexperience and indeed ignorance of the plague, made it questionable why they were called. Granville stated later that his colleagues had turned the medical profession into a laughing stock.[81] Much was made of the plague in British-owned Malta during 1813. Although belief in contagion was widespread, many of the doctors were uncomfortable in assuming that plague was propagated simply by touch, which weakened their enthusiasm for quarantine to remain at the level of strictness which the laws demanded. The Committee were quick to a resolution in June; they decided to 'abstain from giving any opinion on the nature and application of the quarantine regulations as not falling within the scope of their inquiry, but see no reason to question the validity of the principles upon which such regulations appear to have been adopted'.[82] Jackson, however, dissented from that conclusion and felt Maclean was right; he later defended his viewpoint in the House of Commons.[83]

Maclean was contemptuous of the committee's opinion. On 1 July 1819 he told Robinson that while the enquiry was in progress he had forborne from pursuing his claims, as supported by the Levant Company. But as the committee's conclusion 'does not appear to affect the matter of the application', he now wanted his money for research and compensation.[84] The logic of the latter point eluded Robinson, as Maclean had *not* been revealed as the exploder of a costly and useless myth. Three weeks later Maclean wrote another sharp later, stating he would wait only another ten days. The Board of Trade would not be bullied, but the idea of paying off Maclean, simply to get rid of him, had a growing attraction. Accordingly they asked the Treasury whether any fund for such a purpose might exist, but they were told in reply to establish under whose authority Maclean had conducted his researches. Robinson was aware that Government had not been involved, and the matter again stalled. In September, Maclean was notified that the outcome of the parliamentary enquiry did not justify any money for further research becoming available from public funds. The matter of compensation was evaded, but Maclean would not give in. On 29 September, he sent the Board of Trade a 'Remonstrance and Solemn Protest', meandering with anger and prolixity through all the tiresome arguments of

79 More precise details of Granville's Mediterranean experiences were given in his evidence to the 1824 Select Committee.

80 The proceedings of the Committee are well summarized in Mullett, *The Bubonic Plague and England*, pp. 339–43.

81 *Second Report from the Select Committee Appointed to Consider of the Means of Improving and Maintaining the Foreign Trade of the Country. Quarantine* (1824), p. 74.

82 This sentence became widely quoted, for example by Milroy in *British Parliamentary Papers* [*BPP*], vol. 58 (1861), p. 268. The Committee had been encouraged by news that a royal commission in Holland had been appointed to consider quarantine.

83 Hansard, vol. 40, p. 1133.

84 NA BT 6/247, from which all references in this paragraph are taken.

his ineffectual crusade. The president of the College of Physicians was treated to an equally lengthy and aggressive tirade in October. These were the final salvos from a man who knew he was beaten. In January 1820 the Treasury were still minded to procrastinate, telling the Board of Trade that no judgement could be made about Maclean's entitlement to compensation until they had a better understanding of how long he had worked and his actual expenses. And so it would have gone on, had not Maclean exchanged the pen for the printing press in his onslaught on Government and medical jurisprudence.

The 1824 Select Committee

The early years of the 1820s witnessed attempts by the dispirited and enfeebled Levant Company, encouraged by their member Samuel Briggs, to maintain some meaningful existence. Having lost the argument over contagion and made no friends in Government from their association with Maclean, the Company were seriously endangered by *An Act for the Encouragement of Navigation and Commerce ...* passed in June 1822.[85] By this revision to the navigation laws, reciting back to the reign of Charles II, it was lawful, among other provisions, for goods from the Levant to be imported direct in Turkish ships, and for all manner of produce to be imported from European countries in ships of those same nations. This boded well for goods trans-shipped in Holland, where quarantine was less rigid. With their monopoly broken, the Company bluntly informed the Board of Trade, in August 1822, that they could not survive without 'the material diminution of quarantine, and other charges incident to the importation of goods ... in British ships'.[86]

Government had always been aware that the qualified conclusion from the Select Committee in 1819 could only result, sooner or later, in a broader enquiry into quarantine independent of the doctrine of contagion. Commercial unhappiness aside, there were certain aspects of quarantine which were simply anomalous. For instance, a Grand Tourist could travel in a wool-lined carriage from Naples to London in 17 days and escape all detention, while his baggage travelled by ship in a six-week voyage and was subject to quarantine.[87] With new pressure from the Levant Company, there was no reason to delay any longer. In 1824 the Select Committee appointed to consider the improvement and maintenance of foreign trade was charged with making a second report, focused on quarantine. The witnesses comprised merchants, shipbrokers, doctors and the principal quarantine officers at Stangate Creek, Milford Haven and Carlingford in Ireland. The ill-informed and repetitive questioning, verging on hostility in the examination of Dr Newberry, makes it remarkable that the Committee produced such a cogent and sensible report.[88]

85 3 Geo. IV, c.43.

86 *Second Report* (1824), pp. 16–17.

87 *Second Report* (1824), pp. 38, 60, 69. The point had first been made by Dr Harrison in evidence to the 1819 Committee.

88 The Committee appeared to be questioning without prior knowledge or understanding of what the quarantine laws demanded.

There were four main concerns expressed by the commercial lobby. One was the rate of quarantine duty; the second was the way the duty was levied; the third was the apportionment of duty between shipowner and merchant; and the fourth was the long detention of ships and cargoes. With regard to the first point, the duties had been fixed by Parliament in 1800 and unchanged by the quarantine Act of 1805. These duties have been listed earlier in this study, but the two most expensive may be repeated here as they were the focus of discontent. A charge of 7s, 6d per register ton was levied on each ship arrived from Turkey or Barbary with a clean bill of health; this doubled to 15s if the ship had a foul bill. For reasons which the Committee were unable to establish, an extra charge of 1s per register ton was added for ships bound to the port of London. In the case of Stangate Creek, that affected virtually every vessel. The minimum duty payable was 3s (4s for London) by ships with clean bills from Europe. Ironically, it took a doctor rather than a merchant to point out to the Committee that these charges were 25 to 50 times more than those payable in the main Mediterranean lazarettos.[89] The duties had been justified in 1800 by the need to recoup the costs of the lazaret proposed for Chetney Hill. Now that that scheme had 'miscarried', to borrow Granville's tactful description, the view among witnesses, including the doctors, was that the rates might be reduced.[90]

For merchants, the absolute cost of the duties was made more irritating by their being based on the register tonnage of the ship. It made no difference to the payment if the ship were half full or if the goods were enumerated (that is, judged susceptible to carry infection) or totally exempt from quarantine. Neither did it matter how long the ships or their cargoes were detained, or what the value was of the merchandise. Why, the merchants argued, should a ship with a foul bill and a non-susceptible cargo (which gave no work to the quarantine department), be taxed double the amount of a clean-bill ship carrying cotton wool (which would require airing for 15 days)?[91] The register tonnage, being a calculation by set formula of a ship's size, was irrelevant in terms of quarantine. Many ships, especially those built 'very sharp' to bring fruit as quickly as possible, carried a burthen, or deadweight, only half their register tonnage; so, in relation to the cargo carried, merchants were effectively paying a double rate. A ship carrying 150 tons of fruit might pay £260 in quarantine duty, although the cargo was not subject to quarantine.[92] The worst-affected cargoes were those of high density and small value, and judged non-susceptible. Linseed from Egypt fared worst, paying up to 7 per cent of its retail value in duty until the Treasury agreed to reduce it.[93] One merchant knew of a ship carrying linseed from Alexandria which paid duty amounting to 42 per cent of the freight (or hire of space in the hold).[94] The answer for all cargoes, it was suggested, was a flexible payment based on their nature and value, which would bring quarantine in line with other duties collected by the Commissioners of Customs.

89 *Second Report* (1824), p. 83. The comment was made by Granville.

90 *Second Report* (1824), pp. 8, 84.

91 *Second Report* (1824), pp. 13, 18.

92 *Second Report* (1824), p. 24.

93 *Second Report* (1824), pp. 13, 18.

94 *Second Report* (1824), p. 34. The ship had a foul bill.

Quarantine duty was levied from the shipowner as soon as his vessel reported to Customs on arrival. It was then a matter for the owner to recoup from the merchant or importer a share of the duty, in the proportion which the goods bore to the tonnage burthen (not the register tonnage) of the ship. This double system of tonnages led to confusion and conflict between owner and importer. Silk, for instance, was a high-value cargo worth £2,000 a ton, but being relatively light in weight it took up little space in a ship and so represented a small proportion of the deadweight tonnage which the ship could carry.[95] The importer could therefore argue that he owed only a small proportion of the duty payable. This was frustrating for the shipowner, whose vessel might be as much as 500 registered tons and could well have a foul bill of health if it arrived from the Levant. Any silk imported from Italy, the other traditional source, now came overland through France, precisely to avoid quarantine on arrival.[96]

To do away with arguments, which sometimes ended in litigation, the Levant Company drew up a tariff for the reimbursement of duty to shipowners.[97] This was a list of every conceivable item of import, against which the Company set a payment rate, normally per ton of the commodity, according to the status of the bill of health. For instance, taking the example of silk, merchants paid shipowners 17s per ton with a clean bill, and 32s per ton with a foul bill. This was a rough-and-ready formula, not perfect for either side, but 'the ship takes it for better for worse; sometimes she loses by it, sometimes she gains'.[98] There was a proposal that this tariff should be made compulsory by the Treasury, but as its basis was still the inherently bad system of reimbursement set out in the Acts, it was open to the same objections.[99] Also, a problem remained in respect of ships not from the Levant which were nevertheless subject to duty. The practice in these cases was to note the freight, or charge for the hire of the ship, and reimburse the shipowner according to the proportion which the goods of each consignee bore to the total freight.[100]

With regard to the length of quarantine, shipowners and merchants were in accord: the normal 60-day detention for enumerated goods of the first class, with a foul bill, was excessive. This was a third less time than would be expected in the Mediterranean, but the voyages to Malta or Leghorn from the Levant were so much shorter. In time of war, when provisions were dearer, it was reckoned that the cost of maintaining a ship and its crew (and pilot) through full quarantine was as much as £6 a day.[101] A recurrent theme in the questioning was the relative laxity of regulations in Holland, although few witnesses could be specific as to costs and periods of detention. For Britain, however, the facts were clear and hammered home to the Committee. The probationary airings on board ship took 15 days, and another 40

95 *Second Report* (1824), p. 26 (cf. p. 7).

96 *Second Report* (1824), pp. 33, 63.

97 This tariff, reproduced in full in *Second Report* (1824), pp. 107–8, was part of evidence given to the Select Committee by John Hall in 1821.

98 *Second Report* (1824), p. 38.

99 *Second Report* (1824), pp. 14, 17.

100 *Second Report* (1824), pp. 38, 63.

101 *Second Report* (1824), p. 64. There is a brief explanation as to how that figure was arrived at.

were necessary on the floating lazaretto, where the bales of wool or silk were opened and aired more thoroughly. The remaining five, or even six, days, were occupied in transferring bales from ship to lazaretto and then vice versa. Enumerated goods of the second class had no probationary airing, but were quarantined for 30 days. The ship itself (with crew and passengers) would be discharged after 30 days, which led to a dilemma as to whether she should wait for her cargo, if it was to be aired for the full period. If the vessel did not wait, then the onward journey to London in lighters was at the expense and the risk of the shipowner.[102] There were, of course, occasions when detention of both ship and cargo were minimal. If a vessel came from a place against which quarantine was in force, but had a clean bill of health and a non-susceptible cargo, like linseed, her release could be granted in the two or three days it took by post to secure the Privy Council's approval. But then the question re-emerged of the injustice of the duty. The clean-bill rate was based on the register tonnage of the ship, and was therefore the same for harmless linseed as for susceptible cotton wool.

There was disagreement among witnesses as to how far the Privy Council should continue to bear responsibility for the routine release of ships. While an authority for Stangate Creek could arrive by return of post, another for Falmouth or Hull could take five days to materialize, and for a cargo of fruit that delay might be disastrous. As release 'is allowed to be a mere matter of form', said one merchant, it should be a function of the Customs service.[103] That would save six or seven guineas in fees to the Privy Council, as well as so much time. But the Committee heard also from William Pym, who argued that the Council should always be involved, as they had wider intelligence about the outbreak of disease.[104] This might even work in a ship's favour, agreed Charles Sanders, the Superintendent of Quarantine at Stangate Creek, because a ship with a foul bill but unsusceptible goods might be followed in by another ship from the same port which had sailed with a clean one: this could reduce the quarantine period for the ship which had arrived first.[105] The Committee put it to both Sanders and Pym that time might be saved if ships for London anchored in the Lower Hope for an initial inspection, to decide whether or not quarantine were necessary. Both witnesses were against that idea on the grounds that the Thames was narrow and crowded at that point, bringing the risk that infection might be spread by collision.[106]

Some merchants were worried about goods, especially silk, being plundered as well as damaged during the airing process. The Privy Council had been aware of these allegations since 1802, but found them hard to substantiate.[107] Two years later, the Levant Company put forward a six-point plan to put a stop to it.[108] They recommended that no boats should leave Stangate Creek at night; that masters of the

102 *Second Report* (1824), p. 20.
103 *Second Report* (1824), p. 34.
104 *Second Report* (1824), p. 68.
105 *Second Report* (1824), p. 45.
106 *Second Report* (1824), pp. 56, 61.
107 NA PC 2/160/230.
108 NA PC 2/166/130.

floating lazarettos should have no boats for their own use; that silk, wool and similar articles should be weighed on arrival and on leaving the lazaretto; that masters of lazarettos should be responsible for loss or damage while goods were aboard; that a record of the weights should be delivered to Customs when goods were landed in London; that persons possessing goods in suspicious circumstances should prove where they came from; and that in default of proof, the possessor should suffer death as a felon, in accordance with quarantine law.[109] The Privy Council asked the Customs Commissioners to investigate and report. In April 1805 the Council replied to the Levant Company that they could only concede two of their requests: that masters of the lazarettos should not have boats at their disposal, and that the goods should be weighed on arrival and departure.[110] As to punishing persons with goods in suspicious circumstances, that appeared 'to Their Lordships to be quite inadmissible; as the Adoption thereof would subject innocent Persons, in a great variety of Instances to infinite Peril'.[111]

It was against this background that the merchants raised the question of plunder before the Committee.[112] They acknowledged that the Privy Council had approved the system of weighing, but they knew cases where rags, old rope and even a cannon ball had been inserted in a bale to compensate for silk removed during the process of airing. Ostrich feathers were especially prone to disappear. When complaints were made to the quarantine authorities, they denied that plunder had taken place, and the allegations were impossible to prove. The Committee were sympathetic, but wary of being involved in such a delicate issue. They agreed that 'plunder is obviously a vicious addition to the system', but made no recommendations for its prevention.

By coincidence, the Committee sat at the very time when cotton exports from Egypt to Liverpool were dramatically on the increase. The subject was raised by both merchants and doctors. The merchants pointed out that 280 bales had left Alexandria for Liverpool in 1823, the year when imports began.[113] In 1824 Britain was expecting 50,000 bales, nearly half the Egyptian output.[114] The intention of the merchants in mentioning cotton was to emphasize that the foul-bill station at Milford Haven was not well suited for the trade to Liverpool. That was purely a geographical point, and they had no fear of plague being imported in bales. Indeed, Samuel Briggs, a former consul in Alexandria, broke ranks with the doctors by doubting whether the plague was 'really contagious'.[115] Robert Marten, a shipbroker, went even further, asserting to the Committee that merchants were 'without the smallest degree of apprehension' about the spread of infection.[116] It was only when Granville gave evidence later that the threat of an epidemic introduced via the cotton was properly explored. He warned that 'if the plague is to come at all, it will come direct from Egypt, and in precisely

109 Ibid.

110 NA PC 2/167/226.

111 Ibid.

112 *Second Report* (1824), pp. 31–2, from which all references in this paragraph are taken.

113 *Second Report* (1824), p. 29.

114 Ibid.

115 *Second Report* (1824), p. 25.

116 *Second Report* (1824), p. 64.

such goods as cotton'.[117] His words were given extra weight by his knowledge of the trade. It was Granville, not the merchants, who explained to the Committee that it was only four years since a Frenchman named Jumel had introduced cotton into Egypt from Brazil.[118]

Unfortunately, Granville's assessment of British quarantine gave him no expectation that it would keep out the plague. He reckoned the floating lazarettos 'ought to cost nothing [to commerce], as they are good for very little more'.[119] But such sentiments did not solve the difficulty over Milford Haven. If 1,000 cotton bales were removed from a ship to the airing hulk, only 300 or 400 of them could be repacked for the onward voyage to Liverpool, once they had been ripped open and rummaged.[120] The remainder would need to be sent on in another ship. Any bales carried as deck cargo could not be insured.[121] In any event, the insurance between Milford and Liverpool in winter would require an additional premium, because the Irish Sea was so dangerous and the voyage might take up to a month. The cost of this extra travel might be as much as a quarter of the whole freight from Alexandria to Milford.[122] The case for a foul-bill station at Liverpool, preferably on land, was supported by merchants and doctors alike, but not necessarily to be accompanied by the closure of the establishment at Milford, which Pym reckoned was the foul-bill station for Ireland.[123]

The facilities at Milford were scanty to say the least. Whereas Stangate Creek boasted five floating lazarettos, there was only one, the *Triumph* (albeit supported by auxiliary vessels), at Milford.[124] There should have been two, but the *Santa Margaretta* hulk had recently been taken to Liverpool to assist with the airing of cotton from clean-bill ships.[125] On 8 June 1824, after the Acting Superintendent at Milford had given his evidence but before the Committee could report, the *Santa Margaretta* was ordered back to Milford by the Board of Trade.[126] The reason was the advisability of detaining ships with suspected bills in a foul-bill station, but it was evident that a tug of war for possession of the hulk, part of a wider unrest over facilities for airing Egyptian cotton, was about to begin. The Committee would have noted with dismay the dry remark of one of their mercantile witnesses, that 'the whole British navy would scarcely afford sufficient room for a cargo of cotton, if the whole were to be strewed about loose, in order to be aired on board the lazarettes'.[127]

It was perhaps Pym's comment about Milford's importance to Ireland that prompted the Committee to seek an Irish witness. This was James M^c^Neil, tide

117 *Second Report* (1824), p. 85.

118 Ibid.

119 *Second Report* (1824), p. 84.

120 *Second Report* (1824), p. 27.

121 *Second Report* (1824), p. 101.

122 *Second Report* (1824), p. 28.

123 *Second Report* (1824), pp. 62, 67.

124 *Second Report* (1824), pp. 112–13.

125 *Second Report* (1824), p. 98. However, the hulk was recorded as at Milford Haven on p. 113.

126 NA BT 5/32/408.

127 *Second Report* (1824), pp. 36–7.

surveyor at Carlingford, who doubled as pratique master for another £50 a year.[128] The establishment comprised only a 40-ton quarantine 'barge', but McNeil claimed to run a foul-bill station. His evidence as to whether he had ever received a foul-bill ship among the forty vessels handled in the previous three years was confused and contradictory. The reporting system in Ireland (via Customs officers to the Privy Council in Dublin) was very much a copy of the British practice, although it was generally a minimum of five days before permission could be received for a ship's release. McNeil admitted that Carlingford was 'a very detached out of the way place'. That was fine for quarantine, but there was no doctor nearer than Newry, some 12 miles away. When the harbour had been appointed a quarantine station, it was intended that goods would be aired at the old blockhouse guarding the entrance, but it was impossible to land there from the water. Airing, therefore, took place in a token fashion on the deck of the ship. None of this impressed the Committee, who concluded that the Carlingford establishment 'seems to be entirely useless'.[129]

If the mercantile lobby suggested areas where quarantine might be reformed, the medical witnesses, despite their contagionist credentials, heartened the Committee by agreeing that some reform was safe. They were by no means unanimous in every respect: Blane's long-held theory that for eight months of the year Britain was not susceptible to the introduction of plague was not attractive to Pym; and Granville's confidence that a man who swam ashore would rid himself of infection was certainly not shared by Green.[130] Granville wanted 40 days' quarantine to remain against Smyrna for foul-bill ships; Pym would be happy with 35.[131] Blane recommended chlorine as a promising disinfectant for the future, but his attribution of its discovery to Sir Humphrey Davy was delicately denied by the latter, who feared it was inadequately tested and might be damaging to cotton.[132] There was unanimity, however, when it came to enumerated goods of the second class, which might be abolished as a concept. And the doctors were forced to concede, not without some reluctance, that there was not a scrap of evidence that anyone arriving at a British quarantine station or working in a floating lazaretto – even those who rummaged into bales at arm's length – had ever suffered anything worse than passing giddiness.[133]

The Committee made recommendations which were more radical than the merchants had dared to expect.[134] Quarantine should be limited to enumerated goods of the first class, or other goods wrapped or contained in susceptible packaging. Foul-bill or diseased ships bound for London should go to Stangate Creek for their enumerated goods to be aired over 21 days. This period, which would apply also to the ship, was significantly more lenient than the doctors had advised. Cargoes of fruit in foul-bill ships should be delivered after seven days. A foul-bill ship heading

128 *Second Report* (1824), pp. 70–73, from which all references in this paragraph are taken until otherwise stated.

129 *Second Report* (1824), p. 10.

130 *Second Report* (1824), pp. 49, 66, 77, 93.

131 *Second Report* (1824), pp. 66, 86.

132 *Second Report* (1824), pp. 50, 104–5, 121.

133 *Second Report* (1824), p. 43.

134 *Second Report* (1824), pp. 3–10, from which all references are taken until otherwise stated.

elsewhere than London should proceed to wherever the Privy Council might direct. Ships with clean bills from Turkey or Africa, bound for London, should anchor in the Lower Hope 'without other than official communication'. It was envisaged that a rapid report to the Privy Council would result in a certificate allowing the ship to proceed upriver. This bold decision, flouting the advice of witnesses, removed Stangate Creek from the voyage, promising a saving in time and distance. A vague wish was expressed for ships elsewhere in Great Britain and Ireland to 'bring up' according to a similar system. The same procedure was recommended for ships with clean bills from other places in the Mediterranean, but there was another important concession: the Customs service and not the Privy Council should be competent to grant the certificate for the ship to proceed. As for quarantine stations for the outports, the Committee left the locations to the Privy Council, contenting themselves to hope for somewhere more convenient for Liverpool than Milford Haven, which should nevertheless become the foul-bill station for Ireland in place of Carlingford. Having dabbled that far in Irish quarantine, the Committee were disinclined to consider it further.

Another subject to interest the Committee was the punishment of offenders. Despite the claim to have had their attention directed to this topic, it is difficult to find any witness who even touched upon it, and no opinions were sought about the range of offences and penalties. It would appear, therefore, that there were elements within the Committee interested in penal reform, especially in the removal of the death penalty from all offences against quarantine, except the forging or alteration of official papers. Those crimes apart, the Committee recommended a maximum punishment of transportation and, in respect of their own suggested rules, a penalty of £200 for each violation by the master of a foul-bill ship, dropping to £100 if the bill were clean. Although some slackening of the penalties was in keeping with the relaxation being recommended for quarantine procedures, Britain risked being out of step with Continental Europe if the reforms were adopted.

The final recommendation of the Committee, and the measure of their enlightenment, was that the costs of quarantine should be borne by the public purse. This followed recognition that the Levant trade was 'a matter of national interest', and that the abandonment of duty was 'only a return to the former System, which was professedly departed from for the accomplishment of an object long since abandoned'. But it was brave to deny the Treasury a revenue to which they were well accustomed, especially as gross receipts from quarantine in the years between 1800 and 1823 totalled £371,513, providing only 58 per cent of the cost of the service.[135] The Committee were well aware of that, and the 12 appendices to their report (some subdivided) form a compendium of quarantine statistics of considerable importance, although the information is sometimes repetitive.[136] Several of these tables have been mentioned elsewhere in this study and need not now be re-examined. Of the rest, it

135 *Second Report* (1824), p. 111. Expenditure was £483,521 18s, 9d.

136 *Second Report* (1824), pp. 107–21.

will be useful to dwell on the insight they provide into the running and relative size of the various quarantine stations.[137]

Table 12.1 Number of ships performing quarantine in British and Irish stations, 1821–1823 (Ships with foul bills of health are shown in italics)

Q stations	1821	1822	1823	*Total/Agg. totals*	
England/Wales					
Stangate Creek	255 + *18*	223 + *12*	364 + *16*	**888**	
Liverpool (Bro' Pool)	132	108	170	**410**	
Portsmouth (M'bank)	83 + *1*[1]	57	60	**201**	
Falmouth	32 + *1*	44	44	**121**	
Bristol	44	42	34	**120**	
Milford Haven	11	6	6 + *2*	**25**	**1765**
Scotland[2]					
Holy Loch	14	12	13	**39**	
Inverkeithing	3	2	11	**16**	**55**
Ireland					
Cork	29	37	38	**104**	
Dublin	33	24	42	**99**	
Belfast	16	20	20	**56**	
Carlingford	16	12	12	**40**	
Waterford	8	8	2	**18**	
Baltimore	6	7	3	**16**	
Creekhaven	5	4	4	**13**	
Kinsale	2	3	4	**9**	
Beerhaven	2	4	2	**8**	
Kilrush	6		1	**7**	
Londonderry	3	4		**7**	
Drogheda	1	1		**2**	
Sligo			1	**1**	**380**

Notes:
(1) The foul bill at Portsmouth in 1821 was technically a suspected bill.
(2) Dates for Scotland are erroneously given as 1822–4 in the original tables.

Source: Second Report from the Select Committee Appointed to Consider of the Means of Improving and Maintaining the Foreign Trade of the Country. Quarantine (1824)

Table 12.1 raises a surprise. Milford Haven, so much the focus of attention by the Privy Council, Board of Trade and Select Committee of 1824, comes bottom

137 The table below is a synthesis of the figures in Appendices H.1, H.2 and K (*Second Report* (1824), pp. 114–20.

among the English and Welsh stations. The port could evidently go weeks without a quarantine ship in sight. Bristol, which was scarcely mentioned as a station after the turn of the eighteenth century, quarantined nearly five times as many vessels as Milford; so did Falmouth. Another appendix to the 1824 Report lists lazarettos or other vessels attached to the quarantine service, with their personnel, but restricts the coverage to only four stations: Stangate Creek, Motherbank, Liverpool and Milford Haven.[138] This would appear to mean that only those ports had floating lazarettos, but it is difficult to believe there were none at Bristol or Falmouth. There was, it would seem, an official perception of a 'Big Four', with Milford included not for what it was but for what it might become, if cotton imports to Liverpool from Egypt continued to break records.

Facilities at Stangate Creek were far more extensive than anywhere else.[139] There were five floating lazarettos in 1824, as well as a hospital ship and a brig. The four main lazarettos were each manned by a master, mate, two guardians, ten mariners and a boy. The fifth lazaretto, described as temporary, had only four mariners and a boy. The hospital ship was crewed by a master, mate, six mariners and a boy, while the brig housed the Superintendent of Quarantine, a mate and assistant mate, 22 mariners (two deputed) and the inevitable boy. There were also five 'superior guardians'. This gave a total complement for the Creek of 105 men and boys. The second most extensive facilities were, curiously, at Milford Haven, with two floating lazarettos (once one of them had returned from Liverpool), a hospital ship and a pursuit cutter, employing 45 in total. At least some of these men would have been deployed against smuggling in the long interval between ships for quarantine. Liverpool had a complement of 39 men and boys in two floating lazarettos and a guard-ship, purely for the reception of clean-bill ships, which nonetheless carried cargoes in need of airing. Portsmouth came fourth, with 32 men for one floating lazaretto and a cutter. The annual expenses of these stations, in 1823, amounted to some £17,849, of which the sum for each was in proportion to its share of the total personnel. Stangate Creek accounted for £8,502; the other three stations each cost a little over £3,000. As the whole expenditure on quarantine in the outports came to £20,487 in 1823, it will be evident that the service in Falmouth, Bristol and Hull put together cost no more than at Milford, Liverpool or Portsmouth individually.[140]

As well as numbers of ships, the appendices to the Report show their place of departure.[141] Although some of these are difficult to identify, the Levantine (including Black Sea) and African ports, from which foul bills for plague were not unlikely, are reasonably clear. At Stangate Creek, ships from those places amounted to 25 per cent of arrivals; at Bristol 21 per cent; Milford 20 per cent; Portsmouth 18 per cent; Hull 17 per cent; Liverpool 17 per cent; and Falmouth 8 per cent. Again, the unexpected result is Bristol, where the risk of imported disease was greater than at Liverpool,

138 *Second Report* (1824), pp. 112–13, Appendix F.2.

139 Ibid., from which all references in this paragraph are taken until otherwise stated. Stangate Creek appears under the port of Rochester.

140 The totals for expenditure in the outports forms part of Appendix F.1 (*Second Report* [1824], p. 111).

141 This is the final column in Appendices H.1, H.2 and K.

although the argument for Milford being the foul-bill station for Bristol was lost in the frenzy of fear over Egyptian cotton bound for the Mersey. In Scotland, only two of the 39 ships in Holy Loch were from the Levant. Inverkeithing received no ships at all from the Levant or Africa, the arrivals having all sailed from Italy, Spain or Gibraltar.

The position in Ireland is revealed as extraordinary, with nearly twice as many quarantine stations as Britain but only 20 per cent of the volume of business. Many of the smaller stations were probably created by stress of weather, with ships making for anchorages known to be safe from south-westerly gales. Cork, the busiest Irish station, handled only two ships from the Levant; Dublin, only marginally less busy, saw eight ships from the Levant and one from Barbary. Belfast had one ship from Odessa; Carlingford received two from Smyrna and one from Barbary, but not with foul bills. Many of the lesser stations had at least one ship from Zante, Smyrna or Barbary, but they were probably destined elsewhere. There was no attempt by the Select Committee to get figures of quarantine expenses from Irish (or for that matter Scottish) stations, as they had sought for English and Welsh. In 1823 a different parliamentary enquiry had requested the amount of allowances received nationally by Superintendents of Quarantine, with Scotland and Ireland to submit separate returns.[142] There was a nil return from Ireland without explanation, presumably because that title was inapplicable there.[143] This hint of a procedural chasm gave no enthusiasm for any deeper enquiry into how far Irish quarantine was a drain on resources.

Open to attack

Excluded from giving evidence to the 1824 Committee, Maclean circled like a bird of prey, watching for a meal from opinions and judgements which might fatten his case for anti-contagionism. He was emboldened by success in Madrid in October 1822, when he persuaded the Spanish Cortes, against the advice of nine doctors within the assembly and the opinion of most others in the country, not to adopt a code of sanitary laws which was being recommended by a government commission.[144] Having returned to England, he wrote his two hallmark books, *Remarks on the British Quarantine Laws …* , published in 1823, followed a year later by *Evils of Quarantine Laws, and Non-Existence of Pestilential Contagion.* In the first paragraph of *Remarks*, Maclean made his well–quoted comment that quarantine and sanitary laws were ‘perhaps, without exception, the most gigantic, extraordinary, and mischievous superstructure, that has ever been raised by man, upon a purely imaginary foundation’.[145] What followed was a history of British quarantine measures, borrowing to some extent from Russell but with none of his

142 *JHC*, vol. 78, pp. 123, 132.

143 *JHC*, vol. 78, p. 999. As has been shown, the Irish used the term pratique master.

144 There are, of course, many references to this event in Maclean's own writings, but a good summary of his involvement can be found in *Westminster Review*, vol. 3 (1825), pp. 137–8.

145 Maclean, *Remarks on the British Quarantine laws*, p. 2.

objectivity, and an abstract of the sanitary proposals for Spain which he (Maclean) had succeeded in discrediting. The climax of his attack on the British system was, of course, the decision of the 1819 Select Committee to endorse the doctrine of contagion in the face of what Maclean considered overwhelming evidence to the contrary.

In his 1824 publication, Maclean abandoned the historical analysis (except in respect of his own career) and went into even greater detail, with characteristic prolixity, about the 1819 report of the Select Committee and recent events in Spain. This developed into a polemic against J.D. Tully, an army surgeon with experience of plague in the Ionian Islands, who had been one of the prominent contagionists to oppose Maclean's revolutionary thinking.[146] It was natural from this that the plague of 1813 in Malta should come under renewed discussion, but far from predictable that Maclean should raise the question of cholera morbus in the Far East. Europe was much too occupied in 1824 to consider any epidemics other than plague and yellow fever. In another ten years these thoughts on cholera, which he considered a non-contagious disease, would have a chilling relevance. Maclean was especially dismissive of the College of Physicians, the institution whose intransigence, as he saw it, blocked the possibility of an informed and open discussion. He sneered at their shallow experience, 'at a loss to conceive, how a body, whose members, with very few exceptions, have never explored beyond the sources of the Thames, the Cam, or the Isis, can intuitively possess a knowledge of the maladies, which desolate the banks of the Ganges, the Nile, or the Bosphorus …'[147]

In his preface to *Evils*, Maclean confessed 'the support of commerce' for his heretical crusade.[148] His defence for an association which others might think 'culpable' indicates the extent to which mercantile opinion was judged by the public to be incapable of any sentiment beyond self-interest. The merchants' own confessions before the 1824 Committee of insouciance to plague, followed by Ralph Green's testimony to the same body that 'if you give way in one thing the merchants will never stop until they get most of the restrictive regulations done away with', did nothing but reinforce conventional suspicion.[149] But for Maclean, commerce represented a sympathetic platform for anti-contagion and perhaps a source of funding for publications, travel and further research. He would have realized that the Levant Company, his past sponsors, were a spent force, and in fact the Company surrendered their charter in 1825. The future for Maclean lay not in a ship to Turkey but a coach to Liverpool, with its persistent, even militant, pressure groups.

There was coordination of strategy between Maclean and the Liverpudlians during 1824. While the Select Committee were still considering their report, Maclean wrote two memorials, delegated by the Privy Council to the Board of Trade, apparently asking for yet another body to consider whether quarantine was effective.[150] Two

146 For Tully, see Bibliography, and Mullett, *The Bubonic Plague and England*, pp. 349–51.

147 Maclean, *Evils of Quarantine Laws*, p. 21.

148 Maclean, *Evils of Quarantine Laws*, p. xxiv.

149 *Second Report* (1824), p. 95.

150 NA BT 5/32/417.

weeks later, the Board received a letter from Samuel Briggs suggesting a revision to quarantine procedures at Liverpool for ships with cotton; the justification was a letter from the British consul in Alexandria who declared the port had been free of plague for several months.[151] Briggs, who had told the 1824 Committee that plague might well be non-contagious, could now be classed as a follower of Maclean. Within a month, a Mr J. Starbuck had backed the idea for the airing of cotton wool to be modified.[152] Then came the main attack. Aware of the case made to the Committee for a foul-bill lazaretto at Liverpool, the merchants petitioned on 31 July 1824 for such an establishment to be formed at Mostyn, a small port at the mouth of the estuary of the Dee.[153] The Board of Trade replied that charts did not indicate a safe or proper place at Mostyn for lazarettos.[154] While coasts around the Wirral were further examined, the Board sought cooperation from Earl Bathurst, Secretary of State for War and the Colonies, for quarantine to be easier and cheaper at Malta.[155]

In October 1824 Maclean delivered a lecture entitled 'Observations on Quarantine' at the Liverpool Lyceum. The text was then published by the Liverpool Mediterranean Association. This was Maclean's first opportunity to make an attack on the findings of the 1824 Committee, but he did it badly. The paper had none of the eloquent aggression or belittling sarcasm of his work a year earlier. The style was laboured, the long-winded sentences lacking bite and even confidence. Commercial points were taken on trust, such as the allegation that quarantine expenses for cotton at Milford Haven exceeded half the costs of its transmission from Egypt.[156] It was as if Maclean was working with merchants by tactical necessity, whereas only with doctors and politicians did he feel in his element. Yet at the end of this boring paper came the hint of how the next stage of his mission was about to develop. He praised a number of recent Bills which had dared to challenge prejudice and ignorance in fields including warehousing, the silk trade, exportation of machinery, and the emigration of artificers.[157] Maclean had had enough of letters and memorials to the Privy Council and Board of Trade, who obstinately refused to treat him with the respect and seriousness which he felt he deserved. He had now gathered enough high-level support to take his case straight to Parliament.

The Commons had been unsettled about quarantine ever since Sir John Jackson had spoken out in 1819 as a convert to anti-contagionism. In 1821, for no obvious reason, certain statistics were requested for the information of members; these included an account of salaries and contingent expenses at Chetney Hill between 1801 and 1820, a return of gross receipts from quarantine between 1800 and 1820 (updated by the 1824 Select Committee for inclusion in their tables), and a return of quarantine establishments around Great Britain and Ireland, with names of persons

151 NA BT 5/32/434–5.

152 NA BT 5/33/1.

153 NA BT 5/33/59.

154 Ibid.

155 NA BT 5/33/71.

156 C. Maclean, *Observations on Quarantine: being the Substance of a Lecture delivered at the Liverpool Lyceum* (Liverpool, 1824), p. 33.

157 Maclean, *Observations on Quarantine*, p. 38.

receiving more than £100 a year, and contingent expenses in 1790 and 1820.[158] Early in 1823, Parliament was presented with returns, of little significance, showing allowances received by Superintendents of Quarantine for the victualling of ships.[159] None of this material gave Parliament any sense of the direction which quarantine policy should take. Later in 1823 there was a motion brought forward by Joseph Hume for the House to receive copies of correspondence since 1814 between the British merchants at Malta and the Maltese Government about quarantine regulations on the island.[160] This was as much anti-Maitland as pro-trade, and when Robert Wilmot Horton, Under-Secretary of State for War and the Colonies, offered to show Hume papers which proved that the Marseilles Board of Health were satisfied with the Maltese regulations, Hume withdrew his motion.[161] This episode will best be considered more fully in the context of Malta, but it serves here to indicate that a disjointed sequence of quarantine issues maintained the attention of the Commons.

On 2 March 1825 the House resolved to consider the Act of 1822 for the encouragement of navigation and commerce.[162] On the next day the reports of the Select Committee on Foreign Trade, which of course included quarantine, were added to the discussion.[163] Another day later the House resolved to repeal all quarantine duties, in line with the Select Committee's report, and James Brogden, Charles Grant and Thomas Wallace were asked to prepare a Bill.[164] Brogden was a Russia merchant turned parliamentarian; Grant was Vice-President of the Board of Trade, a post he had assumed from Wallace in 1823.[165] Wallace and Grant had taken turns to share the chairmanship of the 1824 Select Committee. But there were wider issues at stake than the repeal of duties, and on 10 March the House decided to resolve itself into a committee to consider all the Acts in force relating to quarantine.[166] This was Maclean's cue. On the following day a petition on his behalf concerning the quarantine laws was presented to the House by John Smith, member for Midhurst and one of a dynasty of Nottingham bankers.[167] Smith had strong philanthropic principles and declared that there was no man's opinion by which he would more readily be guided in matters of quarantine than Maclean's. An immediate intervention by Wallace warned that the initiative by Maclean might well

158 *JHC*, vol. 76, pp. 348, 354, 424, 436, 494. The Chetney Hill statistics, and gross quarantine receipts 1800–1820, were published on p. 1222 and in Sessional Papers. The returns for 1792 and 1820 were published in Sessional Papers alone.

159 *JHC*, vol. 78, pp. 123, 132, 157; published p. 999.

160 Hansard, vol. 9, pp. 1526–8.

161 Hansard, vol. 9, pp. 1528–9; *JHC*, vol. 78, p. 473.

162 *JHC*, vol. 80, p. 153.

163 *JHC*, vol. 80, p. 159.

164 *JHC*, vol. 80, p. 164.

165 History of Parliament [HOP], *The House of Commons 1790–1820* (5 vols, London, 1986), vol. 3, pp. 259–61, notes that Brogden sided with the Whigs and gave up his place on the Treasury Board in 1813 'to become chairman of committees, speaking only in his official capacity thereafter and steadily supporting government until 1826, when he resigned ...'

166 *JHC*, vol. 80, p. 185.

167 *JHC*, vol. 80, p. 193; Hansard, vol. 12, p. 993. For Smith, see HOP, vol. 5, pp. 195–6.

be too radical, but when Smith confirmed that 'he by no means proposed the repeal of the Quarantine laws', members were soothed and the petition was read.[168]

This time Maclean's prose was cogent and to the point. His petition was an attack on the system of quarantine, not a defence of his doctrine. He took anti-contagionism as so manifestly true that systems based on 'the assumptions of the sixteenth and seventeenth centuries' were ridiculous survivals 'of ignorant and credulous times'.[169] If plague were contagious, how could it possibly be that 50,000 ships had not imported the disease over the 244 years in which Britain had been trading with the Levant? What nonsense to ascribe the absence of plague to certain conditions of susceptibility. Quarantine laws increased sickness and mortality in times of pestilence; they impeded science, travel, commerce and discovery, and had sometimes, on the continent of Europe, been 'rendered subservient to the purposes of despotism'. He could guess that losses by the detention of ships, cargoes, crews and passengers since 1720 were 'enormous', with the current figure running at around £200,000 a year. In the colonies, where epidemics were more frequent, the damage from quarantine was even greater and the misery of the people compounded. Maclean, unlike Smith, wanted nothing less than the total repeal of the quarantine laws, as 'being without an object, as an absolutely demonstrated evil, as a code eminently anti-commercial, anti-social, and anti-christian'.[170] Should the House be disinclined to do that, Maclean asked for a new investigation into pestilential contagion. It was ordered that the petition should lie on the table, and be printed.[171]

Against this background, the House went about its business and considered the quarantine Acts in force. On 15 March 1825 Brogden reported from the committee of the whole House that it was expedient to repeal the quarantine laws and make other provisions.[172] This led to a new Bill, which ran into trouble on 30 March, at the second reading.[173] Grant moved the order of the day, but he was evidently inaudible, at least in the gallery.[174] Smith, by contrast, was in good voice. The Bill 'had his most cordial approbation', although it did not go far enough.[175] He showed himself a disciple of whom Maclean could be proud. What followed was the case for the doctrine of anti-contagion, almost without reference to the material harm which quarantine inflicted on commerce. Smith reiterated the hackneyed arguments: Holland, virtually without quarantine laws, had never been infected; Marseilles, where airing of cotton was thorough, had lost only one expurgator since the plague of 1720, and he had probably died of apoplexy; in Turkey, no one caught plague from the clothes of victims, although they were sold in public markets; and plague

168 Hansard, vol. 12, p. 993.

169 Hansard, vol. 12, pp. 993–6, from which remaining references in this paragraph are taken until otherwise stated.

170 This quotation appears also in *JHC*, vol. 80, p. 193.

171 Ibid.; Hansard, vol. 12, p. 996 (with no mention of printing).

172 *JHC*, vol. 80, p. 206.

173 *JHC*, vol. 80, p. 294.

174 Hansard, vol. 12, p. 1315: 'The right hon. Gentleman made a statement to the House, but in so low a tone of voice, that not a single observation reached the gallery'.

175 Ibid.

had never spread to Persia from the caravans leaving Aleppo.[176] If London had been ravaged by plague in 1665, it was owing to filth, overcrowding, bad habits and poor diet. Smith went on to belittle two committees, one rather obscure in 1811, the other notorious in 1819, which had defended contagion. Since the latter, Smith believed many doctors had defected to Maclean, 'whom he was proud to call his friend'. The only other physician he cited was a Dr Armstrong of Russell Square who had found typhus non-contagious, yet its symptoms were decidedly plague-like.

It was only then that Smith advanced a commercial reason to do away with quarantine. A ship had recently arrived in Liverpool with a foul bill of health, which should have subjected it to a lengthy quarantine. But after representation by the owners 'to the proper quarter', the ship was allowed to unload and sail away. The reason, explained Smith, was that the bill was only foul because 'a single old woman' had died of plague at the port of departure, presumably Alexandria. There he rested his case and urged the House to institute a Commission, or another Select Committee, to look at the question of quarantine more closely. Wallace then took the floor and showed less antagonism than might have been expected in his position as Government spokesman.[177] Indeed, he thought 'Government would be a good deal relieved, if any considerable number of medical men concurred in recommending a repeal of the Quarantine laws'.[178] As it was, he felt the anti-contagionists were still well outnumbered. Hudson Gurney, who had been a member of the 1819 Select Committee, despaired at the idea of going over the arguments once again and was convinced that Maclean was wrong.[179] Gurney had little sympathy with the Liverpool merchants and referred to a 'sort of partnership' entered into by 'an English house' with the Pasha of Egypt for the export of cotton.[180] But this merely encouraged John Cam Hobhouse to speak out for 'the enlightened' Maclean.[181] With anecdotes being bandied around the House as to whether or how far Turks and others were or were not infected, the debate was all about whether plague was contagious and the mercantile case against quarantine was never mentioned. Hobhouse ended with a eulogy on Maclean, 'to whom, in future ages, the finger of the historian would point, as one of the greatest benefactors to his species'.[182] After further minor contributions from the floor, the Bill was referred to a Committee of the whole House, but consideration was deferred six times until the middle of May.[183] With Parliament stalling, the debate about contagion transferred to the pages of the literary journals.[184]

In April 1825 there was a move in the Lords to anticipate their discussion of the Bill by calling for, *inter alia*, lists of ships from Alexandria which had arrived

176 Hansard, vol. 12, pp. 1315–20, from which all references are taken until otherwise stated.

177 Hansard, vol. 12, p. 1320.

178 Ibid.

179 Hansard, vol. 12, p. 1320–22.

180 Ibid.

181 Hansard, vol. 12, p. 1322–4.

182 Hansard, vol. 12, p. 1324.

183 *JHC*, vol. 80, pp. 299, 305, 327, 333, 380, 392.

184 Their contribution is usefully summarized in Mullett, *The Bubonic Plague and England*, pp. 359–60.

with clean bills and been admitted to immediate pratique.[185] If this was a sign of impatience, their lordships were destined to wait even longer. The Commons were far from ready to let the Bill go. Not until 13 May did the Committee of the whole House materialize, when John Smith launched a fresh assault on contagion that very much resembled his earlier attack.[186] Once more, Holland was more hero than villain, suffering no epidemics from its lax quarantine, because that quarantine had never been needed. In some areas, Smith's second speech was virtually identical to his first, even repeating the anecdote of the apoplectic expurgator in the Marseilles lazaretto. The next significant speech came from William Huskisson, who had succeeded Robinson as President of the Board of Trade, the body to whom questions of quarantine policy had effectively been delegated by the Privy Council. After some dabbling in medical aspects of contagion, Huskisson became the first speaker to raise the commercial consequences to Britain of a unilateral dilution of the strength of its quarantine laws.[187] Already, Mediterranean countries were placing precautionary quarantines against all British shipping, regardless of port of departure. Huskisson warned that 'we had brought on our commerce a severe infliction, in consequence of the discussion of this question'.[188] A debate with the interests of commerce in mind was turning into an excuse for other countries to cripple that commerce by inordinate delays. But at the same time, the British merchants, by their agitation, had to bear some of the blame. With perhaps one eye on the journalists in the gallery, Huskisson warned merchants that the inconvenience which quarantine brought to their business would not induce the Government to relax quarantine any further than the recent Select Committee had thought safe.[189] Such words, he no doubt hoped, would strengthen representations already made to the authorities at Marseilles and Genoa.

Huskisson could not claim that the suspicions aroused in France and Italy had not been forecast. Granville, one of the few doctors who understood the regulations in foreign lazarettos and the attitude of the Boards who controlled them, had already predicted a bad reaction in his evidence to the Select Committee. He had stressed 'that in proportion as you relax with regard to foul or clean bills of health from Turkey ... so will the other European nations, particularly France, include you in their laws of quarantine ... even on proceeding to Calais'.[190] During the parliamentary debates, Granville resorted to the same device for Huskisson as he had used in 1819 for Robinson. That is to say, he published an open letter refuting the arguments of Maclean. But this time the letter began by claiming his prediction of punitive quarantine abroad had been fulfilled: 'England is declared to be an infected country; she is put on a footing with Turkey at some of the principal ports of the

185 Hansard, vol. 13, pp. 1–2.

186 Hansard, vol. 13, pp. 601–3; *JHC*, vol. 80, p. 414.

187 Hansard, vol. 13, pp. 603–5.

188 Hansard, vol. 13, p. 604.

189 Hansard, vol. 13, p. 605.

190 *Second Report* (1824), p. 85.

Mediterranean …'[191] Although making the same warning as Huskisson, Granville was not taking his side. Indeed, he considered Huskisson as part of the problem. Smith's anecdote of the 'single old woman' whose sickness caused ships to sail with foul bills of health would have troubled Granville profoundly. It was Huskisson who had ordered the arrival at Liverpool to be treated as a clean-bill ship, and this decision was more damaging abroad than all the agitation of merchants. More than 35 years later Huskisson was still being blamed.[192]

In Parliament, the debate of 13 May concluded with a weak, contagionist speech from Wilmot Horton, and the issue of quarantine was then twice again deferred.[193] On 19 May it was again before the House, and Sir Isaac Coffin, a retired admiral, was in no doubt from his experiences in Malta that plague was contagious.[194] Lord Belgrave went even further by declaring it 'really astonishing' that members should think otherwise.[195] He made the interesting comment that a respectable Levant merchant of his acquaintance hoped 'to put into his pocket' some £4,000 or £5,000 if the Bill became law, but he would 'do so with regret, because he considered it as the price of blood'.[196] Belgrave contemplated the harm to the British exports which the current debate was causing, and found it impossible to understand what the promoters of the Bill were trying to achieve, unless they intended 'to establish a joint-stock company for the purpose of extending the burying grounds'.[197] This annoyed Grant, who wished that members had read the 1824 Report of the Select Committee.[198] It was evident from this Report that the doctrine of contagion was accepted, and in the opinion of Sir Gilbert Blane no reforms to the quarantine system were being proposed which would be incompatible with that position. This made Belgrave concede that he was not actually opposed to the Bill; he only wanted to convince members that the plague was contagious.[199]

The last debate in the Commons was on 3 June 1825, the day for the third reading.[200] After predictable comments by Grant and Coffin, it was left to George Canning, Foreign Secretary, to emphasize that the Government were still of a contagionist view and to hope, in view of the damage being done abroad, that the opposing lobby would keep their 'opinions a little more to themselves'.[201] Hume took exception to this and made the pertinent comment that the Bill had been introduced with no ministerial statement that the repeal of the quarantine laws was not intended to be absolute.[202] The last constructive words of the whole debate were uttered by

191 A.B. Granville, *A Letter to the Right Hon. W. Huskisson, M.P. President of the Board of Trade on the Quarantine Bill* (London, 1825), p. 2.

192 cf. Milroy in *BPP*, vol. 57 (1861), p. 269.

193 Hansard, vol. 13, p. 605; *JHC*, vol. 80, pp. 423, 428.

194 Hansard, vol. 13, pp. 788–9.

195 Hansard, vol. 13, p. 790.

196 Ibid.

197 Ibid.

198 Hansard, vol. 13, p. 791.

199 Ibid.

200 *JHC*, vol. 80, p. 489.

201 Hansard, vol. 13, p. 1037.

202 Hansard, vol. 13, p. 1038.

Huskisson, who referred to the responsibility now lying with the Board of Trade, who hoped to have the assistance of an expert on plague and quarantine to guide them towards proper decisions.[203] That expert was to be William Pym, but his name was not mentioned to the House. The Bill finally passed, and Brogden was instructed to carry it to the Lords, where progress was non-eventful.[204]

The 1825 Act

On 27 June 1825 the Bill received royal assent and became *An Act to repeal the several Laws relating to the Performance of Quarantine, and to make other Provisions in lieu thereof.*[205] The preamble also repealed Acts which had authorized the charging of duty on ships which were liable to quarantine, or had performed it. As Hume had hinted, the title was misleading, as the intention was not to replace quarantine by any other system. Indeed, the first provision of the Act was to enable the Privy Council to institute quarantine against arrivals from any place where there was a threat of 'plague or other infectious disease'. If that definition might be construed to include yellow fever in the Mediterranean, it did not extend to yellow fever from America or the West Indies. The Privy Council could order ships from those latter places to be detained for the examination of the crew, but that would not normally constitute quarantine. The Act then, for the first time in Westminster legislation, made particular provision for Ireland, where the Lord Lieutenant with the advice and consent of the Irish Privy Council could issue Proclamations as to the place, duration and manner of quarantine.

There was vague mention, as in previous Acts, of 'goods … more especially liable to retain infection', which could be identified and dealt with as ordered by the King in Council; the same section extended quarantine if necessary to any vessel arriving from anywhere 'under any alarming or suspicious circumstances as to infection'. The theme was maintained in the next section, which also gave the Privy Council emergency powers in an epidemic to isolate infected communities; but, in a somewhat abrupt change of sentiment, it also allowed the Council to release ships from quarantine early, conditionally or absolutely. If plague broke out on a ship 'within or without the Streights of Gibraltar', the master had to make for such place as the Council might from time to time appoint and keep his ship in isolation until further orders. It would have pleased Scillonians that their islands, if still an obvious location for a blighted ship, were no longer the statutory rendezvous. The penalty for disobedience by the master was a fine of £100, a startling leniency when compared with death for the same offence under the Act of 1805. The new Act continued the system of flags denoting liability to quarantine according to the bill of health, and added a new flag (yellow and black, borne quarterly, of eight breadths of bunting) for a ship actually infected. The responsibility of pilots to inform masters of liability to quarantine from their place of departure, and now from the nature of their cargo, was repeated, with the fine for disobedience by the master halved; but penalties were

203 Ibid.

204 *JHC*, vol. 80, pp. 489, 593.

205 *JHC*, vol. 80, p. 603; 6 Geo. IV, c.78.

doubled for the pilot, who was once again enjoined to take a ship liable to quarantine only to an approved port.

There followed the usual instructions for Customs officers to interrogate masters and to force them if necessary to sail on to the right port for quarantine. The penalty for masters who omitted to disclose that they had arrived from an infected place, or wilfully refused to hoist the quarantine signal, was £300 – another significant softening of the law from the death penalty required by the previous Act. There were also fines of between £200 and £400 (in one case with six months' imprisonment) for those who left or boarded quarantined ships or indulged in 'refractory behaviour' (the traditional phrase), another crime which had previously merited capital punishment. On the other hand, the penalty for neglect of duty by a Customs officer (including the embezzlement of goods), which had been curiously low at a fine of £100 in the previous Act, was now doubled. The new Act, however, was coy about the punishment for forgery and giving false certificates, which had traditionally been perhaps the most serious offences in quarantine law: under the new Act they were still classed as felony, but with no specified sentence.

The most significant measure of the new Act (apart from the abolition of duties), and one which followed closely on the recommendation of the 1824 Select Committee, was Section 22: this allowed a ship with a clean bill and a healthy crew from the Mediterranean 'or from any port in Turkey or Africa' to be released from liability for quarantine following approval by the Privy Council of the preliminary report of a 'proper officer'. In other words, the ship could dock immediately after the exchange of formalities. Given the distance to the Privy Council, this was obviously more to the advantage of London than Liverpool, but the advance was nevertheless a milestone in the road to dismantling quarantine altogether. The remaining sections were very much in line with those of the 1805 Act, making no changes to the way ships were discharged by certificate in cases where quarantine was performed, and maintaining the general power of the King in Council to make orders for goods to be aired. There was, however, another major instance of the law being softened, this time in the context of persons removing goods from a ship under quarantine or from a lazaretto. The punishment for this offence, which had been capital under the 1805 Act and was regarded abroad as particularly heinous, was reduced to a mere fine of £100. As usual, the Act took occasion to discourage smuggling, by requiring that during an epidemic the master of a vessel under 100 tons burthen could not sail to such places as would be named in a Proclamation until the master had given a bond in £200.

Britain had now taken a view of quarantine which was, bravely or rashly, at odds with thinking on the Continent. As the Bill became law, few doubted that a new kind of trade war would probably result. What did Maclean make of this Act, destined to give British merchants trouble abroad which outweighed the benefits conceded at home? Was he satisfied, or was he contrite? While the Bill was in Parliament he wished to appear conciliatory, volunteering to investigate a ship at Stangate Creek rumoured to carry plague.[206] But when the Bill became law, he reverted to type. The parliamentary tributes had done nothing but nourish his vanity. On 18

206 NA BT 5/33/442–3.

August, supported by the Ship Owners' Society, Maclean made a new demand for remuneration from the Board of Trade.[207] Their answer was curt and dismissive. The Board did not accept that the recent legislation had resulted from him, and anyway parliamentary awards were not in their province. As for his wish that he be rewarded in proportion to the benefits already conferred on commerce by his exertions, the Board were 'not prepared to admit that the Commerce of this Country has derived any advantages from the promulgation of his doctrines'.[208]

With that final snub, Maclean appears to have given up his claim for money. Mullett concluded that he died later in 1825, as 'it is scarcely conceivable that he would have lived and not written'.[209] But in fact he did write again, and the Board of Trade were once more the target for his impossible demands. In December 1826 they read and then filed more letters, one via an intermediary, requesting an appointment to investigate plague.[210] If Maclean ever wrote after that, it would seem his letters were 'filed' without being read.

---

207 NA BT 5/34/106, 108.

208 NA BT 5/34/106.

209 Mullett, 'Politics, economics, and medicine: Charles Maclean and anticontagion in England', 225.

210 NA BT 5/35/327.

Chapter Thirteen

Malta and the Ionian Islands, 1815–1826

Ionian distractions

In December 1815, when Malta was stumbling to recovery from the consequences of plague, Sir Thomas Maitland was made Commander-in-Chief in the Mediterranean, excluding Gibraltar, and Lord High Commissioner of the seven Ionian Islands.[1] This small archipelago, including the 'Currant Islands' of Zante and Cephalonia, had been taken from the Venetians by the French in 1797. Two years later the islands were united into an independent republic under the protection of Turkey and Russia, but the French regained possession in 1807 by the Treaty of Tilsit. In 1814 the French garrison on Corfu surrendered to British troops who were already in occupation of the islands, and Major-General Campbell was appointed Civil Commissioner.

A system for quarantine had long existed in the islands, but not to the highest standards despite the Venetian control. Hennen argued that 'reformation was most loudly called for' in the years before British rule.[2] He referred to 'absurd and nugatory regulations', with health guardians who were corrupt from poverty and 'among the vilest characters in the community'.[3] The Board of Health at Marseilles began correspondence with Zante in 1725, but did not recognize the *bureau de santé* on Corfu until 1802.[4] Howard noted that in Zante the Health Office decreed 42 days quarantine for arrivals from the Levant or Barbary, but only 21 days for ships from the Morea.[5] From Malta, or indeed elsewhere, ships and passengers were not detained. Howard also described the lazarettos at Zante and Corfu. In fact, Zante had two lazarettos, the old one a building of some consequence run by a prior appointed by Venice, having courtyards, rooms and sheds, as well as Greek and Roman Catholic chapels.[6] Howard explained the layout in some detail as it struck him 'as affording some good ideas for the construction of a house of correction'.[7] The new lazaretto was used by peasants who travelled to the Morea to assist with the harvest and were

1 These were Corfu, Cephalonia, Zante, Santa Maura, Ithaca, Cerigo and Paxos.

2 J. Hennen, *Sketches of the Medical Topography of the Mediterranean: comprising an Account of Gibraltar, the Ionian Islands, and Malta* (London, 1830), p. 201.

3 Ibid.

4 Archives départementales des Bouches-du-Rhône, Marseilles [ADBR], 200 E 465. Correspondence with Corfu on health matters began in 1728, but only with the French consulate.

5 J. Howard, *An Account of the Principal Lazarettos in Europe …* (London, 1789 & 1791), p. 9.

6 Howard, pp. 9–10.

7 Howard, p. 10.

quarantined for seven days on their return.[8] Howard described the lazaretto at Corfu as being 'finely situated on a rock surrounded with water, about a league from the city', but gave no account of its facilities.[9]

When the French were ousted, the management of health in the islands devolved upon the medical officers of the British army. The first army doctor in the quarantine department was J.D. Tully, the diehard contagionist destined to become a protagonist of Maclean. While plague was ravaging Malta, it was also causing havoc in Greece and Albania, and Tully was ordered to the Morea to establish the facts.[10] Before long he was back in Corfu as a worrying sickness had broken out in the low-lying district of Leftimo (or Lefchimo).[11] Campbell set up a committee, followed soon by a full Board of Health under the presidency of Tully, to take control of a rapidly worsening situation.[12] In his history of the outbreak, published in 1821, Tully admitted that he had at first considered the disease to be an 'offspring of the Soil', although his superiors on Malta had already suspected the worst.[13] It was left to Maitland, visiting Corfu in February 1816 against Government wishes, to make the diagnosis of 'the plague, the whole plague, and nothing but the plague'.[14] Luckily for Tully, he and his Board of Health, 'unschooled as we were', had taken measures for isolation, cleansing and inspection which were broadly appropriate.[15]

But these steps, even the quarantine of observation for 14 days on villages outside the cordon, were not enough to contain the disease. Infected clothes and religious vestments were regularly concealed and smuggled between communities, and the progress of the plague was relentless. Tully (who was in quarantine) met Maitland at the barrier of the Health Office, where he was ordered to segregate the infected, the suspected and the healthy with 'the overawing presence of a military force'.[16] Maitland evidently felt dissatisfied with the steps being taken, as control on Corfu was transferred, in March 1816, to Staff Surgeon Andrew White.[17] Unfortunately, Tully did not mention this, or even refer to White, in his book. White became so aggrieved at this omission that he eventually wrote his own treatise on the character and management of the Corfu plague. While he acknowledged that Tully stayed on to fight the disease and that both of them shared contagionist principles, White

8 Howard, p. 9, footnote. He explains that at harvest time the quarantine for others returning from the Morea reduces from 21 to 14 days in the old lazaretto.

9 Howard, p. 10. The site is well described in D. Panzac, *Quarantaines et lazarets. L'Europe et la peste d'orient (XVIIe–XXe siècles)* (Aix-en-Provence, 1986), pp. 158–9, who reproduces the ground plan and elevations of 1870 originally published by Bussolin.

10 J.D. Tully, *The History of Plague as it has lately appeared in the Islands of Malta, Gozo, Corfu, Cephalonia, &c. …* (London, 1821), p. 77.

11 Tully, p. 86. He called the district Leftimo, while his later protagonist Andrew White referred consistently to Lefchimo.

12 Tully, pp. 87, 91.

13 Tully, p. 90; National Archives [NA] CO 158/27 [unpag.], announcement by Maitland, 27 Jan. 1816.

14 Tully, p. 100; A. White, *A Treatise on the Plague …* (London, 1846), p. ix.

15 Tully, pp. 92–8.

16 Tully, p. 108.

17 White, *Treatise on the Plague*, p. vii.

felt a disappointment which festered over time into bitterness.[18] The only benefit of this acrimony to the historian is that the 'police' of the plague in Corfu has been exhaustively covered by both writers.

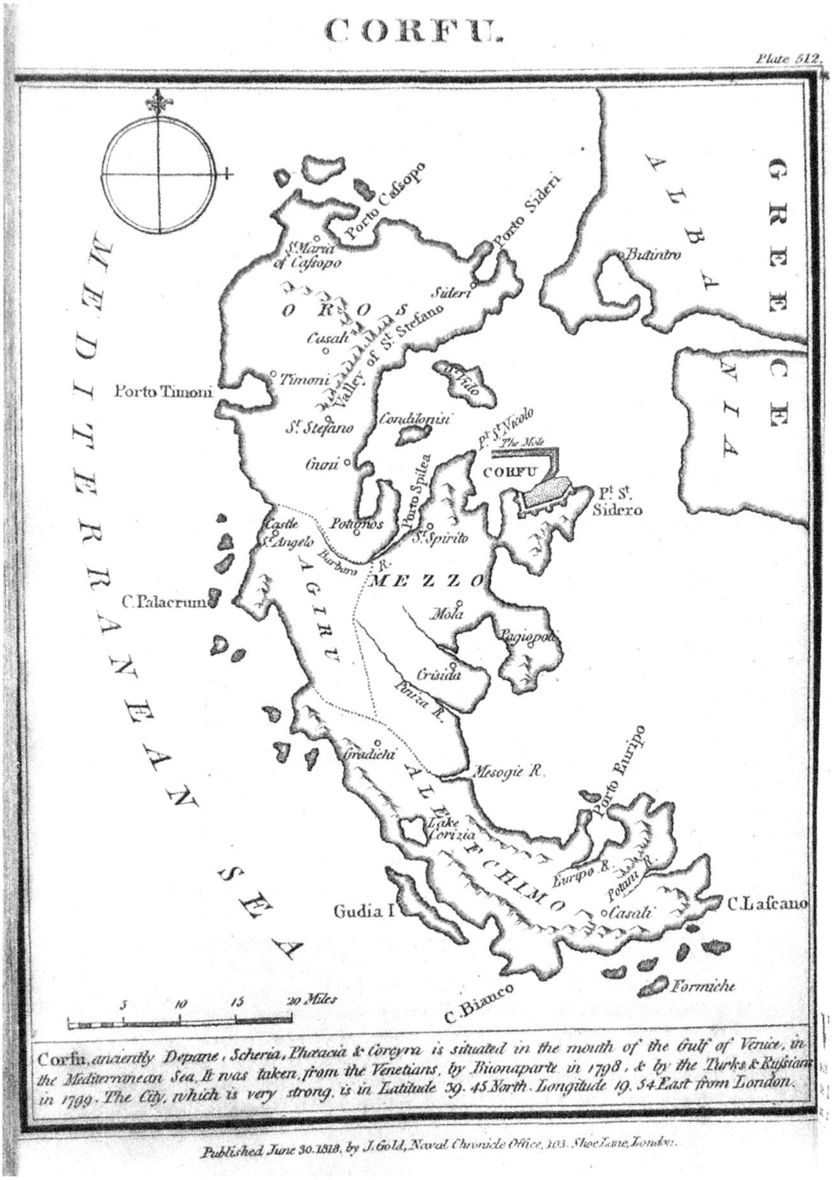

Illustration 13.1 Corfu in 1818. Quarantine was on the island north of the Mole protecting Corfu port.

18 White, *Treatise on the Plague*, pp. v, vi.

Leftimo was rid of infection by Maitland's iron fist. Soldiers were stationed in infected villages and they patrolled night and day; there were daily checks on the health of families; and all intercourse with neighbours was prohibited. Those who seemed likely to break the rules were locked in their homes overnight. Tully's hospitals and camps were removed from their inland sites to the seashore, along with 300 of the sick and suspected.[19] Houses were cleansed, and items considered 'impested' were taken to depots and burnt.[20] Churches were also purified, and plague graves guarded in case effects were stolen or concealed. Priests, accused of consistently flouting the restrictions, were moved with their families to camps of observation.[21] When people were eventually freed from their prison-villages, and survivors returned from the camps, there was a further quarantine of 25 days for those 'highly suspected' of having been infected, and of 17 days for those 'simply suspected'.[22] Convalescents from the pest hospital were quarantined for 50 days.[23] By the end of July 1816 nearly 400 inhabitants had died.[24] The plague on Corfu had been defeated, but not before the military cordon surrounding Leftimo had been progressively weakened by attacks of what was described, perhaps euphemistically, as a remittent fever.[25]

About a month before Corfu was in free pratique, Tully was sent by Maitland to Cephalonia as Inspector of Health.[26] It would appear that he had redeemed himself in the eyes of the High Commissioner, as his mission was to stamp out another outbreak of plague. Again, it was Maitland who made the diagnosis, during a visit to Cephalonia on 21 June 1816.[27] The outbreak was centred on the district of Comitato, which Tully found 'a horrid mass of disease'.[28] On this island, as on Zante, many of the inhabitants worked on the mainland during harvest time, and were also put in a quarantine of observation for seven days on their return. This proved inadequate, as the plague was allegedly introduced by a man (concealing Turkish goods) who managed to hide his developing sickness on the day of release.[29] Tully eradicated the outbreak in 14 days, which involved flocks of sheep and goats, tended by wandering shepherds, being subjected like villagers to Maitland's policy of isolation

---

19 Tully, p. 111.

20 White, *Treatise on the Plague*, pp. 192ff.

21 One of the few points of agreement between Tully and White was that the conduct of the priests was deceitful and highly improper, especially with regard to the concealment of infected cloth.

22 White, *Treatise on the Plague*, pp. 217ff.

23 White, *Treatise on the Plague*, p. 266. This was actually a reduction from 80 days originally ordered.

24 White, *Treatise on the Plague*, p. 115. Total deaths in the Leftimo district were about 375.

25 White, *Treatise on the Plague*, p. 255. Tully, on the other hand, makes little of sickness among troops.

26 Tully, p. 155.

27 Tully, p. 161.

28 Tully, p. 188.

29 Tully, pp. 156–8. Gavin Milroy, in 'Operation and results of quarantine in British ports since the beginning of the present century', *Association Medical Journal*, [1] (1853), 581, found this story 'a very lame one'.

and containment.[30] Unluckily for Tully, his thunder was stolen on Cephalonia as it had been on Corfu. This time, however, the 'thief' did not publish. He was, in fact, Rivarola, a favourite of Maitland and hero of the plague in Malta, who claimed credit for stopping the plague on Cephalonia as part of his campaign for a civil decoration.[31] In his capacity as Inspector General of Police at Malta, Rivarola had played a leading role in enforcing the rules of segregation, especially on Gozo.[32] Maitland had then made him commandant of the Royal Malta Fencibles, before sending him to Zante as civil and military commander.[33] Tully acknowledged that Rivarola had supreme powers over the health departments on Cephalonia and Ithaca and that, on 9 July 1816, they had discussed the outbreak at Rivarola's request.[34] But Tully was perhaps never aware of Rivarola's claim to have eradicated the plague himself.

The other main islands, including Zante, remained plague-free. When Rivarola returned to Malta, the Sanità on Zante was entrusted by Maitland to Staff Surgeon Thomas, who had been acting Superintendent of the Malta lazaretto until relieved by Grieves.[35] Thomas, it will be recalled, was one of the group of army doctors on Malta whom Maitland had initially despised, but soon found useful. Thomas later claimed credit for preventing plague spreading among the garrison and people of Zante in 1819, when a ship arrived from Tunis where plague was known to be rife.[36] Within a few days, crewmen were dead and dying, and a health guardian also succumbed.[37] It was believed in later years that there had not been 'a suitable lazaret ashore', but it seems more likely that Thomas prevented the crew from landing.[38] The success of this episode, in that it kept Zante free of plague, was later used by Thomas as an argument for promotion.[39] It riled him that both White and Tully, his juniors, had reached the rank of Deputy Inspector of Hospitals. This stunted career was no doubt a sign that Maitland's dissatisfaction with Thomas had not entirely gone away.

Army doctors agreed, or perhaps conspired to agree, that the smuggling and concealment of goods rather than any failure of quarantine arrangements had caused the plague to reach Corfu and Cephalonia.[40] In fact, the quarantine restrictions were fully as lax as Hennen suggested, and chaotic between the islands themselves. Maitland discovered that 'Corfu was in quarantine with Ithaca, but not with Zante, Santa Maura and Paxos. Zante was in quarantine with Santa Maura, but not with Ithaca, Corfu or Paxos'.[41] Hennen dated the introduction of effective quarantine in

30 Tully, pp. 190, 200.

31 NA CO 158/38 [unpag.] contains many papers during 1824 resulting from Rivarola's disappointment at not receiving the KCMG which Maitland had promised in October 1816.

32 Ibid.

33 Ibid.

34 Tully, p. 194.

35 NA CO 158/44 [unpag.], memorial of Thomas to Bathurst, 27 Sept. 1824.

36 Ibid.

37 Milroy, 'Operation and results of quarantine in British ports', 582.

38 Ibid. for quote.

39 NA CO 158/44 [unpag.], memorial of Thomas to Bathurst, 27 Sept. 1824.

40 Tully, pp. 141–4; White, *Treatise on the Plague*, p. vi.

41 C.W. Dixon, *The Colonial Administration of Sir Thomas Maitland* (London, 1939), p. 230, quoting [NA] CO 136/389.

the Ionian Islands to 1818, when the first regular tariff was published.[42] The revenue was gathered

> from a per centage on goods expurgated; a certain tax on passengers living in the Lazaretto; a tax on goods brought into the city from the Sanita Barrier (provisions excepted); a tonnage duty on ships and boats in quarantine; a fee on all health patients; a fee on all decisions on subjects litigated by persons in quarantine; and a fee on all contracts, certificates, letters, and other documents relative to the health establishment.[43]

A biographer of Maitland, on the other hand, believed it was 1820 when he 'adopted a general and uniform system of quarantine regulations'.[44] In any event, little was spent on quarantine in the years following the plague. Expenditure on the Health Office during 1818 was less than 1 per cent of the islands' budget, and fell to 0.3 per cent in 1819.[45]

Within a few more years, however, quarantine saw the benefit of the civil engineering agenda which Maitland began, and new lazarettos were built at Cephalonia, Ithaca and Cerigo.[46] Zante, on the other hand, appears to have muddled through with existing buildings, retaining one or perhaps both of the establishments seen by Howard. There was little investment either in Santa Maura, separated from the mainland by the narrowest of channels. There, according to Hennen, was a 'small, sandy islet … fitted up for the purposes of quarantine'.[47] It is unclear whether he meant a permanent building. Hennen praised the 'exemplary' strictness of the guards, but had to admit that the quarantine establishment was 'on a small and mean scale', in keeping with other aspects of the island.[48] A building was erected at some stage because nearly 30 years later, when the island was still under British control, the lazaretto had deteriorated into 'the most miserable shed imaginable'.[49]

The praise bestowed by Hennen on Maitland for his 'paternal care' over quarantine facilities in the islands was far too lavish. Within a few years of his comment that Maitland had brought 'these establishments to the highest state of perfection of which they are capable', the Superintendent of the lazaretto at Malta openly admitted that the regulations in the Ionian Islands were second rate.[50] Other countries had guessed that anyway. Granville told the Select Committee of 1824 that the Tuscan, Austrian and French governments had placed seven, fifteen and twenty-one days' quarantine respectively on arrivals from the islands because their defences against

42 Hennen, p. 202.

43 Ibid.

44 Dixon, p. 231.

45 Dixon, p. 238, has tables for revenue and expenditure, 1817–19. There is no head for quarantine at any date under revenue, and no figure for expenditure on the Sanità during 1817. In 1818, 4,612 dollars were spent on the Sanità, falling to 1,370 in 1819.

46 Dixon, p. 248.

47 Hennen, p. 378.

48 Hennen, pp. 377–8.

49 Milroy, 'Operation and results of quarantine in British ports', 582 footnote. His source added that throughout his travels in Asia and Europe he had 'never met with the equal of this for the utter wretchedness of its accommodation and the insalubrity of the situation'.

50 Hennen, p. 202.

plague from the nearby mainland were inadequate.[51] It would have been noted that Malta, Corfu and Cephalonia had all become infected with plague while the British were in charge of quarantine. The conclusion among Boards of Health was that the British were sloppy, and the lack of a shore-based lazaretto near London suggested that quarantine was not taken seriously, even by central Government. The problem was all too apparent in Malta, which wanted easy communications with Corfu but risked trouble with mainland Europe if arrivals from the Ionian Islands were given free pratique. There were spying eyes in Valletta among the consuls and merchants, and Maitland was to learn that the smallest indiscretion, not least by himself, could add to the quarantine detention of Maltese and British vessels.

Reform and recrimination in Malta

As soon as Malta and Gozo were free of infection, Maitland argued that major ports in the Mediterranean, such as Marseilles and Leghorn, should no longer enjoy a special status in the quarantine arrangements for British shipping.[52] He was annoyed by the reluctance of the Board of Trade to support this view, and hoped they would reconsider.[53] The least Maitland expected was that British ships with foul bills would be forced to perform quarantine in Malta. In view of the bitter relationship he was soon to have with the merchants of Malta, it was ironic that at this stage he feared they would migrate to the mainland.[54] Meanwhile, he set about with customary vigour an overhaul of the island's administration. In the course of this work, he fulfilled his pledge to reform quarantine.

In a long memorandum to Bathurst, sent in October 1814, Maitland made it clear that a well-run lazaretto was a sine qua non for the future of the island.[55] To bring it into sharper focus, he separated the establishments of quarantine and marine police, the former to have control of Marsamxett Harbour and the latter of Grand Harbour.[56] Robert Corner, formerly Harbour Master, was made Intendant of Marine Police at a monthly salary of 416 scudi (about £38) with three assistants and lower ranks.[57] Robert Grieves, confirmed as Superintendent of Quarantine, had a monthly salary slightly exceeding 753 scudi (nearly £70) and a staff of 46, of whom 30 were classed as either 'keepers of the barrier' or boatmen and unnamed in Maitland's return. This was a large reduction (almost wholly among boatmen) from the 95 staff of the plague years, but certain appointments saw significant increases in salary. For instance, the Captain of the Lazaretto would now be paid 210 scudi a month as against the previous 125; and the Captain of the Port would receive 200 scudi as

51 *Second Report from the Select Committee Appointed to Consider of the Means of Improving and Maintaining the Foreign Trade of the Country. Quarantine* (1824), pp. 85–7.

52 NA CO 158/25/73–6.

53 NA CO 158/25/424–8.

54 NA CO 158/25/73–6, 91–2.

55 NA CO 158/25/213–14.

56 Ibid.

57 NA CO 158/25/252–5, from which all details of posts and salaries below are taken.

against the previous 154.[58] Maitland was open with Bathurst that the changes would increase expenditure by 1,018 scudi (approaching £100) a month: the Quarantine Department would now cost 3,121 scudi, which was actually a saving of 26 per cent over the 4,225 scudi of the old undivided department, but the 2,122 scudi being spent on the Marine Police increased the new monthly budget for the combined departments to 5,243 scudi.[59] The salary of Grieves, equating to 9,039 scudi or £800 a year, was outside Maitland's control and therefore unaltered.

'Of all the departments in this Island', wrote Maitland, 'the one most necessary to be paid at least adequately is that of the Lazaretto'.[60] He wanted a career structure for juniors within the quarantine department and a pension for life when they were 'worn out'.[61] If Government would not meet the expense, the lazaretto should be closed. Better no quarantine at all, than a system where the officers were tempted by poverty to embezzle and rob. It was only too easy for a system designed to prevent infection to degenerate into one for introducing it. That, as Maitland saw it, was little short of the current position, as the lazaretto had reached such a 'state of laxness, and in fact non-entity' that improvement would be slow.[62] He informed Bathurst, brazenly, that he would increase the costs of quarantine even further if he thought it necessary; in fact, he was seeking to induce a senior health official at Leghorn to accept a position on Malta.[63] In January 1816 he informed Bathurst that a new post of Registrar, at 4,000 scudi a year, had been created in the quarantine department.[64] This was less than half the salary paid to Grieves as Superintendent but placed the Registrar (who was actually the official from Leghorn) comfortably second in the departmental hierarchy. Maitland had already told Bunbury (now a major-general) that the lazaretto had been enlarged and refurbished, the magazines floored, a new mole built in Marsamxett Harbour, and the existing moles repaired.[65] When Maitland held strong views, he was prepared to back them with money.

Bathurst did not object to these reforms and the only challenge to Maitland's authority came from the Treasury in London in May 1816, during the review of accounts for the previous year.[66] Maitland had persuaded Palmerston, Secretary-at-War, that he was justified in deviating from the establishments approved by Parliament, to the extent of discontinuing some appointments on Malta and instituting three others. One of these was the post of Captain of the Lazaretto, mentioned above. This was not, in fact, a new appointment, but Maitland saw in it scope for the salary to be paid from London. Indeed, the post of Commandant of the Lazaretto (as he called it when writing to Palmerston, to add a military dimension) was absolutely necessary

58 But under the former system there had been two posts of Captain of the Port.

59 NA CO 158/25/213, 253, 255.

60 NA CO 158/25/213.

61 Ibid.

62 NA CO 158/25/214.

63 Ibid. Maitland thought he could even be 'the Head Officer' at Leghorn who was 'at present disgusted with his situation there'.

64 NA CO 158/27 [unpag.], Maitland to Bathurst, 11 Jan. 1816.

65 NA CO 158/26 [unpag.], Maitland to Bunbury, 26 Dec. 1815.

66 NA CO 158/28 [unpag.], correspondence 16–27 May 1816, from which all references in this paragraph are taken until otherwise stated.

to control the quarantine guards, and to administer Fort Manoel once it was free of prisoners of war. Palmerston wrote to the Treasury, hoping they would agree, but the latter informed Bathurst that if these three appointments were judged necessary they should be paid for from the island's revenue. The problem for Government was that no one understood what went on in the Malta lazaretto, or how far Maitland's reforms were justified in the context of the island's administration, and procedures in the Mediterranean as a whole. It was no doubt for these reasons that Grieves, having temporarily returned to London in 1817 on grounds of ill-health, was asked by Bathurst to explain in detail his responsibilities as Superintendent of Quarantine.[67]

During 1815, with the reforms in progress, Maitland had pestered Bunbury with the same case for removing the privileged status of the Italian ports as he had previously presented to Bathurst.[68] As the war had debarred the British from access, and as Malta offered all the facilities for foul-bill quarantine which shipowners had a right to expect, was it not justice to deprive the Continental ports of the revenue from British vessels? But the logic of this argument was let down by an attack, too strongly couched, on the prevailing alternative system of allowing foul-bill ships to sail directly to Britain. Maitland questioned 'the accuracy' of quarantine in England and forecast 'the direst Scene of Confusion' if plague ever got into 'your Lazaretto', by which he presumably meant Chetney Hill. There were, on the other hand, reasons to be grateful for concessions already granted. These included the privilege of direct trade with the British West Indies and the admission of goods depurated in Malta to free pratique in Britain. But Maitland wanted nothing less than the status of 'general Mart' which had been so much a vision of his predecessors.

It was perhaps inevitable that Maitland, like Oakes before him, would see relations with the merchants of Malta deteriorate into a terse hostility. The breakdown was gradual and progressive. In October 1814 he praised the merchants for making a case 'so moderately, and accurately'; in April 1815 he described a letter from them as 'not exactly drawn up in the best manner'; and in October 1817, on receipt of a long memorial, he was angrily dismissive of the whole group.[69] 'I have lived much too long', he told Bathurst, 'not to know the uniform character of all Traders, to wit, that of looking solely to what they suppose their immediate interest, and therefore I am and ever have been equally regardless of their approbation or disapprobation'.[70] Maitland sent the merchants a letter regretting their manner and tone; he would not comment on their views, but informed them he was sending the memorial to London with pertinent observations.[71] In fact, that was what the merchants had requested, if Maitland would not meet their demands.

67 NA CO 158/29 [unpag.], Grieves to Goulburn, 5 Aug. 1817.

68 NA CO 158/26 [unpag.], Maitland to Bunbury, 9 Apr. 1815, from which all references in this paragraph are taken.

69 NAO CO 158/25/177; CO 158/26 [unpag.], Maitland to Bunbury, 9 Apr. 1815; CO 158/29 [unpag.], Maitland to Bathurst, 23 Oct. 1817.

70 NA CO 158/29 [unpag.], Maitland to Bathurst, 23 Oct. 1817.

71 NA CO 158/29 [unpag.], Maitland to merchants, 27 Sept. 1817.

In detail, the memorial followed familiar lines.[72] The merchants blamed the slow decline of the island's trade on import and export duties, port charges, and aspects of quarantine. As before, they wanted a free port which operated by a literal interpretation of the term. Export duties delayed ships and forced owners to manifest outward cargoes, which could lead to complications. The merchants wanted the duties abolished. The 1-per-cent levy on imports not wanted for consumption on Malta was often exceeded and restricted the transit trade on which the island depended. In its place, 'a small Package due' was suggested, but not on goods to be trans-shipped. The merchants felt reform was the more urgent as trade with the West and East Indies was now possible for both Malta and Gibraltar, and as the latter was a free port in a meaningful sense it would engross a greater part of the trade. There were, of course, echoes there of the long-standing jealousy of what merchants considered the privileged position of the Rock. But it was the situation within the Mediterranean which gave most concern. Merchants alleged that Greeks no longer sailed to Malta with speculative cargoes of grain, which had always found a market because the island was closer than the countries of growth and generally more convenient for traders from Spain and Italy. The Greeks, having sold their cargoes, used to buy British and Maltese goods for the return journey. The merchants felt that quarantine regulations on the island had a lot to do with the disquiet of the traders who bought the grain, as they could no longer be sure of returning in free pratique. What was wanted was 'an uniform, and invariable system of Quarantine …, equally calculated to prevent all unnecessary rigour, or impediment to business, and any such occasional laxity as may tend to subject vessels arriving hence in the Continental Ports to quarantine'.

The merchants wanted a reform of the dues, as well as the regulations. Discontent about the 0.5-per-cent rate introduced by Pym on goods admitted to pratique had never gone away, and the merchants alleged that the levy had no parallel in the Mediterranean. Furthermore, costs for the depuration of merchandise were 'equally without Example', rarely falling below 5 per cent *ad valorem*, and often exceeding 10 per cent if the goods were of low value. Charges for ships under quarantine were felt to be just as exorbitant. A small vessel of 50 tons burthen undergoing 40 days quarantine might pay 225 scudi, as well as port charges. If quarantine would fall into line with the other major ports, the merchants were confident that the island would once again attract traders from the Levant, who would exchange their cargoes for the produce and manufactures of Britain and Malta. Another grievance centred on port charges. At Malta, but not at Leghorn and other places, ships in passage could not anchor for 24 hours without paying full dues. The merchants wanted this to stop, with a payment of one-third dues for a stay of 48 hours, and one-half for three days, as long as no goods were discharged or loaded. In their final remarks, the merchants returned to the question of East Indian goods, which were either susceptible by nature or packed in susceptible materials. Unless something were done to get Malta in free pratique with the continental ports, the export of those goods to the mainland

72 NA CO 158/29 [unpag.], merchants to Maitland, 18 Sept. 1817, from which all references in this and the next paragraph are taken.

would be tedious and expensive, and Maltese interests would suffer at the hands of the Americans, whose ships were admitted immediately.

Maitland would not be moved and made it difficult, by the strength of his resentment, for Bathurst to rule against him. With the Governor anxious for revenue and the merchants anxious for themselves, no prospect of a resolution was in sight.

Fighting for acceptance abroad

Discrimination against ships from Malta was particularly bad in Sicily, an island which could, simply by its size and proximity, profoundly affect the Maltese economy. Sicily was a large, fertile granary, and therefore the antithesis of Malta which could never be self-sufficient. It was also a potential market for the Maltese entrepôt, so the prospects for reciprocal trade were theoretically good. But allegations of unnecessary quarantine in Sicilian ports were one of the few grumbles which Governor and merchants were happy to share. In fact, the delays were nothing new, and their reasons were variously explained. It was not a question, as it had been at Marseilles, of a guilty reaction to an outbreak of plague, because the strictness was not impartial. The island was governed with absolute authority by a viceroy appointed by Naples.[73] The British had long had a problem with Sicilian morality, which was considered a corrupting influence on the integrity of local quarantine. In 1766 there had been warnings of 'continual Quarantines that all Neutral Vessels are subject to in this Kingdom, [which] may be considered to be one of the greatest Hardships Trade lies under here, as they are imposed generally upon frivolous Doubts, and probably with second Views ...'[74] The lack of adequate salaries was blamed for venality. The worst port was Messina 'whence it is evident that private Views and particular Interests prevail over the Publick Good'.[75]

When Malta came under French control, Sicily imposed an immediate quarantine on her dependent neighbour.[76] This hurt the starving Maltese at least as much as the French. During the British blockade, Nelson was forced to request Hamilton, in Naples, to get quarantine set aside for ships reaching Sicily for corn; the quarantine was fourteen days and the Maltese stock of bread was only four.[77] After the French Wars, when Malta was firmly British, the Sicilians reverted to a policy of inflexible quarantine which was widely resented. Perhaps Lieutenant-General Cockburn voiced the only dissenting opinion. Cockburn, who had travelled through the Mediterranean in 1810–11, took issue with contemporary censure and described the quarantine laws

73 cf. P. Brydone, *A Tour through Sicily and Malta in a Series of Letters to William Beckford, Esq. of Somerly in Suffolk* (2 vols, London, 1790), vol. 2, p. 85.

74 British Library [BL] Add. MS 38349, fol. 176; *Calendar of Home Office Papers of the Reign of George III* [*CHOP*] (1766–69), p. 77.

75 BL Add. MS 38349, fol. 176.

76 L. de Boisgelin, *Ancient and Modern Malta* (3 vols, London, 1804), vol. 3, p. 115.

77 Sir N.H. Nicolas, ed., *The Dispatches and Letters of Vice Admiral Lord Viscount Nelson* (7 vols, London, 1845–46), vol. 3, p. 163.

as the only ones which the Sicilians exercised fairly and honestly.[78] But Cockburn is unconvincing and his comments would have angered Maitland, if he were ever aware of them. It was still more galling for Maitland that British interests in Sicily were allegedly responsible for the problem. The assumption was that they paid the Sicilians to maintain quarantine so that their own illicit trade with Malta would benefit.[79] In March 1815 Maitland told Bunbury that an Englishman named Gibb was being particularly obstructive.[80] Be that as it may, it was inevitable that the Sicilians would continue a meaningful quarantine against Malta in the aftermath of plague, in case they were themselves punished by the French and Italians for being lax in proximity to a proven weak link in the defensive chain.

On 10 May 1815 the Maltese were informed by Alexander Wood, Chief Secretary to Government, that the quarantine in Sicily was now 'limited' to seven days.[81] No further concessions were made and Grieves put the blame on the Sicilian Board of Health, based in Palermo, who farmed the revenues of quarantine. He complained to Admiral Penrose, in 1819, that the seven-day quarantine was the minimum, often doubled 'on every idle rumour'.[82] Indeed, in July 1817 the quarantine had been increased to 40 days because a ship with plague 'had touched off' Malta; but the Governor had not let it dock. Later in 1817 the same Board of Health had put Malta in double quarantine for receiving Sicilian boats which had been coral fishing off the Barbary coast. And then early in 1819 the quarantine was again doubled for receiving a Sicilian ship with passengers from Tunis. Grieves hoped he had said enough of the 'rankling absurdity' of Sicilian quarantine to induce the Admiral to 'interfere' on the islanders' behalf.

What Penrose was supposed to do is unclear, but the letter from Grieves was part of a concerted effort by Government to bring the Sicilians to their senses. In August 1818 Hector Greig, Acting Chief Secretary in the temporary absence of Richard Plasket (successor to Wood), tried to enlist support from the British Consul General in Palermo.[83] It was, of course, open to Malta to retaliate but, as the smaller island had more to lose, quarantine against Sicily was imposed with reluctance. For instance, in June 1816 a detention of 15 days was introduced, but that was 25 days fewer than the quarantine from the toe of Italy.[84] It was wise, in any case, to demonstrate a good reason. In July 1817, when communication with Messina had reportedly been cut by the Board of Health in Palermo on the grounds of some unexplained disease, Plasket announced that the 'unpleasant' decision had been taken (owing to 'the total absence

78 G. Cockburn, *A Voyage to Cadiz and Gibraltar up the Mediterranean to Sicily and Malta in 1810, & 11* ... (2 vols, London, 1815), vol. 2, p. 85.

79 W.F. Lord, *England and France in the Mediterranean, 1660–1830* (London, 1901), p. 76, and *Sir Thomas Maitland. The Mastery of the Mediterranean* (London, 1897), pp. 146–7.

80 NA CO 158/26 [unpag.], Maitland to Bunbury, 8 Mar. 1815.

81 *Proclamations, Minutes and other Official Notices, published by the Government of the Island of Malta, and its Dependencies, From ... 1813, to ... 1820* (Malta, 1821), p. 100.

82 National Library of Malta [NLM] LIB 843, fols 76–7, from which remaining references in this paragraph are taken.

83 National Archives of Malta [NAM] CSG 7/1, p. 37.

84 NLM LIB 843, fol. 17.

of direct communication from Messina, and of the extraordinary and unaccountable silence' of the authorities) to suspend pratique for all vessels from Sicily.[85]

It was less harmful to the economy to retaliate in the context of a given ship. An opportunity arose in 1819 when the Sicilian consul in Valletta asked permission for a xebec from Tunis to enter Marsamxett Harbour and for her cargo to be depurated in the lazaretto.[86] The same vessel had tried to enter the harbour some time earlier, but had been refused permission because she had come from Tunis at a time of plague. The xebec had then made for Palermo but, in the absence of a lazaretto there, had been sent back to Malta. Plasket, with laboured politeness, informed the consul that the xebec would not be allowed back because the favour being asked was 'neither more nor less than this – that we should for the sake of assisting a Sicilian Vessel subject the whole Island to a heavy additional Quarantine laid on by the very Gov[t] to whom we were affording that assistance – a Measure which His Honor The Lieutenant Governor can never feel it his duty to authorize'.

In the long term this rebuke did little good, and Malta remained exposed for years to the vagaries of Sicilian logic. Nor was she free from vexatious delays elsewhere, but as Maitland and the merchants, despite their differences, shared a common aim in stealing trade from ports such as Leghorn and Genoa, it was not surprising that Boards of Health on the mainland made life uncomfortable for Maltese shipping. It suited the mood of the merchants on Malta to attribute much of the blame to Maitland himself. In a notorious incident during 1815, Maitland made a brief visit to Tunis and excused himself from quarantine on return. At least, that was how it seemed to foreign consuls who had probably expected nothing else when they watched the Governor set sail. Even Maitland's visits to the Ionian Islands were an opportunity for the health police of the diplomatic services to report to their principals about the High Commissioner's attention, or otherwise, to the rules. A quarantine of 15 days was imposed at Marseilles on a ship from Malta, during 1818, when her arrival coincided with news that Maitland had returned from Corfu without quarantine.[87] It mattered nothing that both Corfu and Malta were plague-free at that time.

It fell to Grieves, as Superintendent of Quarantine, to make the best impression possible with the Continental Boards of Health. The way to do that was to invite himself to membership of the clique by sending memoranda to Leghorn, Genoa and Marseilles, and sometimes elsewhere, similar to the circulars which those ports sent among themselves. Such dispatches gave both factual and anecdotal information on the incidence of plague and reported candidly on illnesses within lazarettos and steps being taken, if necessary, to root out infection. It was an understanding between Boards that bad news would be reported no less fully than good, and that the obligation to honesty within the clique transcended the loyalty which a Board felt towards the trade of its own port. Thus if Marseilles, for example, had a case of plague in the lazaretto, the Italian Boards would be notified in the full knowledge

85 *Proclamations* (1821), p. 177.

86 NAM CSG 7/1, pp. 49–50, from which all references in this paragraph are taken.

87 W. Macmichael, *A Brief Sketch of the Progress of Opinion on the subject of Contagion; with some Remarks on Quarantine* (London, 1825), p. 531.

that ships from Marseilles would suffer extended quarantine for weeks on end at ports like Leghorn and Genoa.

This stoical acceptance of pain made the Continental Boards of Health indifferent to pleas from smaller ports, like Malta, that quarantine was ruining their business. The retort would always be that if Malta expected free pratique for her ships, she should be beyond reproach in her quarantine arrangements; and if she experienced disease in her lazaretto, she should expect her shipping to be detained for as long as any one Board felt it necessary. The difficulty for the British, who had long forgotten any lessons learnt in Minorca, was to accept that such rigidity arose from a high-minded concern for public health, and not from an opportunity to settle scores left over from the wars, or from commercial jealousies, or from an administration which was corrupt. In truth, those negative factors contributed both to the severity of quarantine and its continuation into decades when it might otherwise have been abandoned. But underpinning the attitude of the Boards was an idealism which the British, particularly on Malta, never understood, and the differences were about to deepen.

It was a matter of pride for the Maltese Government that Grieves wrote nine times to Boards of Health during 1815, and ten times in 1816.[88] Leghorn, followed by Genoa, were the main recipients, but Trieste and Sicilian Boards were also addressed. In November 1816 Grieves wrote his first multiple warning: the main letter, about suspected plague in the lazaretto at Tripoli, was sent to Leghorn (now recognized in Malta as the senior Board in the brotherhood), with copies to Naples, Genoa, Corfu, Marseilles, Palermo, Rome and Trieste.[89] None of the other 19 letters during the two years above-mentioned was addressed to Marseilles. It would be wrong to deduce from this that Malta and Marseilles were at loggerheads, because to some extent it was a question of language. The lingua franca for Boards of Health was Italian, which was also the first language (other than Maltese, used only in speech) for clerks in the quarantine office on Malta. Grieves would have been hard-pressed to find a clerk who could write to the Marseilles Board in French, and it was evident from experience with Gibraltar that the Board did not welcome letters in English. It might be argued that Grieves could have written to the Board in Italian, which was perfectly understood at Marseilles, where the seniority of Leghorn was recognized. But the understanding between Leghorn and Marseilles was so complete that they (sometimes with Genoa) formed a kind of inner brotherhood within the clique. Grieves could be confident that a letter to Leghorn would suffice for Marseilles, between which Boards there were no secrets.

Managing the department

It must be emphasized that Malta, under the British administration, was still without a system to safeguard public health which was recognized on the European mainland. This was one reason why Grieves, conscientiously sending letters and reports to

88 NA CO 158/31 [unpag.], Plasket to Wilmot, 14 Aug. 1822.

89 Ibid.

foreign Boards, was not rewarded by intelligence in the reverse direction. Malta only received letters when a Board had something specific to impart, usually in response to a question. While Maitland opposed the idea of a Maltese Board of Health, it was a matter of concern for him, as well as for the island's merchants, that every quarantine measure in the island should be acceptable to Leghorn and Marseilles. This meant the imposition of restrictions which were often detrimental to wider British interests. Not only was it impossible to lift quarantine against the Ionian Islands once Maitland became High Commissioner, but it was necessary to impose a quarantine of ten days against Gibraltar, during 1818, when plague was confirmed in Tangier.[90]

One of the earlier measures of Government, announced in April 1814, was a quarantine of 40 days on all ships with clean bills from Barbary, the Levant and the Morea.[91] Arrivals with foul bills would be subject to such additional quarantine as seemed necessary, and ships with plague on board would be refused admittance, or burnt with their cargoes. Vessels from the eastern Adriatic, from Venice to Zante, would be quarantined for 15 days with clean bills, but would be treated as from Barbary, and so forth, if bills were foul. The quarantine of merchant ships was to begin from the date of their arrival or, if they carried susceptible goods, from the date their cargoes were placed in the lazaretto. For warships, however, quarantine was to count from the date they left their port of departure. All merchant ships liable to quarantine were to proceed to Marsamxett Harbour and on no account to enter Grand Harbour. After the lapse of four months 'which must be sufficient time to enable Merchants and others to receive due information on this head', a penalty of 200 dollars was to be levied by the Superintendent of Quarantine on any ship in the wrong harbour.

Another important measure in the same decade concerned the fumigation of mail.[92] It is interesting that Maitland, Wood and Grieves were all away from the island on 6 August 1817, when the Notice was issued by Plasket under the auspices of the Lieutenant-Governor. Their absences had already been long enough to suggest that none of them was privy to the announcement. Indeed, the Notice was issued tentatively 'until the pleasure of… the Governor be known'. Plasket was experienced and standing in for Wood (whom he was destined to supersede within a month), but the office of Superintendent of Quarantine was being temporarily filled by Charles Tucker, who had no previous experience at that level. The new measure appears to have been an initiative by Robert MacNab, agent for the General Post Office in London, and concerned vessels arriving in both the main harbours of Valletta. For Grand Harbour, a system was devised for certifying the number of loose letters carried on a merchant ship, and for conveying them, along with any sealed boxes or bags, to the Post Office. This operation would be overseen by the Captain of the Port before the ship was given pratique. In Marsamxett Harbour, the procedure was for the mail to be delivered from the ship to the lazaretto, under a memorandum from the

90 *Proclamations* (1821), p. 215.

91 *Proclamations* (1821), pp. 33–4, from which all references in this paragraph are taken.

92 *Proclamations* (1821), pp. 177–9, from which all references in this paragraph are taken.

master as to the number of letters and whether they were loose or otherwise. It was expected that if a ship anchored in Marsamxett Harbour during the night, or before 8 a.m. the next day, the fumigation process in the lazaretto would be completed within a few hours, so that the mail would be at the Post Office by 3 p.m. on the same day. But if more than 200 letters were involved, the time would be increased proportionately. If a ship were to anchor between 8 a.m. and 4 p.m., the letters (with the same caveat as to quantity) would be due at the Post Office by 8 a.m. the next morning. The Captain of the Lazaretto would share responsibility for the transit of the letters, after fumigation, to the custody of the Post Office.

It may not be fanciful to see these rules as deliberately imposed while Grieves was in London. Earlier in 1817 he had been forced to defend himself to MacNab against an accusation of opening and fumigating a dispatch from Constantinople to Lord Castlereagh.[93] Grieves argued that as the ship had a foul bill of health he had had no option: unless the rules were indiscriminately followed, the authorities at Leghorn, Genoa and other ports would treat all ships from Malta as foul-bill arrivals. Furthermore, Grieves claimed to know instances when an absence of precautions had resulted in disease. He ended, perhaps too sardonically, with the assurance that if any of His Majesty's ministers wished to receive dispatches which had been fumigated less rigorously, he would be happy to comply. Although the reforms in August concerned speed more than method, they can be interpreted as a further assertion by the Post Office that mail, even in a lazaretto, was not beyond its control.

The episode with MacNab requires that the role of the Superintendent of Quarantine in Malta be more closely examined. It has already been remarked that he enjoyed a salary and status far beyond the dreams of any colleague in Britain. In fact, Grieves did particularly well. After suffering for many months under Maitland's instinctive mistrust, he went about his duties with such confidence and ability that, early in 1816, he was promoted to the military rank of Inspector of Hospitals, and drew half-pay from that position as well as his civil salary of £800 a year.[94] Within Malta, his standing was now higher than that of his predecessors, whom Oakes had rather belittled. The proof of that comes from the order of procession, in 1818, for the investiture in Malta of the first knights of the Order of St Michael and St George. The Superintendent of Quarantine walked immediately behind (and was therefore senior to) colonels of the army and captains of the navy of three years' standing.[95] He was also behind the Advocate of the Crown, the judges and the Inspector General of Police, and only three steps ahead of the Chief Secretary to Government.[96]

It is clear from his correspondence that Grieves used his seniority to good effect. He wrote to presidents of the Boards of Health at Leghorn and Genoa as their equal, and his letter to Admiral Penrose showed not a trace of fawning. He was on cordial terms with Colonel Warrington, the British consul in Tripoli, and

93 NLM LIB 843, fol. 44, from which all references in this paragraph are taken.

94 NA CO 158/28 [unpag.], correspondence with James McGrigor.

95 *Proclamations* (1821), pp. 267–8.

96 Ibid.

had direct communication in Malta with the Chief Secretary to Government.[97] He gave firm advice to Major Carter, military commander on Gozo, and frequent instructions to Robert Corner, Intendant of Marine Police, who was based in Grand Harbour.[98] Grieves also had wider responsibilities. He was a Vice-President of the Maltese Hospitals and later President of the Permanent Committee of the Charitable Institutions.[99] In 1817, and again in 1820, he was made a General Magistrate.[100] Grieves was even respected by Maclean, of all people, who referred to 'my esteemed [and in another place 'worthy'] friend Dr. Greaves [*sic*], in whose house I resided whilst at Malta'.[101]

Within his department, Grieves could rely on expertise from the Protomedico, who was a Maltese doctor, from the Captain of the Port, and from the Captain of the Lazaretto.[102] But they had no standing as a mini-committee and it is difficult, in the immediate post-plague era, to establish how far Grieves was an influence on Government policy. Public notices affecting quarantine were issued by the Chief Secretary and Grieves was never mentioned by name. The impression to the merchants was that Maitland, or a lieutenant-governor during his frequent absences, imposed the rules and restrictions, and the British style of government demanded nothing less. But as time passed, most changes were never the subject of a Government notice and knowledge of them derives usually from letters from Grieves to Corner.[103] It would be unwise, however, to deduce that Grieves had authority to make such alterations himself; any tightening or relaxation of the rules came about with the permission of Government, although it was no doubt Grieves who suggested that some change would be appropriate.[104]

Within the quarantine harbour, procedures were so tightly regulated that Grieves could leave day-to-day matters to subordinates. Grand Harbour, however, presented significant problems. There, Grieves relied on the cooperation and goodwill of Corner to ensure that vessels liable to quarantine were directed to Marsamxett Harbour as quickly as possible. This meant keeping Corner apprised of every change in policy which brought new ports of departure within the scope of restrictions. By Maitland's ruling of April 1814, no merchant ship liable to quarantine should have entered Grand Harbour at all and, when the rule was broken, Corner was expected to detain the ship

97 For relationship with Warrington, see NLM LIB 843, fols 44–5, where Grieves, 8 Mar. 1817, congratulates him 'for Tripoli and the Friends of humanity' on keeping plague out of the town.

98 NLM LIB 843, fols 3, 7, 8 etc.

99 *Proclamations* (1821), pp. 103, 224.

100 *Proclamations* (1821), pp. 187, 278.

101 C. Maclean, *Evils of Quarantine Laws, and Non-Existence of Pestilential Contagion* ... (London, 1824), pp. 347, 366.

102 Under Maitland's reforms, the Protomedico (Dr Luigi Caruana) received a monthly salary of 120 scudi, making him the fourth highest-paid official of the quarantine department.

103 For example NLM LIB 843, fols 38–9, 5 Dec. 1816, Grieves to Corner about the removal of restrictions from Sicily, Sardinia, Naples and the Roman territories.

104 For example NLM LIB 843, fol. 26, 3 May 1816, when Grieves recommends to Lieutenant- Governor Layard that the seven-day quarantine against Sicily be abandoned.

until the fine was paid.[105] There were times, however, when only Grand Harbour was accessible, owing to the direction of the wind; for this reason, and because masters could argue that a recent ruling was unknown to them, the penalty was not enforced unless the breach seemed blatant. The worst offenders were the navy, who sailed into Grand Harbour as a matter of course and were most reluctant to leave it. It was not unusual for Grieves to insist, by recourse to a more senior officer, that a frigate move round into Marsamxett Harbour. In retaliation, the navy could claim that Grieves was hindering the service, as occurred over HMS *Clorinde* during July 1815, when a complaint was laid before the Lieutenant-Governor.[106]

A lesser problem for Grieves was that he did not possess the linguistic skills which had been so much a boon to Eton. Most of his staff were equally disadvantaged in terms of English. It had been one of Bathurst's instructions to Maitland, in 1813, that English should replace Italian as the island's official language.[107] The process proved very slow. If Maltese-born clerks were useful in liaising with the European Boards of Health, their ignorance of English meant that some letters to other departments on the island were still written in Italian. Correspondence in English, fair-copied into the department's letter book, is sometimes so full of mistakes that the meaning is unclear. The recruitment of the Registrar from Leghorn, whose name was P. Armano, did nothing to alleviate the problem as he could (or chose) only to write in Italian to Corner, who had enough problems with difficulties presented in English.[108] In fact, the employment of Armano was soon seen as a significant mistake, and the blame must lie with Maitland rather than Grieves for having enticed him to the island. In 1818 Armano was dismissed from his office on the grounds that he falsified an entry concerning pratique for a warship and was engaged in espionage.[109]

In May 1819 Malta was again on the brink of plague. The bombard *La Trinita* arrived off the island from Susa in Tunisia, after three crewmen had died of plague and with another two showing symptoms.[110] The sick were allowed to land and were successfully treated in the lazaretto. The ship itself was submerged for ten days and the susceptible part of her cargo was burnt. Grieves took credit for the courage shown in allowing plague-stricken sailors to enter the lazaretto, which was contrary to Maitland's stern warning five years earlier, and for the successful containment of the outbreak. This might well have been a repeat of the ghastly events of 1813; that it was not created a bond of confidence among the military doctors, inspiring Tully to publish the reports made by Grieves to Government.[111] Plasket, on behalf of the Governor, was equally keen on the honours and circulated all foreign consuls in

105 For example NLM LIB 843, fol. 25, Grieves to Corner about the ship *Neptune*, 18 Apr. 1816.

106 NLM LIB 843, fols 9–11.

107 cf. H. Luke, *Malta: An Account and an Appreciation appreciation* (London, 1949), p. 101.

108 NLM LIB 843, fol. 7, Armano to Corner, 18 June 1815. Corner died in 1819 and was succeeded by William Symonds (*Proclamations* (1821), p. 240).

109 NA CO 158/31 [unpag.], annotation to letter, merchants to Bathurst, 15 Nov. 1822.

110 There is a summary of the incident in Maclean, *Evils of Quarantine Laws*, pp. 347–9.

111 Tully, *History of Plague*, appendices: reports from Grieves, 9 & 11 May 1819.

Valletta, with particular letters to those from Sicily and Ragusa, trusting that 'even the most timid Minds' would be reassured.[112]

Unfortunately, the satisfaction in Malta was not rewarded by any relaxation of the suspicion in which the island was held by the foreign Boards of Health. With the merchants agitating for rules which conformed more closely to the spirit and letter of regulations in Leghorn and elsewhere, Maitland had little choice but to concede to another overhaul of the system. But as he would not move in his opposition to a Maltese Board of Health, there would have been no confidence among the island's merchants that changes to the rules alone would lighten the quarantine burden on their ships abroad.

On 12 October 1820 Major-General Sir Manley Power, as Lieutenant-Governor, proclaimed new 'Rules and Regulations for the performance of Quarantine in this Island'.[113] He was careful to indicate that Maitland had given his prior approval and referred to the latter's measures of April 1814 which the new regulations were framed to supersede. One feature of the 1814 rules had been their lack of correlation with the *Regulations for the Performance of Quarantine at Malta*, printed in 1812. By altering the periods of quarantine, and making instructions as to the use of the two main harbours at Valletta, Maitland had blundered into aspects to some extent covered by the *Regulations*. It was consistent with Maitland's impatient energy that he should concentrate on measures he considered of strategic importance, regardless of any conflict that would cause with the tedious minutiae of the rules as a whole. In that respect, the Proclamation of 1820 was scarcely an improvement. True, it was followed by detailed regulations superseding those of 1812, but foreigners would have queried why two documents were needed when all the measures could have been included in one. The answer, of course, lay in Maitland's vision of despotic power. While he was content that the lazaretto should issue practical requirements for the performance of quarantine, he saw the basic principles as a matter for himself. But the two aspects were so blurred, that no meaningful division was possible.

In detail, the Proclamation of 12 October confirmed that Marsamxett Harbour was appropriated solely as a quarantine station, and all ships (including warships, by implication) had to proceed there if they were liable. Any merchant vessel entering Grand Harbour 'when it is possible to comply with the foregoing regulation' (a slight softening of the wording) would be fined 200 dollars, as before. In Marsamxett Harbour, the Captain of the Port would indicate an anchorage and interrogate masters, putting to them the questions in the printed rules. Ships with foul bills of health would be subject to 30 days' quarantine, to begin once all susceptible articles were landed in the lazaretto. The goods would 'be exposed in the Lazaretto to thirty-five days expurgation, in the strictest manner – and ten days subsequently for repackage'. Ships with foul bills but unsusceptible cargoes would also be quarantined for 30 days, and the goods would still be unloaded for checking. If the cargo were indeed unsusceptible, the unloading time would be deducted from the quarantine period.

112 NAM CSG 7/1, pp. 52–8.

113 There are two sources for the full text: *Proclamations* (1821), pp. 301–12, and Hennen, pp. 637–52 (the latter without table of fees), from which all references in this and the next three paragraphs are taken.

Ships with touched bills would perform 25 days' quarantine with susceptible goods, otherwise only 20 days. The quarantine for people 'from countries where the plague, or any infectious disease doth exist' would be a maximum of 20 days as long as, after entering the lazaretto, they 'will submit to separate themselves *in toto* from their baggage and clothes, and undergo an ablution with soap and warm water'. People from ships with touched bills would, after the same process, be released after ten days. All communication between ships on the high seas would result in the greater quarantine appropriate for one being visited on the other. Government reserved the right to impose a quarantine of observation on ships and persons, as new circumstances might arise. The Proclamation ended with a quarantine of 15 days for arrivals from the Ionian Islands with susceptible goods, or for 12 days without.

Also on 12 October 1820 Plasket issued the new printed *Regulations* to supersede those of 1812. This time, strangely, they were unnumbered, which must have made comparison and referral quite difficult. At first sight, they seem virtually a restatement of the existing rules, and indeed the questions to be put to masters by the Captain of the Port were identical. In the list of enumerated goods of the first class, the only changes were the inclusion of 'Hoops' rather than hoofs (no doubt a copying error), and the omission of liquor. Among goods of the second class, there was no longer mention of myrrh. More generally, the 1820 rules differed from those of 1812 in four respects: references to the Board of Health were left out, or replaced by ones to the Governor; sections were omitted which referred to bills of health (which were now covered by the Proclamation) and to probationary airing (which was abandoned); some clauses were shortened or simplified; and the rider entitled 'Instructions given to Commanders of Vessels under Quarantine' lost its first five paragraphs, which concerned flags and the use of boats. The regulations ended, as they had in 1812, with a table of Health Office fees. In most respects they were identical, but the charge per day for persons accommodated in the lazaretto fell by one scudo from the previous two scudi and six tari.

When the Proclamation and regulations are taken together, the degree of confusion between what was seen by Maitland as a matter for himself, and what was conceded by him as an ostensible concern for Grieves, must have done nothing to allay the worries of merchants and consuls alike. The measures themselves, regardless of that overlap, were tough and thorough: not only was the concept of a touched bill introduced for the first time in Maltese law, but the possibility of a clean bill from places east was no longer countenanced. The emphasis was now not on the ship, whose bill could not be relied upon, but on the susceptibility or otherwise of the cargo. And if any doubt arose in vaguer circumstances, the quarantine of observation was now a comforting piece of defensive armour. How far Grieves had influenced the new measures cannot be known, but they smack of an attempt by Maitland to arrest and reverse the gradual descent of the initiative to his Superintendent of Quarantine. Such a policy, however, would prove neither easy nor wise in the long run.

More plague, yellow fever and discontent

Now that Grieves had given sanctuary to the plague-stricken crew of *La Trinita*, whether or not Maitland had agreed with good grace, it was difficult to turn away other infected ships, especially if they were locally owned. On 21 March 1821 the Maltese brig *Constanza* limped into harbour with beans from Alexandria and a strong suspicion of plague.[114] A woman, a child and then a boy had perished on the voyage. On 25 March a man from the ship died in the lazaretto. Grieves reported to Plasket that another crewman was ill, and the symptoms gave little room for doubt. A month later Grieves reported to Hector Greig, standing in for Plasket, that in total 13 crew and passengers had been attacked by plague in the lazaretto, as well as one 'depurator' on board the ship. Ten of these people had died, but eight of the crew were still in good health. On 19 May, Grieves informed Greig that the survivors had already performed a quarantine of 42 days and would be admitted to pratique after a final sciorino: 'so the whole of the Depuration, may be said to have terminated without the smallest ... suspicion of any injury to the public health'. There was, however, injury to the budget of the quarantine department, and Grieves asked that 'expurgating' expenses be recovered by legal process.[115] Some 2,764 scudi had already been advanced by Government to put the *Constanza* in a condition for sale.[116]

Costs aside, this episode was an even greater triumph for Grieves than the incident of *La Trinita* two years earlier. As the infection on the second occasion had been greater, with an enhanced risk to the Maltese population, the successful containment within the lazaretto won approval where it mattered most. In June 1821 the French consul in Malta told Greig that the Board of Health at Marseilles were so satisfied with the handling of the crisis by Grieves that no increase would be made in the quarantine laid against ships from Malta.[117] This should have heralded a golden age in relations between the island and the French, but in fact they deteriorated quickly for reasons unconnected with plague. The problem lay in a resurgence of yellow fever in the western Mediterranean where Gibraltar, whether or not it was infected, could not be divorced from the ills of places, both in Europe and Africa, to which it was uncomfortably close.

With General Don as Lieutenant-Governor, Gibraltar was trying hard to ingratiate itself with the Marseilles Board of Health. Late in 1814 Don restarted a correspondence which had lapsed, on account of the war, since Governor Boyd had written about a precautionary quarantine against Corsica in 1792.[118] The auspices, however, were not good, as Don wrote only in English, which was evidently not understood by the recipients.[119] They would have been equally unfamiliar with his manner. Don expected them to take his word about all aspects of health on the Rock, and to accept that a clean bill meant 'no Danger whatever can exist in communicating

114 NLM LIB 843, fols 94–6, from which all references in this paragraph are taken until otherwise stated.

115 NLM LIB 843, fols 101–2.

116 Ibid.

117 NA CO 158/31 [unpag.], Plasket to Goulburn, 12 Jan. 1822.

118 ADBR 200 E 441 embraces both the earlier and later correspondence.

119 Because the letters are always filed against a translation into French.

with the Port and Garrison of Gibraltar'.[120] At the same time, he warned the Board 'that interested and ill disposed people may propagate false reports', and trusted such rumours would be ignored.[121] If that was naïve, it was doubly silly to admit that the 'various measures' he intended 'towards preserving the health of this Fortress ... may create some alarm', especially as he did not explain fully what those measures would be.[122]

Luckily for Don, he was usually supported by one Joseph Viale, who was resident in Gibraltar as 'l'agent du Consulat Général de France'. In that capacity he was below the rank of consul, but in terms of supplying Marseilles with intelligence he fulfilled exactly the same role. In 1816, when Viale began writing to the Marseilles Board of Health, he had cause to be critical of procedures at Gibraltar, which had allowed an American master to make a false assertion that 500 barrels of flour had been offloaded from his ship not there, but at Barcelona.[123] But over the next six years he expressed himself satisfied with the rigour and integrity of Don's control, and the frequent mentions of plague in Barbary, followed by yellow fever in Cadiz, were followed by reassurances that Gibraltar had adequate defences. Viale had access to key officials in the local administration, and Don was increasingly content to let him communicate with Marseilles virtually as a spokesman for Government. On the few occasions when Don himself wrote, it was no longer to explain his own measures but, with studied politeness, to thank the Board for the receipt of intelligence and, more especially, to express his gratitude for the exclusion of Gibraltar from new restrictions imposed on Spanish ports either side of it, as yellow fever gripped both the Atlantic and Mediterranean coasts. For three years, from August 1822, there are no extant letters from Viale, Don or any other person at Gibraltar in the archives of the Marseilles Board of Health, but Silvestre de Sacy, as full consul, began writing in 1825 and was equally well disposed towards Don and his policies.[124]

The satisfaction felt with Gibraltar at Marseilles was not always matched by attitudes on Malta. In July 1821 ships with clean bills were allowed to anchor in Grand Harbour, if from Gibraltar or North America, but on 13 September Greig published a Government minute expressing concern at yellow fever in Spain.[125] In consequence, a quarantine of seven days was imposed on ships from Gibraltar with clean bills, and of fifteen days for arrivals from Spain. But as rumours of the 'most virulent and dangerous nature' of yellow fever gripped the island, along with news that infected ships had reached the lazarettos at Port Mahon and Marseilles, Plasket issued a new and much tougher minute on 18 October.[126] Ships which had cleared direct for Malta from southern Spain were to proceed to St Paul's Bay for a quarantine

---

120 ADBR 200 E 441, 13 Dec. 1814; cf. 23 Nov. 1814: 'when I [Don] issue clean Bills of Health, there can be no danger whatever in communicating with this Port'.

121 ADBR 200 E 441, 16 Mar. 1815.

122 Ibid.

123 ADBR 200 E 441, 16 Sept. 1816.

124 He would appear to be Baron Silvestre de Sacy, the orientalist, but there is no mention of his stint at Gibraltar, or indeed of any similar work for the diplomatic service, in *Nouvelle biographie générale* (Paris, 1862).

125 NLM LIB 843, fol. 97; *Proclamations* (1823), p. 11.

126 *Proclamations* (1823), pp. 14–15.

of observation, before any entry would be admitted to Marsamxett Harbour.[127] Any vessels on which yellow fever existed (unless they were under British or Ionian flag) would be sent back to sea.[128] Arrivals from northern Spain, from Portugal, or from Corsica and Sardinia would be quarantined for between seven and ten days, and indeed any ship from anywhere in the Mediterranean would be examined by the police physician before receiving pratique.[129] On the next day, Plasket announced that the one case of yellow fever at Marseilles had not, it seemed, triggered others, but that ships from there would still undergo a quarantine of observation.[130]

It is significant that neither Maitland nor Grieves was in Malta when the panicky minute of 18 October 1821 was issued. As well as omitting any mention of Gibraltar, which was nevertheless unlikely to have escaped the restrictions, the minute introduced the concept that a ship in dire trouble could expect no mercy in Maltese waters. That was not the policy in cases of plague and Grieves would never have suggested it. For that matter, it was unlikely to have pleased Maitland. As it was, John Locker, who acted as Superintendent of Quarantine until the return of Grieves in February 1822, sent a triumphant memorandum (in English) to the Boards of Health at Leghorn, Genoa, Marseilles, Venice, Trieste, Naples and Palermo, explaining 'the prompt & decided measures' taken by the Maltese Government.[131] Plasket sent a similar note to foreign consuls in Malta.[132] It is not clear when the measure was discontinued, but in August 1822 it was reintroduced against Barcelona only.[133] Grieves was in Malta then, but Maitland was not, and in fact the minute was rescinded three weeks later.[134]

None of these decisions impressed the merchants of Malta, who re-emerged as an active and embittered pressure group, obsessed by the conviction that Maitland was to blame for the quarantine universally inflicted on Maltese shipping in the European Mediterranean ports. In previous complaints, having got nowhere with Maitland, they had asked for their grievances to be considered by ministers in London. Now, in 1821, because Bathurst had previously sided with Maitland, they took the brazen step of petitioning Parliament with a catalogue of their woes.[135] Quarantine aside, these were the constitution of the island's Government, neglect of previous complaints, the monopoly on corn, and the working of the Supreme Council of Justice.[136] On a point of form, the petition could not be considered in the House of Commons, but the merchants had made an impact in London and Maitland was forced into a defensive

127 Ibid.

128 Ibid.

129 Ibid.

130 *Proclamations* (1823), p. 15.

131 NLM LIB 843, fols 100–101. A copy has survived also in ADBR 200 E 464. Locker (who enclosed a copy of the *Malta Government Gazette* for each party) was a magistrate and coroner.

132 NAM CSG 7/1, p. 103.

133 *Proclamations* (1823), p. 53.

134 *Proclamations* (1823), pp. 57–8.

135 P. Cassar, *Medical History of Malta* (London, 1965), p. 293, refers to a copy of the original petition in the possession of a Maltese lawyer.

136 NA CO 158/31 [unpag.], Plasket to Goulburn, 12 Jan. 1822.

position. He was also, of course, deeply offended. In January 1822 he wrote to Henry Goulburn, Under-Secretary to Bathurst, complaining that the merchants 'daily grow worse', but he would meet them and arrange to open up the trade in corn.[137] In the meanwhile, Plasket sent Goulburn a detailed riposte of the merchants' several points, which reveals their particular grievances in regard to quarantine.[138]

The first grievance was the long-standing allegation that Maitland had flouted his own rules in 1815 by returning from Tunis without quarantine. Plasket now explained the official version of events. The Governor, accompanied by Grieves 'as a Matter of precaution', had sailed to Tunis for a meeting with the Bey. He had stayed for two days in the house of the British consul at a time when Tunis had been free of plague for ten years. Under these circumstances, Maitland 'on his return felt himself justified in merely passing thro' the summary process of Quarantine, Viz[t] by stripping off the Cloth[e]s he came in, – washing in vinegar and water, and putting on fresh Clothes from Malta'. Plasket added that Maitland was not in the habit of breaking quarantine and the merchants had failed to mention that on a subsequent return from Corfu he had been in quarantine for 12 days in his own palace. A related allegation of the merchants was that the length of quarantine generally depended on the rank of the individual, but Plasket dismissed this as 'positively false'. The only concession was that passengers on ships with foul bills were allowed to enter the lazaretto where their effects could be purified more easily. This entitled the person to a deduction of no more than six or seven days out of thirty, and Plasket named three dignitaries who could attest to this system. He did not mention that only the better-off could afford to vacate the ship.

Quarantine from the Ionian Islands was another source of complaint. Plasket admitted that merchant vessels were detained 15 days with susceptible cargoes and 12 days with non-susceptible; but that warships were subject to 7 days' quarantine, which was deducted from the sailing time. If the voyage took fewer than seven days, the warships were generally released anyway, being allowed 'a day or two's grace' for bringing favourable reports of the state of public health. Plasket made no attempt to justify the difference in treatment between commercial and military voyages, which had not been announced in the Proclamation of 1820. Instead, he passed quickly to the next allegation of the merchants, which was that no correspondence was maintained, as it had been in earlier years, with the Continental Boards of Health. Here, Plasket was on solid ground and produced a précis of the letters written in the quarantine department since 1815, which showed conclusively that the merchants were ill-informed. This victory gave him confidence to attack their final point, which was that Maltese quarantine would never be respected until it was in the hands of a Board of Health, as at Marseilles. But there were few arguments of any substance for Plasket, who could only ramble about Maitland's sense of duty and bluster against 'chimerical suppositions' for altering a system which was already highly regarded. His trump card was the letter from the French consul, expressing satisfaction felt at

137 NA CO 158/31 [unpag.], Maitland to Goulburn, 12 Jan. 1822. Maitland was unaware that Goulburn had recently been superseded by Wilmot.

138 NA CO 158/31 [unpag.], Plasket to Goulburn, 12 Jan. 1822, from which all references in the next two paragraphs are taken.

Marseilles with the containment of plague in the Malta lazaretto, but he had already played it while denying any long-term damage from Maitland's visit to Tunis. So Plasket ended by inviting Bathurst 'to make himself master of the sentiments of the other Health Establishments in The Mediterranean'.

Long before Plasket's defence had been studied in London, the merchants had come to an understanding with Maitland. First, he wrote to them, promising he would support mercantile interests conscientiously, but he also accused them of gross exaggeration and wilful errors.[139] Then it was their turn to take offence, and the stalemate had to end. On 21 January 1822 Maitland wrote to Bathurst explaining that he had met the merchants as promised: he had withdrawn his letter and they, all 78 of them, had withdrawn their petition to London.[140] But the truce only lasted until the summer, when the merchants took advantage of Maitland's absence to press their case once more. They bypassed Sir Manley Power, once more in the role of Lieutenant-Governor, and sent a memorial direct to Plasket for forwarding to Bathurst in London.[141] This time, quarantine was the only topic of grievance and the principal issues can be glimpsed through another – in fact two – of Plasket's laboured commentaries.[142] The addressee was Robert Wilmot, as Goulburn's successor.

There was little new in the substance of the merchants' complaints. They once more referred to Maitland's trip to Tunis and alleged a 'notorious Partiality' towards certain individuals and ships. Plasket had reported these comments to Power who, 'being perfectly unconscious of any such charge against the Quarantine Department', wanted to know specific cases. With much satisfaction, Plasket told Wilmot that the merchants had declined to provide them on the grounds that it would be invidious, and he suggested that this discredited their personal crusade against Maitland. Quarantine against the Ionian Islands was another resurrected theme, with the usual complaint of disparity between commercial and military arrivals. But Plasket could report that the disparity was not what it used to be, because quarantine for warships had recently been increased to ten days. The reason he gave was that plague had broken out in a village 35 miles inland from the coast opposite Corfu, but it might also be deduced that mercantile pressure had paid off. Warships, however, were subject only to a quarantine of observation.

The aim of the merchants, Plasket explained, was to take quarantine away from Government and vest it in a Board of Health. He was so opposed to this idea that he backed up his letter with a memorandum setting out the wider arguments why such Boards were undesirable. In Naples, Sicily and many other places, officials in the health service were paid not by fixed salary but from the fees, which induced them to inflict as much quarantine as possible on merchant shipping. Furthermore, the two undesirable practices which, according to the merchants, impaired the propriety of Maltese quarantine – that is, partiality towards warships and persons of rank – were

139 NA CO 158/31 [unpag.], Maitland to merchants, 12 Jan. 1822.

140 NA CO 158/31 [unpag.], Maitland to Bathurst, 21 Jan. 1822.

141 This route is explained in NA CO 158/31 [unpag.], Plasket to Wilmot, 14 Aug. 1822, p. 1.

142 NA CO 158/31 [unpag.], Plasket to Wilmot, 14 Aug. 1822, followed by undated memorandum of Plasket, from which all references in the next two paragraphs are taken.

natural by-products of the European systems. In many states, warships were exempt from fees by Government order, so the Boards of Health dismissed them as soon as possible. And any passenger on a warship carrying a letter for Government was immediately given pratique. Even without dispatches, one person at Naples may be detained only three or four days, while another might be quarantined for a fortnight. At Trieste and Ancona it was the same picture. Plasket himself had been given pratique at Genoa after a voyage on a warship of only seven days, and at a time when Maitland's return from Tunis was being openly discussed. He had a similar anecdote concerning his arrival at Messina. Yet if these Governments were asked to intervene about the delay to merchant ships in quarantine, the invariable answer was that Boards of Health were 'perfectly independent … & cannot be interfered with'.

Maitland received a copy of the merchants' memorial while he was passing through Genoa.[143] It is unlikely, however, that he been given a copy of Plasket's responses, because he wrote immediately to Bathurst in terms which did not quite match the sentiments of his Chief Secretary. Dated 12 November 1822, Maitland's letter displayed his usual exasperation with the merchants' motives and misapprehensions, which he took as a personal attack. In ten years of governing Malta, he had 'had more plague and vexation about the Quarantine, and have taken more pains on that subject, than in respect to any of … [his] other duties …' He denied that an independent Board of Health had existed on Malta before 1813 and regarded the case for its reintroduction as 'one of the fashionable revolutionary ideas'. He argued that an independent Board of Health existed nowhere in Europe, but that undermined the point made by Plasket. In all Mediterranean countries, insisted Maitland, the monarch 'interferes' in quarantine, and on Malta he was the representative of a king who would exercise the powers himself if the island were closer to Britain. In terms of partiality, however, Maitland and Plasket made the same point and Maitland's seniority gave him wider scope for personal experience. At Trieste, Ancona, Genoa and Naples he had landed with minimum delay by orders which bypassed the local Board. In any case, he contended, the rules could always be offset by a 'douceur'.

The same letter reveals that Maitland had met Robinson at the Board of Trade to discuss whether quarantine delays at Malta might not be too long. Robinson 'seemed to think' they were and, when Bathurst sent him a copy of the Maltese merchants' memorial, it seemed likely that Robinson would be cast in the role of arbiter.[144] But that was not to be. Bathurst let the merchants know that he was still predisposed towards Maitland's point of view. He did this by asking them, via Wilmot, to justify their allegations of partiality when he already knew from Plasket that they would or could not do so.[145] In their reply of 15 November 1822, the merchants admitted they had kept no record of the infringements and, so far from justifying their claim, conceded that 'the instances we could adduce might be reconcilable with the existing

143 NA CO 158/31 [unpag.], Maitland to Bathurst, 12 Nov. 1822, from which all references in this paragraph are taken.

144 Evidence that Bathurst had written to Robinson comes from an acknowledgement in NA CO 158/31 [unpag.], Maitland to Bathurst, 16 Nov. 1822..

145 Recital in NA CO 158/31 [unpag.], merchants to Bathurst, 15 Nov. 1822.

practice'.[146] But the merchants then made a crafty suggestion: if Bathurst cared to ask the Quarantine Department for a return of all the merchants ships, warships and passengers since 1816, and the number of days' quarantine performed by each, their assertions would be proved correct. In countering other points, they felt more comfortable. Wilmot had quoted Plasket's comment, that Tunis had been free of plague for many years when Maitland made his ill-fated visit. The merchants replied that Tunis was always a 'suspected' country, so quarantine should reflect that. And here they added a new contention: Armano, the professional head-hunted by Maitland from Leghorn, had been dismissed for pointing out an irregularity with regard to the quarantine of a warship. A marginal annotation at this point denied that.

It was in relation to the Ionian Islands that the merchants felt their case was strongest. How far Wilmot had requested their further thoughts is not revealed, but with facts to hand they did not hold back. The *Sonia*, a brig owned by the Ionian Government, had recently arrived in Grand Harbour (not the quarantine harbour of Marsamxett) after only eight days from Corfu and was immediately given pratique. At the same time, after a voyage of nine days, an English merchant arrived in Marsamxett Harbour from Corfu on board an English vessel. He landed in the lazaretto, where he agreed to undergo a spoglio which reduced his quarantine, in theory, to ten days. In fact, he was released a day early, but this was still nine days longer than the detention of the *Sonia*. Furthermore, the circumstances of the brig's arrival reached the Health Office at Syracuse within 48 hours. It was also noted that a British warship, which reached Marsamxett Harbour in eight days from Corfu, was given pratique on the evening of arrival. For such reasons, the merchants feared 'the impracticability of ever obtaining for Malta any alleviation of the Quarantine imposed upon her in the neighbouring Ports'. When told of Maitland's favoured treatment when going ashore on the European mainland, their only comment was 'that the laxity of foreign Institutions should not be admitted as a precedent under a British Government'. The inherent vulnerability of Maltese trade, which had much to do with political and commercial jealousies, made it particularly necessary that quarantine in the island should be beyond reproach. But this could never happen, they stressed, until Malta was re-endowed with a Board of Health.

Bathurst was unimpressed by the merchants, and Maitland and Plasket continued to do all in their power to discredit them. Maitland growled at 'most malicious representations'.[147] Plasket sent Wilmot a request from James Bell, one of the merchants' leaders, to Grieves, requesting an abridged quarantine for his cousin who was returning from Cephalonia.[148] On 1 April 1823 Wilmot wrote to the merchants with the palliative news that the registers of the quarantine department in Malta would be examined as they suggested.[149] But he had also to inform them that Bathurst 'still sees no reason to direct that any alteration should be made in the Quarantine

---

146 NA CO 158/31 [unpag.], merchants to Bathurst, 15 Nov. 1822, from which remaining references in this and the next paragraph are taken.

147 NA CO 158/31 [unpag.], Maitland to merchants, 16 Nov. 1822.

148 NA CO 158/31 [unpag.], Plasket to Wilmot, 18 Nov. 1822.

149 Recital in NA CO 158/34 [unpag.], merchants to Bathurst, 9 June 1823.

Laws which have been established and are now in force in this Island'.[150] That was an unfortunate form of words, as the merchants responded immediately that Bathurst had misunderstood: their complaint was not about the law itself but the 'irregular & partial way in which it has been administered'.[151] There was a definite similarity now between the impasse on Malta and the other one in London, where Maclean had been locking horns for some time with the Board of Trade. In both places a vested private interest had taken on Government, been rebuffed, but refused to back down, while Government for their part would not indulge what they considered impertinence. With neither camp prepared to lose face, the only way forward was to bypass Government and take the argument to Parliament. Maclean did this in 1825, as has been shown, but the merchants had beaten him to it. If their direct petition was technically out of order, there was still another way to get members' attention.

On 10 July 1823 Joseph Hume reported to the House that the Committee of British Merchants on Malta had sent him a recent letter.[152] In it, they reproduced the statement from Bathurst that he would not interfere in the quarantine laws of the island. Adopting the merchants' cause, Hume proposed a motion that correspondence since 1814 between the merchants, the island's Government and the Colonial Office, relating to quarantine, should be laid before the House.[153] This was not the first time that the merchants had been in touch with Hume; he had raised their case earlier in the session, when he was told 'it was to be inquired into'.[154] Evidently, that failed to happen. Hume's free-trade credentials made him an obvious prospective ally, and he did not fail to broaden his speech to cover duty on imported corn.[155] His main points, however, began with the hackneyed arguments which had so long divided the merchants of Malta from their Government. The island, said Hume, had been in free pratique with European ports before 1813. The plague, of course, had altered that, but Genoa and Leghorn had soon intimated that free pratique might return. Unfortunately, 'circumstances arose' to prevent that, and to put matters right Hume suggested that a Board of Health should be established on Malta, replacing the authority of 'Dr. Greaves [*sic*], who was under the control of sir T. Maitland, and who allowed persons from any part of Turkey to land by his directions, without undergoing the usual quarantine'. Then, predictably, came the 'notorious' allegation that Maitland had returned from Tunis and ignored his own rules, which had caused reprisals abroad leading to 'losses and liabilities' among the merchants. Such a thing would never have been allowed at Marseilles, and Hume gave an instance of French punctiliousness. There followed 'some remarks upon the farce of fumigating letters from Malta, while woollens were allowed to pass unnoticed', which carried the debate into new areas. So did a personal attack on Maitland: if the Governor had resided on his island for only 309 days over the last nine years, how, queried

150 NA CO 158/34 [unpag.], merchants to Bathurst, 9 June 1823.

151 Ibid.

152 Hansard, New Series, vol. 9, p. 1526.

153 Hansard, New Series, vol. 9, p. 1528; *JHC*, vol. 78, p. 473.

154 Hansard, New Series, vol. 9, p. 1526.

155 Hansard, New Series, vol. 9, pp. 1526–8, from which remaining references in this paragraph are taken.

Hume, could the courts of justice function effectively, and was it right that important orders concerning Malta should be made from Corfu? One such order, in 1819, had imposed the duty on imported corn, and Hume instanced later Proclamations by lieutenant-governors which had raised it further. The relevance of these commercial issues to quarantine was not explained.

The reply on behalf of Government came from Robert Wilmot Horton (as Robert Wilmot now styled himself).[156] He did not oppose the motion but was keen to speak up for Maitland. Regarding the corn duty, he felt that the island's dependence on a foreign supply might justify exceptional measures. As for the creation of a Board of Health 'instead of the system of regulations', Hume could not have read the correspondence for which he now called, because the merchants admitted that the system at Malta was theoretically as good as anywhere else. Horton mentioned some of the periods of detention and denied that 'any favouritism, in the invidious sense of the word' existed towards warships. It was simply that they were renowned for cleanliness and discipline, and that fumigation and expurgation 'were going on all the while they were at sea'. As for Maitland's trip to Tunis, the place had been free of plague for many years. Hume had alluded to Marseilles, but the Board of Health there were perfectly satisfied with procedures at Malta. Finally, Horton offered to show Hume any correspondence he might call for and on that undertaking, reported Hansard, Hume 'consented to withdraw his motion'.

This parliamentary episode was no more than a piece of theatre. Hume had salved his conscience in a matter which interested him only to a limited extent, perhaps glad to reach a compromise with Horton. Yet the latter had made a poor speech. His point about the corn duty was woolly, while the implication that a Board of Health was somehow a substitute for a set of regulations made no sense at all. The assertion that warships sailed under a continuous process of fumigation was simply wrong (at the best they aired personal effects), and he failed to make the material point that they did not carry susceptible cargoes. Furthermore his defence of Maitland's landing from Tunis was absurdly weak, using none of the facts reported by Plasket to mitigate the Governor's gaffe. In brief, if the parliamentary exchanges were a token of respect for democracy, they did nothing to reconcile the opposing interests, and the year slipped by with no new initiative in London or Malta.

When the stalemate was broken, it was not through negotiation. On 17 January 1824, during a routine engagement on Malta, Maitland died from an apoplectic stroke. His most recent biographer has described him as 'arrogant, imperious, querulous, bad-tempered, and ill-mannered'.[157] These adjectives are consistent with the glimpses of his character provided by his association with quarantine. But an imponderable number of poor people on Malta and Corfu owed their lives to his fearless assault on the plague. In April, Plasket, who had been knighted in 1819, resigned from office and was succeeded by Frederick Hankey, a military man who had served as Private Secretary to Maitland. In the same month Grieves wrote to

156 Hansard, New Series, vol. 9, pp. 1528–9, from which all references in this paragraph are taken.

157 *Oxford Dictionary of National Biography.*

Bathurst for permission to retire.[158] This was not granted immediately but a radically new administration was very much in the offing. The merchants, however, could not wait and devised yet another roundabout route to get their message listened to in England. The ploy this time, revealed in a letter from Hankey to Horton, was for London merchants to lobby the Board of Trade, ostensibly for themselves, about certain aspects of Maltese trade.[159] Hankey dismissed the instigators as 'very inferior to the general class of British Merchants'.[160]

Capitulation

In June 1824 the Marquis of Hastings arrived in Malta as the new Governor and Commander-in-Chief. Although fresh from the East and a brave soldier, he had little else in common with Maitland. Hastings was less combative and more of a statesman. If preoccupied by his own chronic debts, he was nevertheless keen to begin on the right note. Mindful of the sensibilities and importance attached to all aspects of quarantine, he approached the deep-rooted problems with caution and even diffidence. One of his first acts was to ask Hankey to write to Leghorn, but to the British Consul General rather than the Board of Health.[161] Hankey was to make the point that the Government of Malta was now separate from that of the Ionian Islands, which were to be treated to a stricter quarantine. He was to hope, on behalf of Hastings, that this change would earn a diminution of quarantine for Maltese ships at Italian ports, especially as it applied also to warships, for which the days of grace had been abandoned. Hastings now believed that the lazaretto on Malta was 'on a footing hardly Capable of improvement' and formed a basis for reciprocal measures with the European ports. In a postscript, Hankey added that the consul was not to send this letter to the Board of Health, but inform them of its contents in his own words.

If this letter shows that Hastings lacked confidence in his dealings with the Italian states, another indicates that he held them in deep suspicion. Hastings wrote to Bathurst, on 14 August 1824, lamenting that unfair quarantine by 'hostile management' in Italy and France had almost excluded the Maltese from normal trade.[162] He referred to specious excuses to ruin the island's economy, and the mistaken argument that a Board of Health would set matters right. Such a Board, in European eyes, was 'arbitrarily supposed proof against any temptation to deviate from the professed Rules'. Hastings found the assumption offensive that a man in high station (that is, the Governor) would be irresponsible about quarantine while persons of lower rank, such as those who comprised a Board of Health, would be implicitly more reliable. 'Unluckily', he continued, 'it is not an absurd prejudice

158 NA CO 158/38 [unpag.], Grieves to Bathurst, 18 Apr. 1824.

159 NA CO 158/36 [unpag.], Hankey to Horton, 30 Apr. 1824.

160 Ibid.

161 NAM CSG 7/1, p. 171, from which remaining references in this paragraph are taken.

162 NA CO 158/36 [unpag.], Hastings to Bathurst, 14 Aug. 1824, from which all references in this paragraph are taken.

which we have to expose but an unworthy artifice which we have to defeat'. With those cryptic words he prepared Bathurst for the view that a Board of Health, however unwelcome the concept might be, should be attempted in Malta, at least in name. Hastings suggested that the Governor should superintend the Board, but with no brief to relax the laws. His role would be limited to 'dissent and prohibition, and a check against laxity'. If this experiment were not tried, the only recourse, warned Hastings, would be retaliatory quarantine against Europe in which Malta would come off worse.

In the autumn of 1824, before Bathurst could reply, the Hastings–Hankey partnership regained self-confidence and set about a polite but firm confrontation with their European adversaries. Hankey enlisted the help of William Hamilton at Naples in the continuing struggle with the Board of Health in Palermo, who had imposed fresh restrictions on Maltese shipping.[163] This 'extremely vexatious' new burden was 'of a piece with the conduct of the Sicilian Authorities in respect to the Commerce of Malta'.[164] Hankey thought the Neapolitan consul in Malta 'may be at the bottom of this business ... he is full of interference on all occasions, and assumes a very dictatorial style ... which if continued will oblige H.E. to apply for his removal'.[165] Hankey then wrote to British consuls at Leghorn, Marseilles, Naples, Genoa, Ancona and Trieste, informing them of alterations to the quarantine regulations on Malta which he hoped they would forward to the respective Boards of Health. He added the interesting confession: 'It is true that there may have been formerly slight instances of deviation from the Regulations, but this however will never more occur. This I can assure you from His Excellency'.

The next task for Hankey was to write to Sir Charles Stuart, the British ambassador in Paris, for assistance in dealing with the Board of Health at Marseilles.[166] Since the French consul in Valletta had written so soothingly about the Board's satisfaction with Maltese quarantine, the relationship had deteriorated rapidly. Hankey assured Stuart that the lazaretto on Malta 'is certainly the most complete in the Mediterranean, & the whole System of Quarantine more perfect then even Marseilles or Leghorn'. But those ports, wrote Hankey, were treating Malta to a stifling quarantine. He instanced the rule that warships from Malta were being detained for 15 days from arrival, even with a clean bill of health, whereas in many ports the authorities deducted 12 days for the voyage. Stuart was sent a copy of the new regulations at Malta and asked to intervene if he felt able to do so. For good measure, Hankey also sent a copy of the regulations to Horton in London, asking him to forward them to the British Consul General in Paris.[167]

The Board at Marseilles were now under pressure from the French Minister of the Interior and they wrote to Hastings, on 17 October 1824, giving three grounds for the rigorous quarantine imposed against Malta: the island had become an entrepôt

---

163 NAM CSG 7/1, pp. 175–7.

164 Ibid.

165 Ibid.

166 NAM CSG 7/1, pp. 180–81, from which all references in this paragraph are taken until otherwise stated.

167 NA CO 158/36 [unpag.], Hankey to Horton, 9 Oct. 1824.

for goods from the Levant and Barbary; it had been ravaged by plague in 1813; and it admitted warships from the Levant 'après de très courtes épreuves' [after very brief precautions].[168] Hastings was unhappy with that, but had the wisdom to reply in French. His points were that Leghorn was much more of an entrepôt than Malta and yet it was in free pratique with Marseilles; that procedures had tightened since 1813, which the Board had earlier accepted; and that quarantine on Malta was now the same for warships as for merchant vessels, although the former could still deduct their sailing time.[169] This was because crews were regularly examined, clothes and effects were aired, and no susceptible goods were carried.[170] In December 1824 Alexander Turnbull, the British consul in Marseilles, confirmed that the Board of Health were disinclined to relent, but he put that down to their sense of duty, advising Hankey that no 'Political or Commercial Jealousy operates here'.[171] On Malta, that was difficult to accept. Hastings then wrote to Bathurst acknowledging with regret that as long as British warships could abridge their quarantine, the intransigence at Marseilles would not be lifted.[172] But he expected 'too much inconvenience' in making the regulations at Malta compatible with the French.[173]

Another task for Hankey, that of complaining to the Austrian consul about the treatment of Maltese ships at Venice, Trieste and Fiume, underlines how the management of quarantine had changed since the death of Maitland.[174] Letters were now written at a diplomatic level, rather than direct to the Boards of Health, and Hankey had assumed the normal role of correspondent once filled by Grieves. But Grieves was still on Malta and had not yet been replaced as Superintendent of Quarantine. His request for a pension was not straightforward. If he made it via the Governor he would have to resign if the application failed.[175] So Grieves acted through intermediaries, who were Horton and the Honourable George Vernon.[176] By their intervention he was given permission to send a memorial to Bathurst. Dated 18 April 1824, this document summarized Grieves's career on Malta and emphasized that he took no fees in addition to his salary.[177] He referred to 'a service of eleven years in this scorching Island, completing a servitude of forty years to His Majesty', of which 37 had been served abroad.[178] As his sight was now impaired, Grieves asked to retire on terms comparable to those granted to Pym, or be allowed 'a small per centage on the balances of money he has paid into the treasury of Malta monthly, after defraying the expenses of the department, from the quarantine revenues, which

168 NA CO 158/41 [unpag.], letters in French from Health Office, Marseilles; recitals in NAM CSG 7/1, pp. 184–7.

169 NAM CSG 7/1, pp. 184–7.

170 Ibid.

171 NA CO 158/41 [unpag.], Turnbull to Hankey, 11 Dec. 1824.

172 NA CO 158/41 [unpag.], Hastings to Bathurst, 30 Jan. 1825.

173 Ibid.

174 NAM CSG 7/1, p. 189.

175 Recital in NA CO 158/38 [unpag.], Grieves to Horton, 23 June 1824.

176 Ibid.

177 NA CO 158/38 [unpag.], Grieves to Bathurst, 18 Apr. 1824.

178 Ibid.

would rarely amount to half the salary of Superintendent'.[179] Bathurst was in no hurry to reach a view, and Grieves eventually sent Horton a reminder.[180] This was strongly helped by a note from James Maitland, Earl of Lauderdale, to Bathurst explaining that 'there is no better man [than Grieves], nor anyone in whose welfare my Brother [that is, Sir Thomas] was more sincerely interested'.[181] On 20 July 1825 the final decision was sent to Hastings. Grieves was to receive a pension of £362 chargeable to the revenues of Malta, in addition to his half-pay of the same amount as Inspector of Hospitals.[182] This was a generous settlement in that Pym was paid a pension of only £300 from the pratique fees at Gibraltar, but of course Pym had by no means retired.

Hastings learnt by the same letter that Grieves's successor was Hector Greig. The salary, maintained at £800, would raise by £100 his existing pay as Collector of Land Revenue.[183] This was a surprising appointment as Greig was very much an administrator and not a doctor. Had Maitland still been alive, he would no doubt have approved this departure from precedent which ended the domination of army doctors since the departure of William Eton. This change came roughly a year after James McGrigor, Director General of the Army Medical Department, had recommended separate establishments for Malta and the Ionian Islands, with the experienced Dr Hennen in overall command.[184] Greig, as well as his responsibility for the Land Revenues, had regularly deputized for Plasket in his many absences from Malta; he had also served as Acting Treasurer and had once stood in for Rivarola as Inspector General of Police.[185] He was, therefore, well acquainted with most aspects of the administration and had ten years experience of the vulnerability of Malta to disease.

As Grieves played no role in the Hastings administration, and Greig was not yet in office, it also fell to Hankey to deny accusations from merchants that the quarantine charges on Malta were too high.[186] He did this by the somewhat unconvincing dispatch of costings, three years old, showing that the English brig *Castor* from Alexandria paid the equivalent of some 228 scudi in Health Office fees at Leghorn, whereas the charges at Malta would have been 215.[187] The merchants had already lobbied Hastings, predictably, for a total free port; again the Governor left it to Hankey, at his most unctuous, to turn them down.[188] Of more consequence, however, was the depuration of cotton on Malta, now that large quantities were

179 Ibid.

180 NA CO 158/44 [unpag.], Grieves to Horton, received 11 June 1825.

181 NA CO 158/44 [unpag.], Lauderdale to Bathurst, 16 May 1825.

182 NA CO 158/44 [unpag.], undated memo. reciting dispatch, 20 July 1825, to Hastings.

183 Ibid. He had been appointed to that role on 28 July 1814 (*Proclamations* [1821], p. 62).

184 NA CO 158/37 [unpag.], McGrigor to Taylor, 15 July 1824.

185 *Proclamations* (1821), *passim.*

186 NA CO 158/36 [unpag.], Hankey to Horton, 1 Oct. 1824.

187 Ibid. These figures had originally been prepared by Grieves.

188 NA CO 158/36 [unpag.], merchants to Hastings, 21 Sept. 1824; Hankey to merchants, 24 Sept. 1824.

being shipped from Alexandria to Liverpool. The issue was raised by James Calvert, whose exact title was Government Agent and Broker in Grain Transactions.[189] There were possibilities here to interest many parties, among them the Liverpool importers, the merchants on Malta and the Board of Trade in London. Now that the Navigation Act of 1822 allowed goods to be imported direct from Turkey and Egypt, there was no need for produce to be imported via Leghorn, Genoa and the other ports which had for centuries enjoyed a privileged status.[190]

In August 1824 Horton received a letter from the Board of Trade referring to quarantine for ships bound for Liverpool.[191] While Milford was 'expensive & inconvenient', no suitable site for a foul-bill station had been found any nearer.[192] It therefore seemed very appropriate to the Board that Liverpool merchants should have their cotton depurated on Malta, if Bathurst could kindly arrange a reduction in costs and the removal of 'any Inconvenience' – a term which was not explained.[193] When news of this reached Malta, it inspired James Bell & Co., perhaps the leading British merchants on the island, to argue for charges associated with the depuration of cotton to be reduced by one-third to stimulate trade.[194] The Egyptian cotton would arrive in Malta where it would be trans-shipped after depuration to vessels with a clean bill of health for the second leg to England. The view of Bell & Co. gained support in London, where the Board of Trade recommended to Horton that charges for depurating cotton should be lowered to those at Leghorn.[195] This showed that no confidence had been placed in Hankey's out-of-date comparative figures. On 28 February 1825 Hastings confirmed to Bathurst that, as ordered, costs at Malta and Leghorn were now equal.[196] Bell & Co. were now arguing for depuration of Egyptian cotton to be made compulsory on Malta, but the Board of Trade were not interested in dictating policy.[197] It was predictable that the next demand from the Maltese merchants would be the scrapping of all quarantine duties in line with Britain itself, but the annual loss of nearly £5,000 to the island's Treasury was distinctly unattractive to Government.[198]

Such complex and diverse matters distracted both Hastings and Bathurst from the critical, underlying question of whether Malta should have a Board of Health. It was December 1824 before Hastings learnt that Bathurst did not dissent from his view that such a Board was inevitable.[199] But Bathurst had some difficulty with Hastings's sceptical reasoning. The Governor then explained himself more fully

189 NA CO 158/36 [unpag.], memo. 13 July 1824. For Calvert's title, see *Proclamations* (1823), p. 61.

190 Ibid.

191 NA CO 158/37 [unpag.], Lack to Horton, 5 Aug. 1824.

192 Ibid.

193 Ibid.

194 NA CO 158/36 [unpag.], letters and calculations from Bell, 6 Nov. 1824, sent from Hankey to Horton, 23 Nov. 1824.

195 NA CO 158/37 [unpag.], Lack to Horton, 15 Dec. 1824.

196 NA CO 158/41 [unpag.], Hastings to Bathurst, 28 Feb. 1825.

197 NA CO 158/41 [unpag.], Bell to Hankey, 29 Jan. 1825.

198 NA CO 158/42 [unpag.], Power to Bathurst, 13 Sept. 1825.

199 Recital in NA CO 158/36 [unpag.], Hastings to Bathurst, 2 Dec. 1824.

and with even greater cynicism. A Board would show foreign states that Britain was prepared to conform. But the new institution would be 'merely ostensible' and 'wholly superfluous as to our Security'.[200] It was simply that the lack of a Board encouraged neighbouring states to justify a policy of detention 'which operates merely as an interdict on our Shipping'.[201] He then added the new argument that if foreign Boards were to admit that quarantine could be effective without such an institution as theirs, they would put themselves at risk of dissolution.[202]

Bathurst, still unconvinced that a Board of Health should be established for negative reasons, hesitated to make a decision. During 1825 Hastings returned to London, leaving shortly before a letter arrived from Bathurst, dated 5 May, enclosing another memorial from merchants in London who had Maltese connections.[203] This was, as usual, a complex and contentious paper covering eight commercial issues, of which quarantine was number two.[204] In the absence of Hastings it fell upon Power, very experienced as a stand-in governor, to respond.[205] He made fresh and forceful points. If quarantine were being inflicted from commercial or political jealousy, given the excellence of the Maltese regulations, it was surely for the British Cabinet to intervene. The foreign Boards were being hypocritical because Hastings (and his family) had just landed at Nice after only three days' quarantine out of the specified twelve, and Lord Strangford ('with his Baggage and Suite') had recently gone ashore at Trieste after only five days, although coming from Constantinople at a time of plague. Power revealed that Marseilles had now superseded Leghorn as the leading Board of Health in the Mediterranean, and all the requests for pratique which Malta had sent to other bodies were being forwarded to the French for their opinion. Yet among the reasons which that Board had given Hastings for the harsh treatment of Malta, there had been no mention of the absence of a Board of Health. After an allusion to new problems with Sicily, on the grounds that cotton was arriving at Liverpool without depuration, Power begged 'to recommend most strongly that the Quarantine Matters should remain as they stand at present, and no Board of Health be appointed'.

That was not, however, the view of Hastings who saw a copy of the merchants' memorial in July, on his arrival in London.[206] He stated that the Marseilles Board had 'continually urged' the formation of a comparable institution in Malta, and for that reason he still felt a Board – again he used the adjective 'ostensible' – should be created. He then agreed with a point apparently made previously by Bathurst, that 'Commercial Men' should not be eligible for appointment. Indeed, Hastings

200 NA CO 158/36 [unpag.], Hastings to Bathurst, 2 Dec. 1824.

201 Ibid.

202 Ibid.

203 Recital in NA CO 158/42 [unpag.], Hastings to Bathurst, 23 July 1825.

204 The others were: abolition of the Customs House; goods imported in foreign vessels; navigation laws; auction duty or vendue office; corn trade; import UK of Maltese manufactures; lack of notice of changes to commercial regulations.

205 NA CO 158/41 [unpag.], Power to Bathurst, 15 June 1825, from which remaining references in this paragraph are taken.

206 NA CO 158/42 [unpag.], Hastings to Bathurst, 23 July 1825, from which all references in this paragraph are taken.

recommended 'as a Private Condition for Nomination to the Trust [that is, the Board] a Pledge from the Subordinate Members, that they should not interfere unless when specially called upon with the details, but should leave them completely to the Governor & the Superintendant [*sic*]'. Even then, he felt the Board would be of doubtful use in satisfying authorities which were 'acutely jealous' of Maltese trade, but no other option existed.

Whether or not Bathurst was wholly in agreement with these sentiments, which promised no more than a mask for the status quo, he accepted that only one course existed to satisfy both mercantile clamour and international requirements. On 5 April 1826 a minute signed by Hastings vested exclusive control of the sanitary laws of Malta in a new Board of Health.[207] The composition was the Governor as President; Sir Frederick Hankey, as Chief Secretary to Government; Hector Greig as Superintendent of Quarantine; Baron Pasquale Sceberras Trigona, as representative of the Maltese nobility; and Dr Stefano Grillet, First Physician in the Civil Hospitals. On the following day they were sworn to office, and quarantine in Malta entered a new era – one in which the medical arm of the military was no longer to play a role.

207 NLM LIB 847 [unpag.], minute, 6 Apr. 1826; PRO CO 158/50 [unpag.], Hastings to Bathurst, 8 Apr. 1826; Cassar, p. 294.

Chapter Fourteen

Mediterranean Misery, plus Cholera, 1825–1835

Marseilles intransigent

From 1825, in the face of punitive delays to British and Maltese shipping in western Mediterranean ports, the quarantine concerns of London and Valletta coincided. The position for Malta, although increasingly irksome, was roughly the same as it had been for the previous dozen or so years. For Britain, however, this obstacle to trade was an unwelcome new experience, bringing home to Lord Liverpool's administration the unpalatable fact that any violation of the sanctity of quarantine, however much reform might seem justified, risked the displeasure of institutions abroad which for one reason or another were unwilling to agree.

To the Board of Trade fell the melancholy duty of chronicling the steady and unwelcome news of defensive or retaliatory quarantine in the Mediterranean. In late March 1825, when the Bill to amend quarantine barely existed, news arrived from Naples of additional restrictions in Sicily.[1] Clarification followed from Sir Manley Power, Lieutenant-Governor of Malta in the temporary absence of Hastings, that the quarantine against 'England' in Sicily was 21 days for persons and 28 days for goods, because Egyptian cotton was arriving at Liverpool allegedly without depuration.[2] During May and June, when parliamentary proceedings were bogged down in debate, the Board of Trade learnt that Leghorn and Marseilles had joined in the anti-British restrictions, while six ships from Britain (including at least two from Liverpool) were being detained for 15 days on arrival at Genoa.[3] On 22 June the Board learnt that Ancona had joined in the fun, showing equal discrimination against Malta, and other ports in the Adriatic were quick to follow.[4]

There was uncertainty in London about what could be done. The instinct of Government was to lobby at diplomatic level in foreign capitals, but while this might work in Vienna where there was some influence over quarantine at Ragusa, it was less successful in Paris where ministers were reluctant to interfere in the haughty independence of the Marseilles Board of Health.[5] To make matters worse, the Government in London were in a state of extraordinary confusion as to what their quarantine policy really was. The recent Act, following the advice of the Select

1 National Archives [NA] BT 5/33/370.
2 NA CO 158/41 [unpag.], Power to Bathurst, 15 June 1825.
3 NA BT 5/33/426,434–5, 439, 440, 449–50.
4 NA BT 5/33/460. Ragusa quickly followed the lead of Ancona (BT 5/34/37).
5 NA BT 5/34/4, 213.

Committee, had allowed the Privy Council to exempt ships with clean bills from quarantine (subject to a satisfactory preliminary report) wherever they had come from in the Mediterranean. That Act, it will be recalled, received the royal assent on 27 June 1825. Three weeks later – that is, on 19 July – an Order in Council was published explaining how quarantine would be administered.[6] This was normal procedure, but in some respects the new Order was phrased as if the Act which it followed and recited had never existed.

The Attorney-General appears to have anticipated his instructions by virtually reproducing, even to the extent of a typographical error, the Order of 1805.[7] The latter, of course, had been in support of the 1805 Act which the Act of 1825 was declaring out of date. Yet in most respects the two Orders were identical, and when alterations occurred they were mostly limited to the changed background. For instance, references to Chetney Hill were expunged, Milford Haven was added as a foul-bill station, and enumerated goods of the second class were omitted. The term Great Britain was replaced by United Kingdom, so that quarantine stations in Ireland, which had been revealed as prolific and unmanageable in the 1824 enquiry, were now designated along with those in the rest of Britain. As regards England, Wales and Scotland, the quarantine stations were unchanged, with the exception of Cromarty Bay and Carsethorn, which were reintroduced.[8] This seems to have been a careless restatement of the 1805 position, with the drafters unaware that these two stations had been closed in the following year. For Ireland, the number (all clean-bill stations) was reduced to seven, of which three (Ballymastoker Bay near Londonderry, Scattery Bay in the Shannon Estuary, and Killybegs) survived from the original designations of 1711. Stations on the east coast were no nearer Dublin than Carlingford Lough and no nearer Belfast than Larne Lough. Along the south coast, the only station was Baltimore Bay. The west coast of Ireland, between Loop Head and Blacksod Bay, was accorded a station in Clew Bay.

It might be mentioned here, as further evidence of the bad and hurried drafting of the new Order, that further changes to the quarantine stations were made very soon after it was issued. In Scotland, the mistake about Carsethorn and Cromarty Bay was rectified in September 1825 when they were once again closed, leaving only Holy Loch and Inverkeithing Bay in operation.[9] For Ireland, the Privy Council made a radical revision in September 1826.[10] The quarantine stations henceforth were to be Greencastle in Lough Foyle; Garmoyle in Belfast harbour; Warrenpoint; Poolbeg in Dublin harbour; the River Suir at Waterford; Whitegate in Cork harbour; Baltimore;

---

6 NA PC 2/206/281–316. The full text is published in Sir S. Baker, *The Laws relating to Quarantine* (London, 1879), pp. 55–107.

7 The letter to the Attorney-General was dated 30 July, 11 days after the date of the Order (NA PC 2/206/337). The error occurred in Section 33 of the 1805 Order and Section 31 of the 1825 Order: 'And it is hereby further ordered, that if the goods, wares, and merchandises, which shall arrive in vessels with foul bills of health, the articles hereinafter enumerated shall be carried to a floating lazaret ...' The word 'if' is presumably in error for 'in' or 'among'.

8 All the quarantine stations (including Ireland) are detailed in Section 2 of the Order.

9 NA PC 2/206/355, 365; the Order is published in Baker, pp. 108–9.

10 NA PC 2/207/338.

Tarbert in the Shannon estuary; and Black Rock near Galway. This arrangement made better sense for the major ports of Belfast, Dublin, Waterford and Cork.

One of the rare signs in the new Order of original thought was that Milford Haven was now declared the port of arrival for a ship actually infected, rather than the Isles of Scilly.[11] The list of questions to be asked of a ship's master by a Superintendent of Quarantine rose from 26 to 30, but goods enumerated in the new Order were identical with those of the first class in 1805. As regards duration of quarantine, the new Order was also a repeat of the old. Ships with clean bills from the Mediterranean or West Barbary would be quarantined for 15 days, with enumerated goods aired in the floating lazaretto for the same period. Non-enumerated goods would be aired on board the ship itself for one week. In respect of foul-bill ships, probationary airings would continue for 21 days, before airing proper was performed in the lazaretto over 40 days. The ships themselves would be quarantined for 30 days, even if the goods were non-susceptible. Suspected bills would be treated as foul bills, except that the quarantine would be ten days less. The Order (by Section 38) repeated the need for ships from outside the Mediterranean or from the continent of America, carrying enumerated goods, to bring an attested declaration that those goods were not the produce of Turkey or Barbary, which had been a feature of Section 42 in the previous Order. If goods *were* from those places, the ship would be subject to the clean-bill quarantine procedure. Only in one small respect did the Order of 1825 venture to soften the rules of 1805: ships which had performed quarantine in one of the established Mediterranean lazarettos (including, of course, Malta) were now exempt from quarantine in Britain once the Privy Council had given their approval, whereas previously enumerated goods on such ships were subject to a further quarantine of 15 days.

These points appear to demonstrate that despite the findings of the Select Committee of 1824 and the measures passed in the Act of 1825, quarantine restrictions de facto remained virtually unaltered. It was as if Section 22 of the Act, which allowed ships from the Mediterranean, even from Turkey or Barbary, to be excused from quarantine on examination, had never been passed. Was this simply the confusion of a Government insufficiently attentive to a fraught and unyielding dilemma? Or was it a deliberate regression – an acknowledgement that the zeal for reform had gone too far, and that Britain needed to stay in step with Europe until quarantine could be amended under international agreement? The truth embraced both options and created a third: the Order was essentially an authority to act toughly should the dictates of disease or international opinion make it necessary. What the Privy Council chose to do at a more lenient level had nothing to do with the provisions which it was wise to make manifest, demonstrating to Europe that Britain was in earnest. If some of those provisions were kept in reserve, that was seen purely as a matter for the Privy Council. But confusion did exist, especially in Ireland, where the notion was not understood that a clean-bill ship from the Mediterranean should be quarantined for 15 days, simply because she carried enumerated goods. In October the Irish were told not to worry, as the Privy Council, under normal circumstances, were already dispensing with all restrictions against arrivals from Spanish, French,

11 This decision marked the virtual end of quarantine facilities in the Scillies.

Italian and Austrian ports, as well as Malta and Gibraltar.[12] The recommendations of the Select Committee of 1824 had not, after all, been forgotten or abandoned.

On 26 January 1826 George Canning and William Huskisson concluded a Convention of Navigation and Commerce with France.[13] There had been earlier conventions with other nations, but the timing of the Anglo-French agreement gave hope that the stalemate with Marseilles might be resolved by a new diplomatic initiative. In fact, Marseilles had already lifted its quarantine against ships from Britain, but this was no comfort to the merchants of Malta.[14] By article six, the provisions of the Convention were extended to Mediterranean possessions, and therefore to Malta. In essence, these measures ensured that duties based on tonnage, harbour, pilotage and quarantine were reciprocal for ships of either nation in each other's ports. But while that was constructive so far as it went, it did not address the question of unilateral quarantine delays. Hastings, still in London, found little comfort for Maltese shipping. Beginning his return to the island, he wrote to Bathurst on 10 February from his cabin in a warship at Portsmouth.[15] The complaint was the same as ever: quarantine for 'palpably frivolous reasons' in France and Italy, with the blame resting squarely on the Sanitary Committee, as he called it, at Marseilles, which gave the lead to other ports.[16] Hastings did not accept that one municipality could resist the will of the Government in its own country and wanted a more direct intervention at diplomatic level.

Such a forceful stance, however, did not preclude a policy of appeasement by the Board of Health on Malta, of which Hastings was President. On 6 April 1826, the date of their incorporation, the Board took the radical step of making all warships liable to full quarantine at the lazaretto with no deductions for the length of the voyage.[17] This was a significant climb-down by Hastings, who had recently considered such sternness to be impracticable. The Board also imposed a five-day quarantine against arrivals from Spain and Gibraltar, and seven days from the West Indies and North America.[18] They then resolved to circulate all the Health Departments on the Continent with news of the Board's foundation and the measures they had already adopted.[19] Meanwhile, Hastings's wish for a diplomatic initiative had not gone unheeded in London. Canning, as Foreign Secretary, was in correspondence with Augustus Foster, the British Resident in Turin, from whom it was learnt that Sardinia was not averse to putting Malta into free pratique, although it was generally agreed on the Continent, so the Sardinians alleged, that quarantine in Malta had

12 NA PC 7/1/33–6.

13 There is a printed copy in NA CO 158/52.

14 The Board of Trade learnt of the lifting on 8 November 1825 (NA BT 5/34/213).

15 NA CO 158/50 [unpag.], Hastings to Bathurst, 10 Feb. 1826.

16 Ibid.

17 National Library of Malta [NLM] LIB 847 [unpag.], minute, 6 Apr. 1826.

18 Ibid.

19 Ibid. There is a copy of the notification in Italian in the Archives départementales des Bouches-du-Rhône, Marseilles [ADBR], 200 E 464, and another in English in NA CO 158/50.

been less than strict during the recent wars.[20] But the Sardinians conceded that the excellence of the lazaretto on Malta was not widely appreciated.[21] For the information of Bathurst, Canning forwarded other correspondence between Baron de Damas, French Minister of the Interior, and Viscount Granville, British Ambassador in Paris, which revealed that the Board of Health at Marseilles had been invited to modify their stance towards Maltese shipping.[22]

Bathurst was still having difficulty with Hastings's decisions. The Governor had been cynical in his acceptance that a Board of Health was necessary, and now he was being inconsistent in his attitude to the navy. Vice-Admiral Neale, Commander-in-Chief in the Mediterranean, complained immediately to London that Marsamxett Harbour in Valletta was dangerous for large frigates.[23] If he won that argument, Neale was some way towards winning the real prize, which was the setting aside of the Board of Health's decision to remove quarantine concessions for warships. But Hastings engineered a letter from Symonds, as Captain of the Port and Intendant of Marine Police, claiming that quarantine in Grand Harbour set a bad example and posed a significant risk to health.[24] Neale was still defiant, but attention was diverted by a fresh diplomatic move. Canning asked Hastings to send a representative to the various Mediterranean lazarettos, where the problems of Malta could be discussed.[25] The mission fell, predictably, upon Hankey. Granville was requested by Canning to ensure a good reception in Marseilles, and the Resident in Naples was asked to be similarly influential with the Neapolitan Board.[26] While in Paris to meet Granville, Hankey informed Hastings that he intended to reach Marseilles via Genoa.[27]

In the event, Hankey's visits to Naples and Marseilles were unnecessary. It would seem that neither Power nor Hastings was totally correct in assuming that where Marseilles led, others followed. There was pleasing news from Genoa, dated 13 May 1826, that the setting up of a Board of Health on Malta had earned free pratique for the island's shipping in the dominions of the King of Sardinia.[28] Credit for that was due to Foster. Also in May, the Board of Health in Marseilles admitted in a letter to their Maltese counterpart that they were discussing with the Minister of the Interior a reduction of the quarantine against Malta; this would be one of observation only, over seven days, which would be no more than the restriction against Sicily.[29] As the

20 NA CO 158/52 [unpag.], Foreign Office to Hay (for Bathurst), 3 June 1826, with copy letters from Foster.

21 Ibid.

22 NA CO 158/52 [unpag.], Foreign Office to Hay, 8 June 1826, with copy letters from de Damas.

23 NA CO 158/50 [unpag.], Hastings to Bathurst, 12 May 1826, in reply to vice versa, 5 Apr. 1826,

24 Ibid., enclosing copy letter, Symonds to Hastings, 8 May 1826.

25 NA CO 158/52 [unpag.], 3 June 1826, recited correspondence.

26 NA CO 158/52 [unpag.], Canning to Granville, July 1826, and Canning to Naples, 29 July 1826.

27 National Archives of Malta [NAM] CSG 7/1, pp. 238–9.

28 NLM LIB 847 [unpag.], 8 June 1826.

29 NLM LIB 847 [unpag.], 15 June 1826.

two islands were in close contact, they could only be treated equally, and no hopes were extended of a better arrangement.[30]

But in June came a breakthrough, and the crucial move was from Hastings and not Canning. The Maltese Board of Health wrote an excellent reply to Marseilles.[31] They abandoned the traditional use of Italian, and responded in French.[32] While reiterating that quarantine practice on Malta had changed for the better, the Board alluded by implication to the recent international Convention, which inspired hope of an arrangement 'plus analogue à cette franchise et bienveillance mutuelle que nos deux nations ont interêt commun à se témoigner reciproquement' [more in keeping with that mutual frankness and goodwill which our two countries have a common interest to reciprocate]. With similar sentiments emanating from Granville in Paris, the Board at Marseilles were robbed of all pretext to continue discrimination. On 22 July 1826, while Hankey was still fidgeting in Paris, they authorized the acting French consul on Malta, Joseph Borg, to give the good news in Valletta that ships from the island would enjoy free pratique at Marseilles.[33] If Borg was Maltese, as his name would suggest, he nevertheless chose to communicate in French with the island's Board of Health and portrayed every trait of the arrogance which distinguished those whom he represented. He warned the Maltese that only the continuing strict observance of the rules of quarantine, especially with regard to warships and their entry into Marsamxett Harbour, would ensure that free pratique continued.[34] As it was, Borg had noted among other apparent infringements, that the *Revenge*, flagship of Vice-Admiral Neale, was being allowed quarantine in Grand Harbour.

Such impudence, in the days of Maitland, would have been greeted by anger. The emotion, under Hastings, was alarm, leading to a laboured defence by the new Board of Health, backed up by a letter of 6 August from Neale to Greig.[35] In the knowledge that his letter would be copied to Marseilles, Neale was a model of compliance and understanding, stating his 'earnest wish' to conform and promising 'the most prompt attention' to every resolution of the Board of Health. But he would not give in about quarantine for the *Revenge*. The ship, he contested, was as safe from unauthorized contact in its present position as it would be in Marsamxett Harbour, which was too difficult of access in any case for a vessel of that size. Under the Order of St John, all warships had performed quarantine in Grand Harbour and nobody had objected then. His ship was no nearer the shore than it would be if under quarantine in Marseilles, and if her boats left the ship without a sanitary guard, as the consul alleged, that was also the procedure at Marseilles where the ship had 'repeatedly' been quarantined. To

30 Ibid.

31 The Board were so anxious to get the letter right that consideration of the wording was adjourned over three meetings (NLB LIB 847 [unpag.], 22 & 29 June, and 6 July 1826).

32 The text has survived in ADBR 200 E 464.

33 This further correspondence has survived as a file in Marseilles (ADBR 200 E464), but no mention is made of it in the minute book of the Malta Board of Health (NLM LIB 847). This is all the more remarkable as Borg imagined that the Board at Marseilles had also written to Valletta direct.

34 ADBR 200 E 464.

35 Again, the only knowledge of this correspondence is from the copies in ADBR 200 E 464.

mollify any bad reaction to this firm stance, Neale issued a general memorandum to captains and commanders in his fleet enjoining scrupulous obedience to the orders of the Board of Health, pointing out that Malta was now in free pratique with European ports and its continuance depended 'upon an inflexible observance of the rules ...'[36]

The death of Hastings, in November 1826, encouraged Neale to take a stronger line about facilities for the quarantine of warships. On 18 December the Board of Health met solely to consider his request that all warships perform quarantine in Grand Harbour, because of the danger and delay associated with Marsamxett.[37] But the Board would not be bullied. Conceding that Marsamxett Harbour was 'really dangerous' for large vessels, they insisted that it should remain the quarantine station for ships below the size of a frigate. Bigger warships could use Grand Harbour, if they stationed themselves near a new parlatorio opposite the shore at Coradin (or Coradino).[38] Neale would have been unhappy with the divided arrangements because they cut off communication with his sloops, the messenger-ships of the fleet, at a time of tension in the Levant. But it was enough to keep Malta in free pratique with the Continent. Had the Board at Marseilles known that days of grace were being quietly reintroduced, as well as deductions from quarantine for days spent at places like Zante, they might have been less understanding.[39]

Good relations with Europe were put to test by the USS *North Carolina*, which arrived in Grand Harbour from Tunis during January 1827.[40] Commodore Rodgers did not disguise that he had men dead and dying of smallpox. The warship was immediately surrounded by four guard boats and denied access to the parlatorio. Some 15 sufferers and 90 convalescents were removed to the lazaretto, and the ship's senior physician was asked to explain the circumstances and character of the outbreak.[41] Greig proposed immediately that the Board of Health should send a circular to the European Boards, notifying the facts and sending a copy of the physician's report.[42] Smallpox was a new problem which Dr Grillet, the medical member of the Board, felt uncomfortable in tackling alone. Accordingly, an opinion was sought from Dr Gravagna, physician of the Department of Marine Police, as to how long quarantine for the ship should last.[43] Gravagna recommended 15 days to begin once the sick crew and their effects had been landed.[44] The Board were evidently shocked at this leniency and asked a fresh opinion from Dr Calvert,

36 Ibid.

37 NLM LIB 847 [unpag.], 18 Dec. 1826.

38 Ibid. P. Cassar, *Medical History of Malta* (London, 1965) p. 295, dates the parlatorio to 1826.

39 HMS *Seringapatam* from Alexandria was allowed six days' deduction from quarantine for time spent at Zante en route, and given 'the 2 days grace usually granted' (NLM LIB 847 [unpag.], 9 Jan. 1827)

40 NLM LIB 847 [unpag.], 22 Jan. 1827.

41 Reports vary as to the number of casualties: the figures quoted (along with four dead) were those reported to London (NA CO 158/55 [unpag.], copy letter Greig to Hankey, 9 Feb. 1827).

42 NLM LIB 847 [unpag.], 22 Jan. 1827.

43 NLM LIB 847 [unpag.], 7 Feb. 1827.

44 Ibid.

Deputy Inspector of the Military Hospital, who recommended 40 days.[45] Perplexed by the difference, the Board adjourned without a decision. The problem was solved by Commodore Rodgers who decided to re-embark the sick and leave Malta for Mahon without pratique.[46] But the ship had been depurated during its stay, and the Commodore left on good terms with the Board of Health.[47]

Marseilles and the Italian ports seem to have treated smallpox with relative indifference. When, a few months later, the British sloop *Rose* reached Malta with another two cases of the disease on board, the Europeans were unruffled, despite the ship having arrived from Smyrna and Greece.[48] But the Malta Board were always on edge, taking every opportunity to reveal a potential problem and justify its handling. In June 1827 they earnestly asked the Board at Marseilles to believe that an outbreak of 'severe bilious fever' in two small villages was not typhus.[49] This incident, it was claimed, was of no importance, but the French consul had mentioned it and so the Board hastened to reassure the French authorities. They did so in grovelling terms, promising

> no delay shall occur in our acquainting you with any circumstance touching the public health – we can have no wish to conceal anything at any time, and we trust you will continue to place unlimited confidence both in our measures and correspondence, and in the absence of any communication from us, that you will give no attention to any reports that may reach you, as no consideration would induce us to withhold for one moment any information ....[50]

And so on. So urgent was this letter considered that the Board wasted no time in having it translated out of English. In all subsequent letters, they wrote to Marseilles in Italian, still the lingua franca of Mediterranean quarantine.

The Battle of Navarino, fought on 20 October 1827, was indirectly responsible for an interruption to the strained harmony. For Major-General Sir Frederick Ponsonby, who had become Lieutenant-Governor of Malta in February, this was the first quarantine problem to have serious international implications. Navarino was an unplanned battle fought off the Morea between a British, French and Russian fleet on the one hand and a much larger Turco-Egyptian fleet on the other. The former were easily the winners, but they took damage and casualties, and only Malta was in a position to offer repair facilities and medical treatment. There were 20 allied warships involved: 11 British, 7 Russian and 2 French.[51] On 4 November, by which time some of the British fleet had reached Valletta with wounded seamen, Ponsonby

---

45 NLM LIB 847 [unpag.], 8 Feb. 1827.

46 ADBR 200 E 464.

47 Ibid; NA CO 158/55 [unpag.], correspondence following letter, Greig to Hankey, 9 Feb. 1827.

48 Again, there is no mention of this incident in the minute book of the Malta Board of Health. Letters survive in Marseilles (ADBR 200 E 464).

49 ADBR 200 E 464 only.

50 Ibid.

51 The ships were listed in a letter from the Malta Board of Health to Marseilles (ADBR 200 E 464).

was under strong pressure from the navy to waive the normal rules of quarantine, and he convened an immediate meeting of the island's Board of Health. As Navarino was believed free of plague and the Turkish fleet was not known to be infected, the Board agreed on humanitarian grounds, and to facilitate repairs, that ships of the combined fleet would be quarantined for 16 days, to be reckoned from the date 'they ceased to have communication' at Navarino.[52] As it was already 15 days since the battle, most ships would be arriving in immediate pratique.

Losing 'not a moment', the Board transmitted to Marseilles their rationale for suspending normal sanitary regulations for the combined fleet.[53] The letter carried the signatures of Ponsonby and three members of the Board of Health. Despite the small French component of the fleet, the Board were resigned to the expectation that Marseilles would reintroduce quarantine against Maltese shipping. In fact, they virtually suggested that defensive measures should be taken, but felt 'perfectly confident' that once 25 days had passed, representing the period which the fleet ought to have stayed at the lazaretto, free pratique for Malta would be reintroduced as long as 'no accident' had arisen in the meanwhile. On 28 November Ponsonby and his colleagues wrote again, enclosing a list of all the ships in the allied fleet, the date of their arrival in Malta, and when they were granted pratique. The last ship to arrive had been HMS *Glasgow* on 27 November, and of course pratique had been immediate. Ponsonby trusted that as the whole incident was now over, and normal sanitary regulations had been reintroduced, Malta would once again be in free pratique with Marseilles. But the French were unmoved. On 12 December, Ponsonby and Greig sent a copy of the previous letter, allowing themselves to 'entertain no doubt' that the relationship with Marseilles had reverted to normal in the interval. This new letter was entrusted to Vice-Admiral Sir John Gore, who travelled also with important dispatches from Vice-Admiral Sir Edward Codrington, the victor at Navarino, to the British Government. It was explained, with the hint of a threat, that if Gore were detained in quarantine there would be 'the greatest inconvenience'.

But this was all to no avail. Ponsonby was vexed to have to write again, on 7 January 1828, making the point that 40 days had elapsed since the last warship from Navarino was admitted to pratique, yet the Board at Marseilles were still imposing quarantine on ships from Malta. As the weeks passed, it became clear that Navarino was no longer the problem. The French had received intelligence that HMS *Ariadne* might have abridged her quarantine at Malta from Zante and had later put the British Consul General ashore in Algiers, receiving in exchange a tarred box of dispatches allegedly with inadequate precautions.[54] This led to a rapid change of the rules in Malta governing the transfer of boxes between ships and the shore, with reassurance piously sought from Marseilles that the practice now corresponded with theirs.[55] All trace of the pride and self-confidence in quarantine policy which Malta had shown under Maitland and Hastings was now eroded in the overweening desire to appease Marseilles. Ponsonby was in the humiliating position of having to establish

52 NLM LIB 847 [unpag.], 4 Nov. 1827.

53 ADBR 200 E 464, from which all references about Navarino are taken.

54 ADBR 200 E 464.

55 NLM LIB 847 [unpag.], 23 Apr. 1828.

negatives or be denied any likelihood that Malta would regain free pratique. In June 1828 he and Greig wrote to convince the French that Codrington, when he left Malta on his flagship for a cruise towards the Morea, did not call at any port or speak with any vessel during 17 days at sea.[56] Their letter proved an irrelevance when, later in the same month, the Russian frigate *Castor* arrived in Malta from the Morea, having lost four seamen 'after a short illness of a very suspicious nature'.[57] A return to free pratique for Maltese shipping was truly a distant prospect.

Any notion (such as Hastings had harboured) that the French were acting out of commercial or political spite was weakened by the immediate confession from the Board at Marseilles, in July 1828, that their own port was in the grip of smallpox.[58] The hallmark of the French was that they demonstrated the transparent honesty which they expected in return from others. On Malta, the inclination to retaliate was slight, as the commerce of the island would have more to lose than would the French if ships with inbound cargoes were inordinately delayed. But the Board of Health, on 11 August, instituted a ten-day quarantine of observation against arrivals 'from the Meridional Coast of France', which was reduced on 9 October to five days.[59] Other ports, of course, were equally or more severe against the French and for the first time in more than a century the merchants at Marseilles felt the stifling consequences of the interruption to trade which they had been routinely inflicting on others. On 16 October 1828 the Maltese Board of Health had the unusual satisfaction of discussing a letter from the French consul which almost pleaded for the restrictions against the Midi to be lifted.[60] Smallpox, argued the consul, was no longer epidemic in Marseilles but 'reduced to its ordinary course'. Furthermore, the Italian ports had lifted their precautions. But the Maltese board considered that the disease might recover its energy and was still a threat to other countries, and so the quarantine of observation continued.

In the wider history of Boards of Health, this brief defiance by Malta is only of anecdotal importance. Marseilles continued to dictate policy and practice to the satellite Boards, and Malta remained as keen as anywhere to seek the approbation and guidance of the dominant player. But even during the smallpox skirmish, the real attention of both Marseilles and Valletta had been focused on disease in Gibraltar, which was soon to call for a new initiative from London.

56 ADBR 200 E 464. There is no reference in the minute book of the Malta Board of Health.

57 Ibid.; NLM LIB 847 [unpag.], 14 June & 5 July 1828. The full story of the *Castor* incident is recited in G. Milroy, 'Quarantine as it is, and as it ought to be', *Transactions of the National Association for the Promotion of Social Science. 1858* (London, 1859), 64.

58 NLM LIB 847 [unpag.], 11 Aug. 1828.

59 Ibid., and 9 Oct. 1828.

60 NLM LIB 847 [unpag.], 16 Oct. 1812, from which remaining references in this paragraph are taken.

Gibraltar Board of Health

If quarantine in foreign ports was troublesome for merchants on Malta, it was no less irksome for their counterparts on the Rock. General Don, the long-serving Lieutenant-Governor, complained in vain to British consular officials on Sardinia in 1826 that ships from Gibraltar were denied the pratique afforded to vessels from other Mediterranean countries.[61] Enquiries from Turin revealed that the prejudice on Sardinia was 'still stronger than that against Malta', and indeed Malta was part of the problem because it had lately refused pratique to ships from Gibraltar following an outbreak of plague in Morocco.[62] Although quarantine on Malta against arrivals from Gibraltar was not at all unusual, the Sardinian response encouraged Don to retaliate against his colonial colleagues. In June 1827 Hankey complained to the Acting Civil Secretary on the Rock that the quarantine of observation against ships with clean bills from Malta was unacceptable.[63] If Don were to disagree, Hankey wanted the matter referred to the Secretary of State.[64]

The dispute was cut short by the reappearance in Gibraltar, after a 14-year absence, of yellow fever. Malta first became alarmed when Greig read the bill of health of a Russian warship, issued at Gibraltar on 7 September 1828, which referred to several recent 'cases of fever of a highly suspicious Type'.[65] The Maltese Board of Health suspended pratique from Gibraltar immediately and began agonizing once more whether the crowded Marsamxett Harbour was suitable for the quarantine of such a virulent disease. Dr Gravagna attended and was asked to 'convoke a meeting of several classical Physicians' to discuss and advise whether, if an infected ship were in Marsamxett Harbour, there would be 'any danger of the infection reaching Valletta or the shore by means of the air'.[66] In the opinion of Gravagna and eight of his colleagues, such a danger was real.[67] The Board thereupon, on 2 October, allowed ships from Gibraltar with no sickness aboard to enter the quarantine harbour and moor at the usual places allocated for ships under suspicion; but if there were fever aboard, ships had to make for St Paul's Bay, 'there to be subject to the most vigorous Sanitary operations as shall be directed by the Quarantine Department'.[68] On 9 October, when news reached Malta that fever was ravaging the garrison at Gibraltar, the Board ordered a 'rigorous quarantine' of 25 days for the ships in Marsamxett Harbour, and an indefinite quarantine 'according to circumstance' for those in St Paul's Bay.[69]

In London, the alarm was no less acute. A Government Commission was set up with Pym as president, to enquire whether the sickness at Gibraltar could be

61 NA CO 158/52 [unpag.], copy letter Foster to Canning, 11 May 1826.

62 Ibid.

63 NAM CSG 7/1, p. 249.

64 Ibid.

65 NLM LIB 847 [unpag.], 22 Sept. 1828; ADBR 200 E 464.

66 NLM LIB 847 [unpag.], 25 Sept. 1828.

67 NLM LIB 847 [unpag.], 2 Oct. 1828.

68 Ibid.

69 NLM LIB 847 [unpag.], 9 Oct. 1828.

attributed to any failings in quarantine.[70] The outcome of the enquiry, that the disease was imported by a Swedish vessel, was later censured as a contrived attempt to support the doctrine of quarantine and shelter the Gibraltar Government from 'its culpable neglect of proper sanitary measures within the fortress'.[71] There was still no overt acceptance by Pym, the Privy Council or the Board of Trade that quarantine was ineffectual in arresting the spread of yellow fever, despite the fact that the rationale for its use was based on the prevention of contact alone. Doctors on Malta had already concluded that quarantine as traditionally practised was no defence against a disease which, in their opinion, could be transmitted through the air. But the mood in London, where the Board of Trade were still smarting from the rush to judgement in Europe, was that every step should be taken which conformed with the international perception that quarantine worked, and that it should be in the hands of a body whose sole responsibility was the public health. On these grounds, albeit with reluctance, Bathurst had agreed to the Board of Health on Malta; on the same grounds, but with some precipitation, a Board of Health was now ordained for Gibraltar. The administration on Malta were only too pleased to offer guidance with the framework, but the regulations which transpired for Gibraltar show little evidence that Malta was the paradigm.[72]

Whereas the constitution and duties of the Maltese Board had been arranged on the island, with the agreement of the Secretary of State, the establishment of the Gibraltar Board was a matter for the Privy Council in London. The Board was created by an Order in Council of 13 July 1830 which, for the first time, established exact quarantine regulations for a Crown colony.[73] The drafting, however, had been done in the Colonial Office, who had sought advice from the Board of Trade, who had relied heavily on the guidance of Pym.[74] Taking effect from 1 November 1830, the Order set up a permanent Board of Health consisting of the Governor, Civil Secretary, Captain of the Port and Police Magistrate, or any three of them, of whom the Governor had to be one.[75] The Board were instructed to impose quarantine regulations against places which they deemed appropriate, and to make local Orders by Proclamation in the *Gibraltar Chronicle*. The text had normally to be approved beforehand by the King via Sir George Murray, the new Secretary of State for War and the Colonies, but the Board could make emergency Orders which had the force of law. There was clearly no expectation that such Orders would be immediate or frequent, as the Order in Council was explicit in matters of detail. Indeed, it smacked very much of a cross between an Act and an Order, presuming to set penalties as well as regulate practice. These penalties were very weak by Mediterranean standards, most set at £100 for such offences as going ashore without authority, flying the wrong flag, refusing to submit ship's papers, or even concealing goods. The lowest

70 cf. G. Milroy in *British Parliamentary Papers* [*BPP*], vol. 58 (1861), pp. 269–71.

71 *Edinburgh Review*, vol. 98 (1853), p. 207.

72 NAM CSG 7/1, pp. 298–9, for offer of assistance from Malta.

73 NA PC 2/211A/245–70.

74 NA BT 5/37465–6. This was in November 1828.

75 All details of the Board are taken from NA PC 2/211A/245–70.

penalty was £50 for boarding or leaving a ship not yet in pratique, and the maximum £500 for landing or receiving articles in quarantine.

As there was no post in Gibraltar of Superintendent of Quarantine (and it was a sign of the wish to keep the Rock under central control that no such post was now introduced), the administration of the rules was very much a collective responsibility. When a vessel arrived in the harbour it was for the Captain of the Port to ask the preliminary questions. Once the ship was in quarantine, the Inspector of Health made periodic visits and conducted the more searching interrogation. The exact framing of questions was one of the few points in which the Board had discretion. But the Inspector had no seat on the Board, and the bill of health and ship's papers were scrutinized by the Captain of the Port, who could also issue a bill at the ship's departure. The Order was meticulous as to fees, abolishing previous charges for pratique which had been authorized in London in 1809, but maintaining the principle, established in 1816, that part of the shipping dues were to be allocated for the maintenance of the civil hospital. All duties were to be collected by the Captain of the Port, to be paid over weekly to the colony's Collector of Revenues.

The Order established a tariff of fixed charges in both sterling and 'hard' dollars. The highest tariff was £2, 3s, 4d for a square-rigged ship of three masts. This charge, and those for other types of vessel, constituted harbour dues, and a further fixed duty of 8s, 8d was to be levied on any ship liable to quarantine, irrespective of her size or the length of her detention. Other fixed costs included another 8s, 8d for every day's attendance by a health guard, and 4s, 4d for a bill of health. It was evident from these provisions that Gibraltar had no lazaretto in any meaningful sense, that there was no insistence on airing, and that quarantine was the by-product of a brief essentially concerned with the profitable running of a commercial harbour. If Pym can be credited with good work in the administration of quarantine on Malta, his contribution at Gibraltar lacked clarity and innovation. The decisions of the Board were no less suspect. On 4 January 1831 a Proclamation of the Gibraltar Government announced the different periods of quarantine established by the Board for vessels arriving from infected or suspected places. When the details reached Malta, the island's Board of Health found the restrictions against Barbary so far at variance with orthodox practice that they increased the quarantine against Gibraltar to 12 days.[76]

Domestic reforms

Faced with quarantine problems within Britain, the Board of Trade had no interest in procedures on Malta and were involved with Gibraltar only when strictly necessary. The main difficulty at home was steering a route between the recent progressive Act and the more recent reactionary Order. There were still complaints that British ships were unfairly quarantined in Mediterranean ports, grumbles continued about costs and facilities in England and Ireland, and the delays at Milford Haven were getting worse by the month.

76 NLM LIB 847 [unpag.], 31 Jan. 1831.

The priority for the Board of Trade was to solicit three ships of the line from the Navy Board to accommodate 28,000 bales of cotton wool expected at Milford from Alexandria on ships with foul bills.[77] In September 1825 only two old warships, the *Dreadnought* and the *Saturn* had been promised, and when the Admiralty were asked for a sloop to replace the revenue cutter at Milford and act as a guard ship, it had still not materialized nine months later.[78] By then (June 1826) the Board of Trade felt in need of a frigate, and even the larger warships requisitioned for airing were scarcely adequate. The orlop and lower decks were 'nearly useless' without scuttles or air vents, while the upper decks by contrast were too exposed in stormy weather, even when covered by awnings.[79] The royal dockyard at Pembroke was asked to provide the ships with a low roof.[80] With such inadequate facilities, cargoes were detained far longer than necessary, often more than two months, and ships were damaged in winter gales.[81] On 31 December 1825, in a tacit admission that conditions at Milford were unacceptable, the Board of Trade allowed the *Hugh Wallace* from Alexandria to sail on to Bromborough Pool to air her cotton.[82] Similar concessions were not slow to follow.

Attempts to improve facilities for airing were matched by reform of managerial and staffing procedures. From January 1826 the Superintendents of Quarantine at Stangate Creek and Milford Haven were no longer to victual either persons on quarantined ships, who were to be supplied by agents of their choosing, or indeed the personnel of the station, who were to be supplied by contract.[83] The Board of Trade envisaged an establishment of 150 at Milford as against 100 at Stangate Creek, compelling evidence that the Levant trade had now switched from London to Liverpool.[84] Provisions for quarantine staff were to equal those for naval sailors in harbour, in so far as salted meat, either beef or pork, was to be available twice a week.[85] But the navy was not the model in other ways. Table money was now abolished in the quarantine service, and pursers were appointed to manage the buying and distribution of supplies.[86] Beer superseded rum, and tea and sugar replaced flour and suet.[87] The two tiers of health guardian (superior and inferior) were abolished, and the duties reallocated to masters and mates on the floating lazarettos, and to tidewaiters stationed on importing ships.[88] The most significant changes, however, affected the senior ranks. The Admiralty were asked for the names of naval officers who might wish to serve the quarantine service at both Milford and Stangate

77 NA PC 7/1/1.

78 NA PC 7/1/23–6, 128–9.

79 NA PC 7/1/24–6.

80 Ibid.

81 NA PC 7/1/63.

82 NA PC 7/1/74. On the petition of W.A. Brown of Liverpool.

83 NA PC 7/1/58–62.

84 Ibid.

85 Ibid.

86 NA PC 7/1/69–71.

87 Ibid.

88 NA PC 7/1/78–9.

Creek.[89] In April 1826 Captain John Marshall, RN, was appointed Superintendent of Quarantine at Milford at £350 a year; two lieutenants were made his assistants at ten shillings a day; another three lieutenants were appointed masters of the lazarettos actually in use, the *Akbar*, *Santa Margaretta* and *Hannibal*, at 5s, 6d per day.[90]

Before making similar appointments at Stangate Creek, the Board of Trade confirmed Pym as full-time Superintendent General of Quarantine, backdated to 5 January 1826, with a particular brief to oversee the current reforms.[91] He was to receive an annual allowance of £600, instead of the two guineas a day agreed in 1813 when his services were only given when requested.[92] Because he was still allowed travelling expenses, his annual remuneration, already augmented by his pension from Gibraltar, was considerably higher. For instance, Pym claimed more than £130 for one round trip embracing Stangate Creek, Liverpool, Plymouth and Falmouth, and he was continually on the move.[93] He was also conscientious, and it can be assumed that when the Board of Trade reached any decision about quarantine, which they did every few days at this period, the initiative or guidance had come from Pym. He was keen to cement good relations with the naval officers, whose ranks had traditionally been wary of, and even hostile to, the quarantine service. In November 1826 Marshall at Milford was allowed a manservant, while his assistants and the purser were each allocated a boy.[94] The two mates on the guard ship could share a boy servant between them, but the mates on the lazarettos could have one each. The servants themselves fared rather badly, seeing their pay drop from 9d to 6d per day because at that rate, as the Board of Trade noted, 'any Number of Boys may be procured there'.[95]

The policy of employing naval officers led to the removal of Charles Sanders from his long-held post of Superintendent of Quarantine at Stangate Creek. The Admiralty made Captain Henry Bourchier, RN, available, and in December 1826 he was appointed a Superintendent of Quarantine for five years at the annual salary of £350, although the Privy Council were as yet undecided where he should serve.[96] At the same time, the Board of Trade limited all naval appointments in the quarantine service to that duration, having originally thought a seven-year term would be appropriate.[97] Bourchier's salary contrasted with the £100 a year, plus an allowance of £1 for each ship in quarantine, which had been paid to Sanders.[98] A few days later,

89 NA PC 7/1/83–4.

90 NA PC 7/1/105–7. Marshall replaced Dr McMillan, who was then Acting Superintendent.

91 NA PC 7/1/92–4.

92 Ibid.

93 NA PC 7/1/277. For a detailed breakdown of Pym's expenses on a 3-day visit to Stangate Creek in December 1837, see PC 7/5/194: posting allowance to and from Chatham, 64 miles at 2s per mile = £6, 4s; three days' travelling allowance at one guinea a day = £3, 3s; total £9, 11s. Other instances might be cited.

94 NA PC 7/1/197–8.

95 Ibid.

96 NA PC 7/1/245.

97 NA PC 7/1/242–3.

98 NA PC 7/1/272.

Bourchier was sent to Milford from where Marshall was transferred to Stangate Creek.[99] Meanwhile, Lieutenant Archibald Macdonald, First Assistant Superintendent at Milford, had been appointed Superintendent of Quarantine at Bromborough Pool, at a rate of 12 shillings a day plus rations.[100] He was not replaced.[101] When Marshall transferred to Stangate Creek, he found that his deputy, Lieutenant Dixon, was on a salary of £300 a year, plus rations, which seems a generous enhancement of the £85 a year, plus 15 shillings a ship, paid under the 'Old Establishment'.[102]

None of these changes helped with the underlying problem, which was the lack of capacity at Milford Haven and the determined wish on Merseyside that ships should sail there direct, regardless of their bill of health. It does no credit to Pym that Government policy on this issue was ludicrously weak and volatile. The decision to allow some ships to sail on to Liverpool to air their cargoes meant that many masters proceeded to Bromborough Pool in any case, claiming ignorance that Milford was still the foul-bill station.[103] In July 1826 the Board of Trade were worried that congestion was now occurring at the Pool and that lighters being used to supplement the floating lazarettos were unequal to the task.[104] The *Santa Margaretta*, therefore, was once again directed to Liverpool to act as a third lazaretto.[105] Ships queuing in the Mersey were advised to return to Milford, but if they wished to wait their turn at Bromborough Pool, the lighters could only be used at merchant's or shipowner's expense.[106] On 7 September 1826 the Board of Trade were again adamant that all ships from Alexandria with cotton, regardless of their bill of health, had to air their cargoes at Milford.[107] But they were also insisting on the full 40 days of quarantine, and with the *Santa Margaretta* now at Bromborough Pool it was quickly realized that capacity could not match demand. On 18 September, therefore, the brig *Pyrenees* was allowed to proceed to Liverpool, and further concessions were unavoidable.[108] Gradually a compromise formula evolved: all cotton ships from Alexandria had to make for Milford in the first instance; if the facilities were congested, and their bills were clean, they could proceed to Bromborough Pool and air their cargoes in the floating lazarettos; if those were full, lighters could be hired for airing at the ship's expense. Later, airing on the lighters became a matter for the crew, but up to 200 tons of cotton could still be aired on or in the ship itself.[109]

99 NA PC 7/1/249, 252, 254–5.

100 NA PC 7/1/235.

101 From 5 January 1827 the appointments of Assistant Superintendent at Milford Haven and master of the *Santa Margaretta* lazaretto were to remain vacant (NA PC 7/1/236–41).

102 NA PC 7/1/252–3, 272, 274.

103 NA PC 7/1/164.

104 NA PC 7/1/153–5.

105 NA PC 7/1/150–51.

106 NA PC 7/1/153–5.

107 NA PC 7/1/179.

108 NA PC 7/1/184.

109 Thus, NA PC 7/1/170–71. However, elsewhere (PC 7/1/153–5) the amount was given as 200 bales.

Pym was directed to Bromborough Pool to ensure that airing met the necessary standards.[110] He also made changes to the establishment which brought it more in line with Milford. The appointment of Lieutenant Macdonald as Superintendent of Quarantine has already been noticed. He was now allowed the services of a boy at 6d a day.[111] Another boy was allocated to the master of the *Santa Margaretta*, who was made Assistant Superintendent at 8s a day, while his job on the lazaretto was kept vacant. Masters of the other lazarettos, the *Experiment* and the *Perlin*, who had been paid £150 a year under the old system, were now to have 5s, 6d a day. Mates, who been paid £100, now received 4s a day, mariners 2s, and boys 6d plus the usual rations. All table money, fees and other allowances ceased, and while the victualling arrangements were to follow those recently introduced at Milford and Stangate Creek, no post of purser was created and the responsibility for contracts was given to Macdonald.

With so much focus on Liverpool and Milford, Pym had little opportunity to make changes elsewhere. Even the reforms at Stangate Creek seemed a secondary consideration, and there was a reluctance to spend money on its declining facilities. Two floating lazarettos there, the *Valiant* and *Brunswick*, were condemned, and replaced by only one, the *Northumberland*.[112] Elsewhere in England, quarantine stations remained much as they were. The exception was Plymouth, where angry merchants had finally got the better of the Board of Trade. As late as the Order in Council of 1825, ships bound for Plymouth and liable to quarantine were supposed to proceed to St Just's Pool at Falmouth, but that obligation was ignored by masters and shipowners, as it always had been by the navy. In May 1827 the Cattewater at Plymouth was officially declared a quarantine harbour.[113] As the stated reason was the exposed position of the existing station, already at Plymouth, it may be assumed that the Order in Council had been repeating traditional texts and was quite of touch with reality.

Medical Superintendents

Once Malta had been allowed its Board of Health, and Marseilles had reinstated Britain in free pratique, there was a feeling in London that the worst might be over. If 1825 had been a bad year, 1827 looked much better. There had been, after all, time to reorganize the three main quarantine stations, and if the Milford versus Liverpool dilemma was still troublesome, at least a modus vivendi was being established with importers. More significantly, the decades were rolling by and while the Levant and Barbary were beset as always by plague, and Gibraltar and southern Iberia were yet again ravaged by yellow fever, Britain had still escaped any significant epidemic of imported disease. If credit for that escape belonged to quarantine, it would obviously be sanitary madness, as well as commercial suicide internationally, to dismantle the machinery too far. But the Privy Council, acting through the Board of Trade, were

110 NA PC 7/1/201.

111 NA PC 7/1/236–41, from which remaining references in this paragraph are taken.

112 NA PC 7/1/159–60.

113 NA PC 7/1/292–3.

not unreceptive to mercantile pleas for even greater concessions affecting time and expense, and anxious to show the Treasury that establishment costs could be further curtailed. This was not so much complacency as a comfortable, insular feeling that seaborne contagion was under control. But that feeling was not to last.

The Mayor of Liverpool was hopeful that Bromborough Pool could be created a foul-bill station, and it seemed for a while that the Board of Trade agreed: the *Newcastle* and *Akbar* floating lazarettos were transferred there from Milford in July 1827.[114] In fact, the Board began to run down the resources at Milford to a surprising extent. The *Otter* hospital ship and *Nepean* guard ship were declared superfluous, as was the *Lizard* hospital ship at Stangate Creek, and rates of pay were reduced.[115] One month later the Board of Trade came to the startling conclusion that the services of five masters and five mates could be dispensed with altogether at Milford, and another master and mate could be lost at Stangate Creek.[116] Then came the concession that Milford was no longer the compulsory destination for ships with clean bills carrying Egyptian cotton.[117] Although these reductions and relaxations were ostensibly justified by the 'present circumstances' of trade with the Levant, the position was more complex and reflected to some extent a radical new initiative in how the need for quarantine was assessed.

This initiative was sparked by dissatisfaction among merchants with Section 38 of the Order in Council of 19 July 1825. This Section, it will be recalled, required attested declarations that enumerated goods imported from places outside the Straits of Gibraltar were not the product of Turkey or Barbary. Merchants had laboured under a similar constraint for 25 years and the inconveniences were growing as trade with the Baltic was once again on the increase in ports of eastern Britain. The Privy Council forestalled further protest by reducing the number of articles for which declarations were necessary, and extending to European ports outside the Straits the indulgences already granted to Russia and Prussia.[118] By June 1827 only cotton wool, silk, carpets, ostrich feathers, sponges, cotton yarn and mohair yarn required a declaration that they were the produce of the country whence shipped, or not from Turkey or Barbary.[119] Cotton or linen wrappings needed a certificate that they had been washed or otherwise purified.[120] Sensing a belief among ministers that quarantine was still too strict, the commercial lobby sent 'various Petitions' to the Board of Trade that the apparatus might be further dismantled.[121] The result was a collusion between the Board of Trade and the Committee of British Ship Owners which led to an Order in Council, dated 27 August 1827, establishing the post of Medical Superintendent at the principal quarantine stations in Great Britain.[122]

114 NA BT 5/36/218; PC 7/1/326–7.

115 NA PC 7/1/324–5, 328–9.

116 NA PC 7/1/352–4.

117 NA PC 7/1/379. This was promulgated by the Foreign Office, who informed consuls that clean bills need not be endorsed with that instruction.

118 NA PC 7/1/298–9.

119 Ibid. However, the list in PC 7/1/357–65 is rather longer.

120 Ibid.

121 NA PC 7/1/357.

122 NA PC 7/1/357–65; *BPP* (1831), vol. 17, pp. 349–51 (with specimen certificates).

This was a major innovation. Medical Superintendents could give instant release from quarantine to three categories of ships: those with clean bills and non-enumerated goods from ports in the Mediterranean controlled by Britain, France, Spain, Italy, Austria, Sardinia and Greece; ships from those ports with clean bills and enumerated goods from the reduced list, as long as masters carried the necessary declaration that the items were not the produce of Turkey or Barbary; and ships with clean bills from any of the main lazarettos (Malta, Leghorn, Genoa, Ancona, Venice, Trieste, Messina and Marseilles) carrying enumerated goods in free pratique.[123] To pay for these new appointments, the Ship Owners' Society, under the chairmanship of George Lyall, volunteered to pay an additional fee of one guinea for each ship released by a Medical Superintendent.[124] The importance of this scheme was that it did away with the time-consuming referral to the Privy Council in London of ships whose release could be judged as routine. It did not, of course, preclude the referral to the Council of ships for which quarantine was necessary, nor did it mean that other fees associated with the granting of free pratique were dispensed with, even though they were nominal in respect of ships released by Medical Superintendents. To the new fee of one guinea, to be credited to the Customs Service, there had to be added Privy Council fees of £3, 12s, 6d and Treasury fees of one guinea, amounting in total to a standard and inescapable cost of £5, 14s, 6d for every ship excused or released from quarantine.[125] In 1825, following pressure from Liverpool merchants, the Privy Council conceded that the fees could be paid locally.[126]

No time was lost in making the appointments. Before the end of August, Dr W.W. Fraser, Inspector of Hospitals with 15 years' experience at Gibraltar, was made Medical Superintendent at Bromborough Pool on a salary of 10s a day plus rations; Robert Brown, surgeon, associated with quarantine in the Scilly Islands, was given a similar position at Stangate Creek on the same terms; and John Taylor, surgeon, who had served both in Egypt and the Scillies, was appointed to Deal at 7s, 6d a day.[127] The choice of Deal was surprising, and in December 1827 the Board of Trade clarified that the port was not a regular quarantine station, and that Taylor could only act in respect of ships forced to anchor in The Downs by reason of distress or contrary winds.[128] In September 1827 Medical Superintendents were appointed at Portsmouth (W.H. Banks), Plymouth (H.S. Harris) and Falmouth (Dr Fox).[129] They were all paid £50 a year in place of the one guinea per ship allowed under

123 NA PC 7/1/357–65. Greece was entered in pencil, as if still subject to deliberation.

124 Ibid.

125 *Journal of the House of Commons* [*JHC*], vol. 86 (1), p. 512.

126 NA PC 7/1/2. This letter to the Liverpool merchants was published in *BPP*, vol. 17 (1831), p. 349.

127 NA PC 7/1/366–7. There was a local initiative to move Fraser to Liverpool itself. The Privy Council were not averse but insisted that the Superintendent of Quarantine and his Assistant would have to move there as well, as it was not the Medical Superintendent's job to interrogate masters. When the Liverpool Mediterranean Association did not agree that the costs of these removals should be visited on shipping, the idea was abandoned.

128 NA PC 7/1/425–7.

129 NA PC 7/1/380–85.

subsisting arrangements.[130] At Bristol, Hull, Leith and Greenock, the Superintendent of Quarantine could call upon a local doctor, at the customary fee, to act as Medical Superintendent as necessary.[131] Such were the savings expected from the rapid release of ships that the Board of Trade began a new round of cuts. At The Motherbank, the *Prometheus* floating lazaretto, and at Falmouth 'the Old Hulk', were discontinued.[132] These economies were backed by reductions in established staff at both ports, and by a directive to the Superintendent of Quarantine at The Motherbank that he was to communicate in future with Customs and Post Office officials at nearby Ryde, rather than Portsmouth.[133] In December 1827 came yet another significant concession to merchants and shipowners: if the Medical Superintendent were somehow unavailable at Stangate Creek or Milford or Bromborough Pool, the Superintendent of Quarantine could release a ship to prevent her detention by 'even one tide'.[134]

It will be noticed that no new appointment had been made at Milford. This was because the post already existed there, in so far as Dr Quinton McMillan had been appointed Medical Superintendent of Quarantine in 1813 at a salary of one guinea a day.[135] McMillan, who also received half-pay from his army commission as Brevet Deputy Inspector of Hospitals, had really been no more than a Superintendent of Quarantine (sometimes qualified as Acting) who happened also to be a doctor.[136] He had had no powers to release ships without referral to the Privy Council. When Captain Marshall was appointed in his stead, McMillan was awarded three months' pay at a rate pro rata with Marshall's salary.[137] That was apparently consolation for losing his seniority at Milford after so many years, but he retained the abridged title of Medical Superintendent, albeit on a daily payment reduced from one guinea to 7s, 6d on 1 September 1827.[138]

The Medical Superintendent scheme was such an instant success that even greater economies were quickly introduced. In March 1828 the establishment at Milford was severely curtailed by the loss of one Assistant Superintendent, two masters, two mates, fourteen mariners and two boys, and further cuts were made at Stangate Creek.[139] The international reaction was calmer than the Privy Council or Board of Trade might have feared. Part of the rationale for the scheme was to persuade Mediterranean countries to drop quarantine against British ships, as Britain was now prepared, under many circumstances, to give the vessels of those same countries immediate pratique. One problem port was Trieste, where discrimination had led to port and quarantine duties which the consul referred to 'as a very onerous Tax

---

130 Ibid.

131 Ibid. The mention of Leith continued the ambivalent status of that port in relation to Inverkeithing. In March 1828 the Medical Superintendent scheme was extended to Inverkeithing Bay when ships happened to go there. They were not obliged to do so.

132 NA PC 7/1/380–85.

133 Ibid.

134 NA PC 7/1/420–21.

135 NA PC 7/1/451.

136 Ibid.; PC 7/1/110.

137 NA PC 7/1/126–7.

138 NA PC 7/1/366–7.

139 NA PC 7/1/453–4; 463–4.

on British Shipping'.[140] If the Medical Superintendent scheme helped matters there, it did exactly the opposite at Naples, where the Board of Health prescribed seven days' quarantine against British ships; among the reasons given was the contorted logic that, by allowing Neapolitan ships immediate pratique, Britain was exposing herself to a risk of infection from Naples which might then be reintroduced there when the ship returned.[141] But, more generally, the British initiative seems to have escaped defensive retaliation. It certainly gained support in Tunis, where quarantine regulations in some form had recently been introduced, from which ships direct from Britain were exempt.[142]

Only on 24 February 1830, by Treasury Order, was the Medical Superintendent scheme extended to Ireland.[143] It was limited at first to Belfast, Cork and Dublin, and the fee was doubled to two guineas.[144] The scheme was extended to Londonderry in 1834 and to Waterford in 1840, but a request from Newry was turned down.[145]

Cholera: the first pandemic

The advance of cholera morbus towards Britain followed much the same route across Russia towards the Baltic as had been taken 120 years earlier by the plague. In that emergency, perhaps more from luck than quarantine, the plague had stopped short at the North Sea; in the cholera crisis, both luck and quarantine were no match for the inexorable progress of one of the world's most feared diseases. Cholera killed with great rapidity. 'In addition', writes McNeill, 'the symptoms were peculiarly horrible: radical dehydration meant that a victim shrank into a wizened caricature of his former self within hours, while ruptured capillaries discolored the skin, turning it black and blue. The effect was to make mortality uniquely visible ...'[146] Not since the Great Plague had Britain faced such a hideous prospect, but comprehension and terror were slow to dawn.

The first cholera pandemic began in Lower Bengal in 1817.[147] Progress westward was at first very slow, so that not until 1829 were any cases reported in European Russia. But the disease found another route, by which it had reached Astrakhan at the

---

140 NA BT 5/36/45.

141 NA BT 5/37/5. Another ostensible worry in Naples was that ships might be boarded on the voyage back by Barbary corsairs.

142 NA BT 5/36/271. Pym explained that such quarantine was contrary to Mohammedan religion and was only introduced in the North African regencies at the wish of European consuls. He thought fee income was the incentive, and fees continued even when quarantine did not apply (ibid.).

143 *BPP*, vol. 17 (1831), p. 353.

144 Ibid.

145 NA PC 7/1/4/352–3; PC 6/10 [unpag.], 31 Dec. 1835; PC 7/5/1, 316; PC 6/10 [unpag.], 17 Aug. 1839; PC 7/5/300–301, where it is stated Newry received only four or five arrivals annually from the Mediterranean.

146 W.H. McNeill, *Plagues and People* (Oxford, 1977), p. 261.

147 C. Maclean, *Evils of Quarantine Laws, and Non-Existence of Pestilential Contagion* ... (London, 1824), p. 7; C. Creighton, *A History of Epidemics in Britain* (2 vols, Cambridge, 1894), vol. 2, p. 793.

mouth of the Volga in 1823. After some years of marking time, cholera erupted along the Volga valley in 1830, joining forces with the outbreak in the south to ravage the Russian plains. While the disease spread slowly in western Asia, the reaction in Britain was calm. Some clinical papers were published by doctors with experience of cholera in India, but the background was exotic, the threat seemed remote and the public remained unconcerned.[148] During 1830, however, the Privy Council began to feel nervous. It was clear from diplomatic intelligence that the disease was not only in Europe but advancing inexorably from town to town, with no natural barrier to its progress until it should reach the Baltic Sea. If the anti-plague measures of Queen Anne were beyond the scope of human memory, the message from history was nonetheless clear: quarantine had been used then, it had apparently worked, and it would be appropriate now to try it again.

On 11 November 1830, when cholera had reached Moscow, the Privy Council introduced quarantine for ships arriving in Britain from Russian ports.[149] Little was made of the reason, yet this was no orthodox Order as the Council wished to see the answers of masters to the usual interrogatories. Among the shipowners of Hull, the news of the Order went down badly. For their forebears, quarantine against the Baltic had been an expensive and wearisome rigmarole, and with no sense that cholera would succeed where plague had failed, the goodwill was not there to accept a second instalment. Another inherited wisdom was that petitions to the Privy Council were a waste of time, so the merchants addressed their grievances direct to Parliament. On 20 April 1831 the Commons listened to allegations of 'very serious loss' in paying and maintaining crews unexpectedly in quarantine during winter gales which damaged the ships on which they were stranded.[150] Then came a less predictable plea, that the House give relief from the standard fees of £5, 14s, 6d (of which the components have been stated above) for releasing any ship from quarantine.[151] Members were taken unawares by this petition, which excited no reaction.[152]

There followed collusion among east-coast ports, no doubt engineered by the Ship Owners' Society, to harass Parliament into treating the issues more seriously. This resentment was fostered by the refusal of the Privy Council to abandon their reliance on quarantine, but the Council had no other safeguard. Early in 1831 cholera reached Poland, and by May it had arrived at Riga and Danzig and other ports in the Baltic which traded regularly with eastern Britain. Pym (now knighted) was deeply concerned and urged the Privy Council to consider a new Order, hurriedly approved on 23 May, which stressed the 'alarming progress' of cholera morbus.[153] With King William IV absent from the meeting, the Order stressed the powers which had been

148 Creighton, vol. 2, p. 793, lists titles on cholera 'from the English press' between 1821 and 1830.

149 *JHC*, vol. 86 (1), p. 797.

150 *JHC*, vol. 86 (1), p. 512.

151 Ibid.

152 More exactly, it was ordered that the petition lie upon the table and be printed.

153 NA PC 2/212/187–90.

vested in the Lords of the Privy Council by the Quarantine Act of 1825.[154] The Order was brief and blunt, instructing ships arriving from any port in Russia with clean bills to proceed to the most convenient anchorage from among the following: Cromarty Firth; the Firth of Tay, near Dundee; the Firth of Forth between North Queensferry and Lord Elgin's lime kilns; Whitebooth Roads between Hull and Grimsby; Stangate Creek; The Motherbank at Portsmouth; Plymouth; Falmouth; Milford Haven; Bromborough Pool; and Holy Loch. Once at the quarantine station, a ship would be subject to the Order in Council of 19 July 1825. It will be apparent from the above list that two extra quarantine harbours had been created in Scotland. Furthermore, the anchorage in the Firth of Forth, more succinctly known as St Margaret's Hope, was now preferred to Inverkeithing Bay. The omission from the list of Bristol was presumably an oversight.

In June 1831 preparations for cholera from northern Europe reached a frantic level. As the disease had entered St Petersburg, two medical commissioners, William Russell and David Barry, were dispatched to Russia to report back on the symptoms and effects.[155] Traditional concerns for plague and yellow fever, centred on shipping from the Mediterranean, were all but abandoned. For any ship with a foul bill, from a port known to be cholera-infected, only three of the quarantine stations were now available: Cromarty Firth (which became interpreted as Cromarty Bay), Stangate Creek and Milford Haven.[156] At an administrative level, the Government of Earl Grey were persuaded that a Board of Health, such as had been instituted in 1805 in the panicky days of Gibraltar sickness, should be reintroduced. On 18 June the Privy Council asked the College of Physicians to recommend names.[157]

These nervous and rushed instructions were totally at odds with the continuing indifference to danger in the east-coast ports. The only concern there was the detention of vessels, released only after fees which were seen as unjustified in the context of the recent decision that quarantine duties should be borne by the state. In August 1831 the shipowners of Dundee petitioned Parliament for relief against detention and fees, adding weight to the earlier allegations from Hull.[158] Within two weeks, their colleagues in London petitioned specifically against the fees for release.[159] As the City was now involved, Parliament began to take notice and asked for a breakdown of how the fees of £5, 14s, 6d were reached.[160] In fact, the petition from Hull had explained that already. It was then the turn of the shipowners of Montrose to pitch into battle, making exactly the same complaints, with the added information that extra pay and provisions were costing between £20 and £30 per

154 Ibid., from which remaining references in this paragraph are taken.

155 J. Simon, *English Sanitary Institutions* (London, 1890), p. 19; F. Brockington, 'Public health at the Privy Council 1831–4', *Journal of the History of Medicine*, 16 (1961), 162 (who states they were sent to Riga).

156 NA PC 2/212/211–15 (Order, 8 June 1831).

157 Brockington, 'Public health at the Privy Council 1831–4', 162.

158 *JHC*, vol. 86 (2), p. 746.

159 *JHC*, vol. 86 (1), p. 776.

160 Ibid. The answer was given to Parliament on 26 August (*JHC*, vol. 86 [2], p. 788) and the figures were published in *BPP*, vol. 17 (1831), p. 355.

quarantined ship.[161] A week later there was a second petition from Montrose, read on 6 September, at last acknowledging the existence of the 'Contagion which has so fatally ravaged neighbouring countries', on account of which they had 'cheerfully submitted' to quarantine.[162] But perhaps 'the wisdom of Parliament will devise some means of remunerating individuals who have suffered for the public good'.[163] There was no worry shown there that the contagion might actually arrive.

By that time many members of the Commons were hooked on the merits of the shipowners' case, displaying the same disregard as the petitioners for the possibility of an epidemic of awful proportions. On the evidence of Hansard, during the three sittings when quarantine was discussed, the words cholera morbus were never uttered. The first debate was brief, held on 8 August 1831, when the Vice President of the Board of Trade was asked whether any change was being considered in the mode of levying fees on vessels in quarantine.[164] The response was negative, implying that the issue of fees was of little significance as they amounted to only £5,000 a year.[165] But Joseph Hume, ever the shipowners' champion, heard those words 'with regret'.[166] Not only was the figure inaccurate – he put the income at least five times higher – but the principle had been established three years earlier that quarantine should be at public expense. He then made the extraordinary claim that 'England was the only country in the world where such strict regulations were enforced, and where the owners of the ships liable to them were compelled to pay the expense of the constraint they suffered'.[167] He was supported by other members. On 23 August the debate continued when Alderman Thompson presented the petition from the shipowners of London.[168] He alleged that quarantine delays often prevented a ship making a second voyage to the Baltic. As there were some 2,000 vessels on the Baltic run, the income from fees was nearly £16,000 a year from that sector alone.[169] Other speakers agreed with Thompson, among them Hume, who had to present the petition from Dundee. There was regret that no minister was present to defend the Government's position.[170]

The parliamentary proceedings culminated in a debate on 6 September 1831, when Thompson submitted the following motion: 'That it is inexpedient to subject vessels placed under quarantine to the payment of the sum of £5, 14s, 6d for their order of release by the Lords of the Privy Council'.[171] Thompson's point was that the demand was illegal as the 1825 Act had abolished all quarantine payments. In any case, the fixed sum was inequitable. Ships varied greatly in size but paid the same amount. A

161 *JHC*, vol. 86 (2), p. 797.

162 *JHC*, vol. 86 (2), p. 826.

163 Ibid.

164 Hansard, Third Series, vol. 5, p. 935.

165 Ibid.

166 Ibid.

167 Ibid.

168 Hansard, Third Series, vol. 5, p. 455.

169 Ibid.

170 Hansard, Third Series, vol. 5, pp. 455–6.

171 Hansard, Third Series, vol. 5, pp. 1194–6.

vessel might have a cargo worth only £16, of which the fees took a third.[172] Indeed, the mechanics of payment made the true cost of the fees nearer £7 or £8.[173] The imposition of quarantine against the Baltic had been so unexpected that shipowners had been unable to reimburse themselves in the rate of freight. Replying for the Board of Trade, Poulett Thomson announced that Government intended to scrap the fees on 1 January 1832.[174] But they were doing so with reluctance as quarantine establishments cost the country around £30,000 a year, and in future the fees could be recovered from freight, now that quarantine was being continued. He ended by denying emphatically that quarantine fees in Britain were worse than anywhere else. In southern Europe they 'were a horrible exaction'.[175] The debate then centred on when exactly the fees should be abolished, with Hume arguing that the Chancellor should not only act immediately but refund the fees already received since the Baltic crisis began.[176] That was too strong for other members, but Alderman Thompson would not withdraw his motion unless 'the tax was to be abolished instanter', and he pressed for a vote.[177] Despite many speeches in support, the motion was defeated by 64 votes to 20, allowing the fees to continue for the rest of the year.[178]

Before leaving the parliamentary arena of 1831, two further points are worthy of mention. The first is that, as early as 5 August, the House had requested a return of statistics over the previous five years of all ships quarantined in the United Kingdom, whence they had come, at what station they were held, and the amount of fees paid for their release.[179] Parliament had also wanted to know the authority for those fees, its date, to whom the fees were paid, and for what purpose. Finally, they had desired up-to-date figures of ships quarantined, and still in quarantine, since the start of the year. The circumstances of those requests, which were presented on 2 September, are unclear.[180] The returns were apparently unmentioned in the debates which were held before and after that date, yet they would seem to have made unnecessary the request by Alderman Thompson, on 23 August, for details of the fees and how they were applied. The second point is anecdotal, but confirms that some shipowners had serious grounds for disquiet. John London, the part-owner and master of an Ipswich ship, had sailed from Riga on 26 June – when cholera had just reached that port – bound for Hull, carrying 24 tons of hemp and 260 quarters of wheat.[181] For various reasons, including administrative inefficiency, the ship was detained 60 days in quarantine at Whitebooth Roads, which cost London £150 in wages, provisions, pilotage and other charges. What was worse, his ship had missed the

172 Ibid.

173 Ibid.

174 Hansard, Third Series, vol. 5, pp. 1196–7.

175 Ibid.

176 Hansard, Third Series, vol. 5, p. 1198.

177 Hansard, Third Series, vol. 5, p. 1200.

178 *JHC*, vol. 86 (2), p. 827.

179 The date and particulars of the request are known by the recital in the returns. On 5 August *JHC* is silent on the matter.

180 For the presentation, see *JHC*, vol. 86 (2), p. 810. For statistics, see *BPP*, vol. 17 (1831), pp. 347–54, and for comments on some of them see below.

181 *JHC*, vol. 86 (2), p. 874.

chance of another round voyage before winter. The petition, heard on 28 September, was ordered to lie upon the table and be printed.[182]

While the Commons laboured at leisure over a five-pound fee, the physicians agonized about the prevention of a disease which seemed capable of all but depopulating the slums of industrial Britain. On 20 June 1831 a royal Proclamation required the quarantine laws to be strictly enforced and prohibited communication with vessels and crews from the Baltic, or any other designated area, specifically on account of cholera morbus.[183] It also announced the formation of a consultative Board of Health which was formally constituted on the following day. The Board was chaired by the President of the College of Physicians, Sir Henry Halford, supported by five colleagues (Doctors Maton, Turner, Warren, MacMichael and Holland), along with Pym, as Superintendent General of Quarantine, Sir James McGrigor as Director of the Army Medical Department, and Sir William Burnett as his counterpart for the Navy. Membership was completed by the Comptroller of the Navy and the Deputy Chairman of the Board of Customs. Another physician, Dr Seymour, acted as secretary.[184] As in 1805, the brief was advisory and not executive. The Privy Council wished to know if any changes were recommended to the Order in Council of 19 July 1825; to what extent the sick were to be separated from the healthy, should cholera take hold; what measures were needed to assist the infected; and how far the disease was contagious and could be spread by inanimate matter.[185] The Board were particularly asked to suggest ways to prevent cholera spreading.[186]

There were those, from the outset, who had no confidence in the Board's ability. A later commentator, with the benefit of hindsight, called them 'the Board of Death'.[187] The College of Physicians had been damaged by the uncompromising attacks of Maclean and it was evident that the Board had no first-hand experience of the disease they were expected to prevent. 'It is probable', concluded *The Lancet*, 'that a set of men more ill-informed on the subject upon which they will be called upon to report, could not be found in the ranks of the profession'.[188] The journal was sarcastic about 'drones, sycophants and courtiers' which the Grey administration had promised to replace by men of proven ability.[189] Yet here was a Board reporting only to the Privy Council, itself an adjunct of the King, and 'wherever there is the face of royalty', sneered *The Lancet*, 'we are sure to find the nose of Sir Henry Halford'.[190]

---

182 Ibid.

183 Bibliotheca Lindesiana, vol 8: *Handlist of Proclamations issued by Royal and other Constitutional Authorities 1714–1910* … (Wigan, 1913).

184 *Edinburgh Review*, vol. 96, p. 407.

185 Brockington, 'Public health at the Privy Council 1831–4', 163.

186 Ibid.

187 W. White, *The Evils of Quarantine Laws and Non-Existence of Pestilential Contagion* (London, 1837), p. 1.

188 *The Lancet*, vol. 16 (409), p. 434.

189 *The Lancet*, vol. 16 (409), p. 433.

190 Ibid.; *The Lancet* also pilloried Halford as the 'bulletin signer' for the royal family.

On 29 June 1831 the Board sent the Privy Council a draft of the proposed new rules. In the view of the physicians, cholera was 'infectious'.[191] Epidemiology was moving away from the traditional adjective 'contagious', which implied spread by contact alone. But quarantine was only effective against contagion in a literal sense, and the irony of that would not have escaped the Council. *The Lancet* had been worried all along that the spread of cholera by contagion was unproven. The journal supported a European idea that the wearing apparel of those dead and dying from cholera in the Baltic should be rushed to a remote area of north-west France, to be worn by a hundred volunteers.[192] If these people became infected, then the disease would indeed be contagious and quarantine would be vindicated, so that 'the philanthropic merchant will learn to submit with resignation to the restrictions imposed on commerce for the safety of his fellow men'.[193] That conclusion was perhaps naive, but the journal assumed rightly that such an experiment would not interest the College of Physicians.

The Board recommended a national structure of control spreading inland from the coasts, consisting of Local Boards of Health (whose make-up they suggested) supported by District Committees in the larger urban centres.[194] They advised places to be set apart for the compulsory evacuation of the sick, and controlled houses 'in airy and detached Situations' for the isolation of the infected higher classes.[195] Vague guidance was offered on the purification of houses and effects which had belonged to the dead or sick.[196] For the Privy Council, these recommendations were hardly welcome, raising all manner of questions including constitutional authority, overlap with subsisting parochial and municipal government, social discrimination, and the liberty of the individual. Furthermore, the Council's own powers of control and coercion beyond the imposition of quarantine could only legally take effect once an epidemic had erupted. For two months, therefore, as cholera marched from the Baltic to the North Sea coast, the Council procrastinated and the recommendations were suppressed. Meanwhile, many local authorities, mindful that the Proclamation had promised rules and regulations, badgered the Board for details.[197] Only on 8 August 1831 did the Privy Council agree to the circulation of the Board's proposals, as long as they were lawful.[198] But this caveat served to prevent any circulation at all.

As summer turned to autumn and the Continent became ever more infected, the Privy Council could no longer prevaricate. A brief, blunt Order on 13 October extended quarantine to the whole North Sea coast from Skaw, at the tip of Denmark, to Rotterdam, and to ports on the River Weser.[199] On the previous day the Board of

191 The draft is reproduced in Brockington, 'Public health at the Privy Council 1831–4', 163.

192 *The Lancet*, vol. 16 (413), p. 572.

193 Ibid.

194 Brockington, 'Public health at the Privy Council 1831–4', 164.

195 Ibid.

196 Ibid.

197 Brockington, 'Public health at the Privy Council 1831–4', 164–5.

198 Brockington, 'Public health at the Privy Council 1831–4', 165.

199 NA PC 2/212/401–2.

Health had sent new rules and regulations to the Privy Council, and on 20 October 1831 – 'a date', according to Brockington, 'to be feted by the world's army of health administrators' – the Privy Council finally made up their mind.[200] The rules and regulations advised by the Board were to be published in the *London Gazette* that day, together with a statement about the recognition and treatment of cholera.[201]

Enthusiasm like Brockington's for this significant move was not evident at the time. Much of the medical profession beyond the confines of the College of Physicians was gripped by anti-contagionism. Not only were the new procedures prolonging the principle of quarantine which the anti-contagionists rejected, but they harked back to coercive measures, centuries old, which even at their outset had been judged to conflict with civil liberty. The Board, of course, had always been aware that compulsory removal from infected houses or enforced detention within them would be highly contentious. In fact, the original proposals were watered down, to the extent that the sick could only be moved to a hospital if their family consented. But far too many of the rules still copied discredited past procedures. Simon noted that: 'Medically, the *Rules and Regulations* did not represent any advance on what might have been advised in 1720 by Dr Mead'.[202] The Privy Council took no lesson from the Marseilles crisis, when many parliamentarians had taken offence at the suggestion of cordons sanitaires in Britain to isolate infected locations. Perhaps the most severe critic of the rules of 20 October, albeit 20 years later, was the *Edinburgh Review*, which believed that the Board had 'actually revived, and even surpassed, the barbarous counsels which prevailed in the days of King James the First ...'[203] The concept of cordons was especially offensive. Such tactics were 'alike contemptible in the eyes of science and opposed to every sound principle of legislation ...'[204] The journal was also unhappy with a comment by the Board that 'rigorous quarantine' had been found effective against cholera – 'a bold but incautious assumption', and one which underpinned the Government's response.[205]

The onset of cholera morbus in England was insidious. During the summer of 1831 there were many cases around the country, and on board ships in the Medway, of 'dysenteric diarrhoea and cholera'.[206] This was not Asiatic cholera, but an indigenous disease which often erupted during the heat of summer when conditions were even more insanitary than usual. With early symptoms close to those of cholera morbus, attacks of this domestic disease in Port Glasgow, Leith, Hull and other ports associated with the Baltic trade, caused particular worry in July and August. But it was at Sunderland, in late October, where the imported virus was first distinguished from the native strain which had troubled the Wear valley since the summer. Suddenly, cholera morbus lurched through the waterside hovels, shrivelling the strong to an agonized death in the course of only hours. Exactly how the disease reached the

200 Brockington, 'Public health at the Privy Council 1831–4', 169.

201 Simon, pp. 169–71.

202 Simon, p. 170.

203 *Edinburgh Review*, vol. 96, p. 406.

204 *Edinburgh Review*, vol. 96, p. 408.

205 *Edinburgh Review*, vol. 96, p. 407.

206 Creighton, vol. 2, p. 795.

town was not established, but as many Sunderland seamen were engaged in the Baltic trade, it can be assumed that quarantine was evaded or ineffective.[207] Indeed, Sunderland and other north-east ports had no quarantine facilities of their own, and there were doubtless many masters who found an excuse to avoid the authorized station near Hull in Whitebooth Roads. Given the nonchalance towards disease in east-coast ports, preoccupied as they had been with Privy Council fees, the breach was hardly surprising. Nor was it remarkable that many doctors in the Sunderland area rallied to the support of the shipowners, led by the Marquis of Londonderry, when they claimed the outbreak at the worst was 'spasmodic cholera', and probably a form of the indigenous disease.[208]

Once the Privy Council were persuaded that cholera morbus had arrived, they struggled to create a meaningful framework by which the disease might be contained. If local Boards of Health, reporting to the central body, were useful for fighting and monitoring regional infection, they did nothing to ease the disquiet in Whitehall about the legality and efficiency of central control. On 9 November 1831 the Board of Health which had sat under the auspices of the College of Physicians were informed that their services were ended.[209] The Council favoured a new Central Board which promised more immediate and continuous support. The editors of *The Lancet* were, of course, delighted to see the physicians discharged.[210] On 14 November the *London Gazette* announced the formation of the new Board, chaired by Edward Stewart from the Customs Commissioners.[211] The other members were Russell and Barry returned from St Petersburg, two half-pay army officers, and of course Pym as Superintendent General of Quarantine.[212] The physicians, although superseded, were asked to set up an informal committee to advise the Council in strictly medical matters as occasion might arise.[213] Whereas the physicians as a Board had been salaried at £500 a year, their successors, fewer in number, were mostly less expensive individually: Stewart and Pym received no extra salary; Russell was paid £731 a year, Barry £511, the two officers £400, and the Board's secretary, William Maclean, £250.[214] The advantage of the new Board, economies aside, was that it represented experience and administrative skills and an escape from the divided profession of medicine. There was also, perhaps, the thought that if the situation became really out of hand, the military component of the membership could advise on measures of enforcement.[215]

207 cf. Creighton, vol. 2, p. 799.

208 Creighton, vol. 2, p. 798.

209 Brockington, 'Public health at the Privy Council 1831–4', 172.

210 See Brockington, 'Public health at the Privy Council 1831–4', 173–4, for quotations.

211 Simon, p. 171; Brockington, 'Public health at the Privy Council 1831–4', 174. Stewart was Deputy Chairman of the Customs Board.

212 Brockington, 'Public health at the Privy Council 1831–4', 174, refers also to Colonel Rowan, 'head of the police force' who 'seems not to have acted'.

213 Brockington, 'Public health at the Privy Council 1831–4', 173.

214 Brockington, 'Public health at the Privy Council 1831–4', 163, 174.

215 *Edinburgh Review*, vol. 96, p. 409; Simon, p. 171.

In their public face, the Privy Council were at pains to stress that compulsion was not envisaged. They issued through the new Board, on the very day of its creation, a circular trusting that people would be sensible enough to avoid all contact with infected persons or places without having to be forced. They deplored 'all measures of coercion for this purpose which, when tried upon the Continent, have been invariably productive of evil'.[216] This form of words acknowledged that a cordon sanitaire around the north-east of England was neither practicable nor judicious, and the Council retreated to the only measure of defence which they understood. On 28 November they imposed a quarantine of 15 days against ships arriving in British ports from Sunderland, Seaham, Newcastle, and North and South Shields.[217] This was the first time since the sixteenth century that quarantine had been imposed between ports within England, and not since the Great Plague had there been quarantine against England in Scotland. As the hinterland of Sunderland and Newcastle produced much of the coal for southern England, it seemed likely that the winter of 1831 would see a serious shortage of fuel.

The new Central Board gave precise advice to their local counterparts about duties and powers, and recommended a two-tier system of Boards in the larger towns.[218] Inspectors were to be appointed, each with a responsibility for the medical surveillance of around one hundred homes.[219] The Central Board also, in December, circulated *Sanitary Instructions* for infected communities with observations by Russell and Barry on the character and treatment of cholera morbus.[220] On 25 January 1832 the Board warned that winter had not stopped the spread of infection in the north of the country, and London should prepare for an epidemic when the weather turned warmer.[221] Now that Asiatic cholera had arrived, it seemed pointless to continue quarantine against Europe, and during February and March the Privy Council revoked the foul-bill instructions of June 1831, as well as the quarantine against North Sea coasts which they had imposed on 13 October.[222] They were less eager to do away with internal quarantine against ships from the north-east, and made a weak show of tightening procedures by a new Order of 15 March, following cases of cholera among the vessels' crews.[223]

More generally, the Privy Council were occupied with the local Boards of Health, and still worrying how far such essentially royal intervention was lawful. Indeed, fears were enough to warrant an Act of Parliament, given royal assent on 20 February 1832, empowering the Council temporarily to take such emergency measures as they thought appropriate because normal parliamentary procedures would be too slow.[224] Another Act was tailored for Scotland, but the only major difference concerned the raising of money: in England and Wales funds were to

216 *Edinburgh Review*, vol. 96, p. 409.
217 NA PC 2/212/458.
218 Simon, p. 172, gives a list of responsibilities.
219 Ibid.
220 Ibid.
221 Ibid.
222 NA PC 2/213/133, 159.
223 NA PC 2/213/205–6.
224 2 Will. IV, c.10, continued by 3 & 4 Will. IV, c.75.

be applied from the poor rate; in Scotland, they were to come from the police rate paid in urban areas or from special assessments in rural parishes.[225] Despite these concessions, the Commons wanted the Council's Orders laid before Parliament as quickly as possible.[226] The Commons also asked for certain statistics.[227] They wanted to know where the quarantine stations were, the number of ships at each station on 1 December 1831, and on 1 January, 1 February and 15 February 1832. Furthermore, they asked for details of the lazarettos provided since cholera struck and how they were crewed and supported by medical attendants. They were also interested in deaths at each quarantine station, particularly from cholera, and the monthly cost to the public of these stations, of the Central Board of Health, 'and other establishments dependent on it'. It would seem that answers were returned only in respect of costs attaching to the Central Board of Health.[228]

In Sunderland, cholera petered out before the end of 1831, leaving 215 people dead.[229] But the landward spread, checked only by hopeful sentiments from the Privy Council, was inexorable. In December 1831 the disease reached the Tyne valley, erupting in fifty-odd places simultaneously on Christmas Day.[230] During January it threatened Edinburgh, but the main onslaught moved westwards to ravage the outskirts of Glasgow, where the Local Board of Health, supported by district committees, provided 236 cholera beds among five hospitals.[231] From there the northward progress of the disease was relentless, and the epidemic as a whole produced around 10,000 deaths in Scotland, about a third of which were in the region of Glasgow.[232] There was a cynical view that as long as cholera was travelling north, Parliament had little interest in the problem. People in Scotland, it was alleged, 'were left to defend themselves by their own voluntary contributions, their own activity, and their own medical skill, directed by their own good sense'.[233] The Central Board of Health, however, had always realized that cholera would disseminate southwards as well, and in February 1832 it reached the eastern slums of London.[234] But the progress was erratic and faltering, despite gruesome ravages in the metropolis, and by the end of the year the outbreak appeared on the wane. The Central Board was disbanded on 31 December.[235] The *Annual Register* for 1832 (published early in 1833) referred to the epidemic as over.[236] On 1 April 1833 the Privy Council revoked

225 The Act for Scotland was 2 Will. IV, c.11.

226 If Parliament was sitting, they wanted knowledge of the Orders 'forthwith'. If they were not sitting, they wanted knowledge within 14 days of the beginning of the next Session (Section 10 of 2 Will. IV, c.10; Section 12 of 2 Will. IV, c.11).

227 *JHC*, vol. 87, p. 130.

228 *BPP*, vol. 26 (1831–32), p. 475. It is unclear whether even those returns were formally presented to Parliament.

229 Creighton, vol. 2, p. 799.

230 Creighton, vol. 2, p. 803.

231 Creighton, vol. 2, p. 808.

232 Creighton, vol. 2, p. 815.

233 *Annual Review* (1832), p. 305.

234 Simon, p. 173.

235 Brockington, 'Public health at the Privy Council 1831–4', 184.

236 *Annual Review* (1832), pp. 305–6.

all quarantine regulations against the introduction of cholera, unless the disease were actually on board ship.[237] Some 31,000 people in Great Britain are believed to have died in the first pandemic, with as many again infected.[238]

Precise figures survive to show the extent of maritime quarantine during the worst of the outbreak. Whereas the average number of ships in quarantine in British ports in 1826 to 1829 inclusive was 772 (almost all from the Mediterranean), the figure had risen to 1,106 in 1830, and 330 of those ships were from Russia.[239] In Ireland, which had a much smaller trade with the Baltic, the increase was less dramatic: the average of 109 ships (or 120, omitting the freak low year of 1827) rose to 146 in 1830.[240] By 20 August 1831, the date of the return by the Customs Commissioners, the figure for Britain had risen dramatically to 2,556 for the year to that date, although only 153 ships were still being detained.[241] The distribution of those 153 ships is interesting: 65 (or 42 per cent) were at Stangate Creek, which was enjoying a reinvigoration with the crisis being centred on the Baltic. Dundee came second with 41 ships (27 per cent). This was a surprising number for a port which had not been a quarantine station since 1772, but land had been taken in the town for a temporary lazaret and a warship, the *Sybille*, was moored in the Tay estuary until May 1833.[242] The remaining ships in quarantine were at Hull and Plymouth (eleven each), Milford (nine), Liverpool (eight), Leith (six) and Portsmouth (two).

The 2,556 ships were distributed around the country to a wider extent than the totals just quoted would suggest. The figures are particularly misleading for Scotland where the author Hugh Miller, referring to Cromarty Bay, 'became familiar with the site, at first deemed sufficiently startling, of fleets of vessels lying in the upper roadstead, with the yellow flag waving from their mast-tops'.[243] Another eyewitness in Scotland was James Simson, who recalled the disused land lazaret at Inverkeithing being pressed into service in 1832.[244] As at least 28 people died of the disease in the town itself, the building was probably used more for the isolation of infected residents than the crews of ships.[245] When the lazaret was finally sold off in 1835 for £200, the bastion against cholera in the Firth of Forth had moved to St Margaret's Hope, on the other side of the promontory of North Queensferry.[246] Simson recalled that the number of hulks there reached 'five or six' during the cholera epidemic, but

237 NA PC 7/5/24.

238 F.B..Smith, *The People's Health 1830–1910* (London, 1979), p. 230.

239 *BPP*, vol. 17 (1831), p. 348.

240 *BPP*, vol. 17 (1831), p. 352. In 1827 only 76 ships were quarantined.

241 *BPP*, vol. 17 (1831), pp. 351–2.

242 NA PC 7/4/92–3, 170.

243 H. Miller, *My Schools and Schoolmasters* (Edinburgh, 1854), p. 461.

244 J. Simson, *Reminiscences of Childhood at Inverkeithing, or Life at a Lazaretto* (New York, 1882), p. 6.

245 The figures are from W. Stephen, *History of Inverkeithing and Rosyth* (Aberdeen, 1921), p. 378.

246 Simson, p. 5 (followed by Stephen, p. 379) recounts the sale to an Edinburgh lawyer in 1835, but on 18 December 1833 the Privy Council had approved the sale of the lazaret in the following April or May (NA PC 7/4/332–3).

these were reduced to only one in 1835.[247] That remaining hulk was the *Dartmouth* then commanded by a naval lieutenant, an ignominious fate for the flagship of Lord Exmouth during the bombardment of Algiers in 1816.[248] Another naval vessel had apparently been used elsewhere in the Forth estuary during the cholera crisis, presumably at Leith in view of the six vessels noted in quarantine there.[249]

In October 1832 the Privy Council approved a temporary quarantine station at Kirkwall in the Orkney Islands, as long as it was paid for locally.[250] Ships could be detained for up to seven days from infected or suspected places.[251] But the Council were less happy about Holy Loch, where the facilities were becoming gradually disused, despite its inclusion in the official list of quarantine stations in May 1831. For the Council, Holy Loch was an unwelcome distraction, in as much as the shipping magnates in Glasgow who wanted to use it were importing from Egypt, and the risk was therefore from plague. In October 1832 the Council conceded that ships from Alexandria could be aired at Holy Loch if interested parties would bear the expense.[252] This led to the Glasgow Chamber of Commerce joining forces with merchants and shipowners to request that Holy Loch be fully restored as a quarantine station.[253] But cholera had not revived the lazaret at Holy Loch as it had at Inverkeithing, and the Privy Council wanted to backtrack. The station, they replied, was conceived during early worries about yellow fever 'before any Cotton was imported from Egypt'.[254] They were also dismissive of the 'very small number' of ships which cleared annually from Alexandria for the Clyde.[255] If this implied more trade for Milford Haven as the foul-bill station for the west coast, the Welsh were soon disappointed. Milford was also in slump, so little affected by the cholera epidemic, that it received only 43 ships in a year, and most of those from the risk of plague.[256] In December 1832 the port was deprived of two of its warships, the *Hannibal* and the *Dragon*, being used for airing.[257]

Perhaps the busiest foul-bill station in the cholera crisis was Hull, where the warship *Salsette* was anchored in the Humber estuary between 6 December 1831 and 29 February 1832.[258] The journal has survived of the ship's surgeon, named Johnston Hamilton Acheson, who acted as Medical Superintendent for the quarantine station. Acheson reveals that in that short interval of less than three months, exactly 1,125 ships arrived in Whitebooth Roads. Of these, 1,036 were released by Order in Council between five and thirty-five days after arrival. Another 61 were released immediately

247 Simson, p. 6.

248 NA PC 7/4/262 (cf. Simson, p. 6).

249 Ibid.

250 NA PC 7/4/1–3.

251 Ibid.

252 NA PC 7/4/7.

253 NA PC 7/4/49–50.

254 Ibid.

255 Ibid.

256 NA PC 7/4/76–7. The period was 20 November 1831–20 November 1832.

257 NA PC 7/4/78–9.

258 NA PC 6/12, which constitutes the journal of the ship's surgeon, from which all references in this paragraph are taken.

by medical certificate (that is, by Acheson on his own initiative), while 25 were referred to a foul-bill station. Some of these referrals would have been among the vessels glimpsed by Miller in Cromarty Bay. The three remaining ships were judged not liable to quarantine. As the impressive Hull figures did not begin until after the above-quoted total of 2,556 ships had been compiled, it can be safely assumed that quarantine detentions around the country rose hugely as the epidemic continued.

The bills of health issued by Britain had been bland for so many years that the Privy Council now struggled to find meaningful words which expressed the true state of disease, variable as that was. This gave no confidence abroad, and merchants complained that ships trading to Spain with clean, unqualified bills were sent on to Minorca for quarantine as a matter of course; even Gibraltar was fussy about British bills, to the chagrin of the Privy Council.[259] There was, at first, no attempt to impose a national form of words for a foul bill, although on 4 October 1832 the Customs authorities in Liverpool were told to write that cholera had ceased 'as an Epidemic'.[260] That phrase had been used in London from as early as May.[261] On 26 October the Council informed the Customs Commissioners that clean bills could now be issued from London, as there had been no case of cholera reported to the General Board of Health since 15 October.[262] In many countries it would have appeared strange that the Privy Council concerned itself with such matters as the phrasing of bills, but the Customs Commissioners had complained they were much in the dark, having no channel of communication with local Boards of Health.[263]

Anti-cholera measures on Malta

For the Board of Health in Valletta it was difficult to focus on any disease beyond the Scylla and Charybdis of plague and yellow fever. The number of arrivals from the Baltic was low and if cholera threatened from anywhere, the route from the east seemed the most likely. Russian ports in the Black Sea posed as great a danger as St Petersburg, but Malta was indifferent to the risk from anywhere for many months. Not until 18 May 1831 did the Board feel it necessary to impose a quarantine of ten days against Russian ports, which they limited to those in the Baltic.[264] By the same half-hearted measure, paying token respect to concerns in London, arrivals from other ports in the Baltic were quarantined for five days. The Board, with only a quorum attendance, were more concerned with the ritual quarantine against Alexandria and Gibraltar.[265] But on 3 August, cholera won the close attention of a fully attended

259 NA PC 7/4/12–13. In the case of Gibraltar (PC 7/4/22–3), the Privy Council leaned on the Colonial Office to get the Lieutenant-Governor to amend the wording of his regulations, which were in one respect 'more rigid' than even those of the European powers.

260 NA PC 7/4/4.

261 Ibid.

262 NA PC 7/4/20–21.

263 Ibid.

264 NLM LIB 847 [unpag.], 18 May 1831.

265 Ibid.; against Alexandria for plague and against Gibraltar for yellow fever.

meeting.[266] Quarantine against any Russian or Baltic port was increased to 15 days, with a similar period for arrivals from Holland, Belgium, French ports on the Atlantic coast, and from the Adriatic. And for the first time, there were measures against Great Britain and Ireland, from where ships would be quarantined for five days, or for such longer period as would make a total of 30 days since the ship set sail.[267]

By the end of September, any complacency felt by the Board had entirely vanished, with news that cholera morbus had broken out during August in Alexandria and Cairo.[268] As that news came from Tripoli, via pilgrims returning from Egypt, there was suddenly a real fear that Malta was vulnerable from every direction. Within days the Board concluded that normal foul-bill quarantine was insufficient. On 26 September 1831 the Board decreed that any ship from any country where cholera existed, with any infection on board or suspicion of it, 'shall be sent to sea and not be admitted under any pretence whatever to enter any Port in these Islands'.[269] Ships from infected countries which had no sickness on board, and had been fewer than 20 days at sea, were to proceed to St Paul's Bay for a period of quarantine at the discretion of the Board.[270] Only ships with no sickness which had been at sea for more than 20 days were allowed into Marsamxett Harbour.[271] Before this decision was formally minuted, preparations were already in hand to convert St Paul's Bay into a secondary quarantine station, rather than simply an anchorage. Greig, who now had news of cholera at Constantinople, wanted the old Palace of Salomone converted to a lazaretto with money borrowed from the Monte di Pietà.[272] Other expenses would include guard boats and the fitting-out of a building near the shore as a temporary Health Office and a dormitory for the guardians.[273] Greig wanted the Ordnance Department to surrender their keys to the small fort at the entrance to the Bay, where the magazines could accommodate those actually infected if the musket holes were converted into windows.[274] Finally, he wanted bedding, boards, trestles and medicine, and 'some medical Gentleman' to be stationed there.[275]

On 23 November 1831 the Board of Health met to consider the startling news that cholera had broken out in Sunderland.[276] They stopped short of repeating the conditions under which a ship had to make for St Paul's Bay, as if assuming no one would come from Britain and Ireland who was actually infected. But all arrivals would undergo 25 days' quarantine in Marsamxett Harbour and cargoes would be landed in the lazaretto for a vigorous depuration.[277] In December, with better news about Sunderland, the quarantine was reduced to ten days, with a similar

266 NLM LIB 847 [unpag.], 3 Aug. 1831.
267 Ibid.
268 NLM LIB 847 [unpag.], 21 Sept. 1831.
269 NLM LIB 847 [unpag.], 26 Sept. 1831.
270 Ibid.
271 Ibid.
272 NAM C1, pp. 54–5 (17 Aug. 1831). The Monte di Pietà was Malta's savings' bank.
273 Ibid.
274 NAM C1, pp. 58–9.
275 NAM C1, pp. 60–62.
276 NLM LIB 847 [unpag.], 23 Nov. 1831.
277 Ibid.

concession for Roman territories centred on Ancona, following information about cholera precautions on the opposite shore of the Adriatic.[278] But then in March 1832 came news that cholera had reached London and Greig was asked to submit a memorandum detailing every possible scenario of arrival, taking into account bills of health, the susceptibility or otherwise of cargoes, and the good health, sickness or convalescence of crews and passengers.[279] The possibilities were so complicated that the Board needed more than one session to establish rules, but they were now clear that ships from England with foul bills, and with persons sick or convalescent from cholera, should go at once to St Paul's Bay.[280] If a ship with sickness aboard should slip into either Grand or Marsamxett Harbour at night, or in weather so rough that the guard boat could not intervene, she was to be warped or towed back to sea and sent round to the Bay under escort.[281]

The next major scare was a report of cholera in Paris. On 17 April 1832 the Board put a ten-day quarantine of observation on ships with clean bills from all French ports.[282] This measure included Marseilles, which the Board would have preferred to keep in free pratique to ensure reciprocal treatment. With increasing doubts about the ability of quarantine to keep cholera at bay, the Board of Health resolved 'to address a representation to the Governor' to prepare measures to check an epidemic.[283] They recommended the removal of nuisances, the whitewashing and cleaning of rooms in poor districts, the provision of hospitals in towns and villages, the procurement of medicines and beddings, and the allocation of burial grounds. As Governor Ponsonby presided at the meeting, the formality of the resolution was only to justify expenditure. It is doubtful whether any of these precautions were taken, as reports from Europe began gradually to suggest that the worst might be over. On 20 June 1832, with news from both London and Paris that cholera was subsiding, quarantine against all arrivals from Britain was reduced to only three days of observation, while the period against France was shortened to seven days, with depuration of susceptible goods.[284] But suspicions remained about Ireland, from where quarantine remained at ten days.[285] Six days later, the Board heard that cholera had ceased in England, from where they decided to admit ships with clean bills to immediate pratique.[286] At the same time, there was a slight reduction of quarantine against France, as the south of the country seemed largely cholera-free.[287] Ships from Holland and Belgium benefited a few weeks later.[288]

---

278 NLM LIB 847 [unpag.], 14 & 28 Dec. 1831. On the earlier date, quarantine against vessels from Sweden was reduced from 25 to 14 days.

279 NLM LIB 847 [unpag.], 14 Mar. 1832.

280 NLM LIB 847 [unpag.], 21 Mar. 1832.

281 Ibid.

282 NLM LIB 847 [unpag.], 17 Apr. 1832.

283 NLM LIB 847 [unpag.], 16 May 1832.

284 NLM LIB 847 [unpag.], 20 June 1832.

285 Ibid.

286 NLM LIB 847 [unpag.], 26 June 1832.

287 Ibid. The reduction was from seven days to five.

288 NLM LIB 847 [unpag.], 23 July 1832.

By the end of July 1832 the Board concluded that they had been too hasty. It was dawning on them that this was not a disease which would suddenly vanish, and that they might need to treat the West in terms of cholera as they treated the East in terms of plague. During August a quarantine of seven days was reintroduced against 'England' and France, and ships from Belgium and Holland were to be examined before pratique.[289] In October quarantine against England and France was increased to ten days, even with clean bills, and then extended to 14 days later in the month, with susceptible goods to be landed and depurated.[290] This seems to have been a secondary reaction to worries about Amsterdam and New York, both reported to have cholera, and from where ships would now be quarantined for 15 days.[291] It was not until March 1833, on receipt of 'official advice' that cholera had ceased in England and France, that these measures were rescinded; but a quarantine of observation of six days was put in their stead.[292] On 21 April 1833 even this was done away with, but Ireland was still excluded from the relaxation.[293]

Soon cholera was reported on bills of health from Lisbon and Havanna, but more alarming by far was the arrival of a warship, the *Melpomene*, at Toulon with cholera actually on board.[294] New restrictions were immediately put in place against southern France, followed by others against Holland.[295] In September 1833 the inevitable worries about Britain resurfaced. Although it was considered in London that the epidemic was over, ambiguous bills of health suggested otherwise. Ships from Britain with foul bills were to perform 14 days' quarantine, and those with clean bills seven days, with depuration of susceptible cargoes.[296] On 26 October 1833 Ireland was put on the same footing as Britain, and in the following February ships from both countries with clean bills were admitted to immediate pratique.[297] In consequence of 'some reports' of cholera, quarantine was reintroduced against Britain in September 1834, but restrictions were lifted against England on 27 October 'as it does not appear from the public papers that cholera exists in any part ...'[298] On the other hand, the Board of Health at Marseilles confirmed that the disease was in their city.[299] The 21 days of quarantine which resulted was the longest which the Maltese authorities had ever imposed in their agonized relationship with the French port, but it was soon reduced to 14.[300] On 2 March 1835 the Maltese Board finally gave free pratique to ships with clean bills from Ireland and Scotland, the latter being mentioned for the first time in the context of cholera.[301]

289 NLM LIB 847 [unpag.], 7 Aug.1832. 'England' would have encompassed Scotland.
290 NLM LIB 847 [unpag.], 9 & 29 Oct. 1832.
291 NLM LIB 847 [unpag.], 16 Oct. 1832.
292 NLM LIB 847 [unpag.], 11 Mar. 1833.
293 NLM LIB 847 [unpag.], 21 Apr. 1833.
294 NLM LIB 847 [unpag.], 17 May, 10 June & 5 Aug. 1833.
295 NLM LIB 847 [unpag.], 5 Aug. 1833.
296 NLM LIB 847 [unpag.], 6 Sept. 1833.
297 NLM LIB 847 [unpag.], 26 Oct. 1833, 14 Feb. 1834.
298 NLM LIB 847 [unpag.], 8 Sept, 27 Oct. 1834.
299 NLM LIB 847 [unpag.], 27 Oct. 1834, 2 Feb. 1835.
300 NLM LIB 847 [unpag.], 2 & 9 Feb. 1835.
301 NLM LIB 847 [unpag.], 2 Mar. 1835.

It will be convenient to regard the first skirmish of the Maltese with cholera morbus to have ended at this point. The island had escaped infection perhaps more by luck than preparation, and St Paul's Bay, even if the adaptations had been made, was probably never used in the way Greig envisaged. During the 30 months of the cholera scare, scores of sick people had arrived in Marsamxett Harbour and tons of cargo had been offloaded and depurated in the lazaretto. But that was normal and there is no evidence that any of those ships had been visited by cholera. An exception was HMS *St Vincent* which arrived offshore on 13 May 1833, with the captain reporting that six cases had occurred in March.[302] The crisis was short-lived when the ship's surgeon confirmed that the sick then on board were suffering from illnesses which were non-contagious.[303] But in the imperfect state of medical knowledge, such an answer was always an opinion and not a fact. It was the constant risk from many kinds of imported disease, more or less understood, which distinguished the problem of the Maltese from that of the British. In London, during two years of cholera, plague had been almost forgotten. But for Greig it had never gone away. The Levant and North Africa still gave most cause for concern, and if measures against cholera seemed a puzzling succession of strictness and leniency, they were no more than a feeble echo of the war against plague, in which quarantine was relentless and volatile, responsive to every scribbled message on bills of health from Corfu, Greece, Constantinople, Alexandria and Barbary. But for the Maltese Board of Health, cholera had undoubtedly reached second place in the hierarchy of dreaded diseases, displacing yellow fever, smallpox and the occasional rumour of measles. The Board were right to be anxious: the island had escaped the first onslaught, but cholera morbus would soon pay no respect to traditional defences.

Lessons from the epidemic

Cholera killed not only people but the principle of quarantine. The difference was that people died rapidly but quarantine lingered inordinately long while its Establishment nursemaids refused to look death in the face. The first pandemic was the last occasion when Government believed that physical non-contact was enough by itself to prevent the importation of disease. Quarantine had failed to keep cholera out of Sunderland and, once it was on board the colliers, it had failed to isolate it from the eastern slums of London. But the notion that quarantine had kept Britain free of plague for nearly three centuries ensured that its demise would be as dignified and gradual as successive epidemics would allow. And in a curious way, cholera played its own role in maintaining traditional wisdom.

Quarantine might have been wiped out by anti-contagionist arguments as early as 1833 if cholera had taken a less blinkered route through the United Kingdom. The fact that it targeted the poor and weak diverted attention from the inadequacy of quarantine as a line of defence. Had the disease been indiscriminate in its ruthless ravage, there would have been no point in continuing a system which offered no

302 NLM LIB 847 [unpag.], 13 May 1833.
303 NLM LIB 847 [unpag.], 27 May 1833.

benefit. But the focus of attention was elsewhere. There was almost a sense of relief that the fatalities were consistently restricted to areas of poverty and deprivation. The *Annual Review* came near to suggesting that cholera had been a fuss about nothing: 'every where it was much less fatal than preconceived notions had anticipated. The alarm was infinitely greater than the danger; and when the disease gradually disappeared in the course of the autumn [of 1832], almost every one was surprised that so much apprehension had been entertained'.[304] With sentiments like that being bandied around, the reliability of quarantine was an irrelevance.

The same journal noted that 'cholera left medical men as it had found them – confirmed in most opposite opinions, or in total ignorance as to its nature, its cure, and the causes of its origin, if endemic, – or the mode of transmission, if it were infectious'.[305] In such uncertainty, quarantine skulked behind cover and let the doctors argue and the reformers agitate for the sanitary reforms which Britain urgently needed. If cholera taught one major lesson, it was that foetid slums, contaminated water and standing sewage were a national disgrace. Any other lessons, including the one that quarantine was inadequate, did not catch the public mood.

304 *Annual Review* (1832), pp. 305–6.
305 Ibid.

Chapter Fifteen

International Deliberation, 1835–1853

Ingredients for debate

It might appear ironic that, in the years after the first cholera pandemic, quarantine was intensely discussed against a background in which cholera played only a minor role. The reasons for this new debate were varied and complex, but may be summarized under four headings: the first was the resurgence of bubonic plague; the second was the institution of new quarantine restrictions in countries where they were distinctly unwelcome by merchants; the third was the introduction of scheduled steamship services, especially those linking Britain via Egypt with the Indian subcontinent; and the fourth was the growing intolerance to quarantine of the British Mediterranean fleet. These factors must be considered briefly in turn.

The country worst affected by the new scourge of plague was Egypt, which came to be regarded as the hot spot of infection. In a sense, this was nothing new, as Cairo had long been notorious as 'the fountain and granary of plagues', but now it was more dangerous than Smyrna or even Constantinople.[1] In 1835 Egypt 'was visited by one of the most fatal outbreaks of epidemic plague on record', resulting in 33,733 deaths in Cairo and a reputed total of around 300,000 in the port and environs of Alexandria.[2] In only a few other places did deaths from plague exceed those from cholera, but there were worrying developments locally, especially around the northern shores of the Black Sea. Plague made a surprise attack on Odessa in 1837, despite evidence of a slow retreat in preceding years from Turkey, Greece and the Balkans.[3] No port receiving ships from the Levant could afford to treat plague, the original enemy, as in any way less dangerous than it used to be, before the advent of the 'newer' diseases.

This threat from plague, and a realization that virulent epidemics were potentially transmissible from countries (like Britain) long considered healthy, led to quarantine restrictions where none had previously existed. Denmark was a case in point. There

---

1 The quotation is from P. Russell, *A Treatise of the Plague* (London, 1791), p. 313; cf. *Letters, &c. on the Subject of Quarantine* (London, 1799), p. 3: 'Though Egypt, in modern times is considered as the constant abode, and fountain as it were of pestilence …'

2 The quotation is from G. Milroy, *Quarantine and the Plague: being a Summary of the Report on these Subjects recently addressed to the Royal Academy of Medicine in France* … (London, 1846), p. 11; the Cairo death toll is from Hansard, Third Series, vol. 76, p. 1296; the Alexandria death toll is from *British Parliamentary Papers* [BPP], vol. 49 (1847), pp. 580–82.

3 An account of the Odessa plague is in *BPP*, vol. 54 (1843), pp. 149–65. For the retreat of plague elsewhere, see D. Panzac, *Quarantaines et lazarets. L'Europe et la peste d'orient (XVIIe–XXe siècles)* (Aix-en-Provence, 1986), p. 101.

had been a token detention for some years at Elsinore for ships bound for Baltic and Russian ports, usually from Cuba or the Mediterranean.[4] But after the cholera pandemic, and with new fears surfacing from Egypt, the quarantine became longer and more organized. British ships from Liverpool and Hull, bound for Russia with cotton from Alexandria and New Orleans, were sent to a quarantine station at Kyholm, in 1837, for their cargoes to be depurated.[5] The predictable outcry raised problems for the Board of Trade, as Denmark was not the instigator of the quarantine but only the agent. There was no obligation on masters to receive a certificate of health at Denmark, but without one they risked being sent back from their port of destination. It was Russia and Prussia which had engineered the tougher measures and Elsinore, the strategic gateway which had controlled the Sound tolls, was the obvious place to collect the dues. The fear, especially at Hull, was that historic shipping links would be broken; more precisely, that cotton would travel to Hamburg, be taken overland to Lübeck, and then reloaded there for St Petersburg to avoid the 30-per-cent charge at Elsinore on depurated goods.

This was an early test for Palmerston and possibly the first occasion when his office, that of Foreign Secretary, assumed an executive role in a matter of quarantine. In the domestic context, the Lord President of the Council had traditionally been supreme, while quarantine in British possessions had been the province of the Secretary of State for War and the Colonies. That the Foreign Secretary was now poised to make policy decisions augured well for resolving the international difficulties which every extension of quarantine brought about. In July 1838 Palmerston chose not to remonstrate with Denmark, but sought rather to convince Russia and Prussia that quarantine in Britain was so well conducted that cotton trans-shipped in its ports from anywhere in the world could be assumed free of infection.[6] With help from the Board of Trade, he argued that quarantine regulations in Britain were no less vigorous than in Malta. During 1839 Palmerston persuaded both the Danes and their principals that foul-bill goods purified at Stangate Creek, Milford Haven and The Motherbank were perfectly safe – only to make the embarrassing admission a few weeks later that he had been misinformed as to the status of The Motherbank: he meant Bromborough Pool. The Baltic powers were happy with that, and the depuration at Elsinore ceased for cargoes from British ports.[7]

Far greater diplomatic problems were created by new Boards of Health established in Turkey, Egypt and other North African outposts of the Ottoman Empire. The Christian European powers did not understand why these Boards were needed when religious doctrine throughout the Mohammedan world had always demanded a fatalistic attitude towards death by disease. Maclean, writing in 1824, was one of the first westerners to get wind of the new intentions:

---

4 *Second Report from the Select Committee Appointed to Consider of the Means of Improving and Maintaining the Foreign Trade of the Country. Quarantine* (1824), p. 22.

5 *BPP*, vol. 54 (1843), pp. 49–81, from which remaining references in this paragraph are taken.

6 *BPP*, vol. 54 (1843), pp. 49–81, 131–7.

7 Ibid.

> a very few days have elapsed, since I learned that the Pacha of Egypt, in imitation of the Governments of Europe, seriously meditates the introduction of sanitary laws …, not with any view of preventing the spreading of pestilential contagion, in which he can have no belief, but in order to satisfy those Christian countries, with which he has commercial dealings, that they may buy his cottons &c. without the danger or apprehension of being empested.[8]

If this implied that a Board of Health would concentrate on removing the wretched conditions from which plague was thought to emanate, it was all the more baffling to western observers that maritime quarantine was eventually introduced in all Mediterranean ports in the Ottoman Empire. Against whom and what risks, they wondered, was the quarantine intended?

Despite Maclean's disclosure, the Board of Health at Alexandria was not operational until July 1834.[9] The Pasha approached the consular corps asking for representatives, and the great majority of the Board were therefore Europeans. The consuls suggested a lazaretto outside the port, which the Pasha built 'at a very great expense' to accommodate 2,500 people.[10] Two buildings were also constructed, one in each of the port's two harbours, where quarantined individuals could converse and buy provisions.[11] The Superintendent of the Health Office, at 1,200 piastres a month, was Filippo Pulis, probably the former Captain of the Lazaretto on Malta who had been suspended from duty by Greig in December 1831 for embezzling some wheat from a Greek freighter.[12] The Pasha paid all salaries, but the consular Board of Health nominated officials and allocated rates of pay.[13] The Board failed to improve the frightful conditions which led to the great plague of 1835, and one military doctor described the membership as 'inefficient, expensive even to prodigality, [and] tyrannical in its operations.'[14] One of the manifest absurdities, during the epidemic, was the introduction of a quarantine of 21 days for steamers and warships, and 25 days for merchantmen, from Beirut, on the grounds of sporadic plague in Syria.[15]

There was no less dismay at Beirut, where British merchants and traders viewed the introduction of a local lazaretto with alarm. They complained to Consul Moore, late in 1836, that new quarantine charges were disrupting trade with other parts of Turkey and breached the Capitulations agreed with the Porte.[16] The Beirut Board of Health were subordinate to Alexandria, where the consular Board were themselves

8 C. Maclean, *Evils of Quarantine Laws, and Non-Existence of Pestilential Contagion* … (London, 1824), p. 13.

9 A.T. Holroyd, *The Quarantine Laws, their Abuses and Inconsistencies* … (London, 1839), p. 13, quoting letter from Robert Thurburn, British consul.

10 *BPP*, vol. 54 (1843), pp. 387–8.

11 Ibid.

12 Ibid. For the misdemeanour of Pulis, see National Archives of Malta [NAM] C1, pp. 83–5. Pulis was said to be 'deeply remorseful' and Greig asked Hankey for leniency. It would seem he was asked to leave the island in lieu of punishment.

13 *BPP*, vol. 54 (1843), pp. 387–8.

14 Holroyd, p. 19, quoting Dr Thomas Gregson.

15 Holroyd, p. 5.

16 *BPP*, vol. 54 (1843), pp. 388–9.

subject to the Consuls-General at Constantinople.[17] Those dignitaries were reluctant to interfere when quarantine anomalies could be attributed in most part to commercial jealousies within the Ottoman Empire. The detentions at Alexandria, for example, were in retaliation for a quarantine of 14 days for steamers and warships, and 21 days for merchantmen, imposed on arrivals at Beirut from Alexandria.[18] When these problems had been resolved, it was, ironically, the British consul at Damascus who made matters worse. In December 1840 Consul Wood claimed with some satisfaction to have instigated a ten-day quarantine at Beirut against Egypt, solely to embarrass French warships.[19] For this he was denounced in the House of Commons.[20]

But the problems in Egypt and Syria were as nothing compared to those within Turkey proper. Early in 1831, via the British Ambassador in Constantinople, a request reached London for a plan of the lazaretto on Malta and a copy of the regulations for quarantine.[21] When this request reached the island, Greig hurried to comply but wondered how much good they would do. So much depended, he said, on the site of the lazaretto 'and the description of Quarantine to be performed in it'.[22] It would be far better, he argued, if someone from his department were to visit Constantinople to explain principles and practice first hand.[23] G.B. Schembri, Captain of the Quarantine Harbour, whose experience derived from the plague of 1813 volunteered to go there at his own expense, if given three months' leave of absence.[24] This offer was readily accepted and Schembri sailed on the same ship as the Revd Dr Walsh, whose narrative of *A Residence at Constantinople* pays tribute to his 'intelligent' companion 'on his benevolent mission'.[25] Walsh states that Schembri's proposals were 'highly approved of'.[26] They 'embraced the establishment of quarantine offices and lazarettos on the Dardanelles and Bosphorus, and all the maritime towns on the coasts of Asia and Europe, with a board of health to organize a sanitory police, to watch the introduction and appearance of the disease, and take immediate precautions'.[27] The lazaretto for Constantinople was to be in an elevated and attractive location. At 700 feet in length, and costing £20,000, it would 'present to the view an elegant and cheerful abode' and lift the spirits of its inmates.[28] Walsh

17 *BPP*, vol. 54 (1843), pp. 387–8.

18 Holroyd, p. 5.

19 Hansard, Third Series, vol. 61, p. 614.

20 Ibid., by Bowring.

21 National Archives of Malta [NAM] C1, pp. 37–9.

22 Ibid.

23 Ibid.

24 Ibid. P. Cassar, *Medical History of Malta* (London, 1965), p. 295, states that Schembri had been 26 years in the merchant navy.

25 Revd R. Walsh, *A Residence at Constantinople during a Period including the Commencement, Progress, and Termination of the Greek and Turkish Revolutions* (2 vols, London, 1836), vol. 2, p. 303.

26 Ibid.

27 Ibid.

28 Ibid.

guessed that on completion 'it is not impossible that European nations may hereafter adopt this quarantine establishment of the Sultan for their model ...'[29]

Unfortunately, Walsh was comprehensively wrong. Schembri's proposals, if they were ever accepted, had given no more than a blueprint for what might at some point be achieved. It was another six or seven years before Mahmud II made quarantine in Turkey a reality, and his advisers then were from Austria.[30] In 1838 Mahmud set up a Superior Council of Health with a Turk as President and a Frenchman as Director General of Quarantine.[31] Other members of the Council included delegates from European embassies and doctors appointed by Government. 'The duties of this council', commented Dr John Davy, 'are to form regulations; to meet in consultation on all matters of importance connected with the public health; and to give their sanction to all sanatory measures issued for the preservation of the same ... in the French language, in which their proceedings are conducted, and their regulations drawn up'.[32] The strength of the Council was its independence from the Porte, and the protection it anticipated from ambassadors of western states. At least 50 quarantine stations were set up, each run by a doctor (a European) and a Director of Quarantine (a Turk), reporting every 15 days to the Council of Health, and to European consuls in the event of disease. Davy felt the system was 'extensive and costly' and the lazarettos, generally at each quarantine station, were mainly 'of a bad description, totally unfit for the purpose for which they are designed'.[33]

Britain was wary from the outset. Early in 1836 the Privy Council had sought to make quarantine from Turkey less arduous by altering the rules for bills of health. Whereas ships had been calling at Constantinople for a firman, or licence, to pass through the Dardanelles – which brief contact led to a quarantine of observation in Britain – it was decided in future that ships might collect their firman on the outward voyage, by signalling to the British consul at Constantinople or Pera who would send the document out by boat.[34] The system also ensured that the Foreign Office received a regular list of ships which had passed through the Bosphorus; this list was passed on to Customs officers who could normally exempt such vessels from quarantine.[35] There was not the least inclination in London to complicate matters any further, but Britain was expected to contribute to the discussions of the Superior Council about the new arrangements for quarantine. Lord Ponsonby, Ambassador in Constantinople, employed Richard Wood as a dragoman, or interpreter.[36] Wood irritated the Turkish councillors by refusing to agree anything without referral to

29 Walsh, *Residence at Constantinople*, vol. 2, pp. 303–4.

30 *BPP*, vol. 54 (1843), pp. 31–3.

31 J. Davy, *Notes and Observations on the Ionian Islands and Malta ...* (2 vols, London, 1842), vol. 2, p. 451.

32 Ibid.

33 Davy, *Notes and Observations on the Ionian Islands and Malta ...* , vol. 2, pp. 450–53.

34 National Archives [NA] PC 7/5/5–6.

35 The first list appears to be the one noted in NA PC 6/10 under 4 May 1837. The frequency was usually monthly, but it could be every six weeks or as often as every three.

36 *BPP*, vol. 54 (1843), p. 293.

Ponsonby, who was equally diffident to ratify measures without approval from Palmerston.

There was scarcely any aspect of the Turkish proposals which was not contentious. Neither Smyrna nor Egypt would be in free pratique with Constantinople, leading to inordinate delays for packet boats. Of greater concern to Palmerston were the veiled threats against British nationals. He was outraged that the draft regulations would allow health officers to enter the houses of foreigners and enable guards to fire on alleged transgressors.[37] Ponsonby was to tell the Porte that plague would be prevented more successfully by better cleanliness and ventilation in Constantinople 'than by any such violent interference ... with the domestic arrangements of families'.[38] Early in 1839 Palmerston asked the Board of Trade what quarantine charges they would consider reasonable for British shipping as the Government could not oppose them in principle.[39] The Board responded in March that the new Turkish zeal for regulations had already 'proved a source of never-ending and most harassing embarrassment to trade'.[40] They questioned whether the charges should not be resisted, as Turkey had recently argued for exemption in Britain from light and harbour dues.[41]

As the months passed, Ponsonby found himself under intolerable pressure from the Porte. In July 1839 he instructed the Consul-General to inform British masters that the quarantine regulations should be obeyed until further advice from London.[42] For the first time in history, traders to the Levant faced the prospect of quarantine at either end of the voyage. The only benefit to derive from the British acquiescence, sullen as it was, lay in the favour in which Ponsonby was now held by the Turks. On the application of Governor Bouverie of Malta, Ponsonby secured a promise from the Porte that quarantine would be re-established at Tripoli.[43] Any move which gave the Governor a reason to reduce quarantine delays from Barbary without risking punitive retaliation in France was very welcome to the merchants of Malta.

The mention above of packet boats raises the third new dimension in the debate about quarantine, as these vessels were now steam-powered. Malta was deeply affected by the new technology and in a pivotal position to benefit. As early as August 1824 Hastings was interested in a steamship service with the Ionian Islands, and in December that year he pressed unsuccessfully for a steamer link with Messina.[44] That would have connected with the steam packet already operational between Messina and Naples, which was itself linked by steam power to Marseilles. The advantage to Malta in that instance would have been a faster mail route to and from London, as letters on the land route through Italy and Germany could take up to four months to arrive. In 1829 there was talk of a steam link between Malta and Marseilles via

37 *BPP*, vol. 54 (1843), pp. 39, 115.

38 Ibid.

39 *BPP*, vol. 54 (1843), p. 313.

40 *BPP*, vol. 54 (1843), p. 320.

41 Ibid.

42 *BPP*, vol. 54 (1843), p. 331.

43 *BPP*, vol. 54 (1843), p. 425. It was not, however, very efficient (NA PC 6/10, letter from British Consul General, 21 July 1838).

44 NAM CSG 7/1, p. 173; NA CO 158/3 [unpag.], Hastings to Major General Sir Herbert Taylor, 7 Dec. 1824.

intermediate ports, and in July the following year the records of the Maltese Board of Health have their first reference to the arrival of a steam packet – the *Messenger* from Corfu.[45] In 1833 regular steamship services began from Trieste to the Levant, and state-owned steamers monopolized the carrying of mail from Marseilles.[46]

If the British ceded the main Mediterranean network to the French and Austrians, they did not miss out altogether. Packet steamers were introduced between Falmouth and Malta, where a change to the French line would ensure Athens could be reached from England in 18 days and Constantinople in three weeks.[47] But quarantine problems arose in the opposite direction, because measures were only generally in force against Constantinople. In a letter of 27 July 1833, Greig informed Hankey that passengers and luggage were routinely given free pratique at Falmouth, although some people had embarked at Patras in Greece having travelled overland from Constantinople, and were thus avoiding quarantine altogether.[48] In September this information was under the eyes of the Privy Council, who issued an immediate instruction to the Post Office and Commissioners of Customs: any passenger from the Levant had to ensure that he and his luggage passed quarantine at Malta, or they would be liable to detention at Falmouth.[49]

The next problem for Greig, in December 1834, was the decision to run branch steam packets between Malta and Alexandria, part of the new route to and from India via the Red Sea. He warned that by existing rules, no one could land from Alexandria unless he underwent quarantine in the Malta lazaretto.[50] In this context, it was a question of quarantine being too severe. Was it acceptable, he asked, that the chain of steam communication should be suspended for 17 days on such a strategic route?[51] Early in 1835 the Privy Council decided it was not. In a rare intervention into Maltese procedures, they decided that passengers from the Alexandria packet boats with clean bills of health could embark directly on the connecting packets to Falmouth.[52] But if bills were not clean, passengers would have to do ten days' quarantine at Malta. There was an overwhelming wish to maintain all arrivals at Falmouth in free pratique, to ensure a speedy turn-round for the outward leg. Mailbags from Malta and India (if kept separate from bags collected at Alexandria) could be landed at Falmouth without fumigation; but mail from Patras and Alexandria had to be fumigated in the Malta lazaretto.[53] But even this regime, liberal as it was, had its critics. In 1837 an open letter was sent to Viscount Melbourne, the new Prime

45 NAM CSG 7/1, pp. 288–9; National Library of Malta [NLM] LIB 847 [unpag.], 6 July 1830.

46 Panzac, p. 108.

47 Many details of Mediterranean services, including a timetable of departures from Marseilles, are contained in the review of Edward Giffard's *A Short Visit to the Ionian Islands, Athens, and the Morea*, in *Quarterly Review*, vol. 59 (1837), pp. 220–21.

48 NAM C1, pp. 169–71.

49 NA PC 7/4/292, 294, 297–8.

50 NAM C1, pp. 206–8.

51 Ibid.

52 NA PC 7/4/394–5.

53 NA PC 7/4/426–8. In 1840 it was ordered that the exterior of boxes of mail from Egypt, arriving at Falmouth in contract steamers, were to be mopped with vinegar (PC 7/5/345–7).

Minister, arguing that the India to England run should be independent of the Malta steamers.[54] The reason was the rigorous quarantine at Malta, when the formalities might be more conveniently (and by implication less strictly) performed at Falmouth. Unless the quarantine problem could be solved, it was even suggested that steamers should use the route via the Cape of Good Hope.[55]

Although Malta looked forward to the steam packets as assured and regular business, the cold stare of Marseilles required all quarantine procedures to be strictly enforced. The French had been tolerant when sailing packets were allowed to use a wharf in Grand Harbour for quarantine: after all, much of the mail, some of it urgent, was French and it was recognized that a packet boat in Marsamxett Harbour could not leave port against a strong easterly wind.[56] But for steamers the contrary wind made no difference, and in June 1831 the French consul threatened to inform the Board of Health at Marseilles if steamers and their attendant colliers were not made to use the proper facilities in Marsamxett Harbour.[57] Greig had no doubt that the pratique of Maltese ships at Marseilles rested on compliance, and the French as usual had their way. That incident, however, was no more than an irritation. The wider point was that, while agreed durations of quarantine could be factored into timetables, schedules could be utterly wrecked by the capricious imposition or extension of delays at any of the ports of call. As early as 1837 one guidebook was publishing the sailing dates from Marseilles to Leghorn, Civita Vecchia, Naples, Malta, Syra, Athens, Smyrna, Constantinople and Alexandria; the reader was given the length of the voyage and the duration of the stops, all to the nearest hour.[58] If Boards of Health continued as they had always done – that is, increasing the tariff of quarantine against every rumour of plague here or misconduct there – any advantage from steam power would be nullified. And it was not just delay in the western ports to consider; the traveller was now equally liable to quarantine in the Ottoman Empire, especially in the approach to Constantinople. Clearly, there was scope here for common cause among nations.

Malta was at the hub of steamship routes, but it was for another reason that the island provided the impetus for international deliberation on the future of quarantine. The Royal Navy had always preferred Grand Harbour at Valletta to Marsamxett Harbour, but the complaint now was not about the location for quarantine but the length of it. On 29 May 1838 Admiral Stopford complained to the Admiralty that 25 days' quarantine at Malta was ridiculous. 'It appears to me most unnecessary and unreasonable', he wrote,

> to subject Her Majesty's ships, with all their good order, cleanliness, and medical skill, to the same periods of quarantine as merchant-vessels with cargoes, or steam-packets with

54 D. Lardner, *Steam Navigation with India by the Red Sea; advocated in a Letter to the Right Honourable Lord Viscount Melbourne* (London, 1837), pp. 42–3.

55 Lardner, *Steam Navigation with India by the Red Sea*, p. 100.

56 NAM C1, pp. 45–7.

57 Ibid.

58 *Quarterly Review*, vol. 59 (1837), p. 220 (quoting Giffard, as footnote 47).

passengers. Officers are bound by the ties of honour, as well as the risk of forfeiting their commissions, to make a true and correct statement of the health of their crews ...[59]

When Stopford had made these points to Bouverie in April, the Governor had replied that both he and the Board of Health had no scope for leniency, as Malta's free pratique with the Continent depended on warships and merchant ships being treated alike.[60]

The Admiralty relayed the complaint to the Privy Council who could only wring their hands.[61] Pym offered the view that 15 days' quarantine would probably be enough, but that was no consolation for Stopford or Bouverie.[62] It was decided by the Melbourne administration, in a somewhat pathetic display of impotency, to ask the governments in France, Austria and Tuscany to state the shortest period of quarantine which could be allowed to warships in Malta so as to maintain the island in free pratique with the Continent.[63] There was no hint there that the British had a wider agenda, and certainly no signal that they were seeking an international meeting to thrash out the dreadful mess into which quarantine had descended. But the historical importance of Stopford's complaint is that it led indirectly to a series of conferences by which quarantine was eventually dismantled.

Franco-Austrian jealousy

It was Sir Frederick Lamb, British Ambassador in Vienna, who put the thought of a conference or congress into Palmerston's mind. Lamb was charged with imparting to Prince Metternich, the Austrian first minister, the question about quarantine for warships at Malta. But in a letter to Palmerston of 6 July 1838, Lamb ruminated about the wider picture.[64] He was struck by so many bizarre events and anomalies bringing quarantine into disrepute. Trieste, for instance, had been in quarantine with Toulon and Marseilles for six months, as punishment for admitting the Turkish ambassador to premature entry; yet France was giving free pratique to Algiers, a traditional exporter of plague, on the grounds that French 'customs and regulations' were now in force there. Lamb had also noted the growing interest in quarantine in the East. For example, the new state of Greece had imposed regulations and Turkey was about to do so. Lamb had mentioned these points to Metternich who had confided that Austria would join England and France (if the latter were so disposed) in discussing how quarantine should be managed.

59 *BPP*, vol. 54 (1843), pp. 16–18.

60 *BPP*, vol. 54 (1843), p. 18.

61 Ibid.; NA PC 7/5/225–6. More precisely, the Privy Council expressed themselves reluctant to interfere with the rules at Malta, as they appeared to conform with the practice on the Continent.

62 *BPP*, vol. 54 (1843), p. 18.

63 *BPP*, vol. 54 (1843), pp. 21–2, 99, 260–61.

64 *BPP*, vol. 54 (1843), p. 20, from which all references in this paragraph are taken.

In Britain, this idea was well received by Palmerston, the Admiralty and the Board of Trade.[65] But before any initiative could be suggested to France, it became evident that the French had been thinking independently along much the same lines. Indeed, it was now some years since Count Molé, the French Minister of Commerce, had asked M. Ségur-Dupeyron, Secretary of the Supreme Council of Health, to look at the 'reprisals' and 'misunderstanding' among sanitary bodies which were bringing the concept of quarantine into disrepute.[66] From that background, Molé instructed Baron Langsdorff, the French chargé d'affaires in Vienna, to get in touch with Metternich about a conference, possibly in Italy. At that stage, there was no thought of writing to the British, as Molé envisaged only delegates from the Christian states bordering the Mediterranean. Six key questions should be decided: maximum and minimum quarantine terms for plague, yellow fever or cholera; methods and expense of purification; distinctions between susceptible and non-susceptible goods; the role of health guardians; the pay and expenses of guards; and ways to alleviate quarantine for countries 'suspected'. The idea was that France and Austria, as possessors of the two main quarantine ports of Marseilles and Trieste, should get together beforehand to agree basic points.

On 13 July 1838 Metternich replied enthusiastically to Langsdorff, but pointed out that the British had approached him first.[67] The Austrian Premier was as bewildered as anyone by developments in the Levant. 'Religious fanaticism, inveterate prejudices, and the carelessness of Oriental Governments, have hitherto opposed the introduction of sanitary precautions ...' But that was no longer so. Even Egypt had its regulations, 'however imperfect and defective their execution may be'. In such a changing world, Metternich felt the French brief was too limited. The conference should include Britain, not only for 'the priority of the overtures', but because she controlled Malta and the Ionian Islands. (The latter, although Metternich did not mention it to the French, were thought not well disposed towards Austrian ships.)[68] Greece should be represented as well, and Russia for her Black Sea interests. Not unnaturally, Metternich suggested Vienna as the meeting place. He agreed with the six points on the French agenda, but not with the inclusion of cholera, about which doctors still held 'discordant' views, or of yellow fever, which was 'too little known in Europe'.

The Austrians were so keen on a British presence that Metternich arranged for Palmerston to have copies of his correspondence with Molé and Langsdorff.[69] The French had little option but to acquiesce in British participation. On 2 July 1838

65 *BPP*, vol. 54 (1843), pp. 23–4, 99.

66 *BPP*, vol. 54 (1843), pp. 25–6, from which remaining references in this paragraph are taken.

67 *BPP*, vol. 54 (1843), pp. 31–3, from which remaining references in this paragraph are taken unless otherwise stated.

68 On 19 November 1836 Prince Esterhazy complained to Palmerston of 42 days' quarantine in the Ionian Islands against Austrian ships, as well as damage from 'a chemical process' used in fumigation. Masters were alleged to 'prefer remaining at home without employ ...' (*BPP*, vol. 54 [1843], pp. 13–15).

69 *BPP*, vol. 54 (1843), p. 34 (letter of thanks from Palmerston to Esterhazy, 2 Oct. 1838).

Molé wrote to Earl Granville, British ambassador in Paris, imparting that France had proposed 'a kind of Congress, in which the basis of an uniform sanitary system, may be particularly examined'.[70] Other letters were sent to Palmerston in London, and to the Governments on Malta and the Ionian Islands, soliciting representation at a date and place to be decided. Bouverie knew of the French plan before word came from London, as the French consul had already written to Greig with the full proposals, including the six points to be used as terms of reference.[71] Greig assured the consul of the Governor's 'most lively satisfaction' at the news, and Bouverie, writing on 11 June 1838, appeared no less enthusiastic in his answer to Lord Glenelg, Secretary of State for War and the Colonies.[72] The excitement on Malta was in contrast to the mood in Corfu, where Sir Howard Douglas sent a weak and evasive letter to Glenelg, pointing out that any initiative for the Ionian Islands had to come from London.[73]

By then, Bouverie and Greig would have realized that none of the three powers asked to comment about minimum quarantine for warships at Malta (to ease the burden of Admiral Stopford) was prepared to take a view. The first response was from France, in a letter of 14 July 1838 from Molé to Granville, stating that the problem could only be resolved by international conference.[74] The reply on behalf of Tuscany, two weeks later, came from the Board of Health at Leghorn, who insisted that journey times were irrelevant and quarantine could only begin once a ship was in port.[75] It was probably an indication that Leghorn had wind of the French proposals, when they added that only the principal magistrates of health in the Mediterranean could collectively agree to any change.[76] It was 5 November 1838 before Metternich replied to Lamb. He confessed that he 'dare not' make any helpful remarks as the French insisted that warships and their passengers were not to receive special treatment.[77] He cited the case of Lord Strangford who had arrived at Trieste in a British frigate, on the way to Vienna. When the 'courtesy' of preferential treatment reached French ears, health authorities at Marseilles and the Italian ports retaliated, and it took the best part of a year to get punitive quarantine rescinded.[78]

Palmerston, in line with his policy of rapprochement between Britain and France, was keen on the proposed conference but disagreed with the Board of Trade about its make-up. The latter favoured the participation of Sweden, Russia and Prussia because of the difficulties at Copenhagen.[79] Palmerston, however, rejected the inclusion of the Northern Powers as that 'might give the conference too wide a range'.[80] It was certainly the case that Palmerston had more than enough problems over quarantine in the Mediterranean basin without introducing a Baltic dimension.

70 *BPP*, vol. 54 (1843), p. 91.
71 *BPP*, vol. 54 (1843), pp. 93–5.
72 Ibid.
73 *BPP*, vol. 54 (1843), pp. 101–2.
74 *BPP*, vol. 54 (1843), p. 91.
75 *BPP*, vol. 54 (1843), pp. 260–61.
76 Ibid.
77 *BPP*, vol. 54 (1843), pp. 36–7.
78 Ibid.
79 *BPP*, vol. 54 (1843), p. 100.
80 *BPP*, vol. 54 (1843), p. 105.

As well as the Turkish issue, he was supporting Bouverie and Glenelg in yet another manifestation of the eternal dispute between Malta and Sicily, where quarantine policy was dictated by a truculent Naples. In January 1837 Bouverie, on behalf of his merchants, complained that clean bills from Malta were unrecognized and that out-of-date rumours from Leghorn about the island's health were given greater credence than first-hand reports from ships which had sailed to Naples or Palermo direct.[81] Naples even put Malta under quarantine against smallpox when the port was itself infected.[82] Bouverie alleged trading rivalry: 'The conduct of the Neapolitan Government towards this island, on the score of quarantine, is generally ascribed here to other motives than those which solely concern the preservation of the public health ...'[83]

British merchants in Sicily joined forces with their colleagues on Malta. They called the quarantine tariff at Messina 'unlawful', a tax of 2 or 3 per cent on Maltese goods.[84] It was then the turn of British master mariners to join battle. Seven of them were so incensed at being given an arbitrary quarantine of 40 days at Messina, after a ballast run from Naples with clean bills of health, that they implored the 'interference and protection' of Admiral Sir Josias Rowley.[85] The quarantine, in their view, was 'for the private emolument of these pretended guardians of health'.[86] Matters came to a head when Naples imposed a quarantine of 14 days for people and 21 for goods against 'England' because of typhus fever in Glasgow.[87] Palmerston responded to these various irritations with speed and vigour, demanding 'a distinct explanation' from Naples, and earning praise for his 'energetic remonstrances' through the British Resident.[88]

It was soon obvious to Palmerston that the fragility of Maltese trade, entwined with the dissatisfaction of a navy forced to conform to mercantile requirements, made an overwhelming case for international deliberation on the future of quarantine. His position was not made easier by Bouverie who, in autumn 1838, under extreme pressure from Stopford, became slightly more accommodating to the navy than his rules allowed.[89] The disapproval at Marseilles was echoed by the Minister of Commerce, who instructed the French ambassador in London to warn Palmerston of repercussions if such laxity continued.[90] Before Palmerston had time to investigate, Bouverie confessed his mistake to Glenelg, regretting that the incident had 'certainly given a handle to the Board of Health at Marseilles, which they were sure to make use of'.[91] If Palmerston was excused involvement in that instance, he was less fortunate with Gibraltar, where Governor Woodford was confused and unhappy with

81 *BPP*, vol. 54 (1843), pp. 194–5.
82 Ibid.
83 Ibid.
84 *BPP*, vol. 54 (1843), p. 204.
85 *BPP*, vol. 54 (1843), pp. 210–11.
86 Ibid.
87 *BPP*, vol. 54 (1843), p. 196.
88 *BPP*, vol. 54 (1843), pp. 196, 215.
89 *BPP*, vol. 54 (1843), pp. 109–11.
90 Ibid.
91 Ibid.

the quarantine arrangements of the Spanish.[92] For once, it was not a question of quarantine in Spain against Gibraltar, but dissatisfaction in Gibraltar at the standards of Spain. The problem lay at Algeciras, across the bay, where there was an apparent notion that Vigo in northern Spain had been granted a foul-bill lazaretto, so that ships which called there were being given immediate pratique. Enquiries revealed that the San Simón Islands, off Vigo, had been designated in June 1838 as the site for a lazaretto, but it was not yet built and Port Mahon was still the only one under Spanish control.[93]

The French-led idea for an international conference came to nothing. Panzac attributes the failure to war between Egypt and Turkey and tensions between the major powers, especially France and England.[94] But relations between the two last-named countries were better than they had been for years, and as the conference was to be restricted to the Christian Mediterranean powers, squabbles within the Ottoman Empire are unlikely to have derailed the process. The Earl of Aberdeen, successor to Palmerston as Foreign Secretary, could cite no specific reason for failure: he wrote vaguely in 1843 that the 'plan seems to have met subsequently with obstacles'.[95] In the following year, in the House of Commons, John Bowring 'knew not why it [the conference] came to nought', while Gladstone in the same debate referred cryptically 'to the differences in other matters which had then arisen'.[96] The French view, in 1843, was that the conference had foundered 'par suite de difficultés d'exécution soulevées par l'Autriche' [following practical difficulties raised by Austria].[97] Milroy, writing in 1861, followed the French line when he referred to 'difficulties interposed by Prince Metternich'.[98] But Milroy had the advantage of correspondence not made available to the British until 1844, and not published until 1846. These letters included one from Metternich to Langsdorff, 13 July 1838, in which the Austrian premier set out his detailed objections to the French initiative.[99] These included his determination that Vienna should be the conference venue, and would have been enough to put France and Austria at stalemate.

Anti-contagionist vigour

Another reason why the 1838 initiative failed had nothing to do with differences between nations, such as they were, or the blocking tactics of any one of them: it followed renewed calls to investigate whether the plague was a contagious disease. If these calls were heeded, then any conference would be premature. And if plague were proved non-contagious, then any conference should consider the dismantling of quarantine rather than the conformity of procedure. It would be wrong to suggest

92 *BPP*, vol. 54 (1843), pp. 222–3.
93 *BPP*, vol. 54 (1843), pp. 227, 231.
94 Panzac, pp. 109–10.
95 *BPP*, vol. 45 (1846), pp. 445–6.
96 Hansard, Third Series, vol. 76, p. 1308.
97 *BPP*, vol. 45 (1846), p. 447.
98 *BPP*, vol. 58 (1861), p. 270.
99 *BPP*, vol. 45 (1846), pp. 451–3.

that the conference was deliberately abandoned while these points were under open discussion; but, just as Austria did not want cholera and yellow fever on the agenda because their contagious properties were unproven, there was probably a background feeling among nations that the conference would be inappropriate while any doubts remained about the contagious qualities of plague.

The issue of contagion was resurrected by an Englishman, George Cornewall Lewis, who had returned to London from Malta where had been a co-commissioner of enquiry into the island's affairs. On 26 June 1838 Lewis submitted a memorandum, apparently unsolicited, to the British Government advocating new research into the way plague was communicated.[100] He suggested a doctor should be sent to Egypt and another to Constantinople and Smyrna; these would be supported by two from Malta 'as the educated Maltese can speak both Arabic and Italian'. Lewis proposed five heads of enquiry and wondered whether France and Austria should be asked to join in. His concern was for Malta, which risked losing its status at any time as a hub of the steamship network if Marseilles or some other port objected to procedures there. Lewis ended his paper by suggesting an international conference. This appears to have been a coincidence of thought as, at the date he wrote, Lewis could hardly have had wind of the ideas being discussed in London or on the Continent.

Despite the advantage of topicality, Lewis ran into trouble with the Board of Trade, who considered his suggestions 'too extended to lead to any practical result' and liable to resurrect antipathy between contagionists and anti-contagionists.[101] There were still those in Government who remembered the tendentious persistence of Maclean and there was no wish to live through another such onslaught. That might have been the end of Lewis had not two events conspired to keep his ideas alive. The first of these was a lecture by John Bowring to the British Association for the Advancement of Science, delivered on 24 August 1838 and entitled 'Observations on the oriental plague and quarantines'.[102] The second was a long, open letter to Bouverie published in *The Times* on 8 November 1838.[103] Written by two army officers and three merchants, ten days into their quarantine in the Malta lazaretto, the letter castigated the principle of quarantine and the 'defect of intelligence' which allowed the system to blunder blindly on for year after year. This would have been an exasperating development for Bouverie, but it had less national impact than Bowring's lecture, which was immediately published.

In many respects, Bowring (knighted in 1854) was a latter-day Maclean, but he had several advantages over his professed mentor. For some years he was political

---

100 *BPP*, vol. 54 (1843), p. 95, from which all references in this paragraph are taken. The printed letter bears the apparent signature of J. Lewis, which perhaps points to clerical confusion with John Austin, Lewis's co-commissioner. For the work of Austin and Lewis on Malta, see Chapter 16.

101 *BPP*, vol. 54 (1843), p. 99.

102 Published as *Observations on the Oriental Plague and on Quarantines* … (Edinburgh, 1838)

103 Also published *in extenso* in Holroyd, *The Quarantine Laws, their Abuses and Inconsistencies*, pp. 58–62

editor of the *Westminster Review*.[104] Although sometimes referred to as Dr Bowring, his doctorate was honorary, granted for services to Dutch literature, so he avoided the mistrust often associated with medical doctors – and certainly Maclean – in the years of contagionist division. Furthermore, Bowring came from a mercantile background, which led to his appointment in 1831 as a co-commissioner to examine commercial links between Britain and France. This was the stepping stone to an appointment from Palmerston in 1837 'to inquire into the present state and probable future development of our commercial relations in the East', which gave him a year's travel at public expense to Egypt and Constantinople, and a consuming interest in quarantine.[105] In 1841 Bowring was elected Member of Parliament for Bolton on a free-trade ticket, and was thus able to promote in person an agenda which Maclean had to argue by proxy. He did this with no less passion and verbosity, but distinctly more tact and deference.

Bowring's *Observations* were rampantly anti-contagionist. Having denounced the irresponsibility and 'arbitrary waywardness' of quarantine authorities, which cost mercantile interests 'millions of pounds sterling in delays', he accused them of spreading contagionist theories to suit their own ends.[106] He had been appalled in his travels by the stories of how plague was allegedly spread, in one case by a kite string touched by a bird flying in from an infected neighbourhood, in another by a cat which had sat on a basket of washing.[107] In Egypt, Bowring had put ten questions about the character and spread of plague to an English doctor in the fleet of the Pasha, thus anticipating (and exceeding in number) the interrogatories of Lewis.[108] In his booklet, Bowring had the opportunity to publish correspondence received since his lecture from Dr James Laidlaw in Alexandria, whose recent experiences in that port left him in no doubt that plague was not a contagious disease in the conventional sense.[109] Laidlaw argued for another official enquiry into the question but promised to accept its findings, even in the 'incomprehensible' event that plague should again be judged contagious.[110]

Faced with such pressure, the British Government looked earnestly to Pym for a way out.[111] Another commission of enquiry into the contagious properties of plague would be most unwelcome, but the persistence could not be ignored. Pym arrived at the compromise solution of yet more interrogatories. To avoid a board of enquiry or the expensive dispatch of British and Maltese physicians on a fact-finding journey, Pym devised seven questions about aspects of plague to be sent in the first instance to British consuls in Constantinople, Smyrna, Aleppo, Alexandria, Cairo, Odessa

104 For a summary of his complicated career, see *Oxford Dictionary of National Biography*, from which most facts in this paragraph are taken.

105 The quotation is from Bowring, p. 1.

106 Bowring, pp. 2–3.

107 Bowring, p. 4.

108 Bowring, pp. 29–33.

109 Bowring, pp. 36–45. Davy, p. 330, pointed out that Laidlaw, a central figure in the anti-contagionist campaign, had begun his career as a contagionist.

110 Bowring, p. 45.

111 Milroy, *Quarantine and the Plague*, p. 13.

and Marseilles, and to Governor Bouverie in Malta.[112] On 30 January 1839 the master letter was sent via the Board of Trade to the Foreign Office for Palmerston's approval and for reproduction by lithography.[113] But any satisfaction in Government that the matter was now dealt with was spoilt by the publication, later in 1839, of an open letter from Arthur T. Holroyd to Sir John Cam Hobhouse on the alleged abuses and inconsistencies of the quarantine laws.[114] Central to those issues, of course, was the question of contagion and plague.

Hobhouse was President of the Board of Control whose responsibilities were limited to matters affecting India. He was not, therefore, the most obvious target for a letter, but the point was being reiterated that quarantine impeded the new quick route to India by steamships running from east and west to the coasts of Egypt. Holroyd is an obscure figure.[115] He introduced himself to Hobhouse simply as one 'recently returned from Egypt, Syria, and the Mediterranean, where, amongst other subjects, that of the present system of sanatory regulations occupied my attention'.[116] Holroyd began from the topical conviction that quarantine was 'useless and inefficient' and set about proving it by recounting his personal experiences at Beirut and Alexandria.[117] In the latter port, dismayed at the prospect of a lengthy delay, he petitioned the Board of Health for relief and explanation.[118] In this, he was aided by Robert Thurburn, the British Consul, who also put him in touch with European doctors working locally in both civil and military establishments. To these ex-patriates, Holroyd put a total of 96 separate questions about the local Board of Health, the character of the plague, and arrangements for quarantine and sanitation. All these questions and answers he published, along with another set put to Captain Bonavia, Superintendent of the Lazaretto on Malta, and to two of his colleagues.[119] Holroyd also published correspondence, in September 1838, with Henry Bouverie, in which the unfortunate Governor defended an allegation of favouritism.[120] Indeed, it was Holroyd who brought extra attention to the criticism of Bouverie in *The Times*, by reprinting the original letter.[121]

The influence of Holroyd was considerable. Whereas Bowring's monograph came across as long-winded and rhetorical, Holroyd's book was pithy, thorough, and full of comment and statistics. By comparison, the questionnaires of Lewis and even Pym, still trapped in the narrow issue of contagion, looked brief, stale and irrelevant. The Privy Council viewed Holroyd with mixed feelings. While it was no bad thing for the effectiveness of quarantine to be under such close scrutiny,

---

112 Ibid.

113 *BPP*, vol. 54 (1843), p. 431.

114 See Bibliography.

115 Bowring appears to be alone in referring to him as Dr Holroyd (Hansard, Third Series, vol. 61, p. 614).

116 Holroyd, p. 3.

117 The quotation is from Holroyd, p. 2.

118 This was in June 1838, following ineffective correspondence with the British Vice-Consul. The Consul himself was to prove more amenable.

119 Holroyd, pp. 13–28, 38–44.

120 Holroyd, pp. 56–7.

121 Holroyd, pp. 58–62.

Holroyd offered no ideas as to how the institution could be abandoned altogether. But he did instil a resolution in the Council that quarantine should never get more complex than it was at that time, and that every opportunity to limit it should be sought and taken. This led immediately to a firm hand with Ireland where the local Privy Council were struggling, with some reluctance, to keep in step with policy in London. The resurgence of plague in the Levant and Black Sea, resulting in a quarantine of ten days in Britain for ships with clean bills (unless carrying the firman from Constantinople), caught the Irish by surprise.[122] Pym was dispatched to Dublin and spent much energy in 1842 arguing that a lazaret in Ireland was still not justified, and that differing quarantine regulations would 'give rise to inconvenience & ... afford just grounds of complaint'.[123]

Meanwhile, the strong stand of Holroyd had given new vigour to Bowring. On 15 March 1842 he began the first of a long series of parliamentary initiatives by moving that enquiries into the efficacy of quarantine be continued, and that international negotiations be pursued to modify the system.[124] He also wanted all recent correspondence about quarantine lain on the table of the House. In a classic anti-contagionist speech, Bowring did not disguise his admiration for Maclean his mentor, the 'physician of eminence'.[125] In a later speech he would refer to him as 'a martyr to his zeal'.[126] 'Too much neglected, and too soon forgotten', he 'had preceded his day'.[127] But if Maclean had only antagonized the Establishment, Bowring argued to good effect from within it. He never sought to embarrass the Government or press for more than was realistic. His plea was for the momentum of enquiry to continue, not for quarantine to be abolished at a stroke. In his opening speech, Bowring referred back to his address to the British Association for the Advancement of Science.[128] Many of the original points were repeated or amplified. The vague statement of losses occasioned by quarantine was tentatively strengthened to 'between two and three millions', and 'if the losses in the Mediterranean were added together, they alone would make up that amount'. There were no statistics to make this estimate more than a guess, and in a later speech Bowring reduced the figure to between one and two millions pounds sterling.[129] He explained with energy and precision the anomalies of quarantine in the steam age, and sided openly with the navy who were subjected to 'much tomfoolery'. The root of the trouble in the Mediterranean, in Bowring's view, was that so many families at Naples, Leghorn and Marseilles owed their livelihood to the continuation of sanitary laws and the fees which resulted. It would be cheaper, he argued, if these employees and dependents 'were pensioned off to the third and fourth generation'.

122 NA PC 7/5/418–19, 422–4.

123 NA PC 7/5/422–4, 428–30, 436–7.

124 Hansard, Third Series, vol. 61, pp. 608–18.

125 Hansard, Third Series, vol. 61, p. 609.

126 Hansard, Third Series, vol. 76, p. 1293.

127 Ibid.; Hansard, Third Series, vol. 86, p. 877.

128 Hansard, Third Series, vol. 61, pp. 608–18, from which remaining references in this paragraph are taken unless otherwise stated.

129 Hansard, Third Series, vol. 86, p. 880.

There was nothing in the motion to cause Government concern and Sir Robert Peel, who had succeeded Melbourne as Prime Minister, offered no objection to the papers being tabled.[130] But without Bowring's intervention, it is doubtful whether the new administration would have kept quarantine so much in mind. With France and Austria making no fresh overtures, and the situation in Turkey proper showing no deterioration, it was only Egypt which kept the nuisance of quarantine on the Foreign Secretary's desk. The incumbent now was the Earl of Aberdeen, who showed every sign of continuing the positive stance of Palmerston. With Aberdeen's encouragement, the Board of Health in Alexandria was reconstructed early in 1843, under pressure from Colonel Barnett, the British Consul General.[131] In an attempt to rid the area of its endemic disease, new regulations were formulated embracing both 'exterior' and 'interior' quarantine and the 'sanitary police' of the port.[132] This had more to do with ridding the city of accumulated filth than detaining foreign ships.

In Britain, Bowring's powerful speech had the effect of imparting confidence to Pym and the Privy Council. The former set about suggesting new quarantine times based on what he assumed would be acceptable on the Continent. In September 1843 the authority to release clean-bill ships which had been exercised in certain ports by Medical Superintendents since 1827 was extended to the tide-surveyor (or other Customs official) who received the replies to the printed interrogatories.[133] Excepted, however, from this concession were ships from the Levant, which would be quarantined for five days even with clean bills and a non-enumerated cargo.[134] If the cargoes were enumerated, the ships, even with clean bills, would have to unload all their goods for airing over 15 days.[135] In the case of suspected bills and enumerated cargoes, the airing would be from 20 to 25 days (the longer period specifically for cotton) which was five days longer than Pym had recommended.[136] But the Privy Council were happy with his recommendation of 25 to 30 days for ships with foul bills.[137] Copies of the new rules were sent to the Privy Council of Ireland on 13 October.[138]

Another question for Pym was the new role for The Motherbank, as Southampton had replaced Falmouth as the terminal for steam packets from Malta and Alexandria, and soon from elsewhere. Once the mail cases, weighing on average around 50 hundredweight, had passed through the floating lazaretto, who would pay for their removal to Southampton or Gosport?[139] In March 1844 Southampton petitioned for a lazaretto, but this was turned down on the grounds that trade with the Levant was too small.[140] But the port won a small concession later in the year when the Privy

130 Hansard, Third Series, vol. 61, p. 618.

131 *BPP*, vol. 54 (1843), p. 421.

132 *BPP*, vol. 54 (1843), p. 411–13.

133 NA PC 7/5/486–9; cf. Hansard, Third Series, vol. 76, p. 1309.

134 NA PC 7/5/490–93. This applied also to fruit.

135 NA PC 7/5/490–93.

136 Ibid.; PC 7/5/442–3.

137 Ibid.

138 NA PC 7/5/493.

139 NA PC 7/5/511–12.

140 NA PC 7/5/537–9.

Council agreed to move a floating lazaretto, the *Menelaus*, from Stangate Creek to The Motherbank exclusively for the steamer service.[141] The Solent was also given a larger guard ship, a brig of ten guns, to accommodate extra officers and men.[142] To counterbalance costs, further cuts were made at Milford Haven, where at least one lazaretto had to be surrendered to the dockyard at Pembroke, and one mate, one purser, three mariners and two boys lost their jobs.[143]

The elusive conference

Another result of Bowring's speech was that it rekindled the mood for international consensus. On 27 June 1843 Aberdeen asked the British Ambassadors in Paris (Lord Cowley) and Vienna (Sir Robert Gordon) to suggest an interim agreement between Britain, France and Austria, based on the abortive French programme of 1838.[144] Once these powers had 'come to an understanding … as to their own views and wishes', the Italian states could be invited to participate, with Austria, which had the most influence in Italy, taking the lead role in the conference.[145] Russia, said Aberdeen, should also be included from her international status, and because the debate would cover the Black Sea as well as the Mediterranean.[146] The venue could perhaps be Genoa. The French were the first to respond via Guizot, the Minister of Foreign Affairs. He declared himself in favour but felt the conference should be held in Paris.[147] Aberdeen was amenable to that, as long as the Austrians agreed, but Metternich was slow to respond. Guessing that the venue was an obstacle, Guizot backed down and agreed to Genoa if Metternich preferred it.[148]

But it was proving very difficult to discover the Austrian position. In March 1844 Aberdeen wrote impatiently to Gordon for news, but it was late May before Metternich declared his hand.[149] He wanted, in effect, a moratorium of six months before any conference, which should be in Vienna, took place.[150] During that interval, Metternich wanted information gathered from doctors and quarantine officials on three points: minimum and maximum detention periods for passengers and crew; the same for goods; and the best way to disinfect goods susceptible to contagion.[151] Only plague should be on the agenda. The reaction to this from Pym was that the published replies he had already received from nearly 20 doctors in Constantinople,

141 NA PC 7/5/560–67.
142 NA PC 7/5/557.
143 NA PC 7/5/550, 576.
144 *BPP*, vol. 45 (1846), pp. 445–6.
145 Ibid.
146 Ibid.
147 *BPP*, vol. 45 (1846), p. 447.
148 *BPP*, vol. 45 (1846), p. 448.
149 *BPP*, vol. 45 (1846), pp. 449–50.
150 *BPP*, vol. 45 (1846), p. 450.
151 Ibid.

Smyrna, Alexandria and Cairo satisfied most of Metternich's requirements and the rest could be settled by evidence taken at the conference.[152]

On 13 October 1844 Pym set out to visit the main Mediterranean lazarettos to examine regulations, practice and tariffs.[153] This was more to make Government aware of the current position than to meet any of Metternich's desiderata, and it arose after further pressure from Bowring in another major parliamentary speech. The motion this time, proposed on 23 July, was that the House approved of the various relaxations of the quarantine laws, and urged further concessions at home and abroad.[154] This was a speech no less monumental than the first, making the same medley of arguments both anti-contagionist and anti-quarantine. There was extra emphasis on the incompatibility of quarantine with 'an age of philosophical investigation', and an insistence that detention should last no longer than the period during which plague might be dormant. Bowring contended that this period was 'pretty generally allowed even by contagionists, not to exceed fifteen days'. That point reverted to his previous speech, where he had argued that the length of the voyage should always be deducted from the period of quarantine, and would in most cases make quarantine unnecessary. But Europe was going in the wrong direction. The Board of Health at Marseilles were not accepting any clean bills of health from Egypt or Syria; and from other parts of the Ottoman Empire, a year and a day had to elapse from the last case of plague before the Board would grant free pratique. It was a powerful irony that the Levant was now adopting the sanitary regulations so long practised in the West. 'We sometimes boast', remarked Bowring, 'of the return we make to the East, for the favours our forefathers received from those regions. Our last good gift was the curse of the Quarantine Laws'.

The reply on behalf of Government was from Gladstone, as President of the Board of Trade, who spoke at some length.[155] It was as much the intention of the present administration, assured Gladstone, to tackle quarantine as it had been of the last. But while consultation with foreign powers would continue, it should not be forgotten that unilateral decisions were dangerous and 'might be productive of evil effects on the minds of foreigners' who might retaliate against British shipping. Despite Bowring's passionate case for non-contagion, Gladstone would not admit that the argument was won, although he conceded that the majority were inclined to accept it. He then went into some detail about subsisting quarantine arrangements in Britain and elsewhere and explained the recent initiative for an international conference, and the gist of the responses from France and Austria. Gladstone differed here from Aberdeen, in that he suggested to the House that the start of the conference was merely being delayed for six months, and 'he entertained sanguine hopes' for

152 *BPP*, vol. 45 (1846), pp. 456–7. The replies had been published in *BPP*, vol. 54 (1843), pp. 413–583, as 'Queries and Answers Relative to the Contagion of the Plague'.

153 *BPP*, vol. 45 (1846), p. 457.

154 Hansard, Third Series, vol. 76, pp. 1292–1308, from which remaining references in this paragraph are taken (cf. *Journal of the House of Commons* [*JHC*], vol. 91 [1844], p. 531).

155 Hansard, Third Series, vol. 76, pp. 1308–10, from which remaining references in this paragraph are taken until otherwise stated.

further relaxations in quarantine by the next session of Parliament. Joseph Hume, who had made no contribution after Bowring's previous speech, welcomed the tone of Gladstone's comments.[156]

Given such a positive reply from the President of the Board of Trade, it was not surprising that on 1 April 1845 Bowring returned to the House to ask what progress had been made.[157] It fell to Sir George Clerk, Vice-President of the Board of Trade, to put a brave face on the 'reasonable proposition' of the Austrian Government that the conference should be delayed while a report was awaited 'from medical officers appointed by themselves [that is, the Austrians]'.[158] But Aberdeen knew that Metternich had no intention of organizing anything. It was with some impatience that he informed the Board of Trade a few days later that the Austrians were merely making the condition on which a conference might be held.[159] On 16 June 1845 Pym reported to the Board of Trade on the findings of his recent journey, but they offered no new facts for the appeasement of Bowring.[160] Pym thought the first decision by any conference should be whether or not the plague was contagious, 'without entering into a tedious and contradictory examination of medical men'.[161] The problem for Government was that the replies to Pym's questionnaire of 1839 tended to support the doctrine of contagion, while those of the correspondents of Holroyd and Bowring were decidedly against it. It appeared to Aberdeen, in September, that there was only way forward: leaving aside the question of contagion, he thought the detailed statistics and other information about quarantine recently collected by Pym on his travels should be sent *in toto* to Metternich, in the hope that they would be regarded as the groundwork deemed necessary before a conference could be convened.[162]

It was soon evident that Metternich was unimpressed. Before the end of 1845 the British embassy in Vienna twice reported that Pym's papers were allegedly still in the hands of the Austrian Departments of the Interior and Finance.[163] On 28 March 1846 a frustrated Board of Trade asked Aberdeen to press for a response, but it was June before Gordon could relay any constructive message to London.[164] Metternich was polite about Pym's researches but had a memorandum about quarantine of his own, from a Dr Gobbi, which he wished the British to consider.[165] Although not opposed to the idea of a conference, Metternich had a different proposition: the Austrian regulations, in his view, were the most liberal in Europe and if other countries would agree to adopt them – and France had apparently indicated its willingness – any conference would be unnecessary.[166]

---

156 Hansard, Third Series, vol. 76, p. 1310.

157 Hansard, Third Series, vol. 78, p. 1316.

158 Ibid.

159 *BPP*, vol. 45 (1846), p. 456. The letter was actually from Canning, but gave Aberdeen's view.

160 *BPP*, vol. 45 (1846), pp. 457–62.

161 Ibid.

162 *BPP*, vol. 45 (1846), p. 462.

163 *BPP*, vol. 45 (1846), pp. 484–5.

164 *BPP*, vol. 45 (1846), p. 487.

165 *BPP*, vol. 45 (1846), pp. 568–78.

166 *BPP*, vol. 45 (1846), p. 567.

Palmerston was now Foreign Secretary again, in succession to Aberdeen. He sent Gobbi's paper to the Board of Trade who referred it to Pym, and 'confidentially' to Dr Gavin Milroy, for an opinion.[167] This marked the first involvement with Government of Milroy, who had recently published an essay of a length and thoroughness which outdid even Bowring, on the 'absurdly foolish and most ridiculous principles' underpinning quarantine, and the overwhelming evidence, to his mind, that the plague was non-contagious.[168] The intention in Government was apparently to have recourse to a disinterested anti-contagionist viewpoint to counterbalance the opinions of Pym, who remained loyal to his long-held belief that plague was contagious. But as regards Gobbi, Pym and Milroy arrived at the same conclusion. Gobbi was arguing for more lazarettos along the Turkish coasts and frontiers, to be paid for by the four great powers, which should result within a few years in the virtual extermination of plague in the Levant, and therefore the abolition of quarantine in those parts. Pym and Milroy argued that more lazarettos would be in vain when only a greater attention to cleanliness and sanitation in Turkish cities would rid the Levant of disease.[169] And if that was really Gobbi's view, the Britons could not understand why the same course of action was not being argued for Egypt. It was clear to the British Government that the paper had no future and, on 14 May 1847, Palmerston told the Austrian ambassador in London that Britain would not contribute to the suggested funding.[170] Metternich would not have been pleased with the rejection, and that was effectively the end of the second attempt at a conference.

Quarantine in disrepute

Another comment by Milroy was that Dr Gobbi's plan was 'nearly the same' as one promoted by Dr Mapurgo, from the Board of Health at Constantinople, to the Royal Academy of Medicine in France.[171] This latter body, influenced by Metternich's conditional agreement to a conference, had appointed a commission in August 1844 to enquire into all aspects of plague and quarantine.[172] Composed of doctors and scientists, the commission reported a year later and read their findings at a series of meetings during the spring of 1846. These were virtually reproduced by Milroy, who was in complete agreement with the anti-contagionist sentiments.[173] In his report to the Board of Trade about Gobbi, Milroy added that it was 'an utter fallacy' to assume plague was contagious, when all the evidence indicated that it was actually infectious.[174] This was a rare literal distinction between the methods by which the

167 *BPP*, vol. 45 (1846), pp. 578–9.

168 Milroy, *Quarantine and the Plague*, p. 5. The book is a valuable commentary on contemporary events, publications and ideas.

169 *BPP*, vol. 49 (1847), pp. 578–82.

170 *BPP*, vol. 49 (1847), p. 583.

171 *BPP*, vol. 49 (1847), pp. 580–82.

172 Milroy, *Quarantine and the Plague*, p. 15.

173 Milroy, *Quarantine and the Plague*, pp. 19–61.

174 *BPP*, vol. 49 (1847), pp. 580–82.

disease was transmitted, and followed the French line (not that it was very original) which argued that plague was transmitted by atmospheric conditions.

In London, the whole issue of contagion and quarantine was suddenly out of control. The French had succeeded in producing what the British had deemed impossible, which was a quick, coherent, wide-ranging and authoritative report, which bore little evidence of medical schism, which was the bitter legacy of Maclean. Indeed, to the consternation of Government, long reliant on the wisdom of Pym, it seemed as though Maclean had been right all along. This background discomfort was sharply aggravated by two unrelated incidents, both of which brought quarantine into deep disfavour. The less serious of these occurred in Alexandria, where Barnett had failed to improve the Board of Health to a standard acceptable to the West.

In March 1845 Barnett complained to Aberdeen that he could not prevent the capricious imposition of quarantine on mail steamers arriving from Beirut with clean bills of health.[175] But as the months passed it became evident that the delays of ten to fifteen days had not been instituted or sanctioned by the Superior Board of Health in Turkey. They were being imposed by the Pasha himself in retaliation for the absence of free pratique for his own ships at Constantinople. On 20 September 1845 Barnett reported to Aberdeen that he had confronted the Pasha and warned him that British masters would be advised not to pay the quarantine dues, which came to around £15.[176] The Pasha, wrote Barnett, 'replied that it was a matter of indifference to him whether the duties were paid or not'.[177] From then on, matters got steadily worse. In March 1846 Barnett gave formal notice to the Board of Health at Alexandria that he considered all British and Ionian vessels from Syria to be in free pratique, and the 'Intendance Sanitaire' would be held responsible for any obstacles or hindrances.[178] However unwelcome had been quarantine in the Bosporus, it had at least proved amenable to practical solutions which were unforthcoming in Egypt.

The other incident, which had the most far-reaching consequences, concerned HMS *Eclair*.[179] In November 1844 this warship left England for Sierra Leone where many of her crew fell victim to yellow fever. Despite her condition, she was given free pratique at Boa Vista, one of the Cape Verde Islands, in the following August. The men went ashore but in the summer heat, in primitive and insanitary conditions, the sickness only got worse. In September the *Eclair* departed for Madeira but was refused pratique. On 28 September 1845 she arrived off Portsmouth and was detained at The Motherbank in a pitiful condition. There had been 62 deaths up to then, others were dying, and another 23 men were ill.[180] Sir John Richardson, physician to Haslar Hospital in Gosport, boarded the ship and recommended the immediate removal of

175 *BPP*, vol. 45 (1846), p. 455.

176 *BPP*, vol. 45 (1846), pp. 475–6.

177 Ibid.

178 *BPP*, vol. 45 (1846), p. 488.

179 Of many accounts of this episode, perhaps the clearest is in *Edinburgh Review*, vol. 98 (1853), pp. 208–15, from which most facts below are taken.

180 The figures are from *The Times*, quoted by Bowring in Parliament (Hansard, Third Series, vol. 86, p. 877).

the crew to a clean and well-ventilated wing of his hospital. Pym, however, would not hear of it. He advised the Privy Council

> that the disease from which the crew of the *Eclair* have suffered is one against which Europe generally has established a quarantine, and being aware of the disastrous consequences to the mercantile interests of this country, in the event of the *Eclair* being admitted to pratique … I object most decidedly against the release of the *Eclair* as well as against the landing of the crew.[181]

The warship was ordered, in the state she was, to sail on to Stangate Creek for the due process of quarantine. It was 2 October before the *Eclair* limped into the Medway, and the crew were another six days in their wretched imprisonment before removal to a lazaretto. Another five deaths had occurred before that removal, and two more followed on 8 October. One of these was the pilot who had embarked at Portsmouth.

Reaction was furious and immediate. Sir William Burnett, on behalf of the navy, rounded on Pym for his inhumanity, arguing that the sickness was only 'the usual remittent fever of the [African] coast' and represented no danger in England.[182] But the exact nature of the disease was contested. Pym was convinced it was yellow fever, in which he considered himself an expert, and the diagnosis of 'a fever, between the yellow and the black' had appeared in *The Times*.[183] But the real debate was about compassion. Surely fears of commercial retaliation in Europe could never justify such hideous death and suffering. Decades of pent-up frustration over quarantine spurred the navy to build on their moral advantage. Pym sought other ways to justify his action, protesting that the voyage to Stangate Creek was inevitable, as 'boisterous' autumn weather often made communication with The Motherbank difficult.[184] Burnett sent Dr J. McWilliam to Boa Vista to investigate the nature of the sickness which had ravaged the *Eclair*, and continued to cause many deaths on the island after the ship had sailed.[185] McWilliam concluded that the disease was aggravated by the close proximity of the victims 'in a miasmatic and impure atmosphere' and would ordinarily pose little risk.[186] The discomfort of Pym was all the greater when, despite his precautionary sacrifice of human life, ships arriving at Naples and Ancona from ports on the south coast of England were treated to 21 days' quarantine as if the men had been allowed ashore.[187]

---

181 General Board of Health, *Report on Quarantine. Presented to both Houses of Parliament by Command of Her Majesty* (London, 1849), p. 82.

182 C. Lloyd & J.L.S. Coulter, *Medicine and the Navy, 1200–1900. Volume IV: 1815–1900* (Edinburgh & London, 1963), p. 168.

183 Hansard, Third Series, vol. 86, p. 877.

184 General Board of Health (1849), p. 75.

185 J.O. McWilliam, *Observations on that Portion of the Second Report on Quarantine by the General Board of Health which relates to the Yellow Fever Epidemy on board H.M.S. Éclair* … (London, 1852), p. 1.

186 Hansard, Third Series, vol. 91, p. 151.

187 General Board of Health (1849), p. 83. A summary and timetable of the retaliatory quarantines is given in NA PC 6/10 *sub* 1845.

With quarantine so much in the limelight, it was not unexpected that Bowring moved another address to the Queen on the subject of quarantine. It might have surprised many, however, that the tone of his motion, on 19 May 1846, was not more aggressive. He merely requested copies of correspondence with foreign governments since the last return and moved 'that this House will see with pleasure such relaxations in the existing system' as might be compatible with safeguarding public health.[188] But this was no more than a veneer of good manners and his speech hit hard. He began with the *Eclair* and regretted that the official papers relating to the incident, which he had requested in January, were not yet available to the House.[189] Although less blunt than Burnett, he mourned the loss of life in a ship which 'filled with the miasmata of disease' was nothing more than 'a lazar house'. Widespread contagion, he argued, should not have been feared. He then moved rapidly to the question of plague, in which he felt more comfortable. Thanks to Milroy, Bowring had to hand the results of the enquiry by the Royal Academy of Medicine in France. He took the House through their conclusions in detail: plague arose in the Levant from 'the spontaneous action of local and atmospheric causes'; progress of the disease could be controlled and even prevented by better general sanitation; plague did not lie latent for more than eight days and could not be conveyed by merchandise; and 'plague patients alone could create a focus of infection'. This was very much in line with his conclusion about yellow fever and made a persuasive case against quarantine.

The motion was seconded by Joseph Hume, who made his normal point that quarantine was an impediment to free trade, as the delays were 'expensive, and often ruinous'.[190] Irrespective of commercial losses, he reckoned the implementation of quarantine cost the country £120,000 a year.[191] It was again Sir George Clerk who responded, and again there was no inclination in Government to obstruct the motion. Indeed, Clerk conceded that 'apprehensions which long existed in this country about the supposed contagious character of this disease [that is, plague], were losing ground'.[192] But Clerk ended with the warning that British commercial interests in the Mediterranean basin 'required that we should deal with the matter judiciously and deliberately'.[193] Later in 1846, when Clerk had been succeeded by Milner Gibson, quarantine was again before the Commons. Brownlow Layard, an Irish army captain, asked if the report of Pym's Continental journey could be made available to the House, and called for an official enquiry into the nature of the fever which had devastated the *Eclair*, and whether it 'was transmissible from persons

188 Hansard, Third Series, vol. 86, pp. 877–81, from which remaining references in this paragraph are taken, unless otherwise stated.

189 For the request of papers, see *JHC* (1846, Part 1), pp. 8, 39, 798. They were eventually presented on 30 May.

190 Hansard, Third Series, vol. 86, p. 881

191 Ibid. In a later debate, Hume claimed that quarantine cost Britain £190,000 a year to implement, which was less than a tenth 'of the expense to which the country was exposed by them, in consequence of the injury they did to … commerce …' (Hansard, Third Series, vol. 91, p. 159).

192 Hansard, Third Series, vol. 86, p. 881.

193 Ibid.

labouring under it to others in health'.[194] Gibson responded evasively that Pym's report to the Board of Trade was already in the public domain. As to the second point, he was even more elusive: Pym and Burnett had already investigated the fever but disagreed as to whether it was infectious (he did not say contagious). 'With regard to what the Government might think fit to do upon a future occasion, it was not for him to say'.[195]

Under such pressure, Pym was compelled to make concessions to the anti-quarantine lobby. Against the battery of belief that the plague was not, under most circumstances, a contagious disease, he was outgunned to the point of surrender. The battle to maintain quarantine would continue, but the main front would be limited to yellow fever where Pym would eventually make a final stand. The year 1847 witnessed the piecemeal dismantling of quarantine for plague. Bowring hung on whispered words from the agencies of Government, consolidating each step towards success. On 5 March he asked Gibson in the House what changes to quarantine had recently taken place, or were likely.[196] He was gratified by the answer, which he doubtless knew already, that all ships from Turkey, with non-enumerated goods and clean bills would henceforth be exempt from quarantine. Two weeks later Bowring rose again in the Commons to move for the production of recent correspondence on the quarantine laws.[197] Given the victory in terms of plague which now seemed imminent, the speech was curiously long and overfull of mortality in distant lands. Reference to McWilliam suggested that yellow fever might also be the target for Bowring's reforming crusade, but he turned quickly to Milroy, whom he recommended to the House, and plague remained the focus of attack. Bowring was triumphant that the Marseilles Board of Health, which he criticized as 'the very seat of sinister interests and foolish prejudices', now admitted that quarantine needed changing.[198] Gibson replied only briefly. The correspondence could be produced, and quarantine regulations in Britain had already 'been so reduced as in many cases to make them almost nominal'.[199]

The reduction continued. On 17 May 1847 Pym informed Gibson that Turkey had been free of epidemic plague for eight years and Egypt and Syria for nearly three.[200] Was it not time for the Board of Trade to treat clean-bill ships from the Levant, even with enumerated cargoes, the same way as those carrying grain or fruit? Marseilles had made just this concession on 29 April. The Board agreed with alacrity, and on the following day the Privy Council abolished all quarantine for ships from the Levant, whatever their cargo, as long as they carried clean bills and a healthy crew.[201] By coincidence, it was also 17 May when Bowring asked Gibson, in the House, if any new regulations were in mind, following reports 'that a considerable change was to

194 Hansard, Third Series, vol. 88, p. 359.

195 Hansard, Third Series, vol. 88, pp. 359–60.

196 Hansard, Third Series, vol. 90, pp. 948–9.

197 Hansard, Third Series, vol. 91, pp. 150–59.

198 Hansard, Third Series, vol. 91, p. 158.

199 Hansard, Third Series, vol. 91, p. 159.

200 *BPP*, vol. 60 (1847–48), p. 509.

201 Ibid.

take place'.[202] Gibson could not anticipate the Order in Council, but confirmed that new rules were being considered.[203] On 14 June, in response to yet another question from Bowring, he informed the House succinctly that 'the modifications amounted to this – that ships with clean bills were now admitted to immediate pratique, from whatever part of the world they came, and with whatever cargo they were laden'.[204] If quarantine were an edifice, it had lost a wall.

The General Board of Health

With so much attention to plague, and more than a little to yellow fever, it might seem that the ravages of cholera had been forgotten. But that was not the case. On 22 September 1846 the Foreign Office reported to the Privy Council that cholera had broken out in Persia.[205] From then on, not a week went by without a further warning from a British consul that the dreaded disease was creeping westwards. By 1847 it had reached Tabriz, then Baghdad, Mosul and Erzerum. During March it was killing in Syria and in July it laid waste in the Caucasus. The route towards Poland and Russia lay open, and the first case in Moscow was reported on 20 October. The Privy Council weighed the dangers of a second pandemic against the lessons learnt from the first. Cholera had not proved an indiscriminate killer and it could be contained by elementary attention to cleanliness and ventilation. Any decision as to the role of quarantine, ineffective in the first pandemic, was postponed while the administration of Lord Russell grappled with the wider questions of health and sanitation. It so happened that when the second pandemic reached Britain, during 1848, Parliament was at last agreed that a countrywide, albeit permissive, legislation to improve the living conditions of the working class should no longer be delayed.

The road to the Public Health Act of 1848 had been long and rough, running parallel to the highway to quarantine reform, with no association between them. But that lack of contact was about to change. Agitation for improvement to the noisome condition of urban slums had intensified since the first pandemic, inspiring to some extent the Poor Law Amendment Act of 1834, and more directly a Report on the Sanitary Condition of the Labouring Population of Great Britain in 1842.[206] This report was followed quickly by two others from the Royal Commission on the Health of Towns, presented to Parliament in June 1844 and February 1845. Moves by Government to introduce health legislation failed in both 1846 and 1847 following concerns about land ownership and civil liberties, and only the Liverpool Sanitary Act of the former year survived as an earnest of ministerial intentions. In 1848, following the publication of Dr T. Southwood Smith's powerful *Address to the Working Classes …* , Lord Morpeth again took the question of sanitation before

202 Hansard, Third Series, vol. 92, p. 951.

203 Ibid.

204 Hansard, Third Series, vol. 93, p. 472.

205 NA PC 6/10 (by date), from which all references in this paragraph, relating to the progress of cholera, are taken.

206 Most facts in this paragraph are condensed from W.M. Frazer, *A History of English Public Health* (London, 1950), pp. 33–49.

Parliament, and his Bill, introduced in 10 February 1848, received the royal assent on 31 August.[207] The long interval testified to the strength of opposition.

This Public Health Act of 1848, the precursor of many similarly titled Victorian statutes, allowed Local Boards of Health to be established (except in London) to take charge of aspects of local government connected, some rather indirectly, with aspects of health and sanitation. The Act also created a General Board of Health composed of Lord Morpeth (who soon became Earl of Carlisle), Lord Ashley (who later became Earl of Shaftesbury) and a salaried member, Edwin Chadwick.[208] It was a further sign of the irrelevance of quarantine to the domestic debate about public health that such an influential reformer as Chadwick, formerly prominent among poor-law and sanitary commissions, falls only now within the compass of this work. The same might be said of Southwood Smith, who joined the Board on 5 October as their medical member. The reason why issues of quarantine and public health suddenly came together was the second pandemic of cholera. The extent to which that imminent disease facilitated the progress of the 1848 Act is problematical, but there is no doubt that it formed the immediate agenda for the General Board of Health.

It was probably with surprise and annoyance that the Privy Council read a long letter from the General Board, dated as early as 9 November 1848, complaining that quarantine caused suffering in mind and body.[209] Indeed, the Board would have written it sooner, they admitted, had they not been taking urgent precautions against cholera. The substance of their complaint was the way quarantine was conducted in the Humber estuary and to a lesser extent at Stangate Creek. Medical opinion set great store by the theory that 'anxiety and terror act more powerfully in predisposing to cholera than to any other disease'. Yet they had clear evidence of people falling sick on voyages from St Petersburg and Hamburg and being imprisoned on their ship in Whitebooth Roads, seven miles from Hull, in one case with the corpse of a passenger who had been dead for eight days. The revenue cutter serving as a quarantine hulk had no medical personnel on board, and if its boat was sent to Hull for assistance, the return journey might take six hours in adverse conditions, and if wind and tide were both contrary it might not be possible at all. The General Board asked the Council to consider 'whether any evidence can be adduced to show that the public safety requires a vessel in Quarantine should be placed at the distance of eight, four, or even one mile from a port'.

This was not the first communication from the General Board of Health to the Privy Council. On 17 October 1848 the Board confirmed that Asiatic cholera existed in Great Britain but was not yet an epidemic.[210] Learning this news, the Council took the surprising view that quarantine precautions were no longer necessary against cholera, and there was no need to report or detain infected ships, and those under

207 11 & 12 Vic., c.63.

208 Frazer, pp. 56–7.

209 Published in General Board of Health (1849), pp. 131–43, from which all references in this paragraph are taken.

210 NA CUST 58/307/30.

detention could be immediately released.[211] Evidently Pym had confidence in the opinion of Milroy, whose book arguing that quarantine could not prevent cholera had been published in 1847.[212] But this was a brave decision on the part of the Council, by no means followed on the Continent, and not entirely consistent with earlier policy as the epidemic approached. In June 1848 they had initially been confident: if a vessel should arrive with a foul bill, on account of cholera, it might be immediately released without medical visit, provided there had been no case of cholera on board for the previous ten days.[213] But by two Orders in early October, the rules were tightened: the quarantine period for steamers and sailing ships coming from cholera-infected areas was fixed at six days from the date of sailing, after which all healthy people could land; and any persons suffering from cholera had to stay on board for six days after they had been pronounced convalescent.[214] The body of anyone who died on board had to be weighted and disposed of at sea, an instruction which, on the evidence from the Humber recited above, had not been issued soon enough to prevent some harrowing experiences. It can be assumed that the General Board lobbied hard for the concession which followed.

For Customs officers, particularly those who remembered the quarantine between English ports of the first pandemic, the new policy announced on 17 October must have seemed strange indeed. In February 1849 a Russian barque arrived at The Motherbank, bound for the Mediterranean, with a cargo of coal from Newcastle.[215] Three of her crew had died of cholera before she reached the quarantine station, and another died after arrival. Two more men were ill, but thought likely to recover. The Superintendent of Quarantine noted in disbelief: 'I have an order not to detain Vessels arriving with Cholera on board consequently she is not under my directions and … [the] surgeon at Ryde attends on the sick'.[216] For the Privy Council, there was soon disbelief of another kind. As they had indulged the anti-contagionist lobby over cholera, the paper from the General Board pointing out the hardships and inconsistencies of quarantine, especially in the Humber, would hardly have been welcome. But that was nothing compared with the Board's next offering: an anti-contagionist polemic denouncing the futility of quarantine and suggesting new procedures to supersede it.

This document was a printed *Report on Quarantine* addressed to the Queen, on whose instructions (via the Privy Council) it was presented to Parliament on 11 May 1849.[217] Running to 128 pages without the appendices, the *Report* was an astonishing feat in such a short time and testified to the strength and unanimity

211 Ibid.

212 G. Milroy, *The Cholera not to be Arrested by Quarantine: a Brief Historical Sketch of the Great Epidemic of 1817, and its Invasions of Europe in 1831–2 & 1847 …* (London, 1847).

213 NA CUST 58/307/18–19. On 13 September 1848 the Privy Council ordered that if a ship arrived on which cholera had occurred, she had to remain in quarantine until the bedding and clothing of the deceased had been thoroughly immersed in water (CUST 58/307/21).

214 NA CUST 58/307/27–9.

215 NA CUST 58/307/35.

216 Ibid.

217 *JHC*, vol. 49 (1849–50), p. 288.

of feeling among its authors. The title, however, was a slight misnomer, in that the procedures of quarantine were little discussed, and the intention was more to discredit the principles upon which those procedures were founded. Also, the title did not make it immediately clear that the *Report* was produced in the context of cholera, rather than plague. The doctrine of contagion was rejected. Much was made of 'epidemic atmosphere' and the subtle effects of temperature, electricity and magnetism (which the authors admitted were not wholly understood) and the onset of 'premonitory symptoms'.[218] Drawing on facts and opinions throughout the long history of anti-contagionist belief, including evidence to the parliamentary enquiries of 1819 and 1824, the Board were further encouraged by the significant findings of their contemporaries. The opinions of Bowring, Milroy and Holroyd were being happily confirmed by the latest research of Professor Sigmund of Vienna, who was recommending to the Austrian Government a radical curtailment of quarantine which would include its removal from all merchandise.[219]

The Board put their full faith in improved drainage, paving and ventilation, of which quarantine took no account. 'Blindly intent on accomplishing an impossible object, it overlooks the circumstances on which the existence and extension of disease really depend; and after the experience of centuries has shown the inutility of the securities it offers, it still proposes to go on reposing implicit confidence in them and in them only'.[220] The solution put forward by the Board was the abandonment of the entire process and the substitution of sanitary regulations. These were not so much aimed at checking the spread of disease as alleviating conditions where disease existed, especially on ships. The Board had a deep concern for the foul conditions endured at sea, especially by crew, and sought to build on their own precedent of April 1849, when they instructed the civic authority in Aberdeen to board and examine an infected ship and treat it no differently from an infected house.[221] As one appendix to their *Report*, the Board included a 'Draft Order for Sanitary Regulations proposed to be enforced on Merchant Seamen Vessels for the prevention of the spread of epidemic diseases amongst Passengers and Seamen arriving in Port'.[222]

In the aftermath of such a radical *Report*, many parliamentarians and shipowners no doubt feared the kind of backlash from Europe which had followed the half-hearted attempt at reform in 1825. This was, after all, the opinion of a Government agency rather than some doctor or politician on some personal crusade. It was exactly this official status which worried the College of Physicians, whose contagionist policies had long been influencing Pym and the Privy Council. *The Lancet* targeted Southwood Smith as the compiler of the 'gibberish' which had influenced his lay colleagues.[223] But on the Continent, the passage of a quarter of a century had taken

218 These were summarized as 'terrestro-aërial causes' (General Board of Health (1849), p. 19).

219 General Board of Health (1849), p. 78.

220 General Board of Health (1849), p. 16.

221 The Board's Order is reproduced in General Board of Health (1849), p. 156.

222 General Board of Health (1849), pp. 167–9.

223 J.C. McDonald, 'The history of quarantine in Britain during the 19th century', *Bulletin of the History of Medicine*, 25 (Baltimore, 1951), 33.

much of the fight out of Mediterranean Boards of Health. The *Report* was translated into French and Italian and was well received in France, Austria and Russia.[224] Anti-contagionism seemed all but invincible.

International Sanitary Conference, Paris, 1851

It caused some satisfaction at Westminster that, following the availability of the 1849 *Report* in Europe, 'the eyes of the French Government were opened to the uselessness of many of the precautions they had theretofore enforced ...'[225] To be fair to the French, their eyes had been opened some time earlier, but it was undoubtedly the *Report* which broke the diplomatic indecision as to what to do next. In the spring of 1851 it fell to Palmerston, well into his second period as Foreign Secretary, to receive a suggestion from the French that an international conference on quarantine should at last go ahead, attended by those countries which had interests around or within the Mediterranean. Parliament were eager that Palmerston should take it seriously, and he reassured the House that Government were 'very anxious' to participate in the conference, having 'appointed a medical man and a consular officer to attend it'.[226] These words suggested proposals less flamboyant than those of 1838: Malta and the Ionian Islands were no longer canvassed directly, and it was evidently felt inappropriate in London for Pym to attend, probably on the grounds that his contagionist leanings would no longer be welcome. Instead, Britain was represented by Dr John Sutherland, Inspector to the General Board of Health, and Sir Anthony Perrier, the British consul at Brest.[227] In total, there were representatives from twelve states: Austria, the Two Sicilies, Spain, Rome, France, Britain, Greece, Portugal, Russia, Sardinia, Tuscany and Turkey.[228]

The conference convened in Paris in July 1851 and lasted into the following year. It became the stuff of legend that the delegates were too engrossed in their discussions to seek either protection or adjournment while gunfire raked the boulevards during the civic disorder of 4 December.[229] The results of the conference were important as a statement of international unanimity and intent, but quarantine was not to be dismantled overnight. There was even an inherent contradiction in the findings. The principle was conceded that sanitary precautions should supersede the compulsion and isolation of quarantine, but many delegates had been sent with instructions that quarantine was to be amended and not abolished. One journal commented darkly that 'there are unfortunately other and latent considerations connected with quarantine besides the mere question of the public health'.[230]

---

224 cf. comments in Hansard, Third Series, vol. 121, p. 1268, and *Edinburgh Review*, vol. 96 (1852), p. 432.

225 Hansard, Third Series, vol. 121, p. 1268.

226 Hansard, Third Series, vol. 118, p. 567.

227 *Edinburgh Review*, vol. 96 (1852), p. 434.

228 *Edinburgh Review*, vol. 96 (1852), p. 432; Hansard, Third Series, vol. 121, p. 1269.

229 *Edinburgh Review*, vol. 96 (1852), p. 432.

230 *Edinburgh Review*, vol. 96 (1852), p. 434.

There were, nevertheless, significant steps taken towards reform, and the French were given due credit.[231] Quarantine was to be reduced and standardized throughout the Mediterranean, although it could still apply to cholera and yellow fever as well as to plague. Suspected bills were abolished and the issue of foul bills made subject to greater control. All clean bills would be given immediate pratique. The concept of susceptible and non-susceptible goods was abolished, although cargoes like wool, silk, rags and skins would still need depuration in the event of an epidemic. The cleansing of cotton, hemp and flax was made optional. Much was made of the incompatibility of quarantine with the advantages of propulsion by steam, but no stronger remedy could be suggested than the appointment of medical officers to steamers carrying passengers. As for the introduction of sanitary measures, there was agreement that the sick should be cared for in proper establishments, and that measures of general hygiene should be applied in the same way to infected ships as they were to diseased ports.

In Britain, the outcome, for all its limitations, was judged 'commercially … next in importance to Free Trade'.[232] A dissenting view came from the Manchester Chamber of Commerce, who were impatient for something more radical, but the Mancunians were out of step with events.[233] Yellow fever was re-emerging as the greatest worry in British ports, while in Manchester, and indeed in Paris, quarantine was still being assessed primarily in the context of plague. The year 1852 witnessed the Privy Council in disarray as to how yellow fever should be dealt with. The somewhat complacent attitude which had traditionally been adopted, trusting that the disease could not propagate in the cool British climate, was no longer good enough for many politicians. This was because precautions still relied on some element of quarantine. While this was generally token, the *Eclair* incident had revealed that in a serious outbreak isolation could be long and merciless. Opinion was moving firmly towards sanitary measures, including the evacuation of a sickly ship, as the only humane response. This strength of feeling had little to do with the Paris conference, and more with a Report of the Central Board of Health of Jamaica, also in 1852, which concluded that quarantine in their island was 'an irksome encumbrance, interrupting commerce, obstructing national intercourse, perilling [*sic*] life, fostering and engendering disease, and squandering large sums of public revenue'.[234] Such sentiments, of course, had been voiced elsewhere and earlier, but not in a place so ravaged by yellow fever.

In Parliament, the mantle of Bowring in the Commons had been assumed by the Earl of St Germans in the Lords. On 28 May 1852 he moved for the production of the minutes of the Paris conference and regretted that Shaftesbury, as the

---

231 cf. Shaftesbury's comments to Parliament, 28 May 1852: 'They [the French] had not … attained all that was desirable, but a great deal had been done to remove the intolerable shackles which the quarantine system imposed upon commerce and social intercourse along the shores of the Mediterranean' (Hansard, Third Series, vol. 121, p. 1272). The fullest account of the conference (there called the 'International Quarantine Conference') is in *BPP*, vol. 60 (1860), pp. 186–9, with comments by Gavin Milroy.

232 *Edinburgh Review*, vol. 96 (1852), p. 434.

233 *Edinburgh Review*, vol. 98 (1853), p. 191.

234 *Edinburgh Review*, vol. 98 (1853), p. 192.

Chief Commissioner of the General Board of Health, had not already arranged their availability.[235] St Germans made a classic anti-contagionist speech, weak in historical accuracy but well informed on the opinions of the Academy of Medicine in Paris and more especially of the College of Physicians in New Orleans, who had shown that yellow fever was retreating south as sanitary measures improved in the north. Indeed, he was already well briefed on the Paris conference and wanted the Foreign Secretary to explain how the recommendations were being implemented. It was St Germans's belief that most of the states which had sent delegates to the conference 'were prepared to carry their recommendations still further than they had done, if public opinion were ripe for the change'. He went on to contrast the difference in treatment between two British warships, the *Arethusa* and the *Eclair*. The former had arrived in Plymouth in February 1852, with several men suffering from smallpox. But the *Arethusa* was not placed in quarantine. Instead, she was admitted to immediate pratique and the 12 sick sailors were transferred to the Royal Naval Hospital. Two of them died but no epidemic broke out in Plymouth. Having praised this brave and enlightened step, St Germans moved briefly into commercial issues of cost and depreciation. Finally, he asked Shaftesbury when the General Board intended to make a Third Report on Quarantine, this time centred on plague.

Shaftesbury was soothing, but non-committal about the Third Report. He outlined the results of the Paris conference and supported the request of St Germans for the production of papers.[236] But the new Foreign Secretary, the Earl of Malmesbury, was less enthusiastic and thought the problems of international agreement were still significant, with 'difficulties of a technical character', especially with the Italian states.[237] Britain was working towards a convention over quarantine with France, and possibly other countries, and it would be unusual to present papers to Parliament until such a convention were more precise. It was then agreed between Malmesbury and St Germans that only such papers would be produced as the former thought appropriate.[238] But on 19 November 1852 St Germans returned to the subject in a tone distinctly grumpy, as no papers had been produced.[239] Why was this? And had the convention been ratified? If it had not been, what were the obstacles? He reminded Malmesbury that an overhaul of quarantine procedures had been sought by successive Foreign Secretaries for the previous 16 years. He referred to an unfortunate impression 'abroad that persons interested personally in the retention of the quarantine system had prevailed upon … Government to recede from the position occupied by their predecessors'.

St Germans then accosted Lord Lonsdale, wondering why, on 2 September, the Privy Council had instructed the Customs Commissioners to detain under precautionary quarantine, for as long as seemed necessary, any ship carrying cholera

235 Hansard, Third Series, vol. 121, pp. 1267–72, from which remaining references in this paragraph are taken.

236 Hansard, Third Series, vol. 121, p. 1272.

237 Hansard, Third Series, vol. 121, pp. 1274–5.

238 Hansard, Third Series, vol. 121, p. 1275.

239 Hansard, Third Series, vol. 123, pp. 224–8, from which remaining references in this paragraph, and all in the next, are taken.

sufferers or on which cholera had been manifest within five days of arrival. This was a reversal of recent policy. As such severity was not the recommendation of the General Board of Health, on whose advice was it ordered? He could have assumed the answer was Pym, but St Germans was concerned for the rhetorical point. He also queried whether a passage in the same Order, which allowed healthy people 'free communication with the shore', actually allowed them to land, and whether medical facilities existed for persons who fell sick while quarantine was in progress. This brought him to the specific case of the steamer *La Plata* from St Thomas, which had very recently arrived at Southampton in the grip of yellow fever. Had she now been freed from quarantine? If not, what arrangements had been made for the reception of the sick? The *Arethusa* must be the model for the future, and not the *Eclair*.

The first apologist was Malmesbury, who cautioned St Germans against believing 'that contagion was altogether impossible ...'[240] The Government were working towards a European convention on quarantine, but progress was slow and erratic. Portugal, Sardinia, France and probably Russia were prepared to sign along with Britain, but the Italian states, Spain and Austria 'either refused their signature ... , or else put forth such difficulties ... as they had not been able to overcome'.[241] Lonsdale spoke next, but was much less comfortable.[242] Quarantine had been ordered in September because of 'malignant cholera' in the Baltic, and on the advice of 'one of the most skilful physicians of the present day' – a circumlocution for Pym. He sought to make a virtue of the Order by pointing out that, in limiting detention on board to those who were sick, it was in effect a mitigation of the 1825 Act which had empowered the Customs Commissioners 'to send to any quarantine station any vessel arriving from a foreign port with any infected person on board'. Lonsdale said he would not enter into a debate with St Germans on the subject of contagion, but in fact the two peers jousted with evident ill-feeling. It was remarkable that Lonsdale defended his case with such vigour, arguing 'that not merely three-fourths but nine-tenths of the [medical] profession advised all who consulted them to avoid contagion'.[243] That was an unusual speech to hear in Parliament in the mid-nineteenth century.

A propos of the *La Plata*, Lonsdale lacked the courage of his conviction. He claimed to have had details of the case only that morning (although they were known to St Germans) and had immediately consulted with Pym.[244] The sick would be 'relieved from quarantine'.[245] It would appear that, sensing trouble, Lonsdale had asked Pym to go down to Southampton and find a reason why the ship should be released. St Germans still wanted to know whether there was any accommodation for the sick on shore, and his exchanges with a stubborn Lonsdale, backed by a patronising Malmesbury, became increasingly sharp. But St Germans was supported

240 Hansard, Third Series, vol. 123, pp. 228–9.

241 Ibid.

242 Hansard, Third Series, vol. 123, pp. 229–30, from which remaining refs. in this paragraph are taken until otherwise stated.

243 Hansard, Third Series, vol. 123, p. 229.

244 Hansard, Third Series, vol. 123, p. 230.

245 Ibid.

by Lord Stanley of Alderley and Lord Wharncliffe, and the anti-contagionists got the better of the contest.[246] The House of Lords went on, in June 1853, to request copies of all quarantine papers concerning Southampton over the previous 18 months.[247]

For Pym, the problems were mounting. Fast, new steamers threatened Southampton with diseases which had all but petered out when the same packets, under sail, had formerly arrived in Falmouth. And with new railway links to London, news from Southampton reached London in the same number of hours as intelligence from Falmouth took days. Pym would have been aware of the army of anti-contagionists watching and criticizing his every decision. One influential journal joined the camp of St Germans, sneering at quarantine for the *La Plata* and the 'rites' and 'mummeries' of tongs and fumigation before her mail could be landed.[248] On 20 November 1852, the day after the parliamentary exchanges, Pym issued a certificate jointly with John Wiblin, the local Quarantine Officer.[249] Having boarded the ship, they had learnt of no new cases of yellow fever during the previous week, and had 'consequently' lifted the quarantine. The use of this adverb in their certificate was felt by the *Edinburgh Review* to be 'as little creditable to our fair dealing as the performances with the tongs had been to our science'.[250] Their point, of course, was that quarantine should not have been required in the first place, and this argument was strengthened by what happened next. One of the crew went ashore into lodgings, while still working by day in the ship. He proved the last victim to succumb to yellow fever, dying on land on 5 December 1852.[251] But Southampton was spared an epidemic. Then, on 9 December, the mail steamer *Medway* arrived with several sufferers from yellow fever and some reported deaths.[252] The Privy Council appeared to have learnt their lesson: the ship escaped all quarantine measures and the sick were immediately landed.[253]

These two cases had been monitored by Sutherland for the General Board of Health, and before the end of 1852 the Board brought out their Second Report on Quarantine, which concentrated wholly on yellow fever.[254] This, too, was a blast of anti-contagionism, timed to follow the mood of Parliament. But Lonsdale and Pym were still not convinced that quarantine was inappropriate, and began to vacillate between what they deemed was necessary and what would appease their critics. Late in December 1852 when the furore over the *La Plata* had somewhat diminished, the steamer *Orinoco* was quarantined, but the *Magdalena*, arriving at Southampton on 8 January, was given free pratique despite ten deaths from yellow fever on the voyage and another once the ship had docked.[255] The next arrival in January, the *Parana*,

246 Hansard, Third Series, vol. 123, pp. 230–31.

247 *Journal of the House of Lords (JHL)* vol. 85 (1852–53), pp. 347, 421. The papers were presented on 4 July 1853.

248 *Edinburgh Review*, vol. 98 (1853), pp. 194–5.

249 Published in *Edinburgh Review*, vol. 98 (1853), p. 195.

250 *Edinburgh Review*, vol. 98 (1853), p. 195.

251 *Edinburgh Review*, vol. 98 (1853), pp. 195–6.

252 *Edinburgh Review*, vol. 98 (1853), p. 196.

253 Ibid.

254 J. Simon, *English Sanitary Institutions* (London, 1890), p. 218.

255 *Edinburgh Review*, vol. 98 (1853), p. 196.

was quarantined for four days despite only one sick person – who was not allowed treatment on shore.[256]

Such inconsistency could not continue and, on 31 January 1853, the Privy Council issued new instructions for the Southampton port authorities.[257] A covering letter explained that the Council had three priorities: the protection of public health; the danger of Southampton being declared an infected port by other European countries; and the least possible detriment to passengers and crew. Of these, the second reveals the true motive for the reactionary stance. Despite declared initiatives and international debate, the British Government were still as obsessed by the fear of retaliation as they had been in 1825. The instructions, therefore, were more to ingratiate the Government with countries which would not subscribe to the proposed convention, than to endear the Privy Council to Parliament. If yellow fever had existed on any ship within six days of her arrival at Southampton, she should proceed to The Motherbank, where quarantine would last for not less than six days after the date of the last case, or the date of that patient's removal. All sick persons were to be transferred to the *Menelaus*. This frigate, which had been at The Motherbank for several years as a general purpose lazaretto, was to be converted at Portsmouth Dockyard into a hospital ship; another warship was to be provided by the Admiralty as a place of refuge for those 'who not being themselves attacked, may be desirous of removing themselves from the influence of Contagion or Infection …'[258] With such a compromise, the Council hoped in vain to make quarantine acceptable for the second half of the nineteenth century.

256 Ibid.

257 NA CUST 58/307/67–9, from which remaining references in this paragraph are taken unless otherwise stated.

258 NA CUST 58/307/67–70, 74. The fitting-up of the Menelaus cost around £1,500 (CUST 58/307/100–101).

Chapter Sixteen

Malta, 1826–1851, and the Demise of Quarantine

Malta modernizes

By 1851, the year of the Paris conference, quarantine on Malta had completed 25 years under the control of a Board of Health established by Britain. During that interval the system had been managed at a level which corresponded with the standards of the key lazarettos in mainland Europe. While this severity was sometimes to the detriment of British interests – as Admiral Stopford had made clear – the commercial activity of the island was no more impeded in foreign ports, by and large, than ships of other countries were inconvenienced in Malta. It was, of course, this reciprocated misery which the Paris conference was seeking to address, but it was actually a tribute to the Maltese Government that quarantine at Valletta was widely considered on a par with arrangements at Marseilles and Leghorn.

Such favoured reports would not have been possible without demonstrable activity by the Maltese Board of Health. It must, however, be questioned whether the Board were more than a front for the Maltese Government – the token compliance which Governor Hastings, with some cynicism, had recommended to London as the only salvation for Maltese trade. It was fortunate that foreign consuls, the quarantine spies of Europe, were not in the same position to witness the workings of the Maltese administration as they were to observe sanitary procedures in the harbours and creeks of Valletta. The Board of Health, as promulgated, was to meet every Wednesday for routine business, but the Superintendent of Quarantine could 'wait upon the President' (that is, the Governor) for urgent instructions between meetings.[1] Thus there was, from the outset, a means of bypassing the Board proper, and it was only natural that it should develop over time. On 11 August 1828, 20 months after the Board had been created, the frequency of meetings was reduced to every second Monday.[2] In fact, the meetings quickly reverted to a weekly cycle following the arrival of a Russian warship carrying a fever deemed 'highly suspicious', but within a few more months the regularity collapsed.[3] The Board did not meet between 13 March and 19 August 1829, or between 8 December 1829 and 21 June 1830. It became normal thereafter for a month or even longer to elapse between sessions. Only during 1832, with the future of Malta as a steam packet depot at stake, did the

1 National Library of Malta [NLM] LIB 847 [unpag.], 6 Apr. 1826.

2 NLM LIB 847 [unpag.], 11 Aug. 1828.

3 NLM LIB 847 [unpag.], 22 Sept. 1828.

Board assemble punctiliously every week, even when (on two rare but consecutive occasions) they had nothing to do.[4]

The frequency of meetings can be gauged from the Board minute book, which contains a running number against every session. There are, however, reasons for questioning its credibility as an accurate record. Many original letters of the Maltese Board of Health have survived at Marseilles and at least three of them were dated in Malta two days before a minuted meeting.[5] On other occasions Marseilles received important letters signed only by Ponsonby and Greig under the printed rubric of the Maltese Board of Health. One such letter was dated 4 June 1828, eighteen days after the last meeting of the Board and ten days before the next.[6] Moreover, the substance of the letter (the voyage of Admiral Codrington's flagship) was not discussed at either. These facts suggest that routine matters were considered and approved by the Board, but the Superintendent of Quarantine placed important issues directly before the Lieutenant-Governor, taking advantage of the 'urgency' clause in the Board's terms of reference. Responses were then sent as necessary under the Board's letterhead, giving the impression that the Board were always responsible. And unfortunately there is a further complication: of the information given to Marseilles, some of it was routine and varied, exactly the material which the Board of Health would have considered, and the letters were indeed signed by all members of the Board. But, according to their minute book, the Board had not met to consider those issues, and there is no official record of the decisions.[7]

The conclusion from these anomalies is that quarantine policy in Malta was run by the Superintendent of Quarantine in consultation with the Chief Secretary of Government, who was the bridge to the Lieutenant-Governor. In line with perceived urgency, decisions were implemented at three levels: priority letters were sent direct by the Lieutenant-Governor and Superintendent; if time were rather less pressing, they were carried around to members of the Board, wherever they might be, for a full complement of signatures; and if time were unimportant, the matter was taken to a scheduled meeting of the Board, and the letter followed a minuted resolution. Support for this theory is provided by the copy-letter book of the Superintendent of Quarantine, which overlaps significantly with the minute book of the Board.[8] It is evident from the latter that Greig frequently wrote to William Sim and Frederick Hankey, for the attention of the Lieutenant-Governor, about matters which the Board never discussed. Sometimes, this was in response to an enquiry which Greig had

4 Those occasions were 5 and 13 November 1832.

5 For example, the arrival of the Russian warship noted above was discussed by the Maltese Board of Health on 22 September 1828, but the letter to Marseilles was dated 20 September (Archives départementales des Bouches-du-Rhône, Marseilles [ADBR] 200 E 464).

6 ADBR 200 E 464; NLM LIB 847.

7 For example, all members of the Maltese Board of Health signed a letter dated 3 April 1827, received at Marseilles (ADBR 200 E 464), but the Board did not meet between 9 March 1827 (meeting no. 39) and 4 June 1827 (meeting no. 40) (NLM LIB 847).

8 See Bibliography, Primary Manuscript Sources. The Board minute book is in the National Library, Malta [NLM]; the copy-letter book is in the National Archives, Malta [NAM].

received direct. In 1831, for instance, he was asked by Ponsonby why a warship was admitted to pratique despite a smallpox scare, and he was requested to give information about Anthony Surtees, a well-connected Englishman who arrived on another ship with the same disease and died in the lazaretto.[9] A little later it was to Ponsonby (via Sim), and not to the Board, that Greig reported the intention of the French consul to make trouble about the berthing of packet boats, and bad relations between the Quarantine Department and the Marine Police were always reported to Hankey and never raised before the Board.[10]

The make-up of the Board gives insight into its lightweight role. It will be recalled that the three main members were the Lieutenant-Governor, the Chief Secretary to Government and the Superintendent of Quarantine. As this was the triumvirate who made the decisions, their two other colleagues were needed only for subordinate reasons. Trigona was the token representative of the Maltese aristocracy and Grillet was occasionally useful for a medical opinion. The minutes were taken by G.B. Schembri, who had the title of Registrar; but after his visit to Constantinople to advise on quarantine procedure, he was given a place on the Board.[11] This increased the membership to six without altering the balance of power. Thereafter, the minutes were taken by Vincenzo Borg, who had been made First Clerk in the Quarantine Department in 1826.[12] Borg now earned the title of Secretary, and it must be said that the English of the minutes was a lot better for his appointment. Early in 1831 Dr G.P. Portelli succeeded Grillet, but Trigona was still on the Board as late as 1853.[13] Trigona and both doctors had a good attendance record, and indeed the Board was seldom without its President, or the Chief Secretary to Government.

Greig's attendance was more erratic, and his absences explain to some extent why the Board had long gaps between meetings in the early years of their existence. On 29 May 1830 Greig gave eight days' notice for six months' leave of absence.[14] Colonel Bathurst, the island's Treasurer, stood in for him, but the Board met only twice while Greig was away. As Bathurst had no obvious experience of quarantine, policy in the interval was presumably a matter for Ponsonby advised by Hankey. On 1 August 1832 urgent private affairs in France led Greig to solicit another two months' leave, and he sought a similar period, also in France, a year later to attend his 'family'.[15] In January 1835 Greig received news of the death of his eldest brother in Oporto and requested three months' leave of absence to visit another brother there.[16] On this and the previous occasion, he asked for salary in advance. Greig never reached Oporto, for reasons which suggest that certain steam-packet companies were less reliable

9 The smallpox scare concerned HMS *Asia* (NAM C1, pp. 29–31).

10 NAM C1, pp. 45–7 (French consul), and pp. 74–82 (replies to alleged charges of breach of quarantine laid by the Intendant of Marine Police).

11 NLM LIB 847 [unpag.], 21 Aug. 1832.

12 Borg's appointment to First Clerk was noted in NA CO 158/51 [unpag.], 20 Oct. 1826.

13 NLM LIB 847 [unpag.], 31 Jan. 1831; *British Parliamentary Papers* [*BPP*], vol. 60 (1852–53), p. 493 (which reveals that Portelli and Schembri were also still members).

14 NAM C1, pp. 18–19.

15 NAM C1, pp. 125, 172.

16 NAM C1, pp. 212–13.

than their ships.[17] On the last three occasions when Greig left Malta, his stand-in was a Major Holmes, who became sufficiently experienced to run the Quarantine Department almost normally.[18]

On 23 October 1837 Greig was promoted to Chief Secretary to Government and his role as Superintendent of Quarantine passed to Emanuel Bonavia, Captain of the Lazaretto, the first Maltese to hold the top post. Thus Bonavia was reporting to his predecessor in office, which promised an informed control of the lazaretto. The change can be attributed to the recommendations of the Royal Commission of 1836, set up to investigate aspects of the civil governance in Malta following many complaints by the islanders, especially about Hankey.[19] The Commission, whose arrival roughly coincided with that of the new Governor, Sir Henry Frederick Bouverie, comprised the jurist John Austin and his former pupil George Cornewall Lewis. The latter, whose future career would elevate him to the level of Secretary of State, has already been mentioned in this study as a protagonist for quarantine reform. It was a strong recommendation of the Commissioners that Greig should be succeeded, if possible, by a Maltese subordinate. While that promotion would be well received by the Maltese people, the Commissioners also pointed out that a local man 'could afford to perform those duties for a salary considerably lower than that of the present Superintendent'.[20] Indeed, the salary was halved from the £800 enjoyed by Greig, although Bonavia saw a doubling of the £200 he had been receiving as Captain of the Lazaretto.[21]

Despite the subsequent interest of Lewis, the working of quarantine was not part of the Commissioners' brief. But while investigating the work of the Marine Police Department, they concluded that its integration with the Quarantine Department would be very advisable.[22] This was because the Intendant of Marine Police, in his other role as Captain of the Port (that is, Grand Harbour), granted pratique to ships which arrived in his jurisdiction unless the bill of health or other reasons demanded otherwise. Greig confessed himself happy with this delegation as the Intendant was given regular updates and instructions, but the Commissioners felt strongly that all quarantine matters should be within one department. Probably, they had also had wind of bad relations between the Intendant and Greig. Thus, some 23 years after they had been divided, the departments were unified from 25 July 1837, leaving Greig with three months for the integration.[23]

Independent of the Royal Commission, Greig initiated improvements in the lazaretto which Bonavia saw through to completion. No part of the extensive

17 NAM C1, pp. 217–18. Greig had left Malta on the Falmouth packet, hoping to change at Cadiz for Oporto. On finding there was no connection, he proceeded to England for a Post Office steamer, but was told that ships on the Oporto and Lisbon run had been diverted to serve the West Indies.

18 For example, Holmes wrote to Hankey recommending measures to be taken on the death of a barrier keeper, early in 1835 (NAM C1, pp. 215–16).

19 *BPP*, vol. 29 (1838), pp. 311–445, and vol. 17 (1839), pp. 755–875.

20 *BPP*, vol. 29 (1838), p. 72.

21 NAM C1, pp. 184–7.

22 *BPP*, vol. 29 (1838), pp. 366–70.

23 Ibid.; NAM C1, pp. 297–300.

negotiations with Government was ever mentioned in the minutes of the Board of Health. In April 1833 Greig informed Sim that the rooms and magazines needed whitewashing, that the passenger apartments needed proper privies, that another building (known as number nine) should be converted for passenger use, and that the largest apartments should be subdivided to increase accommodation generally.[24] With the advent of steam power and constant worries about a variety of diseases, there were often more people for quarantine than the lazaretto could hold.[25] As money had recently been spent on a new parlatorio, Ponsonby hesitated.[26] A month later Greig returned to the attack, urging that the Director of Works be at least instructed to convert building number nine, which would create three extra rooms.[27] Another urgent expense, but no more than £15, would provide each room in the lazaretto with a table, bedstead and two chairs.[28] A further £20 would make space for 20 new graves in the burial ground, which was virtually full, and improve access; the current entrance was only three feet wide 'which makes it almost impossible to get a coffin through'.[29]

By April 1834, with only token improvements authorized, Greig was getting desperate. He informed Hankey of the 'absolute necessity' for more accommodation 'and this is the more urgent as the number of persons arriving here from India by way of Alexandria is daily increasing and of late it has frequently happened (as at the moment) that individuals cannot be received into the lazaretto for want of room. This is an inconvenience that passengers loudly complain of ... both for comfort and as their quarantine is shorter by being separated from the ship'.[30] And there were other problems, as well as capacity. In December, Greig reminded Hankey that part of the lazaretto had been turned into a coal store two years earlier for the benefit of steamers.[31] This arrangement was not working 'owing to the penetrating nature of the coal dust. Not only are rooms for passengers completely covered but what is of more consequence, goods in depuration are soiled and damaged'.[32] In such cases, Government would be liable for reparation. His solution was for the coal store to be moved to the shore under the bastion of Floriana, but Government were in no hurry to oblige.[33]

---

24 NAM C1, pp. 159–60.

25 Ibid.

26 The reference to the parlatorio (in the context of spare beams having been found too large to use in it) is in NAM C1, pp. 165–6.

27 NAM C1, pp. 162–3.

28 NAM C1, pp. 164–5.

29 NAM C1, pp. 167–8.

30 NAM C1, pp. 182–3.

31 NAM C1, pp. 209–12.

32 Ibid.

33 Ibid.

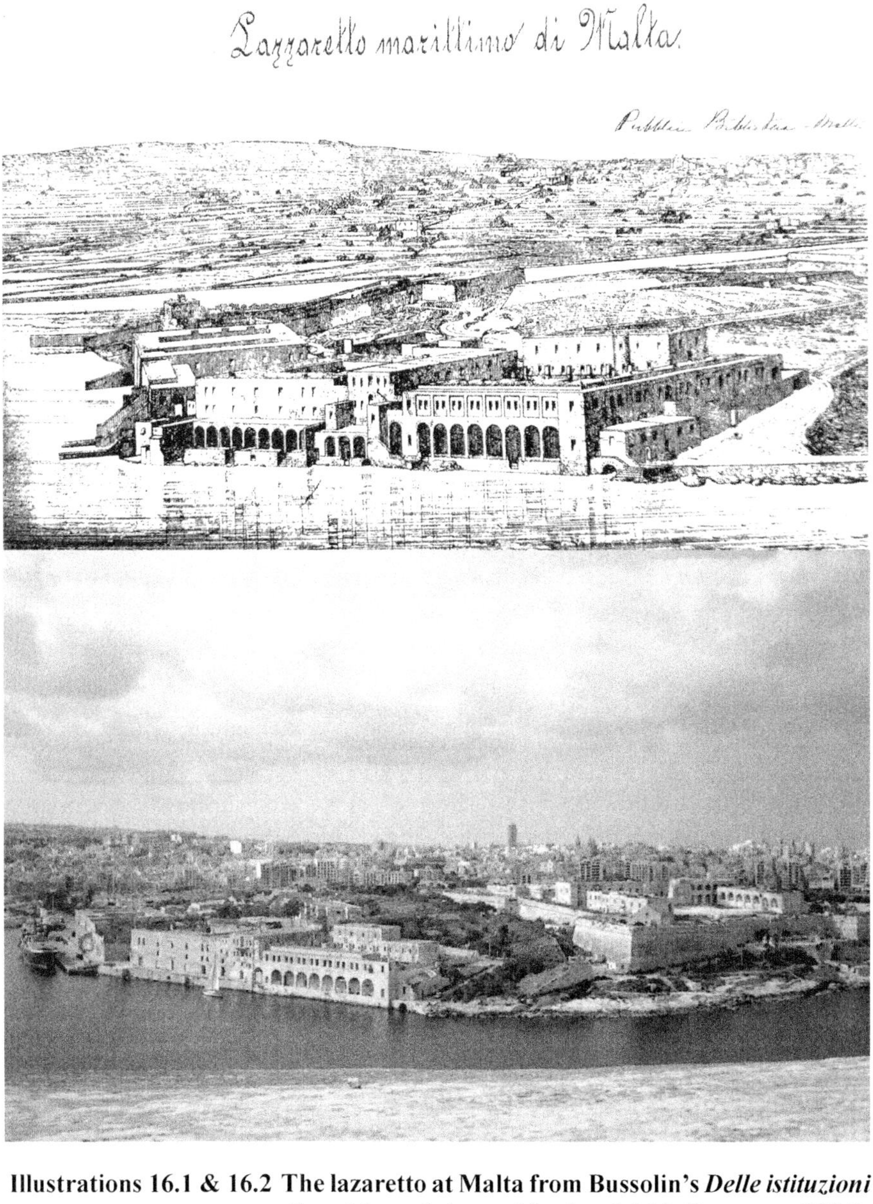

Illustrations 16.1 & 16.2 The lazaretto at Malta from Bussolin's *Delle istituzioni di sanità marittima nel bacino del Mediterraneo* (1881), and the same view today.

During the summer of 1835, with the prospect of French steamers making greater and regular use of the lazaretto, the case for expansion and refurbishment was irresistible. Building works began in August and were completed by June in the following year.[34] The largest rooms were 19 feet by 15 feet and the smallest half that size.[35] Their height was around 17 feet, which seems very generous, yet Greig had to prevent the Acting Director of Works from making them even higher.[36] The main body of the lazaretto, known as the Palazzo Grande, was provided with a covered walk or loggia along the wharf.[37] There were still improvements, however, which Greig felt desirable: the lazaretto office needed another room, for the reception of letters from foul-bill ships, and the landing places were still difficult in bad weather.[38] Some of the passenger quarters had running water, supplied from a reservoir fed by a forcing pump, and Greig wanted the same facilities extended to buildings eight and nine.[39] But the most important desideratum for Greig was now the refurbishment of the kitchen in the Palazzo Grande, as he planned to create the kind of trattoria for passengers which existed at Marseilles and Leghorn. He alluded to constant complaints that dinners brought out from Valletta were invariably cold on arrival.[40]

The success of the trattoria would depend on the removal of the coal depot. In August 1836 Greig played his trump card, which was the imminent arrival of the French steamers, three times a month from the East.[41] Government in Malta were still terrified of bad reaction at Marseilles about any aspect of the lazaretto and when the French consul, also in August, drew up a series of questions about quarantine practice (with the arrival of the steamers dependent on satisfactory answers), Greig was in the unusual position of having the French as his allies.[42] In September he wrote to Hankey about 'the total impossibility' of the coal depot staying where it was.[43] Recent cargoes of coal from England had been landed in a south-easterly wind, and every passenger room was filled with dust. The other problem for Greig was the pollution of cargoes, which was now worse than before. Because of the cholera scare, ships from Genoa and Trieste were not allowed into Sicilian ports, and were being diverted to Malta for their cargoes to be depurated. When the coal was landed, goods on shore were hastily covered by tarpaulins and old sheets, but that practice could not continue.[44]

Coal was also needed by the navy and, in February 1837, Greig reached an agreement with Rear-Admiral Briggs about a new site, which appears to have won Government approval.[45] This was not where Greig had originally intended,

---

34 NAM C1, pp. 234–5, 245–7.

35 NAM C1, pp. 234–5.

36 Ibid.

37 NAM C1, pp. 245–7.

38 Ibid.

39 Ibid.; J. Galea, 'The quarantine service and the lazzaretto of Malta', *Melita Historica*, 4/3 (1966), 198, explains that the roofs of the lazaretto supported a large cistern for rainwater.

40 NAM C1, pp. 247.

41 NAM C1, pp. 249–52.

42 The answers to the queries of the French consul are in NAM C1, pp. 253–6.

43 NAM C1, pp. 260–63, from which remaining references in this paragraph are taken.

44 In a postscript to his letter, Greig warned that a ship had just arrived from Smyrna with a cargo of raw silk valued at £6,000 or £7,000.

45 NAM CI, pp. 272–3

and involved converting an area on the new mole, formerly used for storing the measures of the Grain Department.[46] There was now no reason to delay the trattoria, but it became a matter for Bonavia after Greig's promotion. On 15 April 1838, at the request of Bouverie, the new Governor, Bonavia submitted the proposed tariff: 1s, 8d bought a breakfast of unlimited tea, coffee and milk plus a one-pound loaf of bread, two newly laid eggs, butter and one pound of hot or cold meat.[47] The same breakfast without the meat was 6d cheaper. Dinner could be purchased for 4s and comprised soup, garnished fish or beef (ragout or roast), two dishes of dressed vegetables, sweets, cheese, fruit, bread and a bottle of common Sicilian wine. For 2s, 6d, a lesser meal could be had without fish, vegetables, sweet dish and cheese. The trattoria carried a large cellar: the 27 items included champagne at 5s, 4d, hock at 5s, 10d, claret Lafitte at 5s, 6d, Dutch Curaçao rum at 6s per flask, and ale at 1s, 2d a bottle. This last-named item was 2d more expensive than the cheapest drink, a bottle of Faro wine.

As soon as Bonavia took over, he argued that basic accommodation in the lazaretto was still inadequate. In November 1837 he advised Greig (then Chief Secretary to Government) that new agreements with France meant that rooms were needed at any one time for up to 60 people, many of them ladies 'and generally all of them persons of condition'.[48] This was because, from 1 December, the French steamers between Malta and Marseilles were to run in free pratique; to maintain that status, passengers on the branch Levant steamers would all need a quarantine of 21 days before continuing their voyage. Bonavia's immediate solution was that Fort Manoel be reattached to the lazaretto (as it had been during the plague of 1813) and fitted out with divisions and water closets.[49] The Fort was already being used for overspill accommodation: in March 1837, mainly because of the threat of plague from Tripoli, the lazaretto and Fort together housed over 600 people 'separated into as many as 31 different quarantines'.[50] But the Fort could not be relied upon. Despite being still 'given over for lazaretto purposes' in 1838, the military were keen to have it back.[51] By 1842 Bonavia was resigned to pleading for repairs and alterations to the Palazzo Grande and Palazzo Vecchio, the main components of the traditional lazaretto.[52] Again, improvements to water closets were much on his mind.[53]

Another major development at the lazaretto, initiated by Greig and concluded by Bonavia, was a new plague hospital. On 16 December 1836 Greig informed Hankey that plague was at Tripoli, and Malta could expect infected ships and refugees.[54] The lazaretto already had a plague hospital but it consisted of only 12 small rooms, was

46 Ibid.

47 NAM C1, pp. 314–16, from which remaining references in this paragraph are taken.

48 NAM C1, pp. 304–6.

49 Ibid.

50 NAM C1, pp. 280–84.

51 The quotation is from NAM C1, pp. 321–2.

52 NAM C1, pp. 440–51.

53 Ibid.: 'The necessaries to be so altered that the filth may fall perpendicularly from the seat into the Canal, which at present it cannot do thereby rendering the Canals extremely obnoxious and offensive'. He also requested an extension to the burial ground.

54 NAM C1, pp. 267–9.

being used by ordinary passengers, and was unsuitable in any case as it adjoined the rest of the complex. Greig wanted a 'proper' hospital on a more remote part of Manoel Island.[55] Work began in 1837 and took nearly three years to complete. In April 1839 Bonavia sent Greig (recently knighted) a memorandum of alterations and additions. These centred on the privies, for which Bonavia requested a constant flush of water, 'as this building is intended for the occupation of the lower orders of persons, who can never be expected ... [to] take the necessary precautions for keeping these places properly cleansed'.[56] The request appears to have been granted, and the plague hospital cost over £3,000 to complete.[57] It was barely used. The Ordnance Department had regained a footing on Manoel Island in 1836, and the military turned the new hospital into married quarters.[58]

Galea suggests that cholera played a part in justifying the new hospital but, when the disease struck, building work was well under way.[59] There seems no reason to conclude that the hospital was meant for treating any but contagious diseases, among which plague was still deemed a greater risk than cholera. Certainly, the first cholera pandemic brought great suffering and mortality to Malta, with 4,152 deaths in only four months, but it was relatively late in arrival.[60] Cassar notes that the epidemic began on 9 June 1837, although a few isolated cases may have occurred earlier.[61] Galea states that 'for some reason or other' patients were not transferred to the lazaretto, which harks back to the question of whether cholera was deemed contagious, as the lazaretto was specifically for isolation.[62] On the contagious properties of cholera, opinion on Malta was more divided that it was in Britain.[63] It remained that way in the second pandemic, even though the received wisdom in Europe by that time was that cholera was non-contagious. In fact, the 1848 pandemic did not reach Malta, and there were undoubtedly those who argued that the island's unrelenting, if unfashionable, attachment to quarantine had much to do with it. In 1847, with cholera on the horizon, there were requests for quarantine measures to be strengthened.[64] The response of the Maltese Government was to refuse entry to any ships which had had any contact with cholera within the previous 12 days; such vessels had 'to remain cruising in and off the harbour's mouth for such a number of days as the Board of Health decided'.[65]

The establishment of the Quarantine Department was composed largely of guardians stationed to watch over ships, crews and passengers, both in the harbour and within the lazaretto. The post of guardian comprised three classes, introduced

55 Ibid.

56 NAM C1, pp. 337–9.

57 *Malta Government Gazette* [*MGG*], 25 Apr. 1838, p. 163, and 19 Apr. 1839, p. 118.

58 Galea, p. 198.

59 Ibid.

60 The total is given *BPP*, vol. 60 (1860), p. 247, which is repeated in Galea, p. 198. P. Cassar, *Medical History of Malta* (London, 1965), p. 198, gives 4,252 deaths.

61 Cassar, p. 192.

62 Galea, p. 198.

63 Cassar, p. 195.

64 Cassar, p. 199.

65 *BPP*, vol. 58 (1861), p. 271.

in 1814 to make a clearer distinction from boatmen, who ferried people and goods between ships, and sometimes the shore, and the lazaretto.[66] At that time, the total establishment of boatmen was 18 and of keepers of the barrier 12.[67] In 1835 Greig argued that the number of guardians in the second class (those employed on merchant ships, rather than in the lazaretto) might drop from 59 to 50.[68] The grounds for this reduction was that around eight of them were 'totally unfit for duty', and from then on it became normal, at intervals, for the Superintendent of Quarantine to submit to the Governor a list of guardians of the first and second class in various stages of decrepitude. The returns give useful insight into ages and years of service. In the list prepared by Bonavia in 1838, there were 14 names: the average age was 67 (the oldest 84) and the average length of service was 32 years (the longest 46).[69] In later lists, ages remained roughly the same but the average length of service increased to 36 years.

If Greig's main reason for raising the issue of infirmity was to reduce the number of guardians, he was also motivated by concerns for their welfare. Austin and Lewis praised his 'prudence, conciliatory manners, and knowledge of the opinions and feelings of the Maltese'.[70] He hoped the Government would agree pensions for those unfit for work, but benefits for lower ranks had not been conspicuous in the past. When a boatman or guardian died in office, the widow received only the salary for the last month of service, and even then each case was submitted to the (Lieutenant-) Governor.[71] In exceptional circumstances, however, the Superintendent could plead for more generosity. In 1836, when a guardian of the first class died of typhus fever contracted in the lazaretto from persons arrived from Tunis, Greig argued for a pension of £1 a month to be paid to the widow from charitable institutions, so she could bring up her four children.[72] The 1842 estimates indicate that the 61 guardians of all classes were paid on average £21 a year; the 28 boatmen received around £31.[73] At a slightly higher level were 13 keepers of the barrier, receiving £32.[74] The higher ranks at that time, in roughly ascending order, comprised: keeper of the lazaretto parlatorio (£36); fumigator (£50); guardian in the fumigating office, and head keeper of the Coradino parlatorio (both £55); three junior clerks (£185 in total); Captain of the Lazaretto (£250); Captain of the Ports (£300) and his Assistant (£200); four senior clerks (£255 in total) with two messengers (£66 together); Chief Clerk and Secretary to the Board of Health (£200); and the Superintendent of Quarantine (£400).[75] This was a total salary bill of £6,107, nearly 80 per cent of the quarantine budget.[76]

66 NA CO 158/25/252–5.

67 Ibid.

68 NAM C1, pp. 214–15.

69 NAM C1, p. 311. The list was superseded by another a year later (pp. 342–4).

70 *BPP*, vol. 29 (1838), p. 72; A.V. Laferla, *British Malta* (2 vols, Malta, 1938), vol. 1, p. 158 (who made the contrast with Hankey).

71 For example NAM C1, pp. 208, 241–2.

72 NAM C1, pp. 248–9.

73 *Malta Government Gazette*, 14 Jan. 1842, p. 2.

74 Ibid.

75 Ibid.

76 Ibid.

During 1851 there was a further rationalization of marine and quarantine functions with the creation of a Port Department.[77] The head officer was now designated Superintendent of the Ports; he had two Assistant Superintendents (one each for Grand and Marsamxett Harbours), supported by eight clerks and one messenger. Beneath this level there was a distinction between the 'Force' and the Lazaretto. The former was very much a fusion of elements of the old Marine Police and Quarantine Departments, and comprised one adjutant, two inspectors, two sub-inspectors, one keeper of the powder magazine (who was also a sub-inspector), one searcher, six sergeants of the first class, twelve of the second class, 52 guards of the first class, 26 of the second, and 27 of the third. The lazaretto staff proper were now seen as managerial and clerical: Vincenzo Borg became the Director of the Lazaretto and Secretary to the Board of Health on £200 a year, while Edward Carleton became Assistant Superintendent of the Port and Lazaretto on £150.[78] They were supported by two letter sorters.[79] Carleton was particularly experienced in quarantine work. Between 1827 and 1829 he had been a teacher of navigation in the university and became Captain of the Quarantine Harbour on 1 April 1832 at a salary of £200 a year, which equated at that time with that of Bonavia.[80] When the Marine Police and Quarantine Departments had been merged, it was Carleton who had become Captain of the Ports at a salary of £300, deputizing as necessary for Luigi Casolani who had succeeded Bonavia as Captain of the Lazaretto.[81] Although his salary in the new Port Department was halved, Carleton was aged around 67 in 1851 and was perhaps anxious for a lesser load. He also had private interests in Barbary.[82]

Milroy and the National Association

Despite bureaucratic changes in Malta, the concept of quarantine on that island was barely changing. Within Britain, by contrast, there was a lobby seeking to ensure that it did. Milroy, who in 1853 had sought to publicize his views through the Epidemiological Society, was indirectly responsible for a new body known as the Sub-Committee of Quarantine appointed by the Public Health Department of the National Association for the Promotion of Social Science (NAPSS).[83]

Milroy might never have bothered to pursue his cause had not Pym and the Privy Council recently taken measures to meet the worst plague scare for many decades. The old enemy had a tiresome habit of reasserting itself while medical debate wished

77 *Malta Government Gazette*, 30 May 1851, p. 31, from which remaining references in this paragraph are taken unless otherwise stated.

78 *BPP*, vol. 60 (1852–53), p. 493.

79 Ibid.

80 NAM C1, pp. 184–7; C2, p. 532.

81 NAM C1, p. 365; C2, p. 532.

82 On 4 May 1843 Carleton applied to Greig for two months' leave to attend to private affairs in 'Barbary' (NAM C2, p. 18).

83 Milroy's paper 'Operation and Results of Quarantine in British Ports since the Beginning of the present Century' (see Bibliography) was read before the Epidemiological Society on 6 June 1853.

to move on to other diseases. The seat of the latest outbreak was Benghazi, but the epidemic was initially considered to be typhus. In July 1856 it was realized in Malta that a better diagnosis would be plague, and a fierce quarantine of 21 days was immediately imposed.[84] In London, little was known about this outbreak until, as late as June 1858, the British consul in Marseilles reported extra precautions being taken locally against Benghazi, Tripoli and Alexandria.[85] The reason was 'a fatal Epidemic – a species of malignant Typhus, if not Plague (for Medical opinions appear to be divided on the subject) … Deaths are very sudden, and the cases are attended with Boils or Buboes'. The Privy Council were alarmed; extra care was immediately requested in the examination of bills of health, passengers and crews from the Mediterranean.[86]

Pym was reluctant to appear too harsh. In a letter of 19 August 1858, he reminded the Lord President of the Council that in 1847, following the cessation of epidemics in Egypt three years earlier, he had recommended the abolition of all quarantine against plague.[87] Consequently, the Government had kept 'a mere nucleus' at the three remaining stations of Stangate Creek, The Motherbank and Liverpool.[88] The establishment of Milford Haven had been virtually abandoned during 1844.[89] Pym expressed his 'greatest confidence' in the Boards of Health in Turkey and Egypt, but suggested that the Admiralty should be asked to make up to six old warships available as hulks: two for Stangate Creek, two for Liverpool and one each for The Motherbank and Hull.[90] Pym was directed to visit the existing stations, as well as the ports of Southampton, Hull, Leith and Greenock to report on their awareness of the problem and the case for floating lazarettos at those locations.[91]

It struck Milroy that not only was plague resurgent, but yellow fever was still taking a fearful toll in southern Europe and potentially further north, with opinion as divided as ever about the ability of quarantine to contain it. His sympathies were specifically for Lisbon, which had suffered badly from cholera in 1856, and was then ravaged by yellow fever in 1857–58.[92] The ports of Vigo and Malaga fared little better.[93] Milroy was moved to suggest new ideas. He read a paper entitled 'Quarantine as it is, and as it ought to be' to the Public Health Department (over which Lord Shaftesbury presided) of the NAPSS, and it was published in the Association's *Transactions* for 1858.[94] This was less of an anti-contagionist diatribe than might

84 *BPP*, vol. 60 (1860), pp. 246–7.

85 NA CUST 58/307/126.

86 NA CUST 58/307/127.

87 NA PC 1/4534.

88 Ibid.

89 In July 1844, following 'the great diminution of Quarantine at Milford', the Privy Council authorized one or two lazarettos to be released to Pembroke Dockyard (NA PC 7/5/550).

90 NA PC 1/4534.

91 NA CUST 58/307/128.

92 G. Milroy, 'Quarantine as it is, and as it ought to be', *Transactions of the National Association for the Promotion of Social Science. 1858* (London, 1859), 528.

93 *The Lancet* (1861, vol. 1), p. 45 (letter from Milroy).

94 See Bibliography.

have been expected, and borrowed from the findings of the 1851 Paris conference. Commenting on a range of diseases, among which plague, yellow fever and cholera were foremost, Milroy allowed that quarantine was necessary when a noxious ship arrived with disease actually on board.[95] But the sick should be transferred to a floating hospital or airy rooms on shore. He dismissed the idea of lazarettos for the healthy 'upon the mere speculative apprehension that the disease may be dormant in their systems'. Neither did he accept that most goods were susceptible to convey infection, although he followed the fashionable line that commodities like 'foul rags, putrid hides, rotten meat and vegetables, guano, &., should be landed under special regulations …' Milroy's greatest worry was danger from diseased ships, rather than from the state of their cargoes or the sickness of their crew or passengers. He favoured lime-washing and fumigation, especially of bilges, and suggested that bills of health would do better to describe the condition of the ship than the existence or otherwise of disease at her port of departure. The paper was well received and it was on the Department's recommendation that the Sub-Committee was formed 'to consider the whole subject' and report to the next meeting of the Association.[96]

The value of the Sub–Committee was that, despite unofficial status, it united various interests into a forum of authority and experience which had almost the respectability of a royal commission. Among the membership of 18 were the Directors-General of the Medical Departments of the Army and Navy, Pym in his capacity as Superintendent of Quarantine, and T. Southwood Smith as a member of the late General Board of Health. M^c^William, the yellow fever investigator, attended as Medical Inspector to the Board of Customs. Milroy was described as late Medical Commissioner in the West Indies and in the Crimea; John Davy, famed for his influential comments on quarantine published in 1842, was included as Inspector-General of Army Hospitals; and John Wiblin earned a seat as Medical Superintendent of Quarantine at Southampton.[97] *The Lancet* welcomed the membership as 'a sufficient guarantee that the subject will be treated with the strictest impartiality and the greatest ability', although among its correspondents there were reservations.[98] The Sub-Committee wasted no time in preparing a truly vast number of questions, finalized in 1859, for putting to consuls, colonial governors and military doctors in various foreign stations.[99] There had, of course, been many questionnaires about quarantine and contagion over the previous 25 years, but nothing on such a comprehensive scale. With Palmerston as the new Prime Minister, Shaftesbury leaning hard on the Secretaries of State in the Foreign and Colonial Offices, and the military doctors under orders from their heads of department, there were hopes for a monumental compendium of empirical evidence and informed opinion.

---

95 Milroy, 'Quarantine as it is, and as it ought to be', 528–30, from which remaining references in this paragraph are taken unless otherwise stated.

96 *Transactions of the National Association for the Promotion of Social Science. 1858* (London, 1859), p. 543.

97 *The Lancet* (1859, vol. 1), p. 473.

98 Ibid.; in *The Lancet* (1859, vol. 2), p. 496, is a letter from 'Viator' who thought that a number of the members had an interest in quarantine's continuance.

99 These questions are revealed in the parliamentary papers (see below) which contain the responses.

These hopes were not dashed, but the structure of questioning led to findings so vast, repetitious and complicated that parliamentarians were bewildered by the outcome. In the first instance, the NAPSS sent abstracts of the garnered information to the Board of Trade. In May 1860 Parliament did the dutiful thing by asking for these returns, along with completed questionnaires received at the Foreign Office, to be laid before the House.[100] These were then printed, but not *in extenso*, the abstracts being prefaced by letters of explanation from Milroy.[101] *The Lancet* felt that so much information must surely be the prelude to something momentous, but was not sure what it was: each reader should come to his own conclusion.[102] But for Parliament the mass of paper was simply overwhelming. Despite 85 pages of evidence, consisting of replies and 'Observations', the House still only had access to an edited version of the findings, along with an abstract of quarantine regulations in force in foreign countries. In July 1861 Milroy sent the Board of Trade what he called 'the complement' to the papers they had already received.[103] These additions, which were also printed, included more abstracts of information from consuls and the colonies, followed by a 28-page report on the overall findings drafted by the NAPSS.[104] To round off the report, Milroy produced a long Appendix entitled an 'Historical Sketch of Quarantine Legislation and Practice in Great Britain'.[105]

The report of the NAPSS contained several recommendations, prefaced by their recognition of 'the great importance of an official sanitary supervision in all great seaports ...'[106] Their aim, they admitted, was 'to amend and utilise, not to discontinue or to abolish the existing machinery of action'. This was a significant softening of the line taken a few years earlier by Bowring and Lord St Germans. The recommendations which followed added little to the opinions already expressed by Milroy, and not one was presented without an amending or dissenting caveat from as many as five members of the Sub-Committee. This considerably weakened their impact. There would have been those who shuddered both in Whitehall and Westminster to read the sixth and final recommendation, which was that Government should institute 'an investigation into the results of quarantine, and the working of quarantine establishments, in the chief ports of the south of Europe and of the Mediterranean where the system is still in greatest force, in order to ascertain the actual truth by personal observation on the spot'. For more than a quarter of a century it seemed that Governments and individuals at home and abroad had been doing little else but probe the rationale and workings of the system. If the NAPSS could not arrive at a definitive strategy after exhaustive questioning, what point was there in enquiring further? As *The Lancet* could be relied upon for making just such a point, Milroy wrote the editor a long pre-emptive letter setting out what the NAPSS

100 *JHC*, vol. 115, pp. 224, 484.

101 *BPP*, vol. 60 (1860), pp. 155–276.

102 *The Lancet* (1860, vol. 2), p. 171.

103 *BPP*, vol. 60 (1861), pp. 225.

104 *BPP*, vol. 60 (1861), pp. 225–62 (there are inconsistencies in the original numeration).

105 *BPP*, vol. 60 (1861), pp. 263–71.

106 *BPP*, vol. 60 (1861), pp. 235–62, from which all references in this paragraph are taken until otherwise stated.

were trying to achieve.[107] He now appeared mildly critical of the Paris conference, using the 'disaccord and even contrariety of opinion' among the medical delegates to strengthen the case for the Association's enquiry.[108]

In 1858 the General Board of Health was disbanded and responsibility for public health was transferred to the Privy Council, whose workload in other areas had been steadily passing to ministers and the Cabinet.[109] The enabling Act enjoined the appointment of a Medical Officer, charged with submitting annual and ad hoc reports to the Council and ultimately to Parliament. This officer was John Simon, already a respected physician. He had been Medical Officer to the General Board of Health, following several years working in a similar capacity for the Corporation of London. Simon was destined to become one of the most honoured and influential sanitary reformers of the Victorian period. He served the Privy Council from 1858 to 1871.[110]

The appointment of Simon did not initially undermine the status of Pym. The latter, as a member of the Sub-Committee of the NAPSS, would have been privy to its conclusions. Thus even before the report of the Association had been produced, Pym was aware that the relentless antipathy towards quarantine which had marked the anti-contagionist fervour of the early 1850s was no longer in evidence. That was not to say quarantine was welcome. There was a prevalent view that sanitary measures should be used in a complementary way, that the healthy should not be trapped in a diseased ship, and that the sick should be removed to a place of care and treatment, preferably on land. But there was equally an acceptance that ships themselves, particularly hot, dirty steamers with stagnant bilge water, were transmitters of infection. Such ships needed to be kept at a distance, which meant that quarantine in some circumstances was acceptable and indeed advisable. Pym, always a contagionist, could interpret this change of heart as a qualified endorsement to the tough rules introduced a few years previously for packet steamers arriving at Southampton with cases of yellow fever.

In July 1859 Pym sought and obtained from the Privy Council a slight amendment of the regulations for steamers reaching Southampton 'in a sickly state'.[111] While it was still the rule that such ships would not be released from quarantine until the sixth day after the last patient had fallen ill, if those circumstances meant a quarantine of only two days, it could be passed at the buoy where steamers were accustomed to bring up for medical examination. But for any longer period of quarantine it was still necessary for the steamer to anchor at The Motherbank, as close to the floating lazaretto as possible. Until those few days had passed, all aboard the steamer had to be supplied by the ship's steward, as they could not receive rations from the shore. The only people to escape the ship immediately would be those who could

107 *The Lancet* (1861, vol. 1), pp. 45–6.

108 Ibid.

109 This was under the Public Health Act, 1858 (21 & 22 Vic., c.97). See W.M..Frazer, *A History of English Public Health* (London, 1950), p. 77.

110 See *Oxford Dictionary of National Biography.*

111 NA CUST 58/307/139, from which all references in this paragraph are taken.

swear that they had suffered a previous attack of yellow fever, as the disease was not reckoned to strike twice.

In the following month the Privy Council were persuaded to issue a circular to Customs about cholera.[112] In the third pandemic (1853–54), quarantine had played an insignificant role while doctors continued to debate and investigate how the disease was spread. In 1854 Dr John Snow had demonstrated to the satisfaction of his peers that cholera was transmitted via drinking water contaminated by the excretions of those affected.[113] Five years on, under the influence of Simon, the Privy Council felt able to take general precautions. They acknowledged a definite risk, but were 'desirous to refrain from an interference with the interests of Trade'.[114] Customs officers were ordered 'to use their utmost influence' to persuade sufferers to enter a hospital or other establishment provided by the local authority. They could not, the Council wrote, overestimate the importance of isolating cholera patients, and crewmen should be warned about 'common, and too often dirty' lodging houses in the main ports. Masters should be advised to clean, ventilate and disinfect their ships.

The tone here was softer and more constructive than that used a month earlier for the yellow-fever orders, and pinpoints the difference between Simon and Pym. It is difficult to see how their two roles could have existed in harmony for any length of time, but the problem was resolved in March 1861 by the death of Pym, aged 84.[115] Briefly lamented by the NAPSS, he did not live long enough to see their report published in the parliamentary blue books.[116] The greatest tribute to be paid to Pym is that he was constantly true to his principles. He was widely travelled, well experienced in the practice of quarantine, and knowledgeable about the running of lazarettos both floating and on land. It goes without saying in the Victorian culture that he was conscientious in his duties and attentive to his superiors. He was, however, in the words of Ackernecht, a 'violent contagionist' and even the deaths on the *Eclair* did nothing to shake his belief in the virtues of quarantine.[117] It is difficult for posterity to forgive principles which flouted the tenets of basic humanity.

The Privy Council had always been comfortable with the recommendations of Pym and, Simon notwithstanding, were in no hurry to depart from his extreme caution. It should also be understood that Simon was only responsible to the Privy Council within the limits of the Public Health Act of 1858, which did not qualify him necessarily to be involved with measures taken under quarantine legislation. He can be deemed *hors de cause* when, in September 1862, *The Lancet* criticized

112 NA CUST 58/307/142–3.

113 cf. Frazer, p. 65.

114 NA CUST 58/307/142–3, from which remaining references in this paragraph are taken.

115 *The Times*, 21 Mar. 1861, has an uncritical notice of which the slightly later mention in the *The Lancet* is a copy.

116 *BPP*, vol. 60 (1861), p. 235, for reference to his death.

117 E.H. Ackerknecht, 'Anticontagionism between 1821 and 1867', *Bulletin of the History of Medicine*, 22 (1948), 574.

how the steamer *Melita* had been treated in London's Victoria Docks.[118] Arrived from Nassau, the ship had dropped the master and two passengers at Dover before receiving quarantine clearance off Gravesend. But it transpired, despite her clean bill of health, that eight deaths had occurred on the voyage with symptoms of yellow fever. The ship was pushed into the centre of the basin and port officers and dockers already on board were not allowed to land. Three days later medical opinion conveniently decided that the diagnosis of yellow fever might not have been right. *The Lancet* argued that if the diagnosis had been confirmed, and the ship were still infected, 'a frightful sacrifice of valuable lives' would have resulted. The incident moved the journal to side squarely with the findings of the NAPSS, particularly their recommendation that the healthy in such circumstances should not be detained, and the sick should be removed from the ship as soon as possible.

The resurgence of quarantine

It seemed at long last that, in the face of sanitary reform and the march of reason, the Privy Council could no longer delay in bringing quarantine to a fast conclusion. But within a few years the behaviour of both cholera and yellow fever caused doubt about the wisdom of change. In the summer of 1865 a violent outbreak of cholera in Mecca spread quickly to Alexandria and then to other parts of the Levant and Barbary. The British consul in Alexandria was so late in passing the news that many pilgrims had landed at Malta before proper quarantine could be introduced.[119] By then the island was infected, and the disease reached Sicily and Italy with equal ease. In Britain, reaction by the Privy Council was calm. On 23 June 1865 Customs officers were advised that vessels which arrived with cholera on board need not be detained, but notice should be given to the local authority.[120] In July the Privy Council made it clear that they still wished copies of the interrogatories, when masters arrived with foul bills of health from a cholera-infected port.[121] One month later a correspondent to the *The Lancet* raised the grim prospect of another pandemic and wondered whether in countries around the Mediterranean where quarantine was still used as a defence against cholera, it might not have been introduced sooner and more stringently.[122]

By the spring of 1866 it was evident that Britain was in the grip of the fourth pandemic. On 7 May the Privy Council concluded that the recommendations of Milroy and the NAPSS should be broadly implemented. By the historic process of Order and Proclamation, no person would be allowed to leave a cholera-infected ship within three days of arrival without permission from the Local Board of Health

118 *The Lancet* (1862, vol. 2), pp. 262–3, from which remaining references in this paragraph are taken.

119 Cassar, p. 201.

120 NA CUST 58/307/175.

121 NA CUST 58/307/176.

122 *The Lancet* (1865, vol. 2), pp. 516–17.

or other statutory body.[123] The same authority was to send on board a doctor, who would allow the healthy to go ashore. Persons certified as sick would be taken, if their condition allowed it, to a hospital or other place provided, where they would remain until certified fit to leave. If a cholera death occurred on board, the body would be weighted and disposed of at sea, and effects would be disinfected or destroyed. Offences against the Order would be punished under terms of the 1825 Quarantine Act, which was the legal basis of the new provisions.

It will be noted that the Order, by implication, allowed for three days' quarantine on the ship if the local authority wished. This was a toughening of procedure and put the direction of policy in doubt. The confusion was evident in an editorial, a week later, in *The Lancet*, which accepted that any 'tendency … to repose less and less faith, or altogether to disbelieve, in the efficaciousness of quarantine as a defence against cholera has been rudely shaken by the circumstances attending the diffusion of the disease since the beginning of 1865'.[124] The writer could not bring himself to acknowledge that quarantine was anything more than 'a means of official exaction and commercial loss'.[125] Yet he seemed to suggest there was some elusive formula for the protection of the public which did not omit quarantine altogether. Should 'the presumed well', as *The Lancet* referred to them, really be allowed ashore immediately? Was that not a risk to the public health? Should there not be greater enquiry into the incidence of diarrhoea aboard 'as well as to cholera commonly so called'?[126] A correspondent to the journal soon put the editor in greater uncertainty by pointing out that at Marseilles and Malta, when quarantine was eventually rigorous, the virulence of the disease diminished.[127]

Simon, in his *Eighth Report* to the Privy Council (1865), conceded that 'if I speak to the dry question of medical practice, I have no hesitation in saying that England ought to resist cholera by quarantine'.[128] But it would only work if 'conducted with extreme vigour, and with the precision of a chemical experiment …' The problem was that quarantine as it then existed in Britain was nominal, and Simon suspected that it had always been relatively lax. He alleged that the quarantine stations had become so run down, 'that, at the present moment England has not in readiness the means of properly quarantining even a single ship'. He ridiculed 'the ceremonies to which, under the name of quarantine, certain trans-atlantic ships are subjected', which were only in place 'as part of an international obligation contracted for commercial reasons'. Simon believed, in summary, that even if Britain had the political will to impose a quarantine of European severity, it could not be effective. He might not have been aware of figures, published in 1867, which justified his slighting comments:

123 The printed text is in NA PC 8/326 (under 1884 entries), from which remaining references in this paragraph are taken.

124 *The Lancet* (1866, vol. 1), pp. 516–17.

125 Ibid.

126 Ibid.

127 *The Lancet* (1866, vol. 1), p. 556.

128 J. Simon, *Public Health Reports* (2 vols, London, 1887), vol. 2, pp. 244–5, from which all references in this paragraph are taken until otherwise stated.

between 1850 and 1866, only 28 ships were quarantined at British stations.[129] But the interesting point is that Simon was moving towards contagionism, and if the Privy Council disliked his criticism of quarantine management, at least they were not at odds over doctrine.

By this stage in the debate, a new alarm about yellow fever had already made a significant change in how quarantine was perceived. On 9 September 1865, towards the end of a summer noted for tropical heat, the ship *Hecla* arrived at Swansea from Cuba.[130] One man was dying from yellow fever and two others were convalescent. In themselves, those incidents were unremarkable. But what proved 'unparalleled' in Britain in Simon's belief, and 'of extreme importance', was that the disease jumped ship.[131] The odd case of yellow fever on land had been recorded before, notably in Southampton, but nothing on this scale: 20 inhabitants of Swansea living in the vicinity of the wharf were attacked, of whom 15 died.[132] In France, however, a more complicated outbreak had resulted in 26 deaths from yellow fever, mainly at St Nazaire and Lorient, in the summer of 1861.[133] There was, therefore, no longer a case for assuming categorically that yellow fever could not, to some extent, propagate itself lethally in a relatively cool northern climate. If Pym were still alive, he would have felt his caution (if not his tactics) of prevention had been vindicated.

The deep alarm of the Privy Council about events at Swansea led to immediate precautions against all diseased ships from the West Indies, even in winter. In November 1866, intelligence that the royal-mail steamer *Atrato* would arrive imminently at Southampton, prompted an 'Electric Telegraphic Message' from Wiblin to G.R. Cassé, Superintendent of Quarantine at The Motherbank, based in Ryde.[134] Wiblin ordered the hospital ship *Menelaus* to be prepared for the reception of up to 160 people. He added, 'I shall be there with a tug to advise'.[135] Wiblin's authority was confirmed by a telegram to Cassé from the Privy Council.[136] On 18 November the bodies of two people from the *Atrato*, and a boy who died on the *Menelaus*, were 'secured in new canvas, properly weighted, and sunk at the Quarantine red buoy'.[137] Both ships were strictly guarded by two gunboats, and as Cassé was still on board the *Atrato* he found it difficult to inspect other ships. He recounted that the schooner *Electra* arrived at The Motherbank from Haiti, for orders. 'The master died from Consumption. I went along side in my Boat under Quarantine and granted a Certificate but this [practice] must be discontinued'.[138] He

129 The ships are listed in *BPP*, vol. 64 (1867), p. 619. It is surprising that as many as 20 of them were detained in Liverpool. For the request of the return, see *JHC*, vol. 123, p. 78.

130 Simon, *Public Health Reports*, vol. 2, pp. 230–31; see also *The Lancet* (1866, vol. 2), pp. 581–2.

131 Simon, *Public Health Reports*, vol. 2, pp. 223, 231.

132 Simon, *Public Health Reports*, vol. 2, pp. 230–31; *The Lancet* (1866, vol. 2), pp. 581–2.

133 Simon, *Public Health Reports*, vol. 2, p. 234; NA CUST 58/307/151.

134 NA CUST 58/307/185.

135 Ibid.

136 NA CUST 58/307/187.

137 NA CUST 58/307/185.

138 NA CUST 58/307/187.

later claimed to have been 'fired into' by a gunboat, and the Privy Council agreed to appoint a deputy 'in the present emergency' to assume the duties of Superintendent when Cassé was quarantined.[139]

Another ship, the *Parana*, was used as accommodation for passengers deemed healthy.[140] Once they had been transferred, Cassé was ordered by Wiblin to remove their heavy baggage to the forecastle of the *Atrato* for fumigation.[141] He was to find four jars, put 20 ounces of copper shavings into each, followed by 4 ounces of nitric acid. The portholes were to be closed for up to three hours while the resulting gas was given off, and the baggage could then be removed to the *Parana*. A further six or eight jars were to be used in the holds of the *Atrato* to disinfect the cargo. 'I shall be down tomorrow', wrote Wiblin, 'to give further directions'.[142] On 23 November, ten days after the *Atrato* had arrived, Cassé received a telegram from the Privy Council at 5 o'clock in the morning authorizing the release from quarantine of the *Atrato* and *Parana*, with all people on board, as well as those convalescent on the *Menelaus*.[143] None of this impressed *The Lancet* which, while recognizing the new problem with yellow fever after the outbreak at Swansea, made the customary accusation of 'needless cruelty' towards those confined on shipboard when they would have been better off on land.[144]

For their part, the Privy Council were still inclined towards tough measures and had found in Wiblin a staunch contagionist and virtual successor to Pym. On 24 November 1866, only a day after the release of the *Atrato*, the steamer *Tyne* from St Thomas was sent to The Motherbank following four deaths from yellow fever on the voyage.[145] Cassé was ordered to transfer the sick to the *Menelaus*, and Wiblin sent him another batch of chemicals for the fumigation.[146] These included four gallons of carbolic acid to be diluted with 200 gallons of water for sprinkling over the steamer's coal and pouring into the bilges. But there was a concession to mercy, with the healthy being sent to the *Aeolus*, another hospital ship made available by the Admiralty, from which they were released with their disinfected baggage after only three days.[147] The sick, however, remained on the *Menelaus* from which a boat, at intervals, made legitimate trips to shore. Unfortunately, these runs were never properly explained to the navy, and the boat was again fired upon, prompting an exasperated plea from the Privy Council that Cassé and the officers of the gunboats should 'talk to each other'.[148] On 30 November 1866 the gunboats were withdrawn as no longer necessary, and the potential for a tragic misunderstanding was removed.[149]

139 NA CUST 58/307/191–2.
140 NA CUST 58/307/190.
141 Ibid.
142 Ibid.
143 NA CUST 58/307/191.
144 *The Lancet* (1866, vol. 2), pp. 581–2.
145 NA CUST 58/307/192–3.
146 Ibid.
147 NA CUST 58/307/193–4.
148 NA CUST 58/307/195.
149 NA CUST 58/307/196.

The incidence of yellow fever did not diminish and so the pattern of detention and fumigation continued. In December 1866 the arrival of the *Seine* heralded a slightly revised system.[150] Although the sick were sent to the *Menelaus*, the ship's crew were transferred to the *Aeolus* and the *Parana* was again pressed into service for passengers and their belongings. The sick and convalescent were fumigated before transfer, along with the baggage. Wiblin impressed upon Cassé that the fumes produced by nitric acid reacting with copper filings were too strong for use against people, who would be fumigated instead by sulphur.[151] Even the healthy did not escape the treatment, but it was to be carried out 'in the most careful respectful & least possible offensive manner'.[152] Ladies were to be fumigated as lightly as possible, and children not at all. Within three days, nearly everyone was allowed ashore, but not before a further 'purifying ordeal' involving sulphur.[153] More fortunate were certain imported turtles, which suffered no more than an immersion in sea water.[154] Once the *Parana* had been vacated, the ship was swabbed with chloride of limewater and then fumigated with nitric acid for up to eight hours.[155]

Towards medical inspection

Such activity, although not unlawful, pushed the acceptability of quarantine to its limits. The Privy Council were careful to reinforce every Order with a Proclamation: these were mainly used against named ships (the *Atrato* was subject to further Proclamations in 1867 and 1869), but also for general instructions, and occasionally to allow individuals to visit ships in quarantine without being detained themselves.[156] The legal basis for the management of infected ships had changed with the passing of the Sanitary Act of 1866, which in some respects amended the Quarantine Act of 1825 from which the Privy Council drew their authority.[157] For instance, the penalties under the 1825 Act were reduced 'to such sum as the justices or court think just'.[158] But the scope of the 1825 Act was enlarged to cover diseased vessels not necessarily bound from or to the United Kingdom.[159] It also confirmed the power of the Privy Council to deal with 'cholera and epidemic, endemic and contagious disease' and to announce 'by what Nuisance authority … such orders, rules, and regulations shall be enforced and executed'.[160] This 'Nuisance authority' (in most cases a Local Board of

---

150 NA CUST 58/307/197.

151 Ibid.; but nitric acid and copper filings were still to be used to fumigate baggage.

152 Ibid.

153 NA CUST 58/307/199–200.

154 Ibid.

155 Ibid.

156 Bibliotheca Lindesiana, vol 8: *Handlist of Proclamations issued by Royal and other Constitutional Authorities 1714–1910* … (Wigan, 1913).

157 29 & 30 Vic., c.90; Sir S. Baker, *The Laws relating to Quarantine* (London, 1879), pp. 52–3.

158 29 & 30 Vic., c.90, s.51.

159 29 & 30 Vic., c.90, s.52.

160 Ibid.

Health) had the power to remove to and to detain in hospital 'any Persons ... infected with a dangerous and infectious Disorder' who might arrive on a ship.[161] The specific mention of cholera had echoes of Simon's belief, quoted above, that the disease could be theoretically prevented from spreading by a harshly conducted quarantine. Arrangements for Scotland were broadly similar, set out in the Public Health Act (Scotland) of 1867, but this measure made infected ships specifically subject to the Quarantine Act of 1825.[162]

Although the 1866 Act heralded an alternative approach to seaborne disease (through local government), it still seemed to many in the medical profession that quarantine had re-established an unacceptable foothold. In March 1868 a deputation comprising the President of the College of Physicians, the Director-General of the Navy and a few influential doctors (among them, Sir William Jenner and Milroy), sought to convince the Duke of Marlborough, Lord President of the Council, that a royal commission should be appointed to investigate this very point.[163] His Grace was sympathetic but the appeal was no more than a final push by the NAPSS to complete their long-standing agenda; the Privy Council had no intention of spending public money on yet another round of question and answer, against the background of a medical profession which was still divided. In any event, there were signs that international deliberation was making unilateral investigation unnecessary. In 1856, with cholera very much in mind, several European countries had agreed to work towards a common system of quarantine and an International Commission was formed to draw up a draft convention for the Mediterranean basin.[164] The Commissioners met in Paris, over many months in 1859, but their proposals did not meet universal approval, not least in Britain, and no country ratified the convention.[165] In 1866 a third forum was held in Constantinople, again in the context of cholera.[166] After another lengthy and exhaustive session, in which only 14 of the 37 delegates were medical, the conference concluded that traditional restrictions ought to be maintained and enhanced, leading to a quarantine of ten days (double the time recommended at the Paris conference of 1851) for ships with foul bills.[167] This trend alarmed the anti-contagionist lobby in Britain, although they were not the strident voice which they had been a decade or so earlier.

The year 1871 is another milestone in the history of British quarantine in that it witnessed the passing of the Local Government Board Act on 14 August.[168] The purpose of this Act, the preamble explained, was 'to concentrate in one department ... the supervision of the laws relating to the public health, the relief of the poor, and local government'. This bit deeply into the powers of ministers and of the Privy Council (who lost the services of John Simon) in matters including sanitation and

161 29 & 30 Vic., c.90, s.29.

162 30 & 31 Vic., c.101; Baker, pp. 53–4; cf. NA PC 8/326 (under 1884).

163 *The Lancet* (1868, vol. 1), p. 420; J.C. McDonald, 'The history of quarantine in Britain during the 19th century', *Bulletin of the History of Medicine*, 25 (1951), 37.

164 NA PC 8/326 (under 1882).

165 Ibid.

166 NA PC 8/326 (under 1882); McDonald, pp. 39–40.

167 Ibid.

168 34 & 35 Vic., c.70.

the prevention of disease. In the following year the Local Government Board were empowered to establish Port Sanitary Authorities in England and Wales, a move which seemed likely, eventually, to bring the question of quarantine outside the royal prerogative for the first time in two hundred years.[169] By the Public Health Act, 1875, the powers of the Local Government Board were confirmed, and any infected person on shipboard could be compulsorily removed.[170] The Act gave further impetus to the creation of Port Sanitary Authorities, of which only 50 existed in 1874 among the 88 ports recognized by the Commissioners of Customs.[171] But as the statutory powers of the Privy Council in respect of quarantine continued, the de facto position was that the United Kingdom had a dual policy for dealing with diseased ships. The choice was between quarantine, administered by central government through the Privy Council, and medical inspection, run by local authorities, now with the backing of the Local Government Board. Among other obvious differences, the former relied on fixed rules, while the latter left steps to be determined by circumstance.

Britain was not alone in worrying about the introduction of disease by transatlantic steamers. At Le Havre, precautions were established on the lines of those at Marseilles, where the Board of Health had been superseded by a sanitary department.[172] A new lazaretto was planned for Tatihon in Manche, useful also for Cherbourg, and others were mooted near the mouths of the Loire and Gironde.[173] These developments underlined the importance of The Motherbank, which had slowly become the only working quarantine station in the United Kingdom. During the cholera scare of 1865, hospital ships had been hastily provided for Liverpool and Cork, and soon Plymouth, never happy with its quarantine lot, was arguing for better facilities.[174] But only The Motherbank was fully operational. In 1872 the establishment was 16, led by Cassé, aged 54, who had transferred from Stangate Creek in 1863.[175] He was paid £160 a year, almost double the salary of his deputy (given the rank of mate), who had been in office for 20 years. There were eight mariners paid 3s, 6d a day, and a boy at 2s a day.[176] The mariners' pay had recently increased by 6d, following a petition that they had been relatively better off 25 years earlier.[177] The remaining five personnel constituted the crew (a mate at £105 and four mariners) of the *Edgar*, a former line-of-battle ship used for the reception of passengers.[178] The money for these salaries and wages was recovered by the Customs Commissioners from the Privy Council Office.[179] The hospital ship *Menelaus* and receiving ship *Aeolus*, both ex-frigates

169 35 & 36 Vic., c.79, s.20.

170 38 & 39 Vic., c.55; A. Hardy, 'Cholera, quarantine and the English preventive system, 1850–1895', *Medical History*, 37 (1993), 258.

171 *The Lancet* (1874, vol. 1), p. 555.

172 *The Lancet* (1867, vol. 2), pp. 651–2.

173 Ibid.

174 *The Lancet* (1866, vol. 1), p. 525; (1868, vol. 2), p. 648.

175 NA CUST 58/308/49–50.

176 Ibid.

177 NA CUST 58/308/21–2. Another grievance of the mariners was that they lived most of the time away from their families.

178 NA CUST 58/308/49–52.

179 NA CUST 58/308/46.

(the latter used for convalescents from steamships) were still on station along with a sailing wherry 'necessary for the Service'.[180] The costs of these other vessels were met by the Admiralty, only the *Edgar* being 'lent' to the Board of Customs.[181]

The 3,000–ton *Edgar* was equipped with a saloon dining room and small bedrooms to accommodate 150 passengers and 100 crew.[182] The 1,200-ton *Menelaus* had two dining cabins 'and could accommodate (in sick bay Cabins, 30 in Number) at least 40 patients'.[183] The *Aeolus*, at 1,100 tons, could hold 40 more. Water closets were 'freely distributed at different parts of the Ships for the use of 1st and 2nd Class Passengers & Crews'.[184] Bedding and provisions for passengers were provided by the companies running the mail steamers, but Government provided medical care, drugs and disinfectants.[185] A gunboat had been redeployed to maintain security, but Cassé and the commander had now reached an understanding and bullets were a thing of the past.[186] In overall command was Wiblin, as Medical Superintendent of Quarantine at Southampton, who reported daily to the Privy Council giving the state of health and his opinion of the public danger or otherwise, from which the Council decided when quarantine for any ship should terminate.[187]

Over the next few years, the trend was for the volume of work at The Motherbank to increase. It would have been hardly conceivable, 20 years earlier, that quarantine would remain so entrenched and that the outcry against it would be muted and desultory. In Europe, little progress was being made by the continuing conferences, at least as regards quarantine at seaports. At Vienna, in 1873, it was decided that quarantine at river ports (notably along the Danube) should be abolished, and Russia moved for a debate in the following year, in the same city, centred on the familiar topic of cholera.[188] The British response to cholera was now far less coherent, following Simon's assertion that quarantine might not be as useless as Government had once supposed. In July 1873 the Privy Council asked sanitary authorities to inspect every ship which came from a cholera-infected port, and to detain it for up to 48 hours if something were amiss.[189] If cholera were actually on board, the healthy might land immediately but the sick were to be removed to hospital, the ship fumigated, and clothing disinfected or destroyed.[190] This Order was more or less ignored in major ports like Liverpool and London, but it effectively extended around Britain the kind of management which the Privy Council exercised at The Motherbank quarantine station for the prevention of yellow fever.[191] This did nothing

180 NA CUST 58/308/51–2.

181 NA CUST 58/308/14.

182 NA CUST 58/308/153. Different configurations are given in CUST 58/308/334.

183 Ibid.

184 Ibid.

185 NA CUST 58/308/156.

186 NA CUST 58/308/155.

187 NA CUST 58/308/155–6.

188 *The Lancet* (1874, vol. 1), pp. 554–5.

189 Ibid.

190 Ibid.

191 Ibid.: 'It is said that no workable plan of the kind could possibly be devised for Liverpool, and that the system, if attempted in the Thames, would encounter innumerable

to disentangle the confusion between the twin systems of quarantine and medical inspection, although it was the latter process which the British tried to sell to other delegates at the Vienna conference of 1874.

This conference was marginally more constructive than its predecessors. The United States of America did not attend (although they said they would), but the sittings were brisk and businesslike, and limited to one month.[192] All 22 nations felt that quarantine by land was impracticable, but at seaports all except Spain recommended either a system of medical inspection or quarantine, or a combination of both.[193] Quarantine, however, should not exceed seven days.[194] The British Government noted that these recommendations were limited to the prevention of cholera, and that the conference abstained from discussing yellow fever.[195] A report on the proceedings was given to the Epidemiological Society by one of the delegates, Dr Seaton from the Local Government Board.[196] The discussion which followed was hijacked by Milroy, who barely controlled his irritation that quarantine, whatever modifications were recommended, was still on the international agenda.[197] It worried him especially that British colonies would take the findings as an excuse to continue their 'follies of quarantine' in the absence of any incentive towards medical inspection.[198] But many of Milroy's supporters were now abstaining, or joining the contagionist camp.

In 1874 the extra workload at The Motherbank earned Cassé an increase in salary to £180, with corresponding rises for his deputy and the mate of the *Edgar*.[199] If this was intended to win his acceptance for a new duty – the examination of military transports when they arrived at Spithead – it failed. In July 1875 Cassé pointed out that the anchorage was three miles away and he would need a steamboat to ensure regular access in good weather.[200] But it was the principle which bothered him most. Before 1855 transports had indeed been treated like any other arrival, but their inspection had been a matter for Customs officers from Portsmouth, rather than the quarantine staff at The Motherbank. In that year, however, examination moved to Portsmouth harbour as the Customs officers had lost their cutter.[201] Cassé pointed out that he might well be under quarantine himself, if he had just inspected a ship with yellow fever, and he would not know what to do in any case if the transports had no bill of health.[202] But the Privy Council were not interested in these objections, and Cassé assumed the extra responsibility during 1875, albeit with another increase of

difficulties'.

192 McDonald, p. 40.

193 Ibid.

194 Ibid.

195 NA PC 8/326 (under 1884).

196 *The Lancet* (1875, vol. 1), pp. 623–4.

197 Ibid.

198 Ibid.

199 NA CUST 58/308/123–4.

200 NA CUST 58/308/139–40.

201 NA CUST 58/308/141.

202 NA CUST 58/308/141, 143.

£10 to his salary.[203] In the following year a reduced payment to his deputy (justified by the appointment of a less experienced man) allowed the Council to raise Cassé's salary to £200.[204] It never went beyond that, although Cassé argued that he should be paid as an Examining Officer of Customs, which carried a salary of £220.[205]

Parallel systems

In 1878 particularly bad reports of yellow fever in the Gulf of Mexico brought new anxiety to the Privy Council. Their Clerk, C.L. Peel, was sufficiently alarmed to ask local authorities in England, Wales and Scotland, via the Customs Commissioners, whether they could cope if authorized to deal with a sudden outbreak.[206] He did this in the knowledge that all quarantine grounds except The Motherbank had been 'abandoned' despite the obligation, still in force since 1825, that diseased vessels should make for one of the specified stations. It was clear from the replies that most local authorities would send the sick to a hospital on shore, while leaving the healthy on board. But even those who would land the sick had doubts about the wisdom. When the Medical Officer of Dundee mentioned that the public could well object, Peel feared that this worry might be widely shared. Yet it would be 'objectionable' and 'cruel' to leave people, including the healthy, on an infected ship. That, of course, had been the cry of the medical press for many years, but it now dawned on the Privy Council that removal might not actually be lawful, as Section Two of the 1825 Act had made quarantine compulsory when a ship arrived with disease, and the prevention of yellow fever was still subject to that Act.

This problem was put to the Attorney-General who agreed that the sick and healthy could only be landed following a specific Order in Council.[207] But if that course were adopted, it would 'practically abolish' quarantine and medical inspection would be seen to have triumphed. Peel was unhappy with that idea, arguing that 'it may still be considered expedient for international purposes to keep up the appearance at least of a system which is deemed essential by some foreign Governments'. He suggested that in any new Order some compromise wording might be introduced, for instance allowing people to leave only so that the ship and her cargo (still in quarantine) could be efficiently disinfected. Peel thought the Foreign Office should take a view on the international implications, and that the whole matter should then go to Cabinet before any action were taken by the Privy Council. The Local Government Board were kept abreast of Peel's thinking, and drafted a circular to Port Sanitary Authorities asking them to cooperate fully with the Customs service (and therefore the Privy Council) should yellow fever arrive as feared.

203 NA CUST 58/308/173–4.

204 NA CUST 58/308/187–8.

205 NA CUST 58/308/199. His memorial was followed by others from the mates and mariners also asking for pay increases because of extra duties at Spithead (200–201).

206 NA PC 8/240, from which all references in this paragraph are taken. The point about authorization was that yellow fever was still subject to quarantine as opposed to medical inspection, and therefore remained within the remit of the Privy Council.

207 NA PC 8/241, from which all references in this paragraph are taken.

This spirit of cooperation evaporated very quickly. On 25 March 1879, in a startling reversion to historical practice, the Privy Council issued an Order imposing quarantine against all arrivals from the Baltic, the Black Sea, the Sea of Azoff and the Sea of Marmara at such places and for such times as should be appointed.[208] The reason was international panic at reports of bubonic plague in the Volga delta, brief though they were. *The Lancet* reacted with anger at the 'epidemic lunacy' of Europe which resulted 'in reviving obsolete methods of quarantine, maritime and inland, against the compromised country [Russia], and against the uncompromised countries of each other'.[209] In Britain, the journal mocked a decision which transferred authority 'from the skilled medico-sanitary officers of our seaports to the unskilled fiscal officers of the Customs, and the mere routine procedure of the Quarantine Act'.[210] McDonald attributed this move to a deliberate wish by the Lord President of the Council, the Duke of Richmond, 'to flout the wishes of the sanitarians of the Local Government Board'.[211] The grounds for this attribution lay in a move (unsuccessful) by the Council to seek support from the College of Physicians, and more especially from a robust defence made by Richmond to Parliament, which earned him the cheers of the House.[212]

It is hard to disagree with McDonald, despite the cooperation between the Privy Council and Local Government Board which had immediately preceded the news from Russia. The Board were definitely displeased with how the Council were proposing to act. In a letter to the Council of 20 February 1879 (that is, more than a month before the troublesome Order), they wrote of their strong objections to quarantine, their decided preference for medical inspection, and the disquiet among local sanitary authorities who feared their responsibilities were being usurped by central Government.[213] But luckily for the Privy Council, the contagionist voices were now so widespread that the Board, and for that matter *The Lancet*, were far from winning the argument unopposed. In August 1879 a new figure, Sir Sherston Baker, rose to prominence in the quarantine debate, following a speech to the Association for the Reform of International Law.[214] Baker, indeed, was a lawyer and he offered precise ways in which the opposing systems could be harmonized. Disinfection and the running of lazarettos and hospital ships would become a matter for 'municipal regulations', and countries would be divided into quarantine zones so that, in the event of an epidemic, measures need only be taken against specific locations as opposed to the state as a whole. If quarantine were imposed, it would be by local authorities on their interpretation of the ship's bill of health, which would be made more reliable and precise. At first, *The Lancet* welcomed the 'excellent suggestions'

208 The Order was published in Baker, pp. 110–14. Another copy is in NA CUST 58/309/36–7.

209 *The Lancet* (1880, vol. 1), pp. 688–9.

210 Ibid.

211 McDonald, p. 42.

212 Ibid.

213 NA PC 8/319.

214 *The Lancet* (1879, vol. 2), p. 295, from which all references are taken until otherwise stated. For Baker, see also McDonald, p. 41.

in Baker's speech, but as the implications sunk it became less enthusiastic.[215] Baker had not proposed the abolition of the Quarantine Act so as to avoid 'the clash' between 'political and sanitary aspects' of the prevention of disease, and there were too many echoes from earlier conferences. But the journal was pleased that the quarantine debate had been devolved to a select committee of the Association, which they hoped would take evidence from port sanitary officers, none of whom had attended the lecture and subsequent discussion.

As the Privy Council were aware that no quarantine stations existed around Britain, except at The Motherbank, it was probably no surprise to them that *The Lancet* dismissed their Order against plague as 'absurdly impracticable'.[216] Figures suggest that some ships were diverted to The Motherbank as a result of the plague Order, brief though it was, but not that quarantine resulted. In the 20 years from 1860 to 1879, 12 ships were detained there for yellow fever; 254 arrived from ports in the Mediterranean and were 'liberated' after examination; and 722 ships arrived from ports outside the Mediterranean and were visited and examined, but not detained.[217] The interesting point is that medical inspection applied also at The Motherbank, alongside quarantine, when yellow fever was not an issue. Indeed, Cassé found medical inspection very sensible. It had annoyed him when, in 1873, the local authority at Littlehampton had not allowed a smallpox case to be landed from a Shoreham schooner. 'This gross neglect of their duty', he complained to the Collector at Portsmouth, 'will probably cost the poor man's life'.[218] Later, at The Motherbank, four ships with smallpox and one with cholera were reported by Cassé to the local sanitary authority and dealt with by their regulations.[219] When a troopship arrived at Spithead from Bombay with ten children suffering from scarlet fever, he asked the Collector at Portsmouth to be guided by his sanitary authority.[220] In May 1883, in a good example of how slick the system could be, two cases of smallpox from a Mediterranean steamer were transferred to the borough hospital in Ryde, 13 crewmen were vaccinated, and the ship was disinfected and rapidly granted pratique.[221]

Was there any place left for quarantine when medical inspection was so efficient? *The Lancet* was certain there was not. Quarantine only survived because it was 'plausible and seductive' and fitted the reactionary ideas of certain European states.[222] Such backwardness should not be tolerated in Britain:

> Here the general sanitary administration of the kingdom is so devised that every district, inland or coastwise, is enabled to deal with infectious disease, coming from whatever source, by removal of the conditions which would foster its development, by preventing

215 *The Lancet* (1879, vol. 2), pp. 287–8, from which remaining references in this paragraph are taken.

216 *The Lancet* (1879, vol. 2), p. 288.

217 NA CUST 58/308/250–51.

218 NA CUST 58/308/55.

219 NA CUST 58/308/250–51.

220 NA CUST 58/308/301. This was in 1881.

221 NA CUST 58/308/329.

222 *The Lancet* (1880, vol. 1), p. 687.

> reckless dissemination of infection, by isolation of the infected individual, and by disinfection. In addition ... port sanitary authorities are given the power as regards cholera to medically inspect persons arriving in ships from infected places, to remove and isolate the sick found on board (letting the healthy go free), and to use such processes of disinfection as to the vessel and the articles thereon as may be deemed necessary.[223]

What could quarantine offer in its place but a reliance on negative and superstitious dogma grounded in the Middle Ages?

One of the last decisions of the Duke of Richmond, as Lord President of the Council, was to be lukewarm towards a new sanitary conference proposed to be held in the United States, in the context of yellow fever and cholera.[224] The Privy Council were less supportive than the Foreign Office, who solicited the Board of Trade and the Colonial Office for further views. Of these two bodies, the Colonial Office were markedly more keen, suggesting that Australia, the Cape and Canada should also be represented. This enthusiasm by Secretaries of State led to an opposite alignment, not unexpected, between the Privy Council and the Board of Trade, who believed that more details of the agenda were desirable before any delegate were dispatched. In fact, the proceedings were limited to the need for more accurate advice from ports of departure about local sanitary conditions, and did not touch upon preventive measures on arrival. The British delegate to the conference, held in Washington in 1881, was the consul at New York.

During 1884 came real signs of impatience within the Local Government Board for the twin systems of medical inspection and quarantine to be rationalized. In a long memorandum, dated 23 June, to the Privy Council, the Board gave a resumé of events over the previous decades and the measures in force against the main diseases.[225] They pointed out, incidentally, that the Council had never responded to their letter of 20 February 1879 protesting at the quarantine Order against ships which might be infected with plague. But as that scare was short-lived, yellow fever was now the only disease against which quarantine was normally imposed. Was it not time for yellow fever also to be countered by medical inspection? 'Is there any reason for supposing', they asked, 'that foreign countries would not be satisfied, as they are in the case of Cholera, without requiring quarantine to be imposed?' As long as quarantine was in force, it was used simply because it could be. This confused the public and weakened the authority of the Board vis-à-vis the Port Sanitary Authorities, who could argue or believe that a diseased ship should be quarantined, saving them the trouble of disinfecting and removing the sick. In a note to the new Lord President, Lord Carlingford, the Clerk commented that the Privy Council had never doubted that sanitary authorities were best equipped to deal with these matters, but if quarantine were to be repealed it had to be by Government, having taken advice from the Foreign Office and the Board of Trade as to international reaction. Thus in the passage of 50 years, the traditional anxieties of a nation devoted to trade had not diminished.

---

223 *The Lancet* (1880, vol. 1), p. 689.

224 NA PC 8/256; 8/263, from which all references in this paragraph are taken.

225 NA PC 8/319 from which all references in this paragraph are taken.

Dénouement

Before the end of 1884 it appeared to both the Privy Council and Local Government Board that such differences as existed in their respective attitudes to the prevention of disease were amenable to compromise if not reconciliation. After talks at the level of Clerk on one side and Assistant Secretary on the other, the Council conceded that the system of medical inspection should be extended, while the Board accepted that the same system should accommodate certain aspects of quarantine law.[226] For instance, the yellow-flag rules were sensible, and it was proper for Customs officers initially to stop and interrogate ships. There were still, nevertheless, some disagreements. The Board argued that the recommendation of medical inspection by the 1874 conference at Vienna made The Motherbank station unnecessary, while the Council argued that the context of that recommendation had been cholera and not yellow fever.

But with momentum building, the interpretation of advice given a decade earlier was not significant. A more difficult point was that the Privy Council had jurisdiction over the United Kingdom, whereas the Local Government Board had no authority outside England and Wales. This had already led to a disagreement in policy about the import of rags from Spain: the Local Government Board allowed them, but they could not be landed in Scotland following a ruling of the Board of Supervision in Edinburgh.[227] Furthermore, ships arriving in Scotland infected with cholera were still treated under the Public Health (Scotland) Act of 1867, which invoked the Quarantine Act of 1825. But it was the position in England which focused the attention of both the Privy Council and the Local Government Board, and for some years the idea was mooted that local sanitary authorities might take over the hospital ship or ships at The Motherbank.[228] A hospital ship was already being maintained in the Thames by the Port Sanitary Authority of London.[229] As if in anticipation of the final decision, the establishment at The Motherbank was rapidly run down. In 1885 it was recommended to the Privy Council that the station could get by with only one superintendent, one mate and ten mariners.[230]

The transfer of responsibility at The Motherbank from the Council to the Board became an area of vexed legality. Initially, the proposition seemed simple enough. By August 1887 all parties had agreed that the hulks, when not needed for other reasons, should pass to the Port Sanitary Authorities of Southampton and Portsmouth for the reception of cases of cholera.[231] There would be no fee payable, but the ports would meet costs of wear and tear from actual use, and medical expenses. The Local Government Board drew up a draft Order under their own authority, applicable to local medical officers and the masters of affected vessels. But the Law Lords ruled in November that the Board had no powers to make such an Order because it dabbled in

226 NA PC 8/326, from which all references in this paragraph are taken.

227 Ibid. The full title was the Board of Supervision for the Relief of the Poor.

228 Ibid.

229 Ibid.

230 NA PC 8/343.

231 NA PC 8/377, from which all references in this paragraph are taken.

functions of the Customs service which were not covered by the Public Health Acts. The alternatives, suggested the Law Lords, were for the Local Government Board to draft a new Order within their remit or for the 'whole question' to be put before Parliament, with a view to the revision of the quarantine laws.

While Government hesitated to take this final step, quarantine itself was diminishing. At The Motherbank, Cassé reported in 1884 that the *Aeolus* was being damaged by worm and could be returned to the Admiralty.[232] The hulk had served its purpose since 1866, but need not be replaced. The annual return of the establishment became no more than a reiteration of the previous year. In 1890, when Cassé had reached the age of 72 with nearly 55 years' service, the Privy Council agreed to increase the daily pay of mariners with over 15 years' service from 3s, 6d. to 4s, the first rise since 1872.[233] But as there were no more than ten mariners on the whole station, this was not a significant dent in the Council's budget. In 1891 the boarding station in the Mersey, the last vestige of the quarantine establishment of Liverpool, was declared unnecessary.[234] The Privy Council agreed in March that ships reaching Liverpool from Cuba, or any other place in the yellow-fever latitudes after more than 20 days at sea, could proceed direct to the pier-head entrance of each dock to answer the quarantine interrogatories.[235] As the boarding station had been a few miles upriver from the new docks, this was a valued concession which the pilots supported, and had echoes of pleas from earlier years.

In the Port of London, however, there was no tradition of complacency. In the 1870s it had worried Harry Leach, the Medical Officer of Health, that cholera was establishing itself readily in Europe and that London was becoming too exposed to rapid and serious epidemics.[236] His fears were shared by the Medical Department of the Local Government Board.[237] But Leach's successor, William Collingridge, was more pragmatic, and the passage of 20 years weakened confidence in the quarantine system without diminishing the sense of risk. In May 1891 there was an incident involving the steamer *Memphis* arrived at Gravesend from Baltimore.[238] The master, in response to the usual quarantine interrogatories, stated there was no sickness on board when in fact there were cases of typhoid. When similar incidents came to light, Collingridge was incensed and hoped the Privy Council would make an example of the culprits. The last conviction of a master had been in 1877, for concealing a case of smallpox. But now the Law Lords were unhappy. The interrogatories were so geared to plague and yellow fever that they appeared regardless of anything else, and in any event they were too numerous and lengthy. In March 1892 the Customs Commissioners came up with a revised set, but this time there were worries that plague, still the stuff of governmental nightmares, had been omitted entirely. Not

232 NA CUST 58/308/345. The ship was removed on 6 February 1884.

233 NA CUST 58/308/450–51.

234 NA PC 8/422.

235 Ibid.

236 Hardy, p. 259.

237 Ibid.

238 NA PC 8/447, from which remaining references in this paragraph are taken.

until November 1893 was a new set of questions approved by all parties, including the Local Government Board.

In August 1892 the bad cholera epidemic in Europe, especially at Hamburg, encouraged the Privy Council to sanction new instructions to Customs officials. Questions about cholera were to be put to masters in addition to those for plague and yellow fever sanctioned by quarantine law, and if a ship were infected, or suspected of infection, she was to be detained until the local sanitary authority certified her as 'free'.[239] In a case of actual infection, the ship would be moored wherever the Medical Officer directed.[240] Under no circumstances was a Customs officer to detain a ship under his own authority for more than 12 hours.[241] In a paper to the Shipmasters' Society during April 1894, Collingridge summarized the British position.[242] Quarantine was still legally sanctioned,

> but ... only for the purpose of avoiding certain disabilities to which our shipping would be subject in countries where the fetish ... is still worshipped. All diseases, except yellow fever and plague, are now in practice dealt with by the Port Sanitary Authority, and it cannot be long before even these two will pass into their hands.[243]

Collingridge was correct. On 7 August 1896 royal assent was given to *An Act to make further Provision with respect to Epidemic, Endemic, and Infectious Diseases, and to repeal the Acts relating to Quarantine*, a title generally shortened to the Public Health Act, 1896.[244] This repealed, among other legislation, the Quarantine Act of 1825 and sections or schedules in other Acts in which quarantine was mentioned. In their place, the main provision was an alteration in the powers of the Local Government Board so as to allow them to oversee the routine matters of quarantine which, until then, had been within the purview of the Privy Council. These matters concerned the hoisting of flags, the interrogation of masters, the detention of vessels, and 'the duties to be performed' when a ship was infected. Thus the Board were now able to deal directly with Customs officers and masters, removing the doubts as to their competence which had worried the Law Lords a few years earlier. The Act applied, *mutatis mutandis*, to Local Government Boards in Scotland and Ireland, effectively uniting for the first time the maritime sanitary arrangements of the United Kingdom.

There had been no opposition to the measure and the Bill was only delayed by the prorogation of Parliament in 1895. 'One might have expected some show of sentiment', remarked McDonald, 'to mark the passing of this ancient system [that is,

---

239 NA CUST 58/309/352.

240 Ibid.

241 Ibid.

242 W. Collingridge, *Practical Points in the Hygiene of Ships, and Quarantine* (London, 1894), p. 17.

243 Ibid.

244 59 & 60 Vic., c.19. On the same day was passed the Public Health (Ports) Act, 1896 (59 & 60 Vic., c.20), of which the only measure was to empower the Local Government Board to assign to a Port Sanitary Authority any powers and duties under the Infectious Diseases Prevention Act, 1890.

of quarantine]'.[245] His sense of finality was echoed by Mullett, who referred 'to the termination of quarantine' in England [*sic*] in 1896.[246] But the fact was that quarantine was not being abandoned; it was merely passing from the control of one body to the control of another, and being merged with the process of medical inspection. Two years later, the Shipmasters' Society were informed by a master mariner that several instances had occurred to test the new Act's provisions, notably the arrival of the steamer *Nubia* with cases of cholera.[247] But her detention had been minimal and this was the pattern around the country. No restrictions whatever were being placed on the import of merchandise, even direct from Asia.[248] Such liberality was testimony to the confidence of the Board in the harmonious union of systems which promised to make quarantine no more than a defence of last resort.

By repealing the quarantine laws per se, but vesting key aspects of their operation in the Local Government Board, the British Government had done enough to prevent any repercussions abroad. Most states in Europe had long been convinced that the British were disenchanted with quarantine and perhaps the only surprise was that the legislation had not been repealed sooner. In one sense, it was less complicated to dismantle the system in Britain than in some other countries because the quarantine service was not contracted to outside interests. In Spain, for instance, there was a 'monstrous' requirement for ships to perform quarantine in the lazarettos of Vigo and Port Mahon simply, it was suspected, because they were farmed; it was a similar situation in Portugal.[249] But if Europe was resigned to the defection of Britain from traditional quarantine, there were still countries which felt that Parliament had been ill advised. Generally there was a lack of understanding of the British policy which showed a divergence of attitude and practice between London and Valletta. For instance, it was a source of confusion to Giovanni Bussolin, director of the lazaretto at Trieste, that successive governments which had shown themselves so little inclined to take quarantine measures in the United Kingdom should impose them so vigorously in Malta.[250]

A rebuttal to that comment is that London was simply leaving Malta to her own devices. The Privy Council had always been reluctant to interfere in an area where the Maltese knew best, and the island was near enough to the problematical Levant to be influenced by its politics. An International Sanitary Conference in Rome in 1885, and another in Venice in 1892, had dabbled without conspicuous success in the quarantine arrangements for the Suez Canal, exposing Anglo-French divisions

---

245 McDonald, p. 43.

246 C.F. Mullett, *The Bubonic Plague and England: An Essay in the History of Preventive Medicine* (Lexington, 1956), p. 371.

247 W.G. Romeril, *Quarantine: From a Shipmaster's Point of View* (London, 1898), p. 7.

248 Ibid.

249 Collingridge, p. 28 (comment from the floor by a Captain Froud).

250 G. Bussolin, *Delle istituzioni di sanità marittima nel bacino del Mediterraneo* (Trieste, 1881), p. 51; cf. G.P. Badger, *Historical Guide to Malta and Gozo* (improved and augmented by N. Zammit) (Malta, 1879), p. 196: 'Quarantine [in Malta] is rigorously proclaimed against visitations of cholera which gave constant proof of its propagation by infection'.

which could damage trade between Malta and the Midi.[251] It was also the fact that the lazaretto at Valletta remained highly regarded – or as one guidebook put it in 1884, 'by far the least inconvenient and best regulated purgatory of them all'.[252] The management was still under a Board of Health, an institution which was no longer nominal. In 1867 the composition had been changed to: Governor, as President; Chief Secretary to Government; Superintendent of the Ports; Inspector General of Hospitals; Chief Police Physician; President of the Chamber of Commerce; Professor of Anatomy and Midwifery at the University; and the Cashier of the Government Treasury, who acted as Secretary to the Board.[253] In 1885 a new post of Quarantine Medical Officer, at an annual salary of £250, was attached to the Port Department.[254]

The acceptability of the Maltese lazaretto by its users should not disguise that the same debate existed in the island, as elsewhere in Europe, about the efficacy of quarantine as against medical inspection and sanitary reform.[255] But there was no question of abandoning a system which was still countenanced, for one reason or another, in the countries of the Mediterranean basin which maintained the Maltese economy. It would be beyond the scope of this work to follow the practice of quarantine in Malta (and indeed elsewhere) beyond the nineteenth century, but it should be noted that discussion continued, notably at the Paris Convention of 1903, to make quarantine compatible with advances in preventive medicine. Cassar notes that quarantine at Malta 'was resorted to as late as 1929 in the case of arrivals from Tunis when that country was infected with plague'.[256]

In the modern era the quarantine of shipping remains a possibility under exceptional circumstances and the yellow flag is still included in the International Code of Signals.[257] In Britain, under the Public Health (Ships) Regulations, 1979, a master has an obligation to report infectious illness on his ship. But would quarantine ever be used? The irony is that, with the new diseases of the twenty-first century, recourse is sometimes needed to the methods of the Middle Ages. In May 2003, during the SARS crisis, charterers and shipowners were 'urged to weigh up the costs of quarantine', which seemed a fruitful arena for maritime lawyers.[258] The term 'free practique [*sic*]' was resurrected from misread textbooks.[259] If SARS proved a short-lived scare, avian influenza is still a definite threat and the Marburg virus a dreadful reality. *Lloyd's List*, that most ancient and phlegmatic of newspapers, reported on 14 June 2005 that a bulk carrier remained in quarantine off the island of Réunion

251 For a summary of the later sanitary conferences, see McDonald, pp. 40–41, and D. Panzac, *Quarantaines et lazarets: L'Europe et la peste d'orient (XVIIe–XXe siècles)* (Aix-en-Provence, 1986), pp. 120–22.

252 *Handbook for Travellers to Greece*, 5th edn, Part 1 (London, 1884), p. 16.

253 *Malta Government Gazette*, 11 Jan. 1867, p. 9.

254 *Malta Government Gazette*, 17 Sept. 1885, p. 333.

255 cf. Cassar, p. 297.

256 Ibid.

257 P. Kemp (ed.), *The Oxford Companion to Ships and the Sea* (Oxford, 1976), under 'Quarantine'.

258 *Lloyd's List*, 21 May 2003, p. 6.

259 Ibid.

following the suspected death of a sailor from that very virus. 'The corpse is being kept on ice in an airtight bag', reported the same paper, 'and may need to be buried in a lead coffin'.[260] A lead coffin? There must be a dozen or more hidden in the depths of the Solent, but surely the history of quarantine, in the British context, is not going to repeat itself.

260 *Lloyd's List*, 14 June 2005, p. 1. See also D. Osler, 'Infectious disease: avoid it like the plague', *Lloyd's List*, 30 June 2005, p. 7.

Glossary

The following technical terms are used in this study – some rarely, others very frequently. The definitions given are those relevant to the period and may not always be the modern usage.

bill of health: document given to ship's master by consular official at port of departure, explaining whether or not the locality was free of disease. The main types were 'clean', signifying all was well, or 'foul' indicating an active infection. Italian and French ports recognized intermediate bills, known as 'touched' or 'suspected', which allowed for greater precision and were gradually recognized in Britain. See also **Patent**

bill of lading: declaration of cargo undertaken by a ship's master to be delivered to consignees

burthen: ship's carrying capacity, roughly equivalent to the modern term 'deadweight'

charter party: deed between shipowner and merchant confirming hire of vessel

contagionism: doctrine that disease, typically plague, was transmitted more or less literally by touch. The opposite school of thought was **anti-contagionism**, which argued for the influence of atmospheric conditions.

contumacia: Italian word signifying isolation of suspected persons during a plague epidemic, and sometimes used by British writers as a synonym for quarantine

demurrage: compensation payable for undue detention of a merchant ship, usually because cargo to be loaded had been delayed

depurate: to cleanse a cargo by airing, the operator being known as a **depurator**, and the process **depuration**; often used as a synonym for **expurgate** (**expurgator/expurgation**)

dunnage: material, notably cork, used to protect cargo during the voyage

enumerated goods: items specified in quarantine regulations as being particularly prone to harbour infection, and therefore singled out for thorough airing. There were usually two divisions, first and second class, according to the level of perceived risk.

expurgate: see **depurate**

factory: organized expatriate community, typically in the Levant or at Leghorn, who arranged the export of staple products to Britain

free pratique: see **pratique**

freighter: one who charters and loads a merchant ship

intendant: French word, borrowed sometimes by the British, for an official of a Health Department

lazaret: British word for **lazaretto**, used particularly in the context of the abortive undertaking at Chetney Hill in Kent

lazaretto: corruption of Italian word *lazzaretto* (fever hospital), signifying port building used for the quarantine of passengers and the airing of goods

parloir (**parlatorio**): French (and Italian) words, both adopted by the British, for the room in or attached to a lazaretto where inmates could converse at a distance with visitors

patent: early word for **bill of health**, often used when these were issued to individual travellers

placard: official decree emanating in Holland, used *inter alia* to announce quarantine restrictions

pratique: the release or exemption of a ship, cargo or person from all restrictions on account of quarantine; often called **free pratique**

prior: Italian title for the (secular) head of a **lazaretto**

sanità: Italian word for Board of Health (French: *bureau de santé*) much borrowed by British quarantine administrators, for instance on the Ionian Islands

sciorino: corruption of Italian noun *sciorinamento*, meaning airing of goods

sereine: preliminary or probationary airing of goods (derivation uncertain)

spoglio: Italian word meaning vigorous process of **depuration** for persons and their apparel

susceptible: descriptive of goods liable to retain infection

xebec: small Mediterranean sailing ship with two or three masts, originally used for war but common later as a merchant vessel

Bibliography

1. Primary Sources: Documentary

British Library

Additional MSS among the Liverpool Papers are invaluable for putting quarantine into a political context. The following have proved the most rewarding: 38213, fols 15–25 (Q in Holland and Germany); 38234, fols 29–35 (proposals by the Q Committee) and 36–43 (Q in Mediterranean); 38349, fol. 1 (bills of health), 167–75 (Q in Holland) and 176–82 (Q in Sicily); 38351, fols 243–57 (memorial to Pitt from Levant Company); 38352, fols 179–87 (first report of Turkey [Levant] Company re lazaret); 38353, fols 53–82 (second and third reports of Turkey Company etc.) and 176–8 (ideas for English lazaret); 38354, fols 102–6 (Hawkesbury's views on lazaret and its rules, and admission of foul-bill ships); 38355, fols 113–17 (foul-bill ships); 38358, fols 232–7 (report to Privy Council from Royal College of Physicians).

National Archives, Kew (formerly Public Record Office)

Most information comes from the enormous series of register books of the Privy Council (PC 2) as far as 2/213 (1832). Among loose Privy Council papers, the following are the most useful: PC 1/4531, 4534; 1/8/20; 1/9/126; 1/10/56, 64; 1/13/101–3; 1/44/160; 6/10–12; 7/1, 4–5; 8/240–41, 245–6, 249, 256, 263, 319, 326, 343, 377, 391, 422, 447. Early Board of Trade minute books (CO 391/1–89, covering 1675–1782) contain minimal quarantine entries, but the following books from the later series have references of varying importance: BT 5/8–10, 26–8, 31–7. The best material by far is in BT 6/149, endorsed 'Lazarette Papers', which goes some way towards explaining the abortive moves at Stangate Creek. Papers of Dr Charles Maclean are catalogued as BT 6/247. Treasury papers can certainly yield information about quarantine but the bundles can be tedious to examine and references are seldom about policy. The published calendars of Treasury books and papers, although falling short of the heyday of quarantine, are by far the easiest resource to use. Similarly, the published Home Office papers, such as they are, are adequate for the few references which concern that department. The Chatham papers shed light on the dealings of Pitt the younger with quarantine, and especially valuable are PRO 30/8/26/44–5; 30/8/54/277–80; 30/8/83/1–6; 30/8/114/192, 194, 196, 198; 30/8/152/203; 30/8/149/242; 30/8/160/275; 30/8/168/246–9; 30/8/181/11–12; 30/8/259/170, 175–84, 338–43. Among Customs records of individual ports, incidental references to quarantine are not uncommon, but CUST 58/306–9 based on the port of Portsmouth are the most profitable. Also important is the record of ships quarantined 1790–1800 at Hull, under CUST 92/24. For the Baltic crisis, Customs records of Yarmouth (CUST 97/74a), Harwich (CUST 99/1) and Newcastle (CUST

84/122) are worth inspection. State papers are helpful in a variety of ways. The correspondence and papers of Sir Horace Mann are especially interesting under SP 98/47/145, 148–9, 151–2, 154–5, 160–61, 166–8, 173–5, 193–6, 216–17 during the Messina plague. For the earlier Baltic crisis, there is much useful material under SP 100/61, centred on the Swedish Resident in London. The main value of State Papers, however, is that they include records of the Levant Company under SP 105. The out-letter book (SP 105/116) has many quarantine references, and the register of orders (SP 105/332/103) and court books under SP 105/210 and 332 are enlightening. Minutes of the Admiralty Board, especially ADM 3/24–7, are valuable during the Baltic crisis. For the Mediterranean possessions, Colonial Office papers are extremely important, although for Gibraltar and the Ionian Islands the amount of knowledge to be gleaned is small in relation to the bulk of material. It is with Minorca and Malta that the files become truly absorbing. For Minorca, see especially CO 174/1–9, 12, 15–16 and 19. For Malta, the corpus of evidence is vast, and particularly revealing are CO 158/1–5, 7–14, 16–20, 22–9, 31, 34–8, 41–4, 50–52, 55–7.

Other British repositories

In London, the Sir John Soane Museum has the architect's designs for an English lazaret in volume 60 of the Soane drawings. The Institution of Civil Engineers houses the Rennie Manuscripts which are important for a new dimension in the study of the lazaret fiasco. The relevant references are Rennie MSS, First Series, vol. 4, pp. 80–391; vol. 5, pp. 24–363; vol. 6, pp. 225–426; vol. 7, pp. 126–402; and vol. 8, pp. 30–390. All these page numbers are *passim*. In the National Maritime Museum, the Caird Library has Navy Board minutes (unpaginated), among which references to quarantine during the Baltic crisis can be found in SER/62–4.

Elsewhere, the Staffordshire Record Office has the Dartmouth Papers, which shed light on the relative roles of the Cabinet and the Lords of the Committee in questions of quarantine. The refs are D(W)1778/V/188 and D742/U/1/1–139 and D742/U/2/1–77.

In Scotland, the West Register Office has relevant material under Customs circulars (CE 14/1) and individual ports, notably Dumfries during the Baltic crisis (CE 51/1).

Malta

The main repositories are the National Library in Valletta and the National Archives in Rabat, with some overlap between them. In the former, quarantine records are divided between the archives of the Order of St John (classification AOM) giving, *inter alia*, actual ships quarantined between 1654 and 1694 and between 1739 and 1801, and those of the Library proper (classification LIB). The Quarantine Office letter-book, 1815–23, is LIB 843, while minutes of the proceedings of the Board of Health, 1826–36, constitute LIB 847. (Cassar [pp. 291–2] refers to other minutes of the Board, 1832–56, in the 'Medical & Health Archives, Valletta'.) In the National

Archives, the two main sources are the letter-books of the Quarantine Office, catalogued as C1 and C2. These have been researched between 1829 and 1849, when they tend to become perfunctory. The National Archives have most numbers of the *Malta Government Gazette* on open access.

Marseilles

The Archives départementales des Bouches-du-Rhône house the invaluable records of the Intendance Sanitaire, or Board of Health. In-letters are grouped geographically and the most rewarding series are 200 E 463–4, which cover Malta for most years from 1726 to 1865. Letters from Gibraltar, 1753–1850, are catalogued as 200 E 441. For the Ionian Islands, there is correspondence with the French consulate (1728–1850) and the Health Office (1802–50). Letters from Zante survive roughly 1725–1821, but for all series there are certain years with no extant correspondence. Historians studying quarantine more widely will be interested in the huge series of letters from Venice (200 E 433–5), Livourne [Leghorn] (200 E 426–7) and Gênes [Genoa] (200 E 422–4).

2. Primary Sources: Printed

Acts of the Privy Council of England. New Series (32 vols, London: HMSO, 1890–1907).

Acts of the Privy Council of England (14 vols, London: HMSO, 1921–64).

Acts of the Privy Council of England. Colonial Series (6 vols, London: HMSO, 1908–12).

Anderson, A., *An Historical and Chronological Deduction of the Origin of Commerce* (2 vols, London: A. Millar, 1764).

Annual Register (London, 1758–).

Armstrong, J., *The History of the Island of Minorca* (London: C. Davis, 1752).

An Authentic Account of the Measures and Precautions used at Venice, by the Magistrate of the Office of Health ... (London, 1752).

Ayre, J., *A Letter, addressed to the Right Honourable Lord John Russell, M.P. ... on the Evil Policy of those Measures of Quarantine, and restrictive Police, which are employed for arresting the Progress of the Asiatic Cholera* ... (London: Longman & Co., 1837).

Badger, G.P., *Historical Guide to Malta and Gozo* (improved and augmented by N. Zammit), 6th edn (Malta, 1879).

Bailey, N., *An Universal Etymological Dictionary* (London: E. Bell, 1721).

Barclay, J., *A Complete and Universal English Dictionary* .... (London: Richardson & Urquhart, 1774).

Beckwith, C., *A Poet's Bazaar. From the Danish of Hans Christian Andersen* ... (3 vols, London: Richard Bentley, 1846).

Beldam, J., *Recollections of Scenes and Institutions in Italy and the East* (2 vols, London: James Madden, 1851).

Bibliotheca Lindesiana, vol 5: *A Bibliography of Royal Proclamations of the Tudor and Stuart Sovereigns and of Others Published under Authority 1485–1714 … England and Wales* (Oxford: Clarendon Press, 1910).

Bibliotheca Lindesiana, vol 6: ibid, *Ireland and Scotland* (Oxford: Clarendon Press, 1910).

Bibliotheca Lindesiana, vol 8: *Handlist of Proclamations issued by Royal and other Constitutional Authorities 1714–1910 …* (Wigan, 1913).

Blane, G., *Observations on the Diseases Incident to Seamen* (London: Joseph Cooper, 1785).

Blaquiere, E., *Letters from the Mediterranean; containing a Civil and Political Account of Sicily, Tripoly, Tunis, and Malta …* (2 vols, London: Henry Colburn, 1813).

Boisgelin, Louis de, *Ancient and Modern Malta …* (3 vols, London: G. & J. Robinson, 1804).

Bowring, J., *Observations on the Oriental Plague and on Quarantines …* (Edinburgh: William Tait, 1838).

[Boyer, A], *The History of the Reign of Queen Anne, digested into Annals* (11 vols, London: Roper & Coggan, 1703–13).

Bradley, R., *The Plague at Marseilles Consider'd …* (London: W. Mears, 1721).

Brand, J., *The Histories and Antiquities of the Town and County of the Town of Newcastle upon Tyne …* (2 vols, London: White & Egerton, 1789).

British Parliamentary Papers. Some appear in this Bibliography under their originator (for example, General Board of Health), or title (for example, *Second Report …*), or author (for example, Burrell). Among others, the following are the most significant (titles summarized):

1. *BPP*, vol. 14 (1821), pp. 175–96, Return of Q establishments in England and Scotland, 1792 and 1820.
2. *BPP*, vol. 14 (1821), p. 197, Ditto Ireland, in respect of Customs Department expenses.
3. *BPP*, vol. 21 (1821), p. 337, Salaries and expenses at Chetney Hill lazaret, 1800–1820.
4. *BPP*, vol. 21 (1821), p. 301, Q receipts in UK, 1800–20.
5. *BPP*, vol. 17 (1831), pp. 347–54, Five-year return of vessels in Q in UK with fees for clearance, and vessels in Q since 1 January 1831.
6. *BPP*, vol. 17 (1831), p. 355, How Q release fee is appropriated.
7. *BPP*, vol. 29 (1838), pp. 311–455, Report of committee enquiring into affairs on Malta, with correspondence.
8. *BPP*, vol. 17 (1839), pp. 755–875, Ditto, with further correspondence.
9. *BPP*, vol. 54 (1843), pp. 1–427, Correspondence re contagion of plague and Q regulations of foreign countries, 1836–43.
10. *BPP* vol. 25 (1846), pp. 509–13, Return of how money voted for Q expenses was spent, with payments to named officers.
11. *BPP*, vol. 45 (1846), pp. 443–92, Recent foreign correspondence re Q laws.
12. *BPP*, vol. 49 (1847), pp. 565–84, Further foreign correspondence re Q laws.
13. *BPP*, vol. 60 (1847–48), p. 509, Return of recent measures re Q laws.
14. *BPP*, vol. 35 (1850), pp. 411–37, Return of Q expenses in UK, Ireland, Malta and the colonies over previous ten years, continued in *BPP*, vol. 52 (1851), pp. 683–93.

15. BPP, vol. 60 (1852–53), pp. 491–3, Return of officers (with salaries) at Q stations in UK, Ireland and Malta.

16. BPP, vol. 36 (1854–55), pp. 539–55, Q at Gibraltar.

17. BPP, vol. 52 (1857–58), pp. 451–60, Ten-yearly Q returns from colonies, to 1854.

18. BPP, vol. 60 (1860), pp. 155–90, Q regulations in foreign countries, with report of Paris conference, 1851–52.

19. BPP, vol. 60 (1860), pp. 191–276, Q information from National Association for Promotion of Social Science (NAPSS).

20. BPP, vol. 58 (1861), pp. 225–72, Papers re Q, including report by NAPSS.

21. BPP, vol. 64 (1867), p. 619, Vessels sent to English Q stations, 1850–66.

Brydone, P., *A Tour through Sicily and Malta in a Series of Letters to William Beckford, Esq. of Somerly in Suffolk* (2 vols, London: Strahan & Cadell, 1790).

Burrell, W.H., 'Report on the Plague in Malta in 1813', in General Board of Health, Appendix V to Second Report on Quarantine, in *British Parliamentary Papers*, vol. 45 (1854–55), pp. 399ff.

Bussolin, G., *Delle istituzioni di sanità marittima nel bacino del Mediterraneo* (Trieste, 1881).

Calendar of Home Office Papers of the Reign of George III (4 vols, London: HMSO, 1878–99).

Calendar of the Clarendon State Papers Preserved in the Bodleian Library (5 vols, Oxford: Clarendon Press, 1872–1970).

Calendar of State Papers and Manuscripts [Venetian] (38 vols, London: HMSO, 1864–1947).

Calendar of State Papers, Colonial Series, America and West Indies (45 vols, London: HMSO, 1860–1994).

Calendar of State Papers, Domestic Series ... Charles II (28 vols, London: HMSO, 1860–1947).

Calendar of Treasury Books (32 vols, London: HMSO, 1904–62).

Calendar of Treasury Papers (6 vols, London: HMSO, 1868–89).

Calendar of Treasury Books and Papers (5 vols, London: HMSO, 1897–1901).

Clément, P., *Lettres, instructions et mémoires de Colbert* (9 vols, Paris, 1861–82).

Cobbett's Political Register (1802–35).

Cockburn, G., *A Voyage to Cadiz and Gibraltar up the Mediterranean to Sicily and Malta in 1810, & 11* … (2 vols, London, 1815).

Colegate, J., *Guide to Dunoon* … (Dunoon, 1868).

A Collection of the Statutes relating to the Admiralty, Navy, Shipping, and Navigation … (London: Eyre & Strahan, 1810).

Crouch, H., *A Complete View of the British Customs* … (London, 1724 [and later editions]).

Crouch, H., *A Complete Guide to the Officers of His Majesty's Customs in the Out-Ports ...*(London, 1732).

Davy, J., *Notes and Observations on the Ionian Islands and Malta: with some Remarks on Constantinople and Turkey, and on the System of Quarantine as at Present Conducted* (2 vols, London: Smith, Elder, 1842).

[Defoe, D.], *Due Preparation for the Plague, as well for Soul as Body* … (London: Seeley & Burnside, 1722).

[Defoe, D.], *A Plan of the English Commerce Being a Compleat Prospect of the Trade of this Nation, as well the Home Trade as the Foreign* (London: Charles Rivington, 1728).

Dendy, F.W. (ed.), *Extracts from the Records of the Merchant Adventurers of Newcastle-upon-Tyne* (2 vols, Surtees Society, 1895–99).

Dew, D., *A Digest of the Duties of Customs and Excise …* (London: Richards, 1818).

Diderot & D'Alembert, *Encyclopédie* (Neufchastel, 1765).

Dillon, J.J., *A Memoir Concerning the Political State of Malta* (London: J. Booker, 1807).

Dunford, C. & East, E.H., *Reports of Cases Argued and Determined in the Court of King's Bench …* (London: Whieldon & Butterworth, 1792).

Edinburgh Review (1803–74).

Elliott, C.B., *Travels in the Three Great Empires of Austria, Russia, and Turkey* (2 vols, London, 1838).

Eton, W., *A Survey of the Turkish Empire …* , 3rd edn (London: T. Cadell, 1801).

Eton, W., *Authentic Materials for a History of the People of Malta …* (4 parts, London, 1802–07).

'Explainer', *Distinct Notions of the Plague, with the Rise and Fall of Pestilential Contagion* (London, 1722).

Extracts from the Burgh Records of Edinburgh (Edinburgh: Oliver & Boyd, 1927–50).

Faulkner, Sir A.B., *A Treatise on the Plague, designed to prove it Contagious …* (London, 1820).

Field, Revd J., *Correspondence of John Howard, the Philanthropist* (London, 1855).

Galt, J., *Voyages and Travels, in the Years 1809, 1810, and 1811; containing Statistical, Commercial, and Miscellaneous Observations on Gibraltar, Sardinia, Sicily, Malta, Serigo, and Turkey* (London: Cadell & Davies, 1812).

Gee, J., *The Trade and Navigation of Great-Britain Considered …* (London, 1738).

General Board of Health, *Report on Quarantine. Presented to both Houses of Parliament by Command of Her Majesty* (London, 1849).

General Board of Health, *Second Report on Quarantine. Yellow Fever* (London, 1852) (see also under Burrell).

The Gentleman's Magazine (1731–1868).

Granville, A.B., *A Letter to the Right Honorable F. Robinson, M.P. ... on the Plague and Contagion, with Reference to the Quarantine Laws* (London, 1819).

Granville, A.B., *A Letter to the Right Hon. W. Huskisson, M.P. President of the Board of Trade on the Quarantine Bill* (London, 1825).

Hadley, G., *A New and Complete History of the Town and County of ... Kingston-upon-Hull* (Hull: T. Briggs, 1788).

Hancock, T., *Researches into the Laws and Phenomena of Pestilence; ... and Remarks on Quarantine* (London, 1821).

Hansard, T.C., *Parliamentary Debates* (1803–).

Hasselquist, F., *Voyages and Travels in the Levant; in the Years 1749, 50, 51, 52 ... Published, by ... Charles Linnaeus …* (London: Davis & Reymers, 1766).

Hasted, E., *The History and Topographical Survey of the County of Kent* (4 vols, Canterbury, 1778–99).

Hennen, J., *Sketches of the Medical Topography of the Mediterranean: comprising an Account of Gibraltar, the Ionian Islands, and Malta* (London, 1830).

Historical Manuscripts Commission, *Eleventh Report, Appendix, Part IV* (Townshend) (London, 1887).

Historical Manuscripts Commission, *Thirteenth Report, Appendix, Part VIII* (Charlemont), vol. 2 (1784–99) (London, 1894).

Historical Manuscripts Commission, *Fourteenth Report, Appendix, Part IX* (Buckingham) (London, 1895).

Historical Manuscripts Commission, *Calendar of the Manuscripts of the Marquess of Ormonde* … , New Series, vol. 6 (London, 1911).

Historical Manuscripts Commission, *Report on the Manuscripts of J.B. Fortescue, Esq., preserved at Dropmore*, vol. 8 (Hereford, 1912).

Historical Manuscripts Commission, *House of Lords Manuscripts. New Series*, vols 8–10 (London, 1923–53).

Hodges, N., *Loimologia: or, an Historical Account of the Plague in London in 1665 … with Remarks on the Infection now in France, and the most probable Means to prevent its Spreading here. By John Quincy, M.D.* (London: E. Bell, 1720).

Holroyd, A.T., *The Quarantine Laws, their Abuses and Inconsistencies. A Letter addressed to the Hon. Sir John Cam Hobhouse, Bart. M.P. President of the Board of Control* … (London, 1839).

[Hoste, Sir W.], *Service Afloat or the Naval Career of Sir William Hoste* (London: W.H. Allen, 1887).

[Hoste, Sir W.], *Memoirs and Letters of Capt. Sir William Hoste* (2 vols, London, 1833).

Howard, J., *An Account of the Principal Lazarettos in Europe* … (Warrington, 1789, and London: J. Johnson 1791).

The Immediate Necessity of Building a Lazzaretto for a Regular Quarantine, after the Italian Manner, to avoid the Plague, and to Preserve Private Property from the Plunderers of Wrecks upon the British Coast … (London: J. Murdoch, 1768).

Ingram, D., *An Historical Account of the Several Plagues that have appeared in the World, since the year 1346* … (London, 1755).

Jackson, J., *Reflections on the Commerce of the Mediterranean* … (London, 1804).

Jarvis, R.C. (ed.), *Customs Letter-Books of the Port of Liverpool 1711–1813* (Manchester: Chetham Society, 1954).

Jesse, Capt. W., *Notes of a Half-pay in Search of Health: Russia, Circassia, and the Crimea, in 1839–40* (2 vols, London, 1841).

Johnson, S., *Dictionary of the English Language* … (2 vols, London, 1756).

[Jourdan, A.J.L.], *Receuil général des anciennes lois françaises* (28 vols, Paris, 1822–30).

Journal of the Commissioners for Trade and Plantations (14 vols, London: HMSO, 1920–38).

Journal of the House of Commons (1547–).

Journal of the House of Lords (1509–).

The Lancet (1823–).

Lane, J., *The Reports of the Commissioners appointed to examine, take, and state the Public Accounts of the Kingdom, Presented to His Majesty and to both Houses of Parliament, with the Appendixes Complete* (3 vols, London: T. Cadell, 1783–87).

Lardner, D., *Steam Navigation with India by the Red Sea; advocated in a Letter to the Right Honourable Lord Viscount Melbourne …* (London, 1837).

Latham, R. & Matthews, W. (eds), *The Diary of Samuel Pepys* (9 vols, London: Bell & Hyman, 1970–83).

Legh, T., *Narrative of a Journey in Egypt and the Country beyond the Cataracts* (London, 1816).

A Letter to a Friend from a Merchant who had Resided many Years at Leghorn: Giving an Account of the Methods taken by that State to prevent Infection. Together with the Author's Thoughts what we ought to do at this Conjuncture, in order to preserve our Health and Trade (London, 1721).

Letters, &c. on the Subject of Quarantine (London: Philanthropic Reform, 1799).

Lewis, M.A. (ed.), *A Narrative of my Professional Adventures (1790–1839) by Sir William Henry Dillon* (2 vols, London: Navy Records Society, 1953–56).

Lewis, W.S. (ed.), *The Yale Edition of Horace Walpole's Correspondence*, 52 vols (London: Oxford University Press, 1937–83).

Lind, J., *An Essay on Diseases Incidental to Europeans in hot Climates* (London, 1768).

Lloyd, C. (ed.), *The Keith Papers* (3 vols, London: Navy Records Society, 1950).

Lloyd, C. (ed.), *The Health of Seamen. Selections from the Works of Dr. James Lind, Sir Gilbert Blane and Dr. Thomas Trotter* (London: Navy Records Society, 1965).

Lockhart, J.G., *The Life of Sir Walter Scott* (10 vols, Edinburgh, 1903).

The London Gazette (1666–).

The London Magazine: or Gentleman's Monthly Intelligencer [alternative suffix ... *and Monthly Chronologer*] (1732–85).

Luttrell, N., *A Brief Historical Relation of State Affairs from September 1678 to April 1714* (6 vols, Oxford: Oxford University Press, 1857).

Macgregor, J., *Commercial Statistics ...* (5 vols, London: C. Knight, 1844–50).

Maclean, C., *Results of an Investigation, respecting Epidemic and Pestilential Diseases; including researches in the Levant, concerning the Plague* (2 vols, London, 1817–18).

Maclean, C., *Remarks on the British Quarantine laws, and the so-called Sanitary Laws of the Continental Nations of Europe, especially those of Spain* (London, 1823).

Maclean, C., *Evils of Quarantine Laws, and Non-Existence of Pestilential Contagion …* (London, 1824).

Maclean, C., *Observations on Quarantine: being the Substance of a Lecture delivered at the Liverpool Lyceum* (Liverpool, 1824).

Macmichael, W., *A Brief Sketch of the Progress of Opinion on the subject of Contagion; with some Remarks on Quarantine* (London, 1825).

Macpherson, D., *Annals of Commerce, Manufactures, Fisheries, and Navigation …* (4 vols, London: Nichols & Son, 1805).

M[c]William, J.O., *Observations on that Portion of the Second Report on Quarantine by the General Board of Health which relates to the Yellow Fever Epidemy on board H.M.S. Éclair, and at Boa Vista in the Cape de Verde Islands* (London: W. Tyler, 1852).

Malta Government Gazette (1826–).

Martin, R.M., *History of the British Colonies* (5 vols, London: Cochrane & M'Crone, 1835).

McCulloch, J.R., *A Dictionary, Practical. Theoretical, and Historical of Commerce and Commercial Navigation: Illustrated with Maps* (London: Longman, Rees, 1834).

McCulloch, J.R. (ed.), *Early English Tracts on Commerce* [first published London, 1856] (Cambridge: Economic History Society, 1952).

Matthews, H., *The Diary of an Invalid being the Journal of a Tour in Pursuit of Health in Portugal Italy Swizerland and France in the Years 1817 1818 and 1819*, 2nd edn (London: John Murray, 1820).

Mead, R., *A Short Discourse concerning Pestilential Contagion, and the Methods to be used to Prevent it* (London, 1720).

[Meryon, C.L.], *Travels of Lady Hester Stanhope; forming the Completion of her Memoirs. Narrated by her Physician* (3 vols, London, 1846).

Miège, M., *Histoire de Malte* (3 vols, Paris, 1840).

Miller, H., *My Schools and Schoolmasters* ... (Edinburgh: Johnstone & Hunter, 1854).

Milroy, G., *Quarantine and the Plague: being a Summary of the Report on these Subjects recently addressed to the Royal Academy of Medicine in France* ... (London, 1846).

Milroy, G., *The Cholera not to be Arrested by Quarantine: a Brief Historical Sketch of the Great Epidemic of 1817, and its Invasions of Europe in 1831–2 & 1847* ... (London, 1847).

Milroy, G., 'Operation and Results of Quarantine in British Ports since the Beginning of the present Century', *Association Medical Journal* [1] (1853): 579–82, 635–9.

Milroy, G., 'Quarantine as it is, and as it ought to be', *Transactions of the National Association for the Promotion of Social Science. 1858* (London, 1859): 521–31.

Milroy, G., 'Papers relating to Quarantine', in *British Parliamentary Papers*, vol. 58 (1861), pp. 225–72.

Murray, J., *The Plague and Quarantine. Remarks on some Epidemic and Endemic Diseases* ... , 2nd edn (London, 1839).

Napier, C.J., *The Colonies ... Ionian Islands in Particular* ... (London, 1833).

Napier, E., *Excursions along the Shores of the Mediterranean* (2 vols, London, 1842).

The Nature of a Quarantine as it is Performed in Italy; to Guard against that very alarming and dreadful contagious distemper, commonly called the Plague ... (London: J. Williams, 1767).

The Naval Chronicle (1799–1818).

The New Statistical Account of Scotland (15 vols, Edinburgh & London: W. Blackwood & Sons, 1845).

Nicolas, Sir N.H. (ed.), *The Dispatches and Letters of Vice Admiral Lord Viscount Nelson* (7 vols, London: Henry Colburn, 1845–46).

Notes and Queries (1849–).

Papon, J.P., *De la peste, ou Epoques mémorables de ce fléau, et les moyens de s'en préserver* (2 vols, Paris, 1800).

Pardessus, J.M., *Collection de lois maritimes antérieures au XVIII siècle* (6 vols, Paris: Imprimerie royale, 1828–45).

Parke, G., *Letters and Correspondence ... of ... Lord Visc. Bolingbroke* ... (4 vols, London: G.G. & J. Robinson, 1798).

Pasley, C.W., *Essay on the Military Policy and Institutions of the British Empire* (London, 1811; reissued 1847).

[Penn, G.], *The Policy and Interest of Great Britain, with Respect to Malta, Summarily Considered* (London: J. Hatchard, 1805).

Pfeiffer, I., *Visit to the Holy Land, Egypt, and Italy* (trans. from German) (London: Ingram Cooke, 1852).

Plumptre, A., *A Historical Relation of the Plague at Marseilles in the year 1720 ... translated from the French manuscript of Mons. Bertrand* ... (London: Joseph Mawman, 1805).

Postlethwayt, M., *The Universal Dictionary of Trade and Commerc*e ... , 3rd edn (2 vols, London, 1766).

Proclamations, Minutes and other Official Notices, published by the Government of the Island of Malta, and its Dependencies, From ... 1813, to ... 1820 (Malta, 1821); and *1821, to ... 1822* (Malta, 1823).

Pye, G., *A Discourse of the Plague; Wherein Dr. Mead's Notions are Considered and Refuted* (London, 1721).

Quarterly Review (1809–)

Quincy, J., *Of the Different Causes of Pestilential Diseases and how they become Contagious, with Remarks Upon the Infection now in France* ... (London, 1720) [see also Hodges].

Register of the Privy Council of Scotland (22 vols, Edinburgh, 1877–1908).

Report from the Select Committee Appointed to consider the validity of the doctrine of Contagion in the Plague (1819) [*BPP*, vol. 2 (1819), pp. 537ff.].

Rolt, R., *A New Dictionary of Trade and Commerce* ... (London: T. Osborne, 1756).

Roseveare, H. (ed.), *Markets and Merchants of the late Seventeenth Century. The Marescoe–David letters, 1668–1680* (Records of Social and Economic History. New Series 12) (Oxford, for British Academy, 1987).

Russell, P., *A Treatise of the Plague* ... (London: J. Robinson, 1791).

Savary des Bruslons, J., *Dictionnaire universel de commerce* ... (3 vols, Paris, 1723–30).

Scicluna, H.P., *Documents Relating to the French Occupation of Malta in 1798–1800* (Valletta, 1923).

Second Report from the Select Committee Appointed to Consider of the Means of Improving and Maintaining the Foreign Trade of the Country. Quarantine (1824) [*BPP*, vol. 6 (1824), pp. 165ff.].

Sellers, M., *The Acts and Ordinances of the Eastland Company* (Royal Historical Society, London, 1906).
Semple, R., *Observations on a Journey through Spain and Italy to Naples; and thence to Smyrna and Constantinople*, 2nd edn (2 vols, London: Baldwin, 1808).
Sheahan, J.J., *General and Concise History and Description of the Town and Port of Kingston-upon-Hull* (London, 1864).
Simon, J., *Public Health Reports* (2 vols, London: Sanitary Institute, 1887).
Simon, J., *English Sanitary Institutions* … (London: Cassell, 1890).
Simson, J., *Reminiscences of Childhood at Inverkeithing, or Life at a Lazaretto* (New York, 1882).
Slade, Capt. A., *Records of Travels in Turkey, Greece, etc. and of a Cruise in the Black Sea with the Capitan Pacha*, new edn (London, 1854).
Smith, A., *A Month at Constantinople*, 2nd edn (London: D. Bogue, 1850).
Stewart, C., *Travels of Mirza Abu Taleb Khan in Asia, Africa, and Europe, during the Years 1799, 1800, 1801, 1802, and 1803* (2 vols, London, 1814).
Sutherland, Capt., *A Tour up the Straits, from Gibraltar to Constantinople* … , 2nd edn (London, 1790).
Swan, Revd C., *Journal of a Voyage up the Mediterranean; principally among the Islands of the Archipelago, and in Asia Minor* … (2 vols, London, 1826).
Swift, J., *Journal to Stella*, ed. H. Williams (2 vols, Oxford: Clarendon Press, 1948).
Terry, C., *Scenes and Thoughts in Foreign Lands* (London: W. Pickering, 1848).
Thursfield, H.G. (ed.), *Five Naval Journals, 1789–1817* (London: Navy Records Society, 1951).
Two Very Singular Addresses to the People of England: Faithfully printed from the Originals, 'after performing a Quarantine of more than Forty Days.' (London, 1757).
Tully, J.D., *The History of Plague as it has lately appeared in the Islands of Malta, Gozo, Corfu, Cephalonia, &c.* … (London: Longman, Hurst, 1821).
Vanderpoel, S. Oakley, 'Quarantine …', in A.H. Buck, *A Treatise on Hygiene and Public Health* (2 vols, London: Sampson, Low, 1879).
Voyages and Travels of her Majesty, Caroline Queen of Great Britain … (London: Jones, 1821).
Walsh, Revd R., *A Residence at Constantinople during a Period including the Commencement, Progress, and Termination of the Greek and Turkish Revolutions* (2 vols, London, 1836).
Walsh, T., *Journal of the late Campaign in Egypt: including Descriptions of that Country, and of Gibraltar, Minorca, Malta, Marmorice, and Macri; with an Appendix Containing Official papers and Documents*, 2nd edn (London, 1803).
Warburton, E., *The Crescent and the Cross; or Romance and Realities of Eastern Travel* (2 vols, London: Colburn, 1845).
Westminster Review (1824–1914).
White, A., *A Treatise on the Plague* … (London, 1846).
White, C., *Three Years in Constantinople* (3 vols, London, 1845).
White, W., *The Evils of Quarantine Laws and Non-Existence of Pestilential Contagion* … (London, 1837).

Whitworth, Sir C., *The Political and Commercial Works of that Celebrated Writer Charles D'Avenant, LL.D ...* (5 vols, London: R. Horsefield etc., 1771).
Whitworth, Sir C., *State of the Trade of Great Britain in its Imports and Exports, progressively from the Year 1697 ...* (2 parts, London, 1776).
Willis, N.P., *Pencillings by the Way* (3 vols, London, 1835).
Wood, M., *The Importance of Malta considered in the Years 1796 and 1798; also Remarks, which occurred during a Journey from England to India, through Egypt, in the Year 1779* (London: John Stockdale, 1803).

3. Secondary Sources

Ackerknecht, E.H., 'Anticontagionism between 1821 and 1867', *Bulletin of the History of Medicine*, 22 (1948), 562–92.
Albion, R.G., *Forests and Sea Power: The Timber Problem of the Royal Navy, 1652–1862*, Harvard Economic Studies 29 (Cambridge, Mass., 1926).
Åström, S.-E., *From Cloth to Iron. Part 1. The Growth, Structure and Organization of the Trade*, and *Part 2. The Customs Accounts as Sources for the Study of the Trade* (Helsingfors: Societas Scientiarum Fennica, 1963–65).
Baker, Sir S., *The Laws relating to Quarantine ...* (London: Keegan, Paul, 1879).
Ballou, M.M., *The Story of Malta* (Boston & New York: Houghton, Mifflin, 1893).
Bang, N.E., and Korst, K., *Tabeller over Skibsfart og Varetransport gennem Øresund 1661–1783 og gennem Storebælt 1701–1748 ...* (Copenhagen & Leipzig, 1930).
Barbour, V., 'Marine risks and insurance in the seventeenth century', *Journal of Economic and Business History*, 1 (1928–29): 561–96.
Bashford, A., 'Migration, borders and public health: histories of the future?', *Wellcome History*, 26 (Summer, 2004), 2–4.
Basye, A.H., *The Lords Commissioners of Trade and Plantations commonly known as the Board of Trade, 1748–1782*, Yale Historical Publications Miscellany 14 (New Haven & London, 1925).
Baugh, D.A., *Naval Administration, 1715–1750* (London: Navy Records Society, vol. 120, 1977).
Beaven, A.B., *The Aldermen of the City of London* (2 vols, London: Corporation of London, 1908–13).
Bendall, S., *Dictionary of Land Surveyors and Local Map-Makers of Great Britain and Ireland, 1530–1850*, 2nd edn (2 vols, London: British Library, 1997).
Bense, J.F., *Anglo-Dutch Relations from the Earliest Times to the Death of William the Third ...* (Oxford: Oxford University Press, & The Hague: M. Nijhoff, 1925).
Biddle, S., *Bolingbroke and Harley* (London: Allen & Unwin, 1975).
Biraben, J.–N., *Les Hommes et la peste en France et dans les pays européens et mediterranéens* (2 vols, Paris: Mouton, 1975–76).
Blackstone, Sir W., *The Commentaries on the Laws of England*, 4th edn (4 vols, London: John Murray, 1876).
Bonnassieux, P. (ed.), *Conseil de commerce et Bureau du commerce 1700–1791. Inventaire analytique des procès-verbaux* (Paris, 1900).
Boogert, M.H. van den, *Friends and Rivals in the East* (Brill, 2000).

Braudel, F., *The Mediterranean and the Mediterranean World in the Age of Philip II* (2 vols, London: Collins, 1972–73).

Brockington, F., 'Public health at the Privy Council 1831–4', *Journal of the History of Medicine ...* , 16 (1961), 162–85.

Brockington, F., 'Public health at the Privy Council 1805–6', *Medical History*, 7 (1963), 13–31.

Bynum, W.F., & Porter, R. (eds), *Companion Encyclopaedia of the History of Medicine* (2 vols, London: Routledge, 1993).

Carden, R.W., *The City of Genoa* (London: Methuen, 1908).

Carrière, C., Courdurié, M., & Rebuffat, F., *Marseille ville morte. La Peste de 1720* (Marseilles: M. Garçon, 1968).

Carson, E.A., 'The customs records of Portsmouth', *Journal of the Society of Archivists*, 5/7 (April, 1977), 429–36.

Carswell, J., *The South Sea Bubble* (Stroud: Alan Sutton, 1993).

Cassar, P., *Medical History of Malta* (London: Wellcome Historical Medical Library, 1965).

Chance, J.F., 'England and Sweden in the time of William III and Anne', *English Historical Review*, 16/63 (1901), 676–711.

Chance, J.F., *George I and the Northern War* (London: Smith, Elder, 1909).

Chance, J.F., 'List of diplomatic representatives and agents, England and North Germany, 1689–1727', in C.H. Firth (ed.), *Notes on the Diplomatic Relations of England and Germany* (Oxford: B.H. Blackwell, 1907).

Chance, J.F., 'List of English diplomatic representatives and agents in Denmark, Sweden and Russia ... 1689–1762', in C.H. Firth (ed.), *Notes on the Diplomatic Relations of England with the North of Europe* (Oxford: B.H. Blackwell, 1913).

Chart, D.A., *The Story of Dublin* (London: J.M. Dent, 1907).

Checkland, S.G., *Scottish Banking. A History, 1695–1973* (Glasgow & London: Collins, 1975).

Clark, G.N., *Guide to English Commercial Statistics, 1696–1782* (London: Royal Historical Society, 1938).

Coleridge, E.H., *The Life of Thomas Coutts Banker ...* (2 vols, London: John Lane, 1920).

Colledge, J.J., *Ships of the Royal Navy* (London: Greenhill, 2003).

Collingridge, W., *Practical Points in the Hygiene of Ships, and Quarantine* (London: Shipmasters' Society, 1894).

Colvin, H.M. (ed.), *The History of the King's Works* (6 vols, London: HMSO, 1963–82).

Colvin, H.M., *A Biographical Dictionary of British Architects, 1660–1840*, 3rd edn (London & New Haven: Yale University Press, 1995).

Conn., S., Gibraltar in British Diplomacy in the Eighteenth Century (New Haven: Yale University Press, 1942).

Creighton, C., *A History of Epidemics in Britain* (2 vols, Cambridge: Cambridge University Press, 1891–94).

Cunningham, W., *The Growth of English Industry and Commerce in Modern Times. The Mercantile System* (2 vols, Cambridge: Cambridge University Press, 1896–1903).

Davis, R., *The Rise of the English Shipping Industry* (London: Macmillan, 1962).
Dews, N., *The History of Deptford ...*, 2nd edn (London & Deptford: Simpkin Marshall, 1884).
Dixon, C. Willis, *The Colonial Administration of Sir Thomas Maitland* (London: Longmans, 1939).
Dunkin, A.J., *History of the County of Kent ... Deptford* (London: J.R. Smith, 1854).
Earle, P., *Corsairs of Malta and Barbary* (London: Sidgwick & Jackson, 1970).
Epstein, M., *The Early History of the Levant Company* (London: G. Routledge & Sons, 1908).
Fedorowicz, J.K., *England's Baltic Trade in the Early Seventeenth Century: A Study in Anglo-Polish Commercial Diplomacy* (Cambridge: Cambridge University Press, 1980).
Flinn, M.W., *Men of Iron: The Crowleys in the Early Iron Industry* (Edinburgh: Edinburgh University Press, 1962).
Frazer, W.M., *A History of English Public Health, 1834–1939* (London: Baillière, Tindal & Cox, 1950).
Froggatt, P., 'The Chetney Hill lazaret', *Archaeologia Cantiana*, 79 (1964), 1–15.
Froggatt, P., 'The lazaret on Chetney Hill', *Medical History*, 8 (1964), 44–62.
Galea, J., 'The quarantine service and the Lazzaretto of Malta', *Melita Historica*, 4/3 (1966), 184–209.
Gibson, E.C.S., *John Howard* (London, 1901).
Graham, E.J., *A Maritime History of Scotland (1650–1790)* (East Linton: Tuckwell Press, 2002).
Gregory, D., *Minorca, the Illusory Prize ...* (London: Associated University Presses & Rutherford, NJ: Fairleigh Dickinson University Press, 1990).
Gregory, D., *Malta, Britain and the European Powers, 1793–1815* (Madison: Fairleigh Dickinson University Press & London: Associated University Presses, 1996).
Hardman, W., *A History of Malta ...* (London: Longmans, 1909).
Hardy, A., 'Cholera, quarantine and the English preventive system, 1850–1895', *Medical History*, 37 (1993): 250–69.
Healey, E., *Coutts & Co, 1692–1992: The Portrait of a Private Bank* (London: Hodder & Stoughton, 1992).
Herlihy, P., *Odessa: A History, 1794–1914* (Cambridge, Mass.: Harvard University Press, 1986).
Hill, B.W., *Robert Harley. Speaker, Secretary of State and Premier Minister* (New Haven & London: Yale University Press, 1988).
Hinton, R.W.K., *The Eastland Trade and the Common Weal in the Seventeenth Century* (Cambridge: Cambridge University Press, 1959).
History of Parliament, *The House of Commons, 1790–1820* (5 vols, London: Secker & Warburg, 1986).
Holdsworth, Sir W., *A History of English Law* (17 vols, London: Methuen, 1903–72).
Hollaender, A.E.J., 'A London merchant's letter book', *Archives*, 3/17 (1957), 31–8.

Hoon, E.E., *The Organization of the English Customs System, 1696–1786* (Newton Abbot: David & Charles, 1968).

Horn, D.B. (ed.), 'The Board of Trade and consular reports, 1696–1782', *English Historical Review*, 54 (1939), 476–80.

Jackson, G., *Hull in the Eighteenth Century: A Study in Economic and Social History* (Oxford: Oxford University Press, 1972).

Johnston, W., *Roll of Commissioned Officers in the Medical Service of the British Army ... 1727 to ... 1898* (Aberdeen: Aberdeen University Press, 1917) [reproduced as part of *Commissioned Officers in the Medical Service of the British Army, 1660–1960* (2 vols, London: Wellcome Historical Medical Library, 1968)].

Joyce, J.W., *Daniel Defoe and the Plague in Marseilles (1720–1722)* (Leeds, 1957) (adapted from 'La Peste de Marseille de 1720–21 vue par les Anglais', *Provence Historique*, 5 (1955). 146–54).

Keevil, J.J., *Medicine and the Navy, 1200–1900* (4 vols, Edinburgh & London, 1957–63).

Kemp, P. (ed.), *The Oxford Companion to Ships and the Sea* (Oxford: Oxford University Press, 1976).

Kent, H.S.K., 'The Anglo-Norwegian timber trade in the eighteenth century', *Economic History Review*, 2nd series, 8 (1955–56), 62–74.

Kenyon, J.P. (ed.), *The Stuart Constitution, 1603–1688: Documents and Commentary* (Cambridge: Cambridge University Press, 1966).

Laferla, A.V., *British Malta* (2 vols, Valletta: Government Printing Office, 1938).

Lameire, I., *Les Occupations militaires de l'Ile de Minorque pendant les Guerres de l'Ancient Droit* (Paris: A. Rousseau, 1908).

Lavery, B., *Shipboard Life and Organisation, 1731–1815* (Navy Records Society, vol. 138) (Aldershot: Ashgate, 1998).

Lindsay, W.S., *History of Merchant Shipping and Ancient Commerce* (4 vols, London: S. Low, 1874).

Lipson, E., *The Economic History of England. The Age of Mercantilism* (3 vols, London: A. & C. Black, 1943).

Lloyd, C., & Coulter, J.L.S., *Medicine and the Navy, 1200–1900* (4 vols, Edinburgh and London: E. & S. Livingstone, 1957–63).

Lloyd's List (1734–).

Lord, W.F., *Sir Thomas Maitland: The Mastery of the Mediterranean* (London: T. Fisher Unwin, 1897).

Lord, W.F., *England and France in the Mediterranean, 1660–1830* (London: Sampson Low, 1901).

Luke, H., *Malta: An Account and an Appreciation* (London: George G. Harrap, 1949).

McDonald, J.C., 'The history of quarantine in Britain during the 19th century', *Bulletin of the History of Medicine*, 25 (1951), 22–44.

Mackenzie, W.J.M., & Grove, J.W., *Central Administration in Britain* (London: Longmans, Green, 1957).

Mackintosh, J.P., *The British Cabinet*, 3rd edn (London: Stevens, 1977).

McLachlan, J.O., *Trade and Peace with Old Spain, 1667–1750* (Cambridge: Cambridge University Press, 1940).

McNeill, W.H., *Plagues and People* (Oxford: Blackwell, 1977).

Mallia-Milanes, V., *The British Colonial Experience, 1800–1964: The Impact on Maltese Society* (Malta: Mireva Publications, 1988).

Mansel, P., *Constantinople City of the World's Desire, 1453–1924* (London: John Murray, 1995).

Masson, P., *Histoire du commerce français dans le Levant au XV111e siècle* (Paris, 1911).

Moote, A.L. & D.C., *The Great Plague* … (Baltimore & London: John Hopkins University Press, 2004).

Mullett, C.F., 'A century of English quarantine (1709–1825)', *Bulletin of the History of Medicine*, 22/6 (1949), 527–45.

Mullett, C.F., 'Politics, economics, and medicine: Charles Maclean and anticontagion in England', *Osiris*, 10 (1952), 224–51.

Mullett, C.F., *The Bubonic Plague and England: An Essay in the History of Preventive Medicine* (Lexington: University of Kentucky, 1956).

Office-Holders in Modern Britain II, J.C. Sainty (ed.), *Officials of the Secretaries of State, 1660–1782* (London: University of London, Institute of Historical Research, and Athlone Press, 1973).

Office-Holders in Modern Britain III, J.C. Sainty (ed.), *Officials of the Boards of Trade, 1660–1870* (London: Athlone Press for University of London, Institute of Historical Research, 1974).

Office-Holders in Modern Britain IV, J.C. Sainty (ed.), *Admiralty Officials, 1660–1870* (London: Athlone Press, 1975).

Office-Holders in Modern Britain VII, J.M. Collinge (ed.), *Navy Board Officials, 1660–1832* (London: University of London, Institute of Historical Research, 1978).

Oxford Dictionary of National Biography (60 vols, Oxford: Oxford University Press, 2004).

Panzac, D., *Quarantaines et lazarets. L'Europe et la peste d'orient (XVIIe–XXe siècles)* (Aix-en-Provence: Edisud, 1986).

Paris, R., *Histoire du commerce de Marseille* … (5 vols, Paris, 1949–57).

Phelps, Revd W., *The History and Antiquities of Somersetshire* … (2 vols, London, 1835–39).

Plumb, J.H., 'The mercantile interest: the rise of the British merchant after 1689', *History Today*, 5 (1955), 762–7.

Plumb, J.H., 'The organization of the Cabinet in the reign of Queen Anne', *Transactions of the Royal Historical Society*, 5th series, 7 (1957), 137–57.

Pratique (Quarterly Journal of Disinfected Mail Study Circle) (1974–).

Ransom, J.E., 'John Howard on quarantine', *Bulletin of the Institute of the History of Medicine*, 6 (1938), 111–16.

Ritchie, J., 'Quarantine for plague in Scotland during the sixteenth and seventeenth centuries', *Edinburgh Medical Journal*, 55 (1948), 691–701.

Robinson, H., *Britain's Post Office* (Oxford: Oxford University Press, 1953).

Romeril, W.G., *Quarantine: From a Shipmaster's Point of View* (London: Shipmasters' Society, 1898).

Rose, J. Holland, 'Lord Elgin's report on Levantine affairs and Malta, 28 February 1803', *English Historical Review*, 36 (1921), 234–6.

Saul, N.E., *Russia and the Mediterranean* (Chicago & London: University of Chicago Press, 1970).

Schumpeter, E.B., *English Overseas Trade Statistics, 1697–1808* (Oxford: Clarendon Press, 1960).

Shrewsbury, J.F.D., *A History of Bubonic Plague in the British Isles* (Cambridge: Cambridge University Press, 1970).

Skempton, A.W., *A Biographical Dictionary of Civil Engineers in Great Britain and Ireland, vol 1: 1500–1830* (London: Thomas Telford, 2002).

Smith, D.M. (ed.), *A Guide to the Archives of the Company of Merchant Venturers of York* (Borthwick Texts and Calendars 16, York, 1990).

Smith, F.B., *The People's Health, 1830–1910* (London: Croom Helm, 1979).

Smout, T.C., 'Scottish commercial factors in the Baltic at the end of the seventeenth century', *Scottish Historical Review*, 39 (1960), 122–8.

Stanewell, L.M. (ed.), *Calendar of the Ancient Deeds, Letters, Miscellaneous Old Documents, &c., in the Archives of the Corporation* (Hull, 1951).

Stephen, W., *History of Inverkeithing and Rosyth* (Aberdeen: G. & W. Fraser, 1921).

Sultana, D., *Samuel Taylor Coleridge in Malta and Italy* (Oxford: Blackwell, 1969).

Taggart, J. McA., 'On guard at the Gateway', *Ulster Medical Journal*, 36 (1967), 23–32.

Thomson, M.A., *The Secretaries of State, 1681–1782* (Oxford: Clarendon Press, 1932).

Trousset, J., *Nouveau dictionnaire encyclopédique …* (5 vols, Paris, 1884–86).

Turner, E.R., *The Privy Council of England in the Seventeenth and Eighteenth Centuries, 1603–1784* (2 vols, Baltimore: John Hopkins University, 1927).

Vassallo, C., *Corsairing to Commerce: Maltese Merchants in XVIII Century Spain* (Malta: Malta University, 1997).

Velimirovic, B., 'The quarantine stations at Mahon, Menorca', *Pratique*, 17/3–4 (1992), 74–80.

Walford, E., & Thornbury, W., *Old and New London …* (6 vols, London, 1873–78).

Williams, N., *Contraband Cargoes: Seven Centuries of Smuggling* (London: Longmans Green, 1959).

Wilson, C., *England's Apprenticeship, 1603–1763*, 2nd edn (London: Longman, 1984).

Winslow, C.E.A., *The Conquest of Epidemic Disease …* (Princeton: Princeton University Press, 1943).

Wood, A.C., *A History of the Levant Company* (Oxford: Oxford University Press, 1935).

Appendix 1

Quarantine Stations

Appendix 1 (a)

Quarantine stations in Great Britain and the Channel Islands

The map shows the stations appointed by various Orders in Council in a clockwise rotation from the largest and most important establishment, which was Stangate Creek in the Medway estuary. Four points should be noted: (1) until 1754 quarantine was not a continuous legal requirement, but the earlier gap years are too complicated to be shown in the table; (2) virtually any port, particularly in the south-west of England, could be used occasionally and unofficially for quarantine purposes, usually because the condition of the ship or state of the weather made it arguably dangerous to proceed to the appointed place; (3) in the years before 1720 several anchorages in east and south-east England (for example, Sandwich and The Downs) were recognized by the Privy Council but not subject to an Order in Council; (4) during the cholera crisis of 1832, many small ports often in remote areas, e.g. Kirkwall, were authorized to quarantine arrivals. These minor or temporary stations in (2) – (4) are not represented on the map. Other places not shown are the east-coast Scottish harbours (Montrose, Burntisland etc.) and islands (Inchcolm, Inchkeith) which were occasionally used in the seventeenth century and even earlier. A particular problem is Leith, which was never an official station after the Act of Union, except briefly in the cholera crisis, but managed to quarantine ships fairly frequently.

The key shows stations with foul-bill status (not necessarily throughout the period) in bold, and other major stations (especially those with floating lazarettos over several decades) in italics. Dates indicate the years in which a station was officially operative, but terminal dates are woolly unless the station was deliberately closed. Facilities were nominal from around 1840, except at nos 1, 2 and 9. An asterisk indicates the erection of a land lazaret. Other points, as necessary, are explained in footnotes.

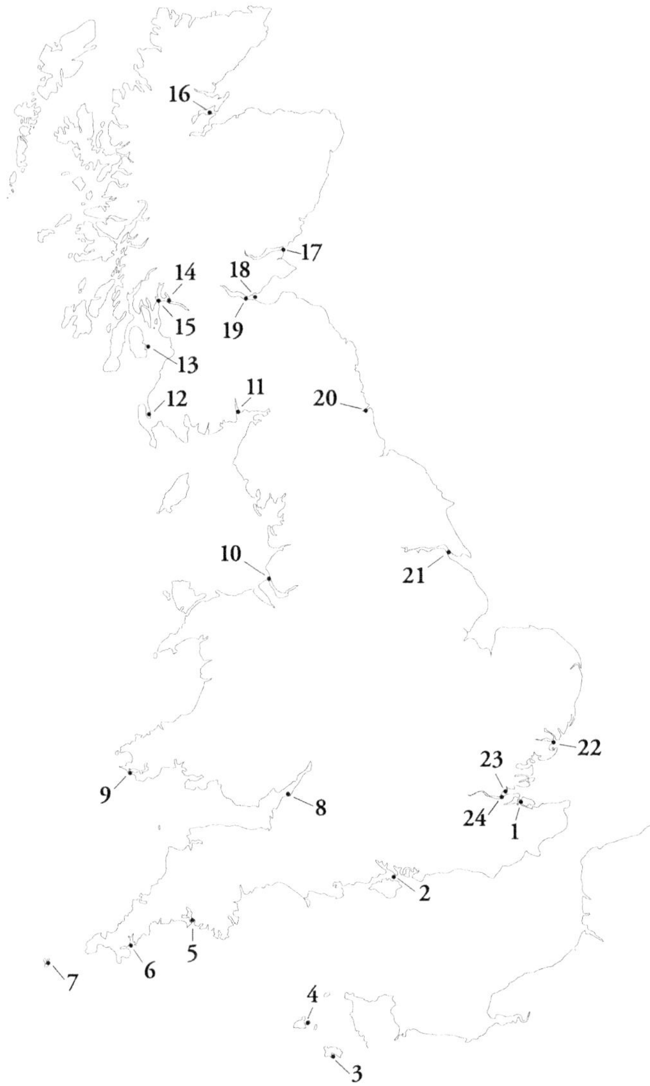

1. Rochester, **Stangate Creek***, 1709–*c.*1870[1]
2. Portsmouth, **Motherbank**, 1709–*c.*1895[2]
3. Jersey, Belle Croute, 1772–1805
4. Guernsey, Little Road, 1772–1805
5. Plymouth, 1720–86; *c.*1827–*c.*1870[3]
6. *Falmouth, St Just's Pool*, 1720–*c.*1850[4]
7. Isles of Scilly, 1753–1825[5]
8. *Bristol*, 1720–*c.*1850[6]
9. **Milford Haven**, 1805–*c.*1870[7]
10. *Liverpool*, 1728–*c.*1891[8]

11. Carsethorn, near Dumfries, 1743–1806[9]
12. Loch Ryan, 1743–72
13. Lamlash, Isle of Arran, 1772–1804
14. Greenock, Tail-of-the-Bank, 1743–72
15. *Holy Loch**, 1804–*c.*1845[10]
16. **Cromarty Firth/Bay**, 1743–1806; 1831–32[11]
17. Dundee, 1743–1772; 1831–33[12]
18. *Inverkeithing**, 1743–1833[13]
19. St Margaret's Hope, *c.*1832–35
20. Newcastle, 1709–14
21. *Hull (Whitebooth Roads)*, 1709–14; 1728 – *c.*1850
22. Harwich, 1709–14
23. Hole Haven, 1663–64; 1668–69
24. The Hope, 1692–93

Notes:

1. The establishment at Stangate Creek embraced, at various dates, Hoo Fort Island and Sharfleet Creek. The lazaret at Chetney Hill, proposed in 1752 and begun in 1764–65, was never completed. The site was abandoned around 1820.
2. The foul-bill station for the navy from 1805, and later for steam packets.
3. Quarantine from c.1768 was in the River Tamar near Saltash. Despite losing its status as a Q port in 1786, Plymouth continued to quarantine warships in Stonehouse Pool or Cawsand Bay and merchant ships in the Cattewater. When Q status was reintroduced, the station was confirmed as the Cattewater.
4. St Just's Pool became the Q anchorage from 1772.
5. This station was reserved for ships actually infected, regardless of their bill of health. The anchorage was New Grimsby (1753–56) and St Helen's Pool (1756–1825).
6. The early anchorage was King Road, backed up by Portshute Pill from 1772.
7. Created foul-bill station in 1813.
8. The early anchorage was at Hoylake, superseded by Bromborough Pool in 1809. From 1772 Liverpool was the Q station for the Isle of Man.
9. Reinstated in error in 1825, but the Order was rescinded within two months. Dumfries itself had been a minor Q port (1709–14).
10. The land lazaret was erected in 1806.
11. In 1825 Cromarty Bay was reinstated in error, but the Order was rescinded within two months. Foul-bill status was not granted until 1831.
12. A land lazaret existed briefly in 1832–33.
13. Inverkeithing Bay had been used occasionally for quarantine in the Baltic and Marseilles crises. The land lazaret was erected in 1806.

Appendix 1 (b)

Quarantine stations in Ireland

The adage 'any port in a storm' explains why virtually any haven in Ireland was used for quarantine purposes at any date. There were, nevertheless, strategically placed harbours where quarantine was encouraged. The earliest of these were the seven appointed by the Lord Lieutenant and Privy Council of Ireland in 1711, which appear in italics in the list below. There was no proper station in Ireland for foul-bill arrivals, although Carlingford Lough claimed that role until 1825, when the Privy Council in London directed that such ships should proceed to Milford Haven. A hospital ship was moored at Cork during the cholera crises, where it is likely that foul-bill ships were occasionally received. There were no land lazarets in Ireland beyond huts on Clontarf Island, off Dublin, in the seventeenth century. Among Irish ports where quarantine was tolerated, but not to the extent that would warrant inclusion in the table, are Drogheda, Sligo and Castlehaven. The numbers are arranged clockwise from Dublin, and where necessary give the exact, alternative, or later anchorage(s) which served the port in question. A final list of nine quarantine stations in Ireland was drawn up by the British Privy Council in 1826: these are underlined. To serve Dublin, Kingstown was substituted for Poolbeg in 1837.

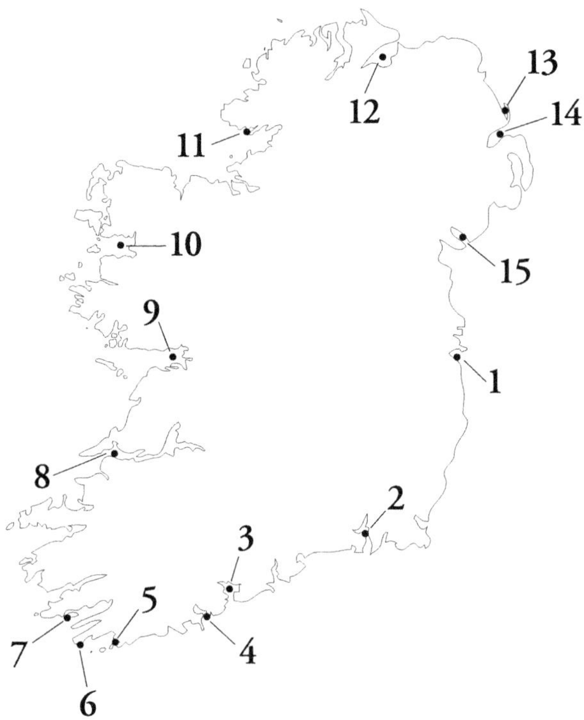

1. *Dublin*: Clontarf; Poolbeg; Dublin Bay; 'Pigeon House'; Kingstown. The sandbank of North Bull was used as an airing ground.
2. Waterford: River Suir
3. *Cork*: Spike Island; Whitegate
4. Kinsale
5. Baltimore
6. Crookhaven
7. Beerhaven
8. *River Shannon*: Scattery Road/Bay; Kilrush; Tarbert
9. *Galway Bay*: Hare Island; Black Rock
10. Clew Bay
11. *Killybegs*
12. *Londonderry*: Ballymastoker Bay; Redcastle Road; Greencastle
13. Larne Lough
14. [Belfast]: *Kilroot*; Garmoyle
15. Carlingford Lough: Warrenpoint

Appendix 2

Summary of Acts of the Westminster Parliament relating wholly or in part to quarantine

Year	Statute	Summarized title (spellings rationalized)
1710	9 Anne, c.10	Act to oblige ships coming from places infected, more effectually to perform their quarantine
1721	7 Geo. I, c.3	Act for repealing the above Act, and for better preventing the plague being brought from foreign parts, and to hinder the spread of infection [to be in force for 3 years]
1721	8 Geo. I, c.8	Act to enable His Majesty effectually to prohibit commerce for one year with any country infected with plague, and for shortening the continuance of 7 Geo. I, c.3 [now to end 25 March 1723]
1721	8 Geo. I, c.10	Act for repealing such clauses in 7 Geo. I, c.3 as give power to remove persons from their habitations, or to make lines about places infected
1721	8 Geo.I, c.18	Act to prevent the clandestine running of goods and the danger of infection thereby, and to prevent ships breaking their quarantine [and for other non-Q purposes]
1728	1 Geo. II, c.13	Act to oblige ships coming from places infected more effectually to perform their quarantine, and for better preventing the plague being brought from foreign parts, and to hinder the spread of infection [to be in force for 2 years]
1733	6 Geo. II, c.34	Act for reviving [for 2 years] so much of 1 Geo. II, c.13 as relates to quarantine and preventing the spread of infection, and to enable His Majesty to prohibit commerce temporarily with any country infected with plague

Year	Statute	Summarized title (spellings rationalized)
1753	26 Geo. II, c.6	Act to oblige ships more effectually to perform their quarantine, and for better preventing the plague being brought from foreign parts
1753	26 Geo. II, c.18	Act for enlarging and regulating trade into the Levant Seas [specifically section 12]
1756	29 Geo. II, c.8	Act to repeal a clause in 26 Geo. II, c.18 whereby New Grimsby was to receive ships infected with plague north of Cape Finisterre, and to appoint a more safe and commodious place
1772	12 Geo. III, c.57	Act to explain and amend so much of 26 Geo. II, c.6 as relates to the establishment of lazarets
1788	28 Geo. III, c.34	Act more effectually to secure the performance of quarantine, and for amending several laws relating to the revenue of Customs
1798	38 Geo. III, c.33	Act to amend 26 Geo. II, c.6 and 28 Geo. III, c.34 respecting the performance of quarantine [and for other non-Q purposes]
1799	39 Geo. III, c.99	Act to encourage trade into the Levant seas by providing a more convenient mode of performing quarantine [and for other non-Q purposes]
1800	40 Geo. III, c.80	Act for erecting a lazaret on Chetney Hill in Kent, and for reducing into one Act the laws relating to quarantine, and for making further provision therein
1800	41 Geo. III, c.30	Act for explaining 40 Geo. III, c.80 as regards payment of tonnage duty in Channel Islands and Isle of Man
1805	45 Geo. III, c.10	Act for making further provision for the effectual performance of quarantine
1805	45 Geo. III, c.97	Act to indemnify all persons concerned in issuing an Order of Council and directions for extending time of certain ships to perform quarantine
1806	46 Geo. III, c.98	Act for making additional and further provisions for the effectual performance of quarantine
1810	50 Geo. III, c.20	Act for removing doubts as to power of appointing Superintendents of Quarantine and their assistants

Year	Statute	Summarized title (spellings rationalized)
1811	51 Geo. III, c.46	Act to authorise officers of the Customs to act for the Superintendent of Quarantine and his assistants
1825	6 Geo. IV, c.78	Act to repeal the several laws relating to the performance of quarantine, and to make other provisions in lieu thereof
1896	59 & 60 Vic., c.19	Act to make further provision with respect to epidemic, endemic, and infectious diseases, and repeal the Acts relating to Quarantine

Note: It should also be noted that many Victorian Public Health Acts were incidentally relevant to the imposition of quarantine and to the gradual substitution of the system of medical inspection.

Appendix 3

Petitioners for the release of ships from quarantine, 1709–1714

Note: This table lists merchants. It does not include other petitioners, e.g. Count Gyllenborg (the Swedish minister), ships' masters, or owners of lobster boats. 'Unspecified' means the exact number of ships is not stated in the record(s). Location of petitioners is unknown when blank. Evidence for 'Scotland' in some cases is only that the referral was to the Customs Commissioners in North Britain (because the ships were quarantined in Scotland). Some London merchants, especially Norris, occasionally petitioned for ships trading to Scottish ports.

The main Swedish merchants are distinguished by (S) after the name.

Petitioner	Location	Ships	Ships in association with other petitioners	Total
Jonas Alberg	London	12	1 with Fullman; 3 with Norris; unspecified with Wallan	16+
Samuel Allison		1		1
James Alstrom	London	9	2 with Thomlinson & Wilkinson	11
Alexander Arbuthnot	Scotland		3 with Farrington	3
William Astell (S)	London	19	1 with Brander & Eastland Company; 1 with Erthman; 1 with Thomlinson; 1 with Bowman & W. Joy; 3 with Taylor; 5 with Benson & T. Coutts	31
Thomas Atkinson	Hull	1		1
Alexander (and/or James) Auchterlony	Scotland	3		3
George Bearance	London		7 with C. Joy	7
Brian Benson (S)	London		5 with Astell & T. Coutts	5
Thomas Bowden		1		1

Petitioner	Location	Ships	Ships in association with other petitioners	Total
William Bowden	Scotland	5	Unspecified with Skinner	5+
Henry Bowman			1 with Astell & W. Joy; 1 with W. Joy & Norris; 3 with Erthman & W. Joy; 6 with W. Joy	11
Charles Brander	London	50	1 with Norris; 1 with Astell & Eastland Company; 1 with Garrett; 3 with A. Crowley; 15 with Erthman	71
Thomas Broadley	Hull	1		1
Robert Bruce	Scotland	1		1
Stephen Bullock	London		Unspecified with Thomas Coutts & Phill	?
William Clayton		1		1
John Cleveland		1		1
Francis Collins	London	6	2 with Taylor	8
Thomas Coore		3		3
William Henry Cornellissen	London	1	3 (and unspecified) with Norris	4+
William Cotesworth			4 with Durley & Erthman	4
Richard Coutts	London		2 with Thomlinson	2
Thomas Coutts	London	6	3 (and unspecified) with Gordon; 5 with Astell & Benson; unspecified with Bullock & Phill; unspecified with Garforth & J. Watson	14+
John Crosby (Crosbie)	Dumfries	4		4
William Crowle	Hull	1	15 with Mowld	16
Sir Ambrose Crowley (S)	London	29	3 with N. Ridley; 3 with R. Ridley; 3 with Brander	38
Executors of Sir A. Crowley and/or John Crowley	London	1	2 with Norris	3
William Davenport	Exeter	1		1
Frederick Dorin	London	22	24 with Meyer	46

Petitioner	Location	Ships	Ships in association with other petitioners	Total
Henry Durley		1	4 with Cotesworth & Erthman	5
Eastland Company	London	4	1 with Astell & Brander; 9 with Green	14
Andrew Endrupe		2		2
Henry Erthman	London	38	1 with Astell; 3 with Bowman & W.Joy; 4 with Cotesworth & Durley; 4 with Reup; 15 with Brander	65
John Farrington	Scotland		3 with Arbuthnot	3
Joseph Fearnley	Hull		1 with Maister & St Quintin	1
Robert Fenwick	N'castle	1	2 with Proctor, Ridley & J. Stephenson (Newcastle)	2
William Fenwick	N'castle	1		1
Leonard Fosbrooke	Hull	1		1
David Fotheringham			2 with Norris	2
William Fullman		8	1 with Alberg	9
William Garforth		6	Unspecified with T. Coutts & J. Watson	6+
Thomas Garrett	London	2	1 with Brander	3
John Gordon	Scotland		3 (and unspecified) with T. Coutts	3+
Edward Go(u)ld		2		2
Richard Green	London	4	1 with R. Knipe, Lyell & Reup; 3 with Wordsworth; 7 with Norris; 9 with Eastland Co.; unspecified with Mowld & Wilkinson	24+
Christian Guliker	?Exeter	1		1
Richard Hardwick	London	8	4 with Joseph	12
Samuel Holden	N'castle		1 with Hutchinson; 1 with Reup, Thornton & Wilkinson; 2 with Reup & Wilkinson	4
Nicholas Hutchin(g)s		1		1

Petitioner	Location	Ships	Ships in association with other petitioners	Total
Jonathan Hutchinson	N'castle		1 with Holden	1
John Jackson			6 with J. Watson	6
Jacob Jacobsen (S)	London	2	12 with Meyer	14
Claudius Johnson	Scotland	1		1
Benjamin Joseph	London		4 with Hardwick	4
Charles Joy (S)	London		7 with Bearance	7
Peter Joy (S)	London	1	5 with Norris; 24 with Martin & Thomlinson	30
William Joy	Sweden		1 with Astell & Bowman; 1 with Bowman & Norris; 3 with Bowman & Erthman; 6 with Bowman; 5 unspecified	16
Sir Andrew King		1		1
Sir Alexander Knipe	London	8		8
Sir Randolph Knipe	London	17	1 with Green, Lyell & Reup; 20 unspecified	37
John Low	Scotland	2		2
Henry Lyell (S)	London	34	1 with R. Knipe, Lyell & Reup; 1 with Travers; 2 with Smallwood	38
William Maister	Hull	2	1 with Fearnley & St Quentin	3
Michael Malton	Scotland	1		1
Joseph Martin	London		24 with P. Joy & Thomlinson	24
Peter Meyer	London	12	24 with Dorin; 12 with Jacobson	48
Alexander Mitchell	Scotland	4		4
William Morden			1 with Pitman & D. Watson	1
George Morley	London		3 with Robinson	3
William Mowld	Hull	3	15 with Crowle; unspecified with Green & Wilkinson	18+

Petitioner	Location	Ships	Ships in association with other petitioners	Total
Henry Norris (S)	London	38	1 with Bowman & W. Joy; 1 with Brander; 1 with Travers; 2 with Fotheringham; 2 with executors. of Crowley; 3 (and unspecified) with Cornellison; 3 with Alberg; 7 with Green; 9 with D. Watson; 5 with P. Joy	72+
Alexander Patterson	Scotland	8		8
Henry Phill	London	1	3 with Pierson; unspecified with Bullock and T. Coutts	4+
(Sir) William Phippard	London	8		8
Thomas Pierson			3 with Phill	3
Thomas Pillens (Pillant)		1		1
William Proctor	N'castle		2 with R. Fenwick, Ridley & J. Stephenson (N)	2
George & Thomas Randall	Cerne Abbas	1		1
Peter Renew		1		1
John Reup	London	29	1 with Green, R. Knipe & Lyell; 1 with Holden, Thornton & Wilkinson; 2 with Holden & Wilkinson; 4 with Erthman	37
Nicholas Ridley (S)	N'castle		6 with A. Crowley; 2 with R. Fenwick, Proctor & J. Stephenson (N)	8
Richard Ridley	N'castle		3 with A. Crowley	3
Richard & Nicholas Ridley (joint)	N'castle	1		1
Ralph Robinson	London		3 with Morley	3
William St Quentin	Hull		1 with Fearnley & Maister	1
Daniel Scarlet			6 with Turner	6
John Skinner		4	Unspecified with Bowden	4+
John Smallwood			2 with Lyell	2

Petitioner	Location	Ships	Ships in association with other petitioners	Total
John Stephenson	Hull	1		1
John Stephenson	N'castle		2 with R.Fenwick, Proctor & Ridley	2
William Stephenson	Hull	1		1
Walter Stuart (Stewart)	Scotland	1		1
Thomas Stiles	London	1		1
John Taylor	London	17	2 with Collins; 3 with Astell	22
Richard Thomlinson (S)	London	25	1 with Astell; 2 with R. Coutts; 2 with Alstrom & Wilkinson; 3 with D. Watson; 7 with Wilkinson; 24 with P. Joy & Martin	64
John Thornton	Hull	3	1 with Holden, Reup & Wilkinson	4
John Travers	London	4	1 with Lyell; 1 with Norris	6
John Turner			6 with Scarlet	6
James Wallan			Unspecified with Alberg	
David Watson (S)	London	39	1 with Morden & Pitman; 3 with Thomlinson; 9 with Norris	52
John Watson			6 with Jackson; unspecified with T. Coutts & Garforth	6+
Robert (Richard) Wightman	Edinb'h	1		1
Philip Wilkinson	Hull		1 with Holden, Reup & Thornton; 2 with Holden & Reup; 2 with Alstrom and Thomlinson; 7 with Thomlinson; unspecified with Green & Mowld	12
Josias Wordsworth (S)	London	12	3 with Green	15
George Yeaman	Scotland	1		1
Thomas York		1		1

Sources: NA PC 2/82–4; Calendar of Treasury Books, vols 24–8; NA SP 44/245 and CUST 99/1; Hull City Archives WB 8, 9; Åström

Appendix 4

Gross receipts and expenses of the quarantine service in Great Britain, 1800–1823 (to nearest £ sterling)

Year	Receipts	Expenses	Year	Receipts	Expenses
1800	1,400	6,921	*1812*	15,212	19,060
1801	5,910	11,489	*1813*	13,311	24,636
1802	7,329	13,188	*1814*	18,327	23,521
1803	15,506	18,250	*1815*	17,298	23,625
1804	13,295	18,104	*1816*	16,316	23,336
1805	23,273	22,670	*1817*	14,998	21,524
1806	13,371	18,975	*1818*	23,499	21,915
1807	10,425	20,408	*1819*	23,393	23,566
1808	12,746	20,172	*1820*	18,288	22,955
1809	22,173	22,694	*1821*	15,921	21,485
1810	20,211	22,099	*1822*	14,419	21,162
1811	12,806	21,279	*1823*	22,082	20,487

Source: Appendices E and F1 forming p. 111 of the Second Report from the Select Committee Appointed to Consider of the Means of Improving and Maintaining the Foreign Trade of the Country. Quarantine (1824) [BPP, vol. 6 (1824), pp. 165ff.]

Appendix 5

Quarantine income at Malta, with breakdown of components (when known)

Year	INCOME (£) Estimate	Actual	BREAKDOWN (£) Docs.	Shipping	Goods	Persons	Cattle
1779		[211]					
1780		[112]					
1781		[142]					
1782		[90]					
1783		[27]					
1784		[169]					
1785		[251]					
1786		[201]					
1787		[165]					
1788		[90]					
1801		1,613					
1802		c.2,000					
25 July 1802 – 24 July 1803		1,321					
25 July 1803 – 24 July 1804		1,961					
25 July 1805 – 24 July 1806		1,052					
1807		?					
1808		?					

Year	INCOME (£)		BREAKDOWN (£)				
	Estimate	Actual	Docs.	Shipping	Goods	Persons	Cattle
1809		8.932					
1810		9,200					
1811		11,555					
1812 6 months		4,844					
1 Oct. 1813 – 31 Dec. 1814		17,925					
1815		11,377					
1816		9,599					
1817		7,294					
1818		7,204					
1819		6,774					
1820		6,521					
1821		5,218					
1822		5,987					
1823		6,319					
1824		4,750					
1825		5,101					
1826		4,933					
1827–31		?					
1832		7,762					
1833		4,212					
1834		3,718					
1835		?					
1836		2,895	151	1463	974	307	
1837		2,848	110	1271	1064	403	
1838		2,896	115	1211	834	736	

Year	**INCOME (£)**		**BREAKDOWN (£)**				
	Estimate	Actual	Docs.	Shipping	Goods	Persons	Cattle
1839		3,027	118	1475	784	650	
1840		3,004	98	1197	862	847	
1841	2900	3,892					
1842	2900	3,854					
1843	3205	3,169					
1844	3335	3,588					
1845	3308	2,283					
1846	3347	2,386					
1847	3214	2,303					
1848	3012	1,784		845	110	480	349
1849	1575	1,070		495	79	214	282
1850	740	1,608		607	76	331	594
1851	700	698		261		96	341
1852	900	449		178		83	188
1853	600	154		117		31	6
1854	220	31		18		13	
1855	nil	31		29		2	
1856	31	33		23		10	
1857	31	2		2			
1858	31	404		155	16	81	152
1859	21	206		104	46	55	1
1860	90	nil					
1861	nil	nil					
1862	nil	nil					
1863	nil	nil					
1864	nil	nil					
1865	nil	479		187	44	248	
1866	nil	877		420	169	229	59

Year	INCOME (£)		BREAKDOWN (£)				
	Estimate	Actual	Docs.	Shipping	Goods	Persons	Cattle
1867	nil	1,219		898	96	151	74
1868	nil	nil					
1869	nil	nil					
1870	nil	148		105	4	21	18
1871	nil	977		883	18	60	16
1872	nil	1,631		1539	13	62	17
1873	nil	650		484	29	107	30
1874	nil	919		745	37	93	44
1875	nil	535		35		2	498
1876	nil	532		7			525
1877	nil	113					113
1878	nil	89					89
1879	nil	408		56	17	135	200
1880	nil	301					301
1881	nil	454		8		15	431
1882	nil	296		7		9	280
1883	nil	?					
1884	nil	1,329		402	50	278	599
1885	nil	360		289	2	53	16
1886	nil	?					
1887	nil	247		152		11	84
1888	nil	562					562
1889	nil	?					
1890	nil	705					

Sources:

1. Figures for 1779–88 are taken from de Boisgelin, *Ancient and Modern Malta*, vol. 1, p. 305, where they are given in Maltese crowns or scudi. The amounts shown in square brackets are the equivalent sums in pounds sterling, calculated at an exchange rate of 9 scudi to the pound.
2. Figures for 1801–34 are gleaned from papers filed under the several volumes for those years catalogued in the National Archives under CO 158.
3. Figures from 1836 are taken from the *Malta Government Gazette*. After 1840 estimates of income were prepared as part of the annual budgeting process. In explanation of the headings: 'documents' means the charge for the issue of certificates and bills of health; 'shipping' means charges for the quarantine of vessels; 'goods' and 'persons' means the charges for airing or detention of cargoes and passengers/crew in the lazaretto. Importers of cattle were charged for a nominal delay and a brief passage of the animals through water.

Appendix 6

Quarantine expenditure under British control on Malta

Year	Expenditure (£)
1801	3,007
25 July 1802 – 24 July 1803	1,683
25 July 1803 – 24 July 1804	1,977
25 July 1805 – 24 July 1806	3,044
1807–8	?
1809	5,648
1810	4,463
1811	5,059
1812	2,634
1 Oct. 1813 – 31 Dec. 1814	12,274
1815	7,693
1816	6,699
1817	5,778
1818	5,581
1819	4,892
1820	4,686
1821	4,465
1822	4,416
1823	4,571

1824		4,470
1825		4,496
1826		4,948
1827–36		?
1837		7,311
1838		6,804
1839		5,213
1840		5,451
1841		6,111
1842		5,574
1843		5,489
1844		5,632
1845		5,117
1846		5,098
1847		5,125
1848		4,473
1849		4,918
1850		5,359

Notes:

1. Early figures are derived from papers in the National Archives under CO 158.
2. Figures for 1837–38 and 1849–50 are from the *Malta Government Gazette*.
3. Figures 1839-48 are taken from *BPP*, vol. 35 (1850), p. 413.
4. The huge outlay in 1813–14 was in response to the attack of plague.
5. The figure for 1837 includes £1,648 towards the cost of the new plague hospital.
6. In June 1851 the quarantine function became part of the new Port Department of Malta and statistics of expenditure become misleading.

Index

Note: (1) there may be more than one entry on a page; (2) references found only in footnotes are marked n, e.g. 290n; (3) ships (italicized) are indexed only if particularly significant to the narrative.

Printed in Great Britain
by Amazon

39448327R00366